Psychiatry
For UKMLA and Medical Exams

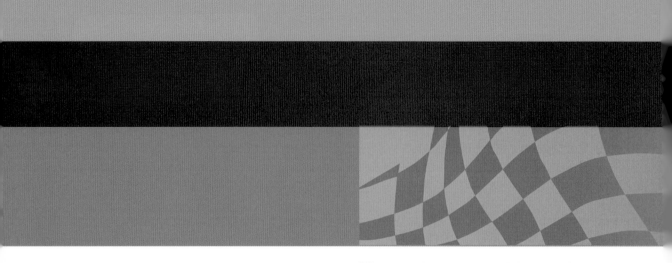

First and second edition authors
Darran Bloye
Simon Davies
Alisdair D Cameron

Third edition authors
Juilius Bourke
Matthew Castle

Fourth edition authors
Katie Marwick
Steven Birrell

Fifth edition author
Katie Marwick

6th Edition
CRASH COURSE

SERIES EDITOR

Philip Xiu

MA (Cantab), MB BChir, MRCP, MRCGP, MScClinEd, FHEA, MAcadMEd, RCPathME

Honorary Senior Lecturer

Leeds University School of Medicine

PCN Educational Lead

Medical Examiner

Leeds Teaching Hospital Trust

Leeds, UK

FACULTY ADVISOR

Steven Birrell

MBChB, FRCPsych, PGCertClinEd, AFHEA

Consultant Liaison Psychiatrist, NHS Fife, Victoria Hospital, Kirkcaldy

Clinical Lead for Training & Education, NHS Fife Mental Health and Learning Disability Service

Honorary Clinical Senior Lecturer, College of Medicine and Veterinary Medicine, University of Edinburgh

Katie Marwick

MA (Hons), MB ChB (Hons), MRC Psych, PhD

Honorary Consultant Psychiatrist, NHS Lothian

Senior Clinical Research Fellow, University of Edinburgh, UK

Psychiatry
For UKMLA and Medical Exams

Robyn Canham

MBChB, MRCPsych

Medical Education Fellow, NHS Lothian

Hollie Craig

BMedSci(Hons), MBChB, MRCPsych

ST4 in General Adult Psychiatry, NHS Lothian

ELSEVIER

First edition 1999

Second edition 2004

Third edition 2008

Fourth edition 2013

Updated Fourth edition 2015

Fifth edition 2019

Sixth edition 2025

Notices

Practitioners and researchers must always rely on their own experience and knowledge in evaluating and using any information, methods, compounds or experiments described herein. Because of rapid advances in the medical sciences, in particular, independent verification of diagnoses and drug dosages should be made. To the fullest extent of the law, no responsibility is assumed by Elsevier, authors, editors or contributors for any injury and/or damage to persons or property as a matter of products liability, negligence or otherwise, or from any use or operation of any methods, products, instructions, or ideas contained in the material herein.

ISBN: 978-0-443-11573-8

Content Strategist: Trinity Hutton
Content Development Specialist: Shivani Pal
Project Manager: Shivani Pal
Design: Miles Hitchen
Marketing Manager: Deborah Watkins

Printed in India

Last digit is the print number: 9   8   7   6   5   4   3   2   1

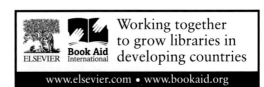

Working together
to grow libraries in
developing countries

www.elsevier.com • www.bookaid.org

Series editor's foreword

With great honour and pride, we present the latest edition of the *Crash Course* series. This series has traversed a journey of nearly a quarter-century, stemming from the vision of Dr. Dan Horton-Szar, and his legacy continues to walk with us on this pathway of knowledge.

The series has been popular with students worldwide, selling over **1 million copies** and being translated into more than **8 languages**, reinforcing our commitment to global learning.

We remain extremely grateful for your unwavering trust. The series has once again been refreshed and fully upgraded in accordance with the rapidly changing medical guidelines, ensuring the content is comprehensive, accurate and fully up-to-date.

This latest series continues our tradition of integrating clinical practice with basic medical sciences, tailored meticulously for today's medical undergraduate curriculum. A central highlight of this instalment is our emphasis on high-yield exam content designed specifically for the UKMLA curriculum.

The addition of the **Rapid UKMLA Index** at the beginning of the book enhances this offering, serving as a valuable aid to students to track their exam preparation efficiently. We have also revised all self-assessment questions to align with the single best answer format in line with the latest UKMLA examination style. We have also added ***High-Yield Association Tables***. These are essential tools designed to aid students in recognizing clinical patterns and acing vignette-style exam questions. By condensing complex medical scenarios into digestible, manageable insights, these tables ensure efficient learning. They connect symptoms, diagnosis and treatment, bolstering understanding and confidence in tackling the rigorous UKMLA exams. This comprehensive approach makes these tables an indispensable asset in your exam preparations.

Utilizing student feedback, we have strived to maintain the core principles of this series: delivering precise and readable text that brings together depth and clarity. The authors are experienced junior doctors who successfully navigated these exams recently, ensuring practical and tested guidance. A team of expert faculty advisors from across the United Kingdom ensures the content's accuracy, making it resilient and reliable.

As we turn a new chapter with the latest edition, we honour the past, cherish the present, and embrace the promise of the future. We wish you every success in your journey of learning and growth and hope that this series adds value to your life, both as students and as future medical professionals.

Philip Xiu

Prefaces

Authors

Just as we all have physical health, which we may struggle with from time to time, we can all face challenges with our mental health. Additionally, we live in a rapidly changing social landscape, where new innovations and challenges arise every day to impact the way we feel and connect to those around us.

While we cannot (yet!) diagnose schizophrenia with a blood test or a CT scan, we hope that this book will help you at the start of your journey into understanding mental disorders, through learning to ask the right questions and provide empathic and supportive care, even when a patient's own mind is working against them.

The way we make diagnoses in psychiatry has once again been updated, with the recent publication of the 11th edition of the International Classification of Diseases (ICD-11). This book has been extensively updated to reflect the changes brought in by this new classification system. We have also included a new chapter on psychiatric emergencies, which provides concise, high-yield information in this critical area. We have also built on the previous edition's chapter on management of intellectual disability and neurodevelopmental disorders, giving both these areas a chapter of their own, reflecting the increasing prominence and recognition of neurodiversity within our population. Lastly, we have mapped the chapters of this book to the content of the new Medical Licensing Assessment, which we hope means this book will be an invaluable tool as you prepare to tackle this new assessment hurdle.

We of course hope that many of you reading this book might consider a career within psychiatry. However, whichever area of medicine you ultimately choose to specialise in, the ability to recognise, assess and support those struggling with their mental health is vital, and has the potential to be as life changing as any other aspect of your clinical care.

As previous editions of Crash Course Psychiatry were for us during our own time at medical school, this book is intended to be a solid foundation upon which to base your exploration of this exciting, impactful, and evolving area of clinical practice. Good luck!

Hollie Craig and Robyn Canham

Faculty advisor

Welcome to the 6th edition of Crash Course Psychiatry! As proud members of the team which wrote and edited the 4th and 5th edition we are delighted that we are both Faculty Advisors for this edition, and it is the best yet. The major change this time round is the incorporation of the revised classification of psychiatric disorders in ICD-11. This revision is a once in a generation event and the changes are still bedding down into clinical practice. We have done our best to relay the new definitions and diagnoses and to highlight key differences between ICD-11 and ICD-10, supporting you in your exams and clinical experience whatever system is used. We have also added a new chapter on Psychiatric Emergencies, making information you may need in a hurry as accessible as possible. I hope this book will be an enjoyable and reliable companion to you on your journey through psychiatry and beyond.

Katie Marwick and Steven Birrell

Acknowledgements

It goes without saying that this book would not exist in its current iteration without the guidance, wisdom and support of our faculty advisors, Dr Katie Marwick and Dr Steve Birrell. Their dedication and encouragement have been invaluable during the process of writing this book. Thank you for all you have done for us.

We have benefited greatly from the advice and opinions of colleagues who have been kind enough to give their time and expertise to the review of some of the book's chapters during the writing process. We are very grateful to Dr Margaret White, ST6 in the Psychiatry of Learning Disability, NHS Lothian; Dr Naomi Entwistle, ST5 in Child and Adolescent Psychiatry, NHS Lothian; Dr Elizabeth Robertson, ST5 in Old Age Psychiatry, NHS Lothian; Dr Sarah Kennedy, Consultant Psychiatrist, Liaison Psychiatry, NHS Lothian and Dr Emily Nelson, ST5 in General Adult Psychiatry, NHS Lothian. For his specific advice around the reform of the England and Wales Mental Health Act we would also like to thank Dr Howard Ryland, Consultant Forensic Psychiatrist, researcher and Honorary Senior Clinical Research fellow at Oxford Health NHS Foundation Trust, Oxford Health Biomedical Research Centre and the University of Oxford respectively. We are particularly grateful to Dr Daryl Whitehall, ST4 in Emergency Medicine, NHS Lothian, who co-authored our new chapter on psychiatric emergencies. We would also like to take this opportunity to acknowledge all the people who have made contributions to the previous editions of Crash Course Psychiatry, whose wisdom and knowledge continue to be reflected in the pages of this book.

When we began writing this textbook the International Classification of Diseases, 11th Edition (ICD-11) was not in widespread use in our health board. Grappling with this new system was a daunting prospect, and we would be remiss not to acknowledge the authors of the 'Training Course on ICD-11 Requirements for Mental, Behavioural, and Neurodevelopmental Disorders', provided by the World Health Organization and the WHO Collaborating Centre for Capacity Building and Training in Global Mental Health at Columbia University. While we have not had direct contact with them, their extensive course informed many of our changes to this new edition.

Writing a textbook is no mean feat, and we would not have been able to succeed without the support of our partners and families. Their patience and understanding have been unwavering throughout this process. Thank you for everything.

Robyn Canham and Hollie Craig

Series editor's acknowledgement

We would like to express our sincere gratitude to those who have provided their support and expertise in preparing this sixth edition of the *Crash Course* series. Our junior doctor contributors' participation in crafting the manuscript has been indispensable. Their first-hand experience and current medical knowledge have infused realism and practicality into our content.

Our faculty editors deserve a special note of thanks. They have extensively validated the correctness of the information, ensuring that the content is not just accurate but also contemporaneous, credible, and aligns with the latest medical standards.

We extend our heartfelt thanks to our publisher, Elsevier. Their staff have demonstrated an unwavering commitment to quality, maintaining the high standards set since the first edition. Their insights have routinely enriched the content and process alike.

Our Commissioning Editor, Jeremy Bowes, deserves a special mention for his consistent support and guiding hand throughout the development process. His directions and advice have bettered this edition and spurred us on our quest for excellence.

We are greatly indebted to Alex Mortimer for her wisdom, practical insights and valuable guidance. A big thank you to our Content Strategists, Trinity Hutton and Cloe Holland-Borosh, who need special acknowledgement for meticulously outlining the direction and scope of the content. They've managed to mix details with a strategic plan, keeping our readers in mind.

Lastly, much gratitude is owed to our Content Product Managers, Taranpreet Kaur, Ayan Dhar, Shivani Pal and Tapajyoti Chaudhuri, who have juggled the numerous day-to-day tasks with utmost dedication and perseverance. Despite the ever-approaching deadlines, they have shown remarkable patience and steadfast determination, ensuring that each step of the book's development was accomplished seamlessly.

In conclusion, we sincerely thank each of these wonderful people for their outstanding contributions and support, without which this work wouldn't have been achieved. Their passion, commitment and collaborative effort have helped us bring this edition together.

Philip Xiu

Dedications

I would like to dedicate this book to my wonderful husband and my parents. Your belief in me and what I can achieve has been the spark behind every accomplishment.

Robyn Canham

To all my family, but particularly my Grandad Peter, who has been waiting to see my name on a book cover. I hope it was worth the wait!

Hollie Craig

To my Clinical Supervisor, Dr Jude Halford, Consultant Liaison Psychiatrist, with respect and gratitude

Katie Marwick

To my wife, children, family, friends, colleagues, trainees, students, and patients who all continue to inspire, challenge, and support me

Steven Birrell

RAPID UKMLA Index

The UKMLA Curriculum Conditions Priority levels have been based on the below:

Level 1: Conditions that a newly qualified doctor should have a good knowledge of and be able to recognise and manage.
Level 2: Conditions requiring knowledge for recognising and confirming diagnosis and planning first-line management in straightforward cases.
Level 3: Conditions where recognition of clinical presentation and describing principles of management are important.

Table 1 UKMLA Conditions and Where to Find Them

Priority List	UKMLA Conditions	Chapter	Page
1	Acute stress reaction	Chapter 14: The patient with a reaction to a stressful event	125
1	Anxiety disorder: generalised	Chapter 3: Psychological therapy	38
		Chapter 12: The patient with anxiety, fear or avoidance	111
		Chapter 25: The anxiety, stress-related, OCD-related and bodily distress disorders	227
2	Anxiety disorder: post-traumatic stress disorder	Chapter 14: The patient with a reaction to a stressful event	125
		Chapter 3: Psychological therapy	38
		Chapter 25: The anxiety, stress-related, OCD-related and bodily distress disorders	230
1	Anxiety, phobias, OCD	Chapter 9: The patient with psychotic symptoms	91
		Chapter 3: Psychological therapy	38
		Chapter 12: The patient with anxiety, fear or avoidance	111
		Chapter 25: The anxiety, stress-related, OCD-related and bodily distress disorders	232
		Chapter 13: The patient with obsessions and compulsions	120
		Chapter 29: Disorders relating to the menstrual cycle, pregnancy and the puerperium	258
3	Attention deficit hyperactivity disorder	Chapter 8: The patient with neurodevelopmental differences	74
3	Autism spectrum disorder	Chapter 9: The patient with psychotic symptoms	87
		Chapter 8: The patient with neurodevelopmental differences	75
		Chapter 32: The neurodevelopmental disorders	275
1	Bipolar affective disorder	Chapter 11: The patient with low mood	107
		Chapter 24: The mood (affective) disorders	222
		Chapter 29: Disorders relating to the menstrual cycle, pregnancy and the puerperium	259
		Chapter 33: Child and adolescent psychiatry	286
1	Delirium	Chapter 9: The patient with psychotic symptoms	90
		Chapter 17: The patient with alcohol or substance use problems	151
		Chapter 10: The patient with elated or irritable mood	195
		Chapter 19: The patient with impairment of consciousness or cognition	171
		Chapter 20: Dementia and delirium	190

continued

continued

Contents

Contents

GENERAL

Psychiatric assessment and diagnosis

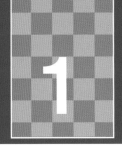

The psychiatric assessment is different from a medical or surgical assessment in that: (1) the history taking is often longer and requires understanding each patient's unique background and environment; (2) a mental state examination (MSE) is performed; and (3) the assessment can in itself be therapeutic. Fig. 1.1 provides an outline of the psychiatric assessment, which includes a psychiatric history, MSE, risk assessment, physical examination and formulation.

INTERVIEW TECHNIQUE

- Whenever possible, patients should be interviewed in settings where privacy can be ensured – a patient who is distressed will be more at ease in a quiet office than in an accident and emergency cubicle.

- Chairs should be at the same level and arranged at an angle, so that you are not sitting directly opposite the patient.
- Establishing rapport is an immediate priority and requires the display of empathy and sensitivity by the interviewer.
- Notes may be taken during the interview; however, explain to patients that you will be doing so as this can be unnerving. Make sure that you still maintain good eye contact.
- Ensure that both you and the patient have an unobstructed exit should it be required.
- Carry a personal alarm and/or know where the alarm in the consulting room is, and check you know how to work the alarms.
- Introduce yourself to the patient and ask them how they would like to be addressed. Explain how long the interview will last. In examination situations, it may be helpful to explain to patients that you may need to interrupt them due to time constraints.
- Keep track of and ration your time appropriately.

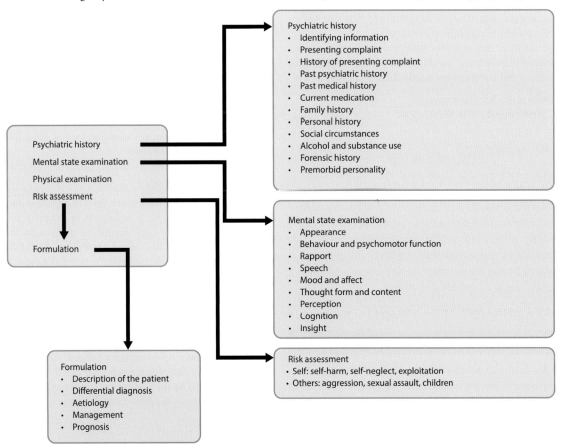

Fig. 1.1 Outline of the psychiatric assessment procedure.

3

- Flexibility is essential (e.g., it may be helpful to put a very anxious patient at ease by talking about their background before focusing in on the presenting complaint).

Make use of both open and closed questions when appropriate

Closed questions limit the scope of the response to one- or two-word answers. They are used to gain specific information and can be used to control the length of the interview when patients are being over-inclusive. For example:

- Do you feel low in mood? (Yes or no answer)
- What time do you wake up in the morning? (Specific answer)

Note that closed questions can be used at the very beginning of the interview, as they are easier to answer and help to put patients at ease (e.g., 'Do you live locally?'; 'Do you have a partner?'; see Identifying Information later).

Open questions encourage the patient to answer freely with a wide range of responses and should be used to elicit the presenting complaint, as well as feelings and attitudes. For example:

- How have you been feeling lately?
- What has caused you to feel this way?

PSYCHIATRIC HISTORY

The order in which you take the history is not as important as being systematic, making sure you cover all the essential subsections. A typical format for taking a psychiatric history is outlined in Fig. 1.1 and is described in detail later.

Identifying information

- Name
- Age
- Pronouns
- Marital status and children
- Occupation
- Reason for the patient's presence in a psychiatric setting (e.g., referral to out-patient clinic by family doctor, admitted to ward informally having presented at casualty)
- Legal status (i.e., if detained under mental health legislation)

For example:

LM is a 32-year-old married teacher with two children aged 4 and 6 years. They were referred by their family doctor to a psychiatric out-patient clinic.

Presenting complaint

Open questions are used to elicit the presenting complaint. Whenever possible, record the main problems in the patient's own words, in one or two sentences, instead of using technical psychiatric terms. For example:

LM complains of 'feeling as though I don't know who I am, like I'm living in an empty shell'.

Patients frequently have more than one complaint, some of which may be related. It is helpful to organize multiple presenting complaints into groups of symptoms that are related; for instance, 'low mood', 'poor concentration' and 'lack of energy' are common features of depression. For example:

LM complains firstly of 'low mood', 'difficulty sleeping' and 'no self-esteem', and secondly of 'taking to the bottle' associated with withdrawal symptoms of 'shaking, sweating and jitteriness' in the morning.

It is not always easy to organize patients' difficulties into a simple presenting complaint in psychiatry. In this case, give the chief complaint(s) as the presenting complaint, and cover the rest of the symptoms or problems in the history of the presenting complaint.

History of presenting complaint

This section is concerned with eliciting the nature and development of each of the presenting complaints. The following headings may be helpful in structuring your questioning:

- Duration: when did the problems start?
- Development: how did the problems develop?
- Mode of onset: suddenly, or over a period of time?
- Course: are symptoms constant, progressively worsening or intermittent?
- Severity: how much is the patient suffering? To what extent are symptoms affecting the patient's social and occupational functioning?
- Associated symptoms: certain complaints are associated with clusters of other symptoms that should be enquired about if patients do not mention them spontaneously. This is the same approach as in other specialties; for example, enquiring about nausea, diarrhoea and distension when someone reports abdominal pain. When 'feeling low' is a presenting complaint, affective, cognitive-behavioural, neurovegetative and psychotic features of depression, as well as suicidal ideation, should be asked about. You can also ask about symptom clusters for psychosis, anxiety, eating problems, substance use and cognitive problems, among others. Also, symptoms such as sleep, appetite disturbance, agitation and memory difficulties are common to many psychiatric conditions, and these should be screened for (e.g., a primary complaint of insomnia may be a sign of depression, mania, psychosis or a primary sleep disorder).
- Precipitating factors: psychosocial stress frequently precipitates episodes of mental illness (e.g., bereavement, moving house and relationship difficulties).

Table 1.1 directs you to the relevant chapters with example questions for different components of the history and MSE.

HINTS AND TIPS

It is useful to learn how to screen patients for common symptoms. This is especially so with patients who are less forthcoming with their complaints. Remember to ask about:

- Low mood (depression)
- Elevated mood and increased energy (hypomania and mania)
- Delusions and hallucinations (psychosis)
- Free-floating anxiety, panic attacks or phobias (anxiety disorders)
- Obsessions or compulsions (obsessive-compulsive disorder)
- Alcohol or substance use
- Thoughts of self-harm or suicide, or thoughts of harming others

Table 1.1 Typical questions used to elicit specific psychiatric symptoms

Questions used to elicit...	Chapter
Suicidal ideas	6
Delusions	9
Hallucinations	9
Mania/hypomania	10
Depressive symptoms	11
Symptoms of anxiety	12
Obsessions and compulsions	13
Dissociative symptoms	14
Somatoform disorders	15
Symptoms of anorexia and bulimia	16
Problem drinking	17
Memory and cognition	19
Symptoms of insomnia	27

Past psychiatric history

This is an extremely important section, as it may provide clues to the patient's current diagnosis. It should include:

- Previous or ongoing psychiatric diagnoses
- Dates and duration of previous mental illness episodes
- Previous treatments, including medication, psychotherapy and electroconvulsive therapy
- Previous contact with psychiatric services (e.g., referrals, admissions)
- Previous assessment or treatment under mental health legislation
- History of self-harm, suicidal ideas or acts

Past medical history

Enquire about medical illnesses or surgical procedures. Past head injury or surgery, neurological conditions (e.g., epilepsy), endocrine abnormalities (e.g., thyroid problems) and chronic pain are especially relevant to psychiatry.

Current medication

Note all the medication patients are using, including psychiatric, nonpsychiatric and over-the-counter drugs. Also enquire how long patients have been on specific medication, any side effects and whether it has been effective. If they are on any depot medications make note of when it was last given and who usually administers it. Nonconcordance, as well as reactions and allergies, should be recorded. Sometimes patients may not know what all of their medications are, and reviewing their notes can be very helpful for a full medication history.

Family history

- Enquire about the presence of psychiatric illness (including completed/ attempted suicide and substance use) in family members, remembering that genetic factors are implicated in the aetiology of many psychiatric conditions. A family tree may be useful to summarize information.
- Enquire whether parents are still alive and, if not, causes of death. Also ask about significant physical illnesses in the family.
- Ask whether the patient has any siblings and, if so, where they are in the birth order.

Personal history

The personal history consists of a brief description of the patient's life. Time constraints will not allow an exhaustive biographical account, but you should attempt to include significant events, perhaps under the following useful headings.

Infancy and early childhood (until age 5 years)

- Pregnancy and birth complications (e.g., prematurity, foetal distress, caesarean section).
- Developmental milestones (e.g., age of crawling, walking, speaking, bladder and bowel control).
- Childhood illnesses.
- Unusually aggressive behaviour or impaired social interaction.
- Who lived in the house when the patient was growing up?

Later childhood and adolescence (until completion of higher education)

- Relationships with close family members.
- Adverse childhood experiences.
- School record (e.g., academic performance, number and type of schools attended, need for special educational support, age on leaving, final qualifications).
- Relationships with teachers and peers. Victim or perpetrator of bullying.
- Behavioural problems, including antisocial behaviour, drug use or truancy.
- Higher education and training.

COMMUNICATION

'Child abuse' can encompass several different types of abuse, which often co-occur. Physical abuse is the intentional causing of physical harm or injury. Emotional abuse is deliberately scaring, humiliating, isolating or ignoring a child, and includes allowing a child to witness domestic violence. Neglect is when a child's basic physical/emotional needs are not met. Sexual abuse is forcing or enticing a child to take part in sexual activities, which can be contact or non contact (e.g., online). Around one in five adults in the United Kingdom were abused in at least one way as children (2020 Crime Survey for England and Wales).

Occupational record

- Details of types and duration of jobs.
- Details of and reasons for unemployment and/or dismissal.

Relationship, marital and sexual history

- Details and duration of significant relationships, including reasons for break-ups.
- Marriage/divorce details.
- Children.
- Ability to engage in satisfactory sexual relationships. Sexual dysfunction, or gender identity problems (only enquire if problem is suspected).

COMMUNICATION

A history of childhood abuse is important to detect, but it can feel awkward to ask about. Most people respond well to being straightforwardly asked, 'Were you ever abused in any way when you were growing up?' In young people, or those you are struggling to build a rapport with, a more graded approach may be preferable (e.g., 'Have you ever been touched in a way you didn't want? When was your first relationship? When was your first sexual experience? Have you ever had an unpleasant sexual experience? Sometimes such experiences are unpleasant because they are unwanted or because the person is too young to understand …?') Leaving the question open allows the patient room to answer freely, rather than simply answering 'yes' or 'no'.

Social circumstances

This includes accommodation, social supports and relationships, employment and financial circumstances and hobbies or leisure activities. It is important to identify if the patient has current frequent contact with children, in case their presentation raises any child protection concerns. It is also important to find out if the patient has any responsibilities for looking after children, vulnerable adults or pets as Social Work may need to be informed.

Alcohol and substance use

This section should never be overlooked, as alcohol/substance-related psychiatric conditions are very common.

The AUDIT questionnaire is a useful tool to screen for alcohol dependence (see Chapter 17). Higher scores suggest more severe alcohol misuse, with ≥8 suggesting hazardous drinking and ≥20 indicating possible alcohol dependence. Try to elicit a patient's typical drinking day, including daily intake of alcohol in units, type of alcohol used, time of first drink of the day and places where drinking occurs (e.g., at home alone or in a pub).

If recreational drugs have been or are being used, record the drug names, routes of administration (intravenous, inhaled, oral ingestion) and the years and frequency of use. Also enquire about possible dependence (see Chapter 17).

Forensic history

Enquire about the details and dates of previous offences and antisocial behaviour, including prosecutions, convictions and prison sentences. It is important to ask specifically about violent crime, the age of the patient's first violent offence and whether the patient has any charges pending. Upcoming court dates may be a source of stress for the patient, and in some cases a reason to report mental health symptoms with a view to secondary gain.

Premorbid personality

The premorbid personality is an indication of the patient's personality and character before the onset of mental illness. It can be difficult to ascertain retrospectively. Indirect evidence of it can be provided from the personal history (e.g., Have they ever been able to hold down a job or been in a long-term relationship? Have their interests changed?). Patients may be asked directly about their personality before they became ill, or it may be useful to ask a close family member or friend about a patient's premorbid personality.

For example:

A young person with schizophrenia, with prominent negative symptoms of lack of motivation, lack of interest and poverty of thought, was described by their mother as being outgoing, intelligent and ambitious before becoming ill.

COMMUNICATION

One way to explore premorbid personality in a patient with some insight is to ask questions such as: 'How would people have described you before?' 'How about now?'.

COLLATERAL HISTORY

Gaining additional information from people the patient knows (family, friends, other staff involved in their care) can be vital to getting an accurate impression of a patient's mental state. This can also be useful for finding out how the patient usually is when they are well. Collateral histories are particularly important if a patient cannot tell you their own history, such as if they have been very guarded in their assessment, they are very thought disordered or they have cognitive impairment.

MENTAL STATE EXAMINATION

The MSE describes an interviewer's objective impression of many aspects of a patient's mental functioning at a certain point in time. Whereas the psychiatric history remains relatively constant, the MSE may fluctuate from day to day or hour to hour. It is useful to try and gather as much evidence as possible about the MSE while doing the psychiatric history, instead of viewing this as a separate section. In fact, the MSE begins the moment you meet the patient. In addition to noting their appearance, you should observe how patients first behave on meeting you. This includes their body language and the way that they respond to your attempts to establish rapport.

COMMON PITFALLS

The MSE, like a physical examination, is a snapshot of a person's presentation during the interview. Only record what the patient demonstrates or experiences during the interview (e.g., if a patient reports having had a hallucination a week ago, that would be described in the history, not the MSE – much as you wouldn't record that someone had abdominal pain the week before your physical examination). Including history in the MSE is a very common mistake in student case reports.

By the time you have finished the psychiatric history, you should have completed many aspects of the MSE and you should just need to ask certain key questions to finish this process off. The individual aspects of the MSE, which are summarized in Fig. 1.1, are discussed in more detail later.

There is some variation in the order in which the MSE is reported (e.g., speech is sometimes described before mood, and sometimes before thought form). As long as you include the information, the exact order is not important.

HINTS AND TIPS

Do not just ask questions and write down answers! Appearance and behaviour are vital to the mental state examination, especially with less communicative patients. Posture, facial expression, tone of voice, spontaneity of speech, state of relaxation and movements made are all important. You may find it helpful to practise with a colleague – try writing down 10 points that describe their appearance and behaviour.

HINTS AND TIPS

The purpose of a mental state examination is to paint a picture of the patient sitting in front of you, with details such as how they look, how they act and what they are saying to you. Ideally someone who has read your MSE should be able to pick your patient out of a room of people.

Appearance

- Physical state: how old does the patient appear? Do they appear physically unwell? Are they sweating? Are they visibly underweight or obese?
- Clothes and accessories: are clothes clean? Are accessories appropriate (e.g., wearing sunglasses indoors)? Are clothes appropriate to the weather and circumstances, or are they bizarre? Is the patient carrying strange objects?
- Self-care and hygiene: does the patient appear to have been neglecting their appearance or hygiene (e.g., unshaven, dirty tangled hair, malodorous, dishevelled)? Does the patient appear to have stopped caring about aspects of their appearance they might have cared about before (e.g., chipped nail varnish, long roots in someone with dyed hair)? Is there any evidence of injury or self-harm (e.g., cuts to wrists or forearms)?

Behaviour and psychomotor function

This section focuses on all motor behaviour, including abnormal movements such as tremors, tics and twitches; displays of suspiciousness, aggression or fear; and catatonic features. Documenting patients' behaviour at the start of, and during, the interview is an integral part of the MSE, and should be done in as much detail as possible. For example:

LM introduced themselves appropriately, although only made fleeting eye contact. They sat rigidly throughout the first half of the interview, mostly staring at the floor and speaking very softly. They became tearful halfway through the interview when talking about their lack of self-esteem. After this their posture relaxed, eye contact improved and there were moments when they smiled. There were no abnormal movements.

The term 'psychomotor' is used to describe a patient's motor activity as a consequence of their concurrent mental processes. Psychomotor abnormalities include *retardation* (slow, monotonous speech; slow or absent body movements) and *agitation* (inability to sit still; fidgeting, pacing or hand-wringing; rubbing or scratching skin or clothes).

Note whether you can establish a good rapport with patients. What is their attitude towards you? Do they make good eye contact, or do they look around the room or at the floor? Patients may be described as cooperative, cordial, uninterested, aggressive, defensive, guarded, suspicious, fearful, perplexed, preoccupied or disinhibited (i.e., a lowering of normal social inhibitions; e.g., being over-familiar or making sexually inappropriate comments), among many other adjectives.

HINTS AND TIPS

Observations of appearance and behaviour may also reveal extrapyramidal side effects from antipsychotic medication (see Chapter 2). It is useful to remember to look for:

- Parkinsonism: drug-induced signs are most commonly a reduced arm swing and unusually upright posture while walking. Tremor and rigidity are late signs, in contrast to idiopathic parkinsonism.
- Acute dystonia: involuntary sustained muscular contractions or spasms.
- Akathisia: subjective feeling of inner restlessness and muscular discomfort, often manifesting with an inability to sit still, 'jiggling' of the legs (irregularly, as opposed to a tremor, which would be regular) or psychomotor agitation.
- Tardive dyskinesia: rhythmic, involuntary movements of head, limbs and trunk, especially chewing, grimacing of mouth and making protruding, darting movements with the tongue.

Speech

Speech should be described in terms of:

- Rate of production: pressure of speech in mania; increased latency, long pauses and poverty of speech in depression
- Quality and flow of speech: volume, dysarthria (articulation difficulties), dysprosody (unusual speech rhythm, intonation or pitch), stuttering
- Word play: punning, rhyming, alliteration (generally seen in mania)

COMMON PITFALLS

Note that disorganized, incoherent or bizarre speech (e.g., flight of ideas) is usually regarded as a thought disorder and is described later in the Thought Form section.

Mood and affect

Mood refers to a patient's sustained, subjectively experienced emotional state over a period of time. *Affect* refers to the transient ebb and flow of emotion in response to stimuli (e.g., smiling at a joke or crying at a sad memory).

Mood is described subjectively (what the patient says they are feeling) and objectively (what your impression of their prevailing mood is during the interview). For example, *her mood was subjectively 'rock bottom' and objectively low.* Mood can also be described as elated, anxious, frightened, angry. Affect is assessed by observing patients' posture, facial expression, emotional reactivity and speech. There are two components to consider when assessing affect:

1. The appropriateness or congruity of the observed affect to the patient's subjectively reported mood (e.g., a woman with schizophrenia who reports feeling suicidal with a happy facial expression would be described as having an *incongruous* affect).
2. The range of affect or range of emotional expressivity. In this sense, affect may be:
   - Within the normal range.
   - Blunted/flat: a noticeable reduction in the normal intensity of emotional expression, as evidenced by a monotonous voice and minimal facial expression.
   - Labile: rapidly fluctuating affect that moves between extremes (e.g., a person with a mixed affective episode alternates between feeling overjoyed, with pressure of speech, and miserable, with suicidal ideation).

Thoughts

Problems with thinking are considered under two headings: thought form (abnormal patterns of thinking) and thought content (abnormal beliefs).

Thought form

Disordered thinking includes circumstantial and tangential thinking, loosening of association (derailment/knight's move thinking), flight of ideas and thought blocking (see Chapter 9 for the definitions of these terms). Whenever possible, record patients' disorganized speech word for word, as it can be very difficult to classify disorganized thinking, and writing it down can help.

Thought content: obsessions, overvalued ideas and delusions

An obsession is an involuntary thought, image or impulse that is recurrent, intrusive and unpleasant and enters the mind against conscious resistance. Patients recognize that the thoughts are a product of their own mind. See Chapter 13 for more information.

An overvalued idea is an incorrect belief that is not impossible, is held with marked emotional investment, but not with unshakeable conviction.

A delusion is the most severe form of abnormal thought content. It is a fixed belief arrived at illogically and is not amenable to reason. It is not accepted in the patient's cultural background.

It is diagnostically significant to classify delusions as:

- Primary or secondary
- Mood congruent or mood incongruent
- Bizarre or nonbizarre
- According to the content of the delusion (summarized in Table 9.1)

See Chapter 9 and Table 13.1 for a detailed description of types of abnormal thought content.

COMMUNICATION

Some psychiatrists include thoughts of self-harm, suicide or harm to others under thought content, while others mention it only under risk assessment. As long as you mention it, it doesn't matter where.

Perception

Hallucinations are often mentioned during the history. However, this is not always the case, so it is important that you specifically enquire about abnormal perceptual experiences (perceptual abnormalities are defined and classified in Chapter 9). If patients admit to problems with perception, it is important to ascertain:

- Whether the abnormal perceptions are hallucinations, pseudohallucinations, illusions or intrusive thoughts.
- From which sensory modality the hallucinations appear to arise (i.e., are they auditory, visual, olfactory, gustatory or somatic hallucinations – see Chapter 9).

- Whether auditory hallucinations are elementary (a very simple abnormal perception; e.g., a flash or a bang) or complex. If complex, are they experienced in the first person (audible thoughts, thought echo), second person (critical, persecutory, complimentary or command hallucinations) or third person (voices arguing or discussing the patient, or giving a running commentary)?

It is also important to note whether patients seem to be responding to hallucinations during the interview, as evidenced by them laughing inappropriately as though they are sharing a private joke, suddenly tilting their head as though listening or quizzically looking at hallucinatory objects around the room.

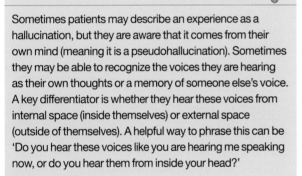

RED FLAG

Elementary hallucinations (simple sounds such as whistling/ buzzing) or simple second-person hallucinations (e.g., single words such as 'Idiot!') are more common in delirium, migraine and epilepsy than in primary psychiatric disorders.

HINTS AND TIPS

Sometimes patients may describe an experience as a hallucination, but they are aware that it comes from their own mind (meaning it is a pseudohallucination). Sometimes they may be able to recognize the voices they are hearing as their own thoughts or a memory of someone else's voice. A key differentiator is whether they hear these voices from internal space (inside themselves) or external space (outside of themselves). A helpful way to phrase this can be 'Do you hear these voices like you are hearing me speaking now, or do you hear them from inside your head?'

Cognition

The cognition of all patients should be screened by checking orientation to place and time. Depending on the circumstances, a more thorough cognitive assessment may be required. Cognitive tests, including tests of generalized cognitive abilities (e.g., consciousness, attention, orientation) and specific abilities (e.g., memory, language, executive function, praxis, perception) are discussed fully in Chapter 19.

Insight

Insight is not an 'all or nothing' attribute. It is often described as good, partial or poor, although patients really lie somewhere on a spectrum and vary over time. The key questions to answer are:

- Do you think you are unwell in any way?
- Do you think you are mentally unwell?
- Do you think you need treatment (pharmacological, psychological or both)?
- Do you think anything might be impacting how you feel right now, such as circumstances or substances?
- Do you think you need to be admitted to hospital (if indicated)?

RISK ASSESSMENT

Although it is extremely difficult to make an accurate assessment of risk based on a single assessment, clinicians are expected, as far as is possible, to establish some idea of a patient's risk to:

- Self: through self-harm, suicide, self-neglect or exploitation by others. Chapter 6 explains the assessment of suicide risk in detail.
- Others: includes violent or sexual crime, stalking and harassment. Also includes the safety of any of the patient's dependents. Chapter 34 discusses key principles in assessing dangerousness.
- Children: includes physical, sexual or emotional abuse, as well as neglect or deprivation e.g., is an alcohol-dependent parent able to provide adequate care for their children? Was a child in the home when an overdose was taken, potentially placing them at risk of finding their parent incapacitated or dead? Child abuse is discussed in more detail in Chapter 33.
- Property: includes arson and physical destruction of property.

RED FLAG

Risk assessment is a vital part of psychiatric assessment. You should always assess risk to self and others.

HINTS AND TIPS

A mnemonic that some find helpful to learn the sections of a mental state exam is ASEPTIC:

A – Appearance and Behaviour

S – Speech

E – Emotion (mood and affect)

P – Perception

T – Thought

I – Insight

C – Cognition

PHYSICAL EXAMINATION

The psychiatric examination includes a general physical examination, with special focus on the neurological and endocrine systems. Always remember to look for signs relevant to the psychiatric history. In patients who misuse alcohol look for signs of liver disease, or if they are withdrawing from alcohol look for signs of Wernicke encephalopathy (ophthalmoplegia or ataxia). In patients with substance misuse issues examine for physical signs of drug misuse such as track marks. In patients with eating disorders look for signs such as lanugo hairs, Russell sign (scars on the back of their knuckles), or any red flag signs (unable to get up from a squatting position without using their hands, bradycardia or hypothermia - see Chapter 16). Also, examine for side effects of psychiatric medication (e.g., parkinsonism, tardive dyskinesia, dystonia, hypotension, obesity and other cardiometabolic sequelae, signs of lithium toxicity).

It may not be possible to complete a detailed physical examination in an exam situation, but you should always recommend that it should be done. Always make a point of mentioning your positive physical findings when summarizing the case.

THE FORMULATION: PRESENTING THE CASE

'Formulation' is the term psychiatrists use to describe the integrated summary and understanding of a particular patient's problems. The formulation usually includes:

- Description of the patient
- Differential diagnosis
- Aetiology
- Management
- Prognosis

Description of the patient

The patient may be described: (1) in detail by recounting all the information obtained under the various headings in the psychiatric history and MSE; or (2) in the form of a case summary. The case summary consists of one or two paragraphs and contains only the salient features of a case, specifically:

- Identifying information
- Main features of the presenting complaint

- Relevant background details (e.g., past psychiatric history, positive family history)
- Positive findings in the MSE and physical examination

See the case summary box for an example and Table 1.2 for a formulation.

HINTS AND TIPS

When presenting your differential diagnosis, remember that two or more psychiatric disorders can coexist (e.g., depression and harmful use of alcohol). It is important to ascertain whether the conditions are independent or related (e.g., poor sleep that followed an increase in alcohol use).

Differential diagnosis

The differential diagnosis is mentioned in order of decreasing probability. It helps your clinical reasoning to provide reasons for and against all the alternatives on your list. Table 1.2 provides an example of a typical differential diagnosis.

Aetiology

The exact cause of most psychiatric disorders is often unknown, and most cases involve a complex interplay of biological, social and psychological factors. In clinical practice, psychiatrists are especially concerned with the question: 'What factors led to this patient presenting with this specific problem at this specific point in time?' That is, what factors predisposed to the problem, what factors precipitated the problem, and what factors are perpetuating the problem? Table 1.2 illustrates an aetiology grid that is very helpful in structuring your answers to these questions in terms of biological, social and psychological factors. The aim is to *consider* all the blocks in the grid, not necessarily fill them.

Management

Investigations
Investigations are considered part of the management plan and are performed based on findings from the psychiatric assessment. Appropriate investigations relevant to specific conditions are given in the relevant chapters. Familiarize yourself with these, as you should be able to give reasons for any investigation you propose.

Table 1.2 Example of a case formulation (differential diagnosis, aetiology, management)

Differential diagnosis	
Diagnosis	**Comments**
1. Schizophrenia	For: symptoms present for more than 1 month For: ICD-11 and first-rank symptoms of delusions of control or passivity (thought insertion); delusional perception; and third-person running commentary hallucinations For: clear and marked deterioration in social and work functioning
2. Schizoaffective disorder	For: typical symptoms of schizophrenia Against: no prominent mood symptoms
3. Mood disorder (either manic or depressive episode) with psychotic features	Against: on mental state examination, mood was mainly suspicious (as opposed to lowered or elevated) and appeared secondary to delusional beliefs Against: no other prominent features of mania or depression Against: mood-incongruent delusions and hallucinations
4. Substance-induced psychotic disorder	Against: long duration of symptoms Against: no evidence of illicit substance or alcohol use
5. Psychotic disorder secondary to a medical condition	Against: no signs of medical illness or abnormalities on physical examination

Aetiology

	Biological	**Psychological**	**Social**
Predisposing (what made the patient prone to this problem?)	Family history of schizophrenia	-	-
Precipitating (what made this problem start now?)	The peak of onset for schizophrenia for men is between 18 and 25 years	-	Break-up of relationship Recently started college
Perpetuating (what is maintaining this problem?)	Poor concordance with medication due to lack of insight	High expressed emotion family	Lack of social support

Management

1. Investigations (bloods including a metabolic screen, ECG, neuroimaging)

2. Management plan below

Term	**Biological**	**Psychological**	**Social**
Immediate to short term	Antipsychotic medication, with benzodiazepines if necessary	Establish therapeutic relationship Support for family (carers)	Admission to hospital Allocation of care coordinator (care programme approach) Help with financial, accommodation and social problems
Medium to long term	Review progress in out-patient clinic Consider another antipsychotic then clozapine for nonresponse Consider depot medication for concordance problems	Relapse prevention work Consider cognitive behavioural therapy and family therapy	Regular review under care programme approach Consider day hospital Vocational training

Prognosis

Assuming PP has a diagnosis of schizophrenia, it is likely his illness will run a chronic course, showing a relapsing and remitting pattern. Being a young man with a high level of education PP is particularly at risk for suicide, especially following discharge from hospital. Good prognostic factors include a high level of premorbid functioning and the absence of negative symptoms.

● Case summary

PP is a 23-year-old single man in full-time education who recently agreed to informal hospital admission. He presented with a 6-month history of hearing voices and maintaining bizarre beliefs that he was being subjected to government experiments. During this time, his college attendance had been uncharacteristically poor, he had terminated his part-time work, and he had become increasingly socially withdrawn. He has no history of psychiatric illness and denies the use of alcohol or illicit substances; however, he did mention that his maternal uncle has schizophrenia. On mental state examination, he appeared unkempt and behaved suspiciously. He had delusions of persecution, reference and thought control, as well as delusional perception. He also described second-person command hallucinations and third-person running commentary hallucinations. He appeared to have no insight into his mental illness, as he refused to consider that he might be unwell. There were no abnormalities on physical examination.

Specific management plan

It may help to structure your management plan by considering the biological, social and psychological aspects of treatment (the *biopsychosocial approach*) in terms of immediate to short-term and medium- to long-term management. See Table 1.2 for an example of this method.

Prognosis

The prognosis is dependent on two factors:

1. The natural course of the condition, which can be predicted based on studies of patient populations; these are discussed for each disorder in the relevant chapters.
2. Individual patient factors (e.g., social support, concordance with treatment, comorbid substance abuse)

See Table 1.2 for an example.

CLASSIFICATION IN PSYCHIATRY

There are two main categorical classification systems in psychiatry:

1. The ICD-11: the eleventh revision of the International Classification of Diseases, Chapter 6 – Mental, behavioural or neurodevelopmental disorders (published by the World Health Organization). ICD-11 came into clinical practice in 2022, and many patient's notes will refer to previous ICD-10 classifications. Individual chapters explain the key differences.
2. The DSM-5: the fifth edition of the Diagnostic and Statistical Manual of Mental Disorders (published by the American Psychiatric Association, 2013).

The ICD-11 and the DSM-5 share similar diagnostic categories and are fairly similar for the most part.

Both the ICD-11 and the DSM-5 make use of a *categorical classification system,* which refers to the process of dividing mental disorders into discrete entities by means of accurate descriptions of specific categories. In contrast, a *dimensional approach* rejects the idea of separate categories, hypothesizing that mental conditions exist on a continuum that merges into normality. This better reflects reality but is harder to put into clinical practice; for example, would someone whose mood is 'one standard deviation lower than normal' be likely to benefit from treatment with an antidepressant? The ICD-11 takes a hybrid approach, with some dimensional options within categorical diagnoses (e.g., for personality disorder traits or schizophrenia specifiers).

The ICD-11 categorizes mental disorders according to descriptive statements and diagnostic guidelines which are not rigid: clinical judgement is required too. The DSM-5 categorizes mental disorders according to *operational definitions,* which means that mental disorders are defined by a series of precise inclusion and exclusion criteria.

The ICD-11 and the DSM 5 share similar diagnostic categories and are fairly similar for the most part. The DSM-5 and the ICD11 take a lifespan approach to diagnoses. Classification begins with neurodevelopmental disorders (autism, psychotic disorders), followed by disorders that often present in early adulthood (bipolar, depression, anxiety) and ending with neurocognitive disorders (dementia).

These classification systems are evolving over time as new evidence about the aetiology of mental disorders arises. Currently, psychiatric disorders are classified by clustering symptoms, signs and behaviours into syndromes. As yet, they are not based on a clear understanding of pathogenesis. As this develops, classification systems will continue to change and improve.

Chapter Summary

- A psychiatric history is like any other history, except that more attention is given to personal and social circumstances, and a mental state examination is conducted during it.
- A mental state examination, like a physical examination, is a snapshot of how the person presents at the time you meet them.
- Physical examination is still important, even in patients who do not report physical symptoms.
- Psychiatric diagnostic systems are evolving in light of new understanding of mental disorder aetiology.

UKMLA Presentations
Auditory hallucinations
Behaviour/personality change
Confusion
Elation/elated mood
Low mood/affective problems
Visual hallucinations

UKMLA Conditions
Depression
Schizophrenia
Self harm

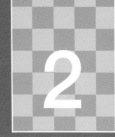

Pharmacological therapy and electroconvulsive therapy

2

Psychotropic (mind-altering) medications can be divided into the following groups:

- Antidepressants
- Mood stabilizers
- Antipsychotics
- Anxiolytics and hypnotics
- Other

Despite its simplicity, this method of grouping drugs by the disorder they were first used to treat is flawed, because many drugs from one class are now used to treat disorders in another class (e.g., antidepressants are first-line therapies for many anxiety disorders, and some antipsychotics also have mood stabilizing, antimanic and antidepressant effects).

ANTIDEPRESSANTS

History

Antidepressants were first used in the late 1950s, with the appearance of the tricyclic antidepressant (TCA), imipramine and the monoamine oxidase inhibitor (MAOI), phenelzine. Research into TCAs throughout the 1960s and 1970s resulted in the development of many more tricyclic agents and related compounds. A major development in the late 1980s was the development of the first selective serotonin reuptake inhibitor (SSRI), fluoxetine (Prozac). There has since been a considerable expansion of the SSRI class, as well as the development of antidepressants such as venlafaxine and duloxetine, which are serotonin and noradrenaline reuptake inhibitors (SNRIs), and also mirtazapine and agomelatine that have different mechanisms of action. More recent developments have included the development of SSRIs with additional actions at serotonin receptors, including vortioxetine. Research is also currently underway focusing on the use of ketamine and psilocybin in treatment-resistant depression.

Classification and mechanism of action

At present, antidepressants are classified according to their pharmacological actions, as there is not yet a complete explanation as to what exactly makes antidepressants work. Although there are many different classes of antidepressants, their common action is to elevate the levels of one or more monoamine neurotransmitters in the synaptic cleft. Some predominantly influence serotonin, some noradrenaline and some dopamine, with many influencing the transporters or receptors for multiple neurotransmitters. It is likely that the combination of effects on multiple neurotransmitter pathways acts synergistically in causing the antidepressant effect. For example, agomelatine is both a melatonin receptor agonist and a 5-HT$_{2C}$ (serotonin 2C) receptor antagonist, but neither of these actions alone have an antidepressant effect. Fig. 2.1 illustrates the mechanism of action of antidepressants at synapses, and Table 2.1 summarizes their classification and pharmacodynamics.

> **HINTS AND TIPS**
>
> When recommending antidepressants to trial in a patient with treatment-resistant depression, it makes sense to try those with different pharmacodynamic properties to antidepressants that have been trialled before. See Table 2.1.

Indications

SSRIs are used in the treatment of:

- Depression.
- Anxiety disorders.
- Stress-related disorders including post traumatic stress disorder.
- Obsessive-compulsive or related disorders.
- Other: chronic abdominal pain including irritable bowel syndrome (IBS).

SNRIs are used in the treatment of:

- Depression.
- Anxiety disorders.
- Panic disorders.
- Other: diabetic neuropathy and urinary incontinence (duloxetine).

Mirtazapine is used in the treatment of:

- Depression (particularly where sedation or increased oral intake is desirable).

TCAs are used in the treatment of:

- Depression.

15

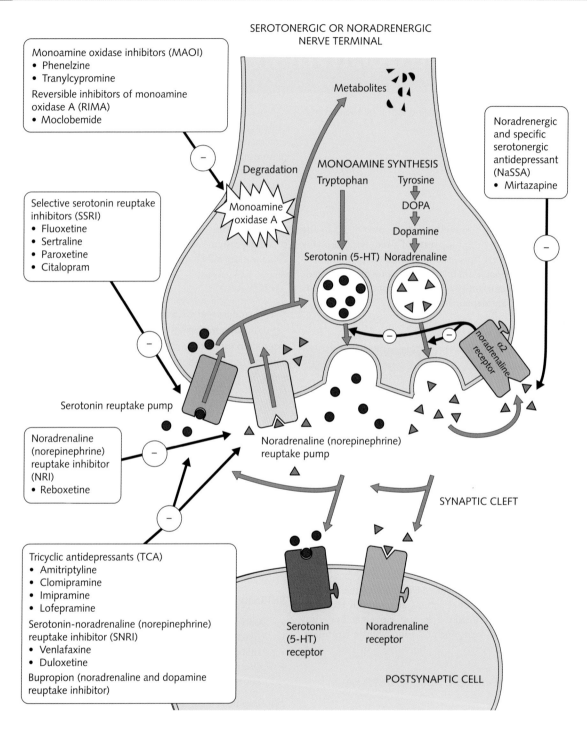

Note: the serotonin and noradrenaline (norepinephrine) pathways are presented together for convenience; they do not occur in the same nerve terminal

Fig. 2.1 Mechanism of action of antidepressants at the synaptic cleft.

Table 2.1 Classification and pharmacodynamics of the antidepressants

Class of antidepressant	Examples	Mechanism of action
Commonly used		
Selective serotonin reuptake inhibitor (SSRI)	Fluoxetine, sertraline, paroxetine, citalopram, fluvoxamine	Selective presynaptic blockade of serotonin reuptake pumps.
Serotonin and noradrenaline reuptake inhibitor (SNRI)	Venlafaxine, duloxetine	Presynaptic blockade of both noradrenaline (norepinephrine) and serotonin reuptake pumps (also dopamine in high doses), but with negligible effects on muscarinic, histaminergic or α-adrenergic receptors (in contrast to tricyclic antidepressants).
SSRI and serotonin modulator	Vortioxetine	Selective serotonin reuptake inhibitor, plus varied effects on different 5-HT receptor subtypes (1A agonist, 1B partial agonist, 1D, 3 and 7 antagonists).
Noradrenergic and specific serotonergic antidepressant (NaSSA)	Mirtazapine	Presynaptic alpha 2 receptor blockade (results in increased release of noradrenaline (norepinephrine) and serotonin from presynaptic neurons). Also 5-HT$_{2A/C}$ and 5-HT$_3$ receptor antagonist and histamine 1 receptor antagonist.
Serotonin antagonist and reuptake inhibitor I	Trazodone	Varied effects on different 5-HT receptor subtypes (1A partial agonist, 2A and 2B antagonist). At high doses acts as SSRI. Also antagonist at alpha 1 adrenergic receptors, histamine type 1 receptors and T-type calcium channels. Which of its actions is important in inducing its sedative and anxiolytic effects is unclear.
Tricyclic antidepressant	Amitriptyline, lofepramine, clomipramine, imipramine	Presynaptic blockade of both noradrenaline (norepinephrine) and serotonin reuptake pumps (to a lesser extent – dopamine). Also, blockade of muscarinic, histaminergic and α-adrenergic receptors.
Monoamine oxidase inhibitor (MAOI)	Phenelzine, tranylcypromine, isocarboxazid	Nonselective and irreversible inhibition of monoamine oxidase A and B.
Reversible inhibitor of monoamine oxidase A (RIMA)	Moclobemide	Selective and reversible inhibition of monoamine oxidase A.
Noradrenaline and dopamine reuptake inhibitor	Bupropion	Dopamine and noradrenaline reuptake pump inhibitor.
Dopamine agonist	Pramipexole, ropinirole	Dopamine receptor agonist (D$_2$, D$_3$, D$_4$).
Selective noradrenaline reuptake inhibitor (NRI)	Reboxetine	Selective presynaptic blockade of noradrenaline (norepinephrine) reuptake pumps.
Melatonin agonist and serotonin antagonist	Agomelatine	Melatonin receptor 1 and 2 agonist and 5-HT$_{2C}$ receptor antagonist.

- Anxiety disorders.
- Obsessive-compulsive disorder (clomipramine).
- Other: some types of pain (neuropathic pain, tension headache, chronic continuous abdominal pain, Irritable Bowel Syndrome (IBS)-related abdominal pain) nocturnal enuresis, narcolepsy.

MAOIs are used in the treatment of:

- Depression (especially atypical depression, which is characterized by hypersomnia, overeating and anxiety).
- Anxiety disorders.
- Other: Parkinson disease, migraine prophylaxis, tuberculosis.

Vortioxetine is used in the treatment of:

- Depression.

Side effects and contraindications

SSRIs, SNRIs and serotonin modulators

SSRIs do not have the anticholinergic effects of the TCAs and are not sedating. The majority of patients find them alerting, so they are prescribed to be taken in the morning. Soon after initiation, or when taken at high doses, some patients can feel alerted to the point of agitation/anxiety. This may be associated with an increased

BOX 2.1 COMMON SIDE EFFECTS OF SSRIS

Gastrointestinal disturbance (nausea, vomiting, diarrhoea, pain) – early[a]

Anxiety and agitation – early[a]

Loss of appetite and weight loss (sometimes weight gain)

Insomnia

Sweating

Sexual dysfunction (anorgasmia, delayed ejaculation)

[a] Gastrointestinal and anxiety symptoms occur on initiation of treatment and resolve with time.

Table 2.2 Common side effects of tricyclic antidepressants

Mechanism	Side effects
Anticholinergic: muscarinic receptor blockade	Dry mouth Constipation Urinary retention Blurred vision
α-Adrenergic receptor blockade	Postural hypotension (dizziness, syncope)
Histaminergic receptor blockade	Weight gain Sedation
Cardiotoxic effects	QT interval prolongation ST-segment elevation Heart block Arrhythmias

risk of suicide, particularly in adolescents (see Chapter 33 for recommendations on use in young people). Due to their relatively low cardiotoxicity, SSRIs are the antidepressant of choice in patients with cardiac disease and in those who are at risk for taking an overdose. However, they do have their own side effects that may be unacceptable to some patients. These are summarized in Box 2.1. SSRIs and SNRIs such as venlafaxine and serotonin reuptake inhibitors and modulators (vortioxetine) have similar side effects to SSRIs. The side effects of SNRIs tend to be more severe than SSRIs.

Contraindications: mania, poorly controlled epilepsy and prolonged QTc interval (for citalopram and escitalopram).

COMMUNICATION

Sexual dysfunction is a common side effect of SSRI medication and may lead to poor concordance. After initiating an SSRI, it is important to sensitively ask about changes in sexual functioning.

Mirtazapine

Mirtazapine is very commonly associated with increased appetite, weight gain and sedation (via histamine antagonism). These side effects can be used to advantage in many patients. It is also associated with headache, dry mouth and, less commonly, dizziness, postural hypotension, tremor and peripheral oedema. It has negligible anticholinergic effects.

Contraindications: mania.

Tricyclic antidepressants

Table 2.2 summarizes the common side effects of TCAs, most of which are related to the multireceptor blocking effects of these drugs. The sedative side effect can be useful if patients have insomnia. TCAs with prominent sedative effects include amitriptyline and clomipramine. Those with less sedative effects include lofepramine and imipramine. Due to their cardiotoxic effects, TCAs are dangerous in overdose, although lofepramine (a newer TCA) has fewer antimuscarinic effects, and so is relatively safe compared with other TCAs.

Contraindications: recent myocardial infarction, arrhythmias, acute porphyria, mania and high risk for overdose.

RED FLAG

Tricyclics can be particularly dangerous in overdose due to cardiovascular and neurological complications. Please see Chapter 7 for further discussion on common features of TCA overdose and management.

Trazodone

Trazodone is a relatively weak antidepressant but a good sedative. It is relatively safe in overdose and has negligible anticholinergic side effects. It is often used as an adjunctive antidepressant in those receiving a nonsedative primary antidepressant (e.g., an SSRI). Its low side effect profile means trazodone is commonly used in patients with stress and distress in dementia (see Chapter 20), although this is an 'off label' use of the medication.

Contraindications: as TCAs (closely related structurally).

RED FLAG

Antidepressants should be used with caution in patients with epilepsy, as they can increase seizure frequency, either by directly lowering the seizure threshold or by interacting with the metabolism of antiepileptics. However, depression is common and often undertreated in patients with epilepsy, so it is important not to avoid antidepressants if they are indicated. SSRIs or SNRIs are usually recommended as first-line treatments.

MAOIs/RIMAs

Due to the risk for serious interactions with certain foods and other drugs, the MAOIs have become much less frequently used in modern psychiatry. Their inhibition of monoamine oxidase A results in the accumulation of amine neurotransmitters and impairs the metabolism of some amines found in certain drugs (e.g., decongestants) and foodstuffs (e.g., tyramine). Because MAOIs bind irreversibly to monoamine oxidase A and B, amines may accumulate to dangerously high levels, which may precipitate a life-threatening hypertensive crisis. An example of this occurs when the ingestion of dietary tyramine results in a massive release of noradrenaline (norepinephrine) from endogenous stores. This is termed the 'cheese reaction' because some mature cheeses contain high levels of tyramine. Box 2.2 lists the drugs and foodstuffs that should be avoided in patients taking MAOIs.

RED FLAG

An early warning sign of a hypertensive crisis is a throbbing headache. Check blood pressure in someone taking an MAOI who feels unwell.

BOX 2.2 DRUGS AND FOODS THAT MAY PRECIPITATE A HYPERTENSIVE CRISIS IN COMBINATION WITH MAOIS

Tyramine-rich foods

Cheese – especially mature varieties (e.g., Stilton)
Degraded protein: pickled herring, smoked fish, chicken liver, hung game
Yeast and protein extract: Bovril, Oxo, Marmite
Chianti wine, beer
Broad bean pods
Soya bean extract
Overripe or unfresh food

Medication or substances

Adrenaline (epinephrine), noradrenaline (norepinephrine)
Amphetamines
Cocaine
Ephedrine, pseudoephedrine, phenylpropanolamine (cough mixtures, decongestants)
L-DOPA, dopamine
Local anaesthetics containing adrenaline (epinephrine)

Note: the combination of MAOIs and antidepressants or opioids (especially pethidine or tramadol) may result in serotonin syndrome. Opioids have some serotonin reuptake inhibitory activity.

The reversible inhibitor of monoamine oxidase A (RIMA) moclobemide reversibly inhibits monoamine oxidase A. Therefore the drug will be displaced from the enzyme as amine levels start to increase. So, although there is a small risk for developing a hypertensive crisis if high levels of tyramine are ingested, dietary restrictions are much less onerous.

RED FLAG

When other antidepressants that have a strong serotonergic effect (e.g., SSRIs, clomipramine, imipramine, vortioxetine) are administered simultaneously with an MAOI, the risk for developing the potentially lethal serotonin syndrome is increased (see Chapter 7). Therefore antidepressant 'wash-out' periods are required if starting or stopping an MAOI – check guidance for the specific switch you are considering.

MAOIs may have further side effects like those induced by TCAs, including postural hypotension and anticholinergic effects.

Contraindications (MAOIs): phaeochromocytoma, cerebrovascular disease and mania.

HINTS AND TIPS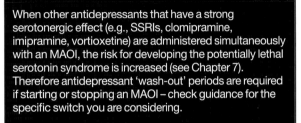

The abrupt withdrawal of any antidepressant may result in a discontinuation syndrome with symptoms such as gastrointestinal disturbance, agitation, dizziness, headache, tremor and insomnia. SSRIs with short half-lives (e.g., paroxetine, sertraline) and venlafaxine are particular culprits. Therefore all antidepressants (except for fluoxetine, which has a long half-life and many active metabolites) should be gradually tapered down before being withdrawn completely.

COMMUNICATION

Although certain antidepressants may cause a discontinuation syndrome, they do not cause a dependence syndrome or 'addiction'. Patients do not become tolerant to them or crave them.

MOOD STABILIZERS

These include lithium and the anticonvulsants valproate, carbamazepine and lamotrigine. Antipsychotics such as quetiapine and olanzapine are also increasingly used in treating episodes of mania and in prophylactic mood stabilization (these are covered in the next section; see also Chapter 24).

History

In 1949, John Cade discovered that lithium salts caused lethargy when injected into animals, and later reported lithium's antimanic properties in humans. Trials in the 1950s and 1960s led to the drug entering mainstream practice in 1970.

Valproate was first recognized as an effective anticonvulsant in 1962. Along with carbamazepine and lamotrigine, it was later shown to be effective in treating patients with bipolar disorder.

Mechanism of action

It is not known how any of the mood stabilizers work. Lithium appears to modulate the neurotransmitter-induced activation of second messenger systems. Valproate, carbamazepine and lamotrigine all inhibit the activity of voltage-gated sodium channels, and also enhance GABA-ergic neurotransmission.

Indications

Lithium is used in the treatment of:

- Acute mania
- Prophylaxis of bipolar disorder (prevention of relapse)
- Treatment-resistant depression (lithium augmentation)

Valproate is used in the treatment of:

- Epilepsy
- Acute mania
- Prophylaxis of bipolar disorder (second line)

Carbamazepine is used in the treatment of:

- Epilepsy
- Prophylaxis of bipolar disorder (third line)

Lamotrigine is used in the treatment of:

- Epilepsy
- Prophylaxis of depressive episodes in bipolar disorder (third line)

HINTS AND TIPS

Valproate is available in formulations as sodium valproate, valproic acid and semi-sodium valproate (Depakote), which comprises equimolar amounts of sodium valproate and valproic acid. Different formulations have different equivalent doses, so prescribe by brand.

Side effects and contraindications

Lithium

Lithium has a narrow therapeutic window between nontherapeutic and toxic blood levels. Lower levels can be toxic in older patients.

- Therapeutic levels: 0.4 to 0.8 mmol/L when used adjunctively for depression; 0.6 to 1.0 mmol/L for treatment of acute mania and for bipolar disorder prophylaxis
- Toxic levels: >1.5 mmol/L
- Dangerously toxic levels: >2 mmol/L

Lithium is taken orally as the carbonate or citrate salt, and is excreted almost entirely unchanged by the kidneys, without hepatic metabolism. Clearance of lithium is decreased with renal impairment (e.g., in older adults, dehydration) and sodium depletion. Certain drugs such as diuretics (especially thiazides), nonsteroidal antiinflammatory drugs (NSAIDs) and angiotensin-converting enzyme (ACE) inhibitors can also increase lithium levels and should ideally be avoided or prescribed with caution and frequent checks of lithium levels during initiation. Furthermore, antipsychotics may synergistically increase lithium-induced neurotoxicity; this is important, as lithium and antipsychotics are often coadministered in acute mania. Table 2.3 summarizes the side effects and signs of toxicity of lithium. See Chapter 7 for further information on identifying and managing lithium toxicity.

RED FLAG

Lithium toxicity can arise rapidly in someone who becomes dehydrated for any reason (e.g., vomiting, diarrhoea, inadequate fluid intake). Always check a random lithium level in someone prescribed lithium who is physically unwell.

Table 2.3 Side effects and signs of toxicity of lithium (see also Chapter 7)

Side effects	Signs of toxicity
Thirst, polydipsia, polyuria, weight gain, oedema Fine tremor Precipitates or worsens skin problems Concentration and memory problems Hypothyroidism Hyperparathyroidism Impaired renal function Cardiac: T-wave flattening or inversion Leucocytosis	**1.5–2 mmol/L:** nausea and vomiting, apathy, coarse tremor, ataxia, muscle weakness **>2 mmol/L:** nystagmus, dysarthria, impaired consciousness, hyperactive tendon reflexes, oliguria, hypotension, convulsions, coma

The following investigations are needed prior to initiating therapy:

- Full blood count
- Urea and electrolytes
- Calcium
- Thyroid function
- Pregnancy test (in women of childbearing age)
- Electrocardiogram (if cardiac disease or risk factors)

Blood levels are monitored weekly, 12 hours postdose, after starting treatment until a therapeutic level has been stable for 2 consecutive weeks. Lithium blood levels should then be monitored every 3 months for the first year, then every 6 months (unless the patient is at high risk for complications from lithium or has poor concordance). Renal function, calcium and thyroid function should be monitored every 6 months or more frequently if there is any evidence of impairment.

Contraindications/cautions: untreated hypothyroidism, heart failure, cardiac arrhythmia, Addison disease.

Valproate, carbamazepine and lamotrigine

Table 2.4 summarizes the side effects of carbamazepine, valproate and lamotrigine. It is important to check liver and haematological functions prior to and soon after starting valproate or carbamazepine, due to the risk for serious blood and hepatic disorders.

Prescribing advice around valproate has tightened significantly recently. The current recommendation is that valproate should not be prescribed to anyone under the age of 55, unless two specialists independently agree that it is absolutely essential. Valproate has a high teratogenic risk and has been linked to developmental disorders (one-third of births) and congenital malformations (one-tenth of births). It has also been linked to male infertility. If it is felt that there is no other alternative to valproate, ensure that the patient is fully aware of the risks, and if female, that they are registered with the pregnancy prevention program. As part of the program, they must sign a risk acknowledgment form prior to commencing the medication, agree to take adequate forms of contraception and agree to consult promptly if they become pregnant while taking valproate.

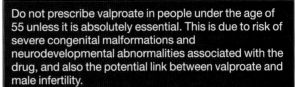

RED FLAG

Do not prescribe valproate in people under the age of 55 unless it is absolutely essential. This is due to risk of severe congenital malformations and neurodevelopmental abnormalities associated with the drug, and also the potential link between valproate and male infertility.

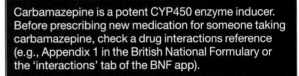

RED FLAG

Carbamazepine is a potent CYP450 enzyme inducer. Before prescribing new medication for someone taking carbamazepine, check a drug interactions reference (e.g., Appendix 1 in the British National Formulary or the 'interactions' tab of the BNF app).

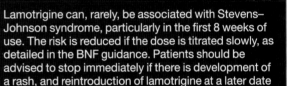

RED FLAG

Lamotrigine can, rarely, be associated with Stevens–Johnson syndrome, particularly in the first 8 weeks of use. The risk is reduced if the dose is titrated slowly, as detailed in the BNF guidance. Patients should be advised to stop immediately if there is development of a rash, and reintroduction of lamotrigine at a later date should be considered only by a specialist.

ANTIPSYCHOTICS

History and classification

Antipsychotics or neuroleptics (originally known as 'major tranquillizers') appeared in the early 1950s with the introduction of the phenothiazine, chlorpromazine. It was synthesized

Table 2.4 Side effects of valproate, carbamazepine and lamotrigine

Valproate[a]	Carbamazepine[b]	Lamotrigine[c]
Increased appetite and weight gain	Nausea and vomiting	Nausea and vomiting
Sedation and dizziness	Skin rashes	Skin rashes (consider withdrawal)
Ankle swelling	Blurred or double vision (diplopia)	Headache
Hair loss	Ataxia, drowsiness, fatigue	Aggression, irritability
Nausea and vomiting	Hyponatraemia and fluid retention	Sedation and dizziness
Tremor	Haematological abnormalities	Tremor
Haematological abnormalities (prolongation of bleeding time, thrombocytopenia, leucopoenia)	(leucopoenia, thrombocytopenia, eosinophilia)	
Raised liver enzymes (liver damage very uncommon)	Raised liver enzymes (hepatic or cholestatic jaundice, rarely)	

[a]Serious blood and liver disorders do occur, but are rare.
[b]Serious blood and liver disorders do occur, but are rare.
[c]Stevens–Johnson syndrome can occur, but it is rare.

by Charpentier and was initially developed as a possible agent to enhance the actions of general anaesthetic agents. A number of antipsychotics with a similar pharmacodynamic action soon followed (e.g., the butyrophenone haloperidol in the 1960s). Their ability to treat psychotic symptoms had a profound impact on psychiatry, accelerating the movement of patients out of asylums and into the community. However, serious motor side effects (extrapyramidal side effects (EPSEs)) soon became apparent with all these drugs.

Clozapine was the first antipsychotic with fewer EPSEs, and thus was termed 'atypical'. It led to the introduction of several other atypical (or 'second generation') antipsychotics, including risperidone, olanzapine and quetiapine. The older antipsychotics such as haloperidol and chlorpromazine became known as 'conventional', 'first generation' or 'typical' antipsychotics. However, this distinction is increasingly viewed as artificial – all antipsychotics can induce EPSEs if given at high enough doses. Clozapine is the only 'true' atypical antipsychotic, in that it has a distinct receptor binding profile and can be effective in two-thirds of the patients for whom other antipsychotics have failed. Table 2.5 lists common antipsychotics.

Mechanism of action and side effects

The primary mechanism of action of the majority of anti-psychotics is antagonism of dopamine D_2 receptors in the mesolimbic dopamine pathway. Clozapine is a comparatively weak D_2 antagonist, but has a high affinity for serotonin type 2 receptors (5-HT$_{2A}$ receptors) and dopamine D_4 receptors, among many other receptor targets. Most second-generation antipsychotics also block 5-HT$_2$ receptors. Aripiprazole is different to other second-generation antipsychotics, as it is a partial D2 agonist. The weaker D_2 antagonism of clozapine is why patients tend to have fewer motor side effects compared to, e.g., older first-generation antipsychotics, which cause a D_2 blockade across the brain. The blockade of dopamine D_2 receptors throughout the brain, results in diverse side effects. In addition, antipsychotics also cause side effects by blocking muscarinic, histaminergic and α-adrenergic receptors (as do TCAs). Fig. 2.2 and Table 2.6 summarize both the useful and

Table 2.5 Commonly used antipsychotics

First generation	Second generation
Chlorpromazine	Clozapine
Haloperidol[a]	Olanzapine[a]
Sulpiride	Quetiapine
Flupentixol (Depixol)[a]	Risperidone[a]
Zuclopenthixol (Clopixol)[a]	Aripiprazole[a]

[a]Can be given in long-acting intramuscular injection (depot) form.

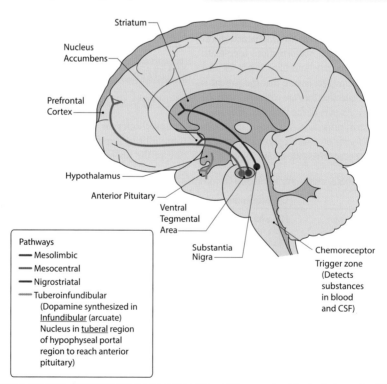

Fig. 2.2 Dopaminergic pathways. See Table 2.6 for consequences of D_2 receptor blockade in each of these regions. CSF, *Cerebrospinal fluid.*

Table 2.6 The clinical effects and side effects of conventional antipsychotics

Dopamine D$_2$-receptor antagonism		
Location of dopamine D$_2$ receptors (see Fig. 2.2)	Function	Clinical effect of dopamine D$_2$-receptor antagonism
[1] Mesolimbic pathway	Involved in delusions/hallucinations/thought disorders, euphoria and drug dependence	Treatment of psychotic symptoms.
[2] Mesocortical pathway	Mediates cognitive and negative symptoms of schizophrenia	Worsening of negative and cognitive symptoms of schizophrenia.
[3] Nigrostriatal pathway (basal ganglia/striatum)	Controls motor movement	Extrapyramidal side effects (see Table 2.7): • Parkinsonian symptoms • Acute dystonia • Akathisia • Tardive dyskinesia • Neuroleptic malignant syndrome
[4] Tuberoinfundibular pathway	Controls prolactin secretion – dopamine inhibits prolactin release	Hyperprolactinaemia • Galactorrhoea (breast milk production) • Amenorrhoea and infertility • Sexual dysfunction
Chemoreceptor trigger zone	Controls nausea and vomiting	Antiemetic effect: some phenothiazines (e.g., prochlorperazine (Stemetil)) are very effective in treating nausea and vomiting.
Other side effects		
Anticholinergic: muscarinic receptor blockade		Dry mouth, constipation, urinary retention, blurred vision
α-Adrenergic receptor blockade		Postural hypotension (dizziness, syncope)
Histaminergic receptor blockade		Sedation, weight gain
Cardiac effects		Prolongation of QT-interval, arrhythmias, myocarditis, sudden death
Metabolic effects		Increased risk for metabolic syndrome
Dermatological effects		Photosensitivity, skin rashes (especially chlorpromazine: blue–grey discolouration in the sun)
Other		Lowering of seizure threshold, hepatotoxicity, cholestatic jaundice, pancytopenia, agranulocytosis

troublesome clinical effects of D$_2$-receptor antagonism, as well as the side effects caused by the blockage of other receptors. Learn this table well; these effects have a big impact on patients' quality of life and concordance (and as such are frequently asked exam questions). See also Table 23.2 for the relative frequency of side effects for some commonly used antipsychotics.

The risk for metabolic syndrome (obesity, diabetes, hypertension and dyslipidaemia) is particularly high with clozapine and other second-generation antipsychotics. Metabolic syndrome is associated with increased cardiovascular mortality, so it is important to monitor and manage the components of this syndrome.

Clozapine is associated with some rare serious side effects such as agranulocytosis, myocarditis and cardiomyopathy, which means it is reserved for treatment-resistant cases.

HINTS AND TIPS

If you can remember the side effects of tricyclic antidepressants, you can remember many of the side effects of antipsychotics, as both are multireceptor blockers. Both groups are anticholinergic (dry mouth, constipation, blurred vision, urinary retention), antiadrenergic (postural hypotension) and antihistaminergic (sedation, weight gain).

Table 2.7 summarizes the antipsychotic-induced EPSEs and treatment. Certain antipsychotics are available in a slow-release form as an intramuscular depot preparation that can be administered every 1 to 12 weeks (e.g., flupentixol (Depixol), zuclopenthixol (Clopixol) and paliperidone). They are used for patients who are poorly concordant with oral therapy or who prefer the simplicity of an infrequent injection.

Contraindications/cautions: severely reduced consciousness level (sedating), phaeochromocytoma, basal ganglia disorders (e.g., Parkinson disease or Lewy body dementia (can exacerbate)), arrhythmias (can prolong QTc, consider baseline electrocardiogram).

Indications

- Schizophrenia, schizoaffective disorder, delusional disorder
- Prophylaxis in bipolar disorder
- Depression or mania with psychotic features
- Psychotic episodes secondary to a medical condition or psychoactive substance use
- Behavioural disturbance in delirium posing a signifcant risk to the patient or others

Behavioural disturbance in dementia (caution is recommended, as there is an increased risk for cerebrovascular events)

Severe agitation, anxiety and violent or impulsive behaviour

Tics (Tourette syndrome)

Nausea and vomiting (e.g., prochlorperazine)

Intractable hiccups and pruritus (e.g., chlorpromazine, haloperidol)

Clozapine

Introduction

Clozapine was first introduced into clinical practice in Europe in the 1970s, but shortly afterwards it was withdrawn by manufacturers due to reports of deaths because of agranulocytosis (bone marrow suppression). Following several trials which studied the use of clozapine alongside regular blood monitoring with positive results, it was reintroduced in the United Kingdom in 1990 alongside compulsory haematological monitoring for all patients taking the medication. Clozapine is only used for patients who have failed to respond to adequate trials of two or more antipsychotics (also known as treatment-resistant schizophrenia), or in those who cannot tolerate the movement-related side effects of other antipsychotics.

Clozapine is effective in around 40% to 50% of patients with treatment-resistant schizophrenia, and it has been linked to a reduction in an all-cause mortality, completed suicides, and aggression in this patient group. Despite the positives of clozapine, there are several side effects that can be problematic for patients, and in some cases life-threatening. Agranulocytosis, life-threatening bone marrow suppression, occurs in approximately 0.8% of patients taking clozapine. With the introduction of monitoring, fatalities from agranulocytosis are very rare, occurring in less than 1 in 5000 patients.

Side effects and monitoring

While it is an extremely effective antipsychotic, clozapine is associated with a long list of side effects including:

1. Agranulocytosis
2. Myocarditis
3. Postural hypotension and tachycardia
4. Hypersalivation
5. Constipation
6. Weight gain and metabolic syndrome
7. Urinary problems (incontinence and urinary retention)
8. Seizures (clozapine lowers the seizure threshold)
9. Sedation

Due to the potential for side effects, clozapine is commonly initiated in an inpatient setting, although it can occasionally be initiated in the community for certain patient groups. It is started at a low dose, and increased in stepwise increments, usually over a 2-week period, although this can be adjusted

Table 2.7 Antipsychotic-induced extrapyramidal side effects and treatment

Extrapyramidal side effect	Description	Treatment
Parkinsonism	Muscular rigidity, bradykinesia (lack of or slowing of movement), resting tremor Generally occurs within a month of starting antipsychotic	Anticholinergics (e.g., procyclidine (i.v. or i.m. if unable to swallow, oral otherwise)) Consider reducing dose of antipsychotic or switching to antipsychotic with fewer extrapyramidal side effects (e.g., atypical)
Dystonia	Involuntary sustained muscular contractions or spasms (e.g., neck (spasmodic torticollis), clenched jaw (trismus), protruding tongue, eyes rolling upwards (oculogyric crisis)) More common in young men Usually occurs within 72 hours of treatment	
Akathisia	Subjective feeling of inner restlessness and muscular discomfort Occurs within days to weeks of starting an antipsychotic	Propranolol or short-term benzodiazepines Consider reducing dose of antipsychotic or switching to antipsychotic with fewer extrapyramidal side effects (e.g., atypical)
Tardive dyskinesia	Rhythmic, involuntary movements of head, limbs and trunk, especially chewing, grimacing and making protruding, darting movements with the tongue Develops in up to 20% of patients who receive long-term treatment with conventional antipsychotics	No effective treatment Withdraw antipsychotic if possible Clozapine might be helpful Consider benzodiazepines Do not give anticholinergics (may worsen tardive dyskinesia)

Neuroleptic malignant syndrome – see Chapter 7

depending on factors such as age and side effect burden. Due to the risk of side effects detailed earlier, close physiological monitoring is done before and during clozapine initiation, and continues, albeit less frequently, once a patient has been established on a regular dose. The following parameters/tests are included as part of clozapine monitoring:

1. Full blood count (FBC): patients who are prescribed clozapine must be registered with the manufacturers mandatory blood monitoring program, due to the association with agranulocytosis. All patients will have a FBC taken as a baseline prior to initiation of clozapine. They will then have FBCs taken weekly for the first 18 weeks, fortnightly for weeks 18 to 52 and monthly after the patient has been taking clozapine for a year and their neutrophil counts have been stable. If neutrophil counts drop, a traffic light system is in place to help decide whether the drug needs to be reduced or stopped.
2. Body mass index (BMI): there is an association with weight gain and metabolic syndrome following the initiation of clozapine. Weight is taken at baseline, 3 monthly for 1 year and then annually. Lifestyle advice around diet and exercise is the first-line recommendation for patients who struggle with clozapine-related weight gain.
3. Fasting glucose: this is measured at baseline, at 1 month and then 3 monthly up to a year and then on a 6-monthly basis.

If there are concerns about a patient developing Type II diabetes, an HbA1c can be checked and discussed with their GP regarding ongoing management.

4. Blood lipids: these are checked at baseline, 3 monthly for a year and then 6 monthly. If they are elevated, consider commencing a statin.
5. Blood pressure and heart rate: these are monitored closely during the initiation period due to the potential for hypotension. If a patient develops tachycardia during initiation, consider whether they are experiencing any other symptoms of myocarditis, e.g., chest pain, shortness of breath, fever; and also consider the results of other investigations such as ECG, the C-reactive protein (CRP) and troponin. If there are any concerns about myocarditis, the patient needs to be transferred urgently for medical assessment and intervention. If the tachycardia is not associated with myocarditis, then consider slowing down the rate of dose increase.
6. ECG: an ECG is obtained at baseline, 3 months and then annually.
7. Urea and electrolytes and liver function tests: these are obtained at baseline and then annually or as clinically indicated.
8. CRP and troponin: these are measured during the initiation phase in some areas – any increase may be suggestive of the

patient developing myocarditis and will require further investigation.

9. Smoking status: the chemicals in cigarette smoke increase the rate of metabolism of clozapine. Therefore, a patient who is a heavy smoker may require a higher dose of clozapine than if they were a nonsmoker. If a patient who has been a heavy smoker quits, there can be a rapid increase in the plasma level of clozapine which can cause toxicity or severe side effects.

10. Pregnancy/contraceptive status (for women of reproductive age): clozapine is contraindicated in breastfeeding and is used cautiously in pregnancy. Women of childbearing potential should be signposted to information about contraceptives and encouraged to engage in pre-pregnancy counselling and tell services promptly if they become pregnant.

Indications

- Treatment-resistant schizophrenia
- Psychosis in Parkinson disease

Contraindications

History of agranulocytosis or neutropenia, paralytic ileus, severe cardiac disorders, e.g., myocarditis, uncontrolled epilepsy, coma

ANXIOLYTIC AND HYPNOTIC DRUGS

A hypnotic drug is one that induces sleep. An anxiolytic drug is one that reduces anxiety. This differentiation is not particularly helpful, as anxiolytic drugs can induce sleep when given in higher doses, and hypnotics can have a calming effect when given in lower doses (e.g., the benzodiazepines, which are anxiolytic in low doses and hypnotic in high doses). This is reflected in the term 'sedative,' which refers to both these effects and is generally used to refer to a drug with hypnotic and/or anxiolytic effects. All such drugs can result in tolerance, dependence and withdrawal symptoms. Furthermore, their effects, when used in combination or with alcohol, are additive. The most important drugs in this group are the benzodiazepines and 'Z drugs' (zopiclone, zolpidem and zaleplon), which have very similar actions and indications.

HINTS AND TIPS

In the past, the antipsychotics have been referred to as the 'major tranquillizers,' and the anxiolytics as the 'minor tranquillizers'. This is misleading because: (1) these drugs are not pharmacologically related; (2) the antipsychotics do far more than just tranquillize; and (3) the effect and use of anxiolytics are in no way minor.

History

In the 1960s, the benzodiazepines replaced the often-abused barbiturates as the drugs of choice for the treatment of anxiety and insomnia. However, this initial enthusiasm was tempered by the observations that they were associated with serious dependence and withdrawal syndromes and had gained a market as drugs of abuse. Z drugs were introduced in the 1990s and were initially thought to be less likely to cause dependence – this is not true. Today, benzodiazepines and Z drugs are recognized as highly effective and relatively safe drugs when prescribed judiciously, for short periods and with good patient education.

Classification

From a clinical perspective, it is useful to group benzodiazepines and Z drugs according to their duration of action and route of administration. Table 2.8 summarizes these qualities in some common drugs.

Mechanism of action

Benzodiazepines potentiate the action of GABA (γ-aminobutyric acid), the main inhibitory neurotransmitter in the brain. They are $GABA_A$-positive allosteric modulators: they bind to specific benzodiazepine modulatory sites on the $GABA_A$ receptor complex, which results in an increased affinity of the complex for GABA, and so an increased flow of chloride ions into the cell. This hyperpolarizes the postsynaptic membrane and reduces neuronal excitability. Z drugs are also $GABA_A$-positive allosteric modulators, binding to a different but neighbouring site to benzodiazepines.

Indications of benzodiazepines

- Insomnia, especially short-acting benzodiazepines (short-term use only).
- Anxiety disorders (short-term use only).
- Alcohol withdrawal, especially chlordiazepoxide.
- Acute mania or psychosis (sedation).
- Akathisia: see Table 2.7.
- Other: epilepsy prophylaxis, seizures, muscle spasm (diazepam) and anaesthetic premedication.

Indications of Z drugs

- Insomnia (short-term use)

Side effects of benzodiazepines and Z drugs

- Risk for developing dependence, especially with prolonged use and shorter-acting drugs.
- Patients should be warned about the potential dangers of driving or operating machinery due to drowsiness, ataxia and reduced motor coordination.

Table 2.8 Classification of the benzodiazepines and Z drugs

Drug	Dose equivalent to 5 mg diazepam (mg)	Duration of action	Time to peak effect	Half-life (h)	Routes of administration
Benzodiazepines					
Midazolam	2.5	Short	5–10 min	2	Oromucosal solution, s.c., i.v.
Temazepam	10	Short	2–3 h	11	Oral
Lorazepam	0.5	Short	1–4 h	15	Oral, i.m.[a], i.v.
Nitrazepam	2.5	Medium	1–2 h	30	Oral
Chlordiazepoxide	15	Long	1–4 h	100	Oral
Diazepam	5	Long	5–10 h	100	Oral, per rectum, i.v.; i.m. only if no alternative
Clonazepam	250 µg	Medium	1–4 h	30	Oral
Z drugs					
Zaleplon	5	Very short	1 h	1	Oral
Zolpidem	5	Short	1 h	2	Oral
Zopiclone	3.75	Short	2 h	5	Oral

[a]Lorazepam is the only benzodiazepine that has predictable absorption when given intramuscularly.

- Use with great caution in older adults where drowsiness, confusion and ataxia can precipitate falls or delirium.
- Use with caution in patients with chronic respiratory disease (e.g., chronic obstructive pulmonary disease, sleep apnoea), as they may depress respiration.

RED FLAG

Benzodiazepines or Z drugs (zopiclone, zolpidem and zaleplon) are seldom fatal in overdose if taken alone, but can be when taken in combination with other sedatives. Flumazenil is an antagonist at the benzodiazepine site on the GABA$_A$ receptor and can reverse the effects of both benzodiazepines and Z drugs (which bind close by). It can precipitate acute benzodiazepine withdrawal and lower the seizure threshold, so must only be used in an acute hospital setting when the benefits outweigh the risks.

RED FLAG

Alcohol, opiates, barbiturates, tricyclic antidepressants, antihistamines and other sedatives may all enhance the effects of benzodiazepines and Z drugs; therefore moderate doses of benzodiazepines in combination with some of these substances can result in respiratory depression.

Other hypnotic and anxiolytic agents

- Pregabalin is used to treat generalized anxiety disorder. It is structurally related to GABA but does not act directly on receptors or enzymes that recognize GABA. Rather, it reduces the release of a range of neurotransmitters through binding to an auxiliary subunit of voltage-gated calcium channels. Gabapentin's mechanism is very similar.
- Buspirone is a 5-HT$_{1A}$ receptor agonist that is used to treat generalized anxiety disorder. It is unrelated to the benzodiazepines; does not have hypnotic, anticonvulsant or muscle relaxant properties; and is not associated with dependence or abuse. Response to treatment may take up to 2 weeks, unlike the benzodiazepines, which have an immediate anxiolytic effect.
- Melatonin is a synthetic version of the natural hormone produced by the pineal gland which triggers sleep initiation. It is commonly used in CAMHS and learning disability settings but is also licensed for short-term use in the management of insomnia in over 55 s and in jet lag. It promotes sleep initiation only, not maintenance.
- Sedating antihistamines (e.g., diphenhydramine (Nytol), promethazine (Sominex)) are available for insomnia without a prescription. Unfortunately, their long duration of action may lead to drowsiness the following day.

- Promethazine may also be used in the management of agitation and acute behavioural disturbance in psychiatric inpatients, often in combination with haloperidol. It is increasingly used as part of local 'rapid tranquilization' policies.

OTHER DRUGS USED IN PSYCHIATRY

- Alcohol dependence: acamprosate, disulfiram, naltrexone.
- Opiate dependence: methadone, buprenorphine, lofexidine, naltrexone.
- Dementia: cholinesterase inhibitors (donepezil, rivastigmine, galantamine), memantine.
- Attention deficit hyperactivity disorder: *stimulants:* methylphenidate, dexamfetamine; and *nonstimulants:* atomoxetine, guanfacine.
- Antipsychotic-induced weight gain: metformin.

ELECTROCONVULSIVE THERAPY

History

The possibility that seizures could improve psychiatric symptoms arose from the observation that convulsions appeared to lead to an improvement of psychotic symptoms in patients with comorbid epilepsy and schizophrenia. This led to seizures being induced pharmacologically with intramuscular camphor in the early 1930s. An electric stimulus was later discovered to be an effective way of inducing seizures. Modern-day anaesthetic induction agents and muscle relaxants make electroconvulsive therapy (ECT) a highly safe and nondistressing procedure. ECT is a highly effective and often life-saving treatment for patients with serious mental illness. It is the most effective treatment known for severe depression (with an effect size of 0.9).

Indications

ECT is predominantly used for depression and can be particularly effective in older adults and postpartum women. Although antidepressants are usually tried first, ECT is considered for the following features of depression:

- Life-threatening poor fluid intake
- Strong suicidal intent
- Psychotic features or stupor
- When antidepressants are ineffective or not tolerated

ECT is an effective treatment for severe mania (although in rare cases it can precipitate a manic episode in patients with bipolar disorder). ECT is also an effective treatment for certain types of schizophrenia: catatonic states, positive psychotic symptoms and schizoaffective disorder. ECT is also used for puerperal psychosis (see Chapter 29) with prominent mood symptoms or severe postnatal depression where a rapid improvement is necessary to reunite the mother with her baby.

In 2018 to 2019, 68% of people who had been treated with ECT were 'much-improved' or 'very much improved' at the end of treatment (1361 courses out of a total of 2004).

Administration and mechanism of action

ECT is usually administered 1 to 2 times per week. Most courses of ECT last for between 3 and 6 weeks, with typical numbers of treatments required ranging between 6 and 12. An anaesthetist administers a short-acting induction agent and muscle relaxant that ensure about 5 to 10 minutes of general anaesthesia. During this time, a psychiatrist applies two electrodes to the patient's scalp, in a bilateral or unilateral placement, and delivers an electric current of sufficient charge to cause a generalized seizure of at least 15 seconds in duration.

It is still not clear how ECT works. It causes a release of neurotransmitters, as well as hypothalamic and pituitary hormones; it also affects neurotransmitter receptors and second messenger systems, and results in a transient increase in blood–brain barrier permeability.

Side effects

The mortality rate associated with ECT is the same as that for any minor surgical procedure under general anaesthesia (i.e., around 1 in 100,000). Loss of memory is a common complaint, particularly for events surrounding the ECT. Some patients also report some impairment of autobiographical memory. Unfortunately, studies that examine the long-term effects of ECT are difficult to perform. Memory impairment can be reduced by unilateral electrode placement (as opposed to bilateral).

Minor complaints such as confusion, headache, nausea and muscle pains are experienced by 80% of patients. Anaesthetic complications (e.g., arrhythmias, aspiration) can be reduced by a good preoperative assessment. Prolonged seizures may occur, especially in patients who are on drugs that lower the seizure threshold (e.g., antidepressants and antipsychotics). In contrast, benzodiazepines increase the seizure threshold, making it more difficult to induce a seizure of adequate length.

Contraindications

Absolute contraindications to ECT:

- phaeochromocytoma

Relative contraindications include:

- Heart disease (recent myocardial infarction, heart failure, ischaemic heart disease)
- Raised intracranial pressure
- Cerebral or aortic aneurysm
- Risk for cerebral bleeding (hypertension, recent stroke)
- High anaesthetic risk

ETHICS

Media portrayals of ECT have included its use as a punishment, given without patient consent. In modern practice, a patient with capacity will make their own decision about commencing ECT or not. A patient who lacks capacity may be given ECT without their consent if it is felt to be in their best interests; however, this requires a second opinion from an independent psychiatrist.

Chapter Summary

- Psychotropic medications are classed by the indication for which they were first licensed, but many medications are of benefit in other disorders.
- Antidepressants mainly influence the serotonin, noradrenaline and dopamine systems.
- Many antidepressants are well tolerated.
- Lithium requires regular monitoring of blood levels because high levels are toxic.
- Antipsychotics exert their effect at dopamine receptors.
- Clozapine is a very effective antipsychotic but due to some rare but potentially life-threatening side effects it requires close monitoring.
- Antipsychotics often have unpleasant and debilitating side effects.
- Benzodiazepines and Z-drugs both increase the activity of $GABA_A$ receptors.
- Medications with shorter half-lives are more likely to cause discontinuation symptoms.
- Electroconvulsive therapy is a highly effective and safe treatment for severe mental illness.

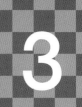
Psychological therapy, or 'talking therapies' as they are commonly known, involves the interactions between a client and a therapist with a view to influencing the thoughts, feelings and behaviours they are experiencing in a positive way. The therapy can be targeted at specific difficulties that the client is experiencing (e.g., systematic desensitization therapy in phobias), or might be more generally about trying to improve a client's sense of wellbeing (e.g., counselling). Psychological therapy can be delivered by people from many different disciplines including clinical psychologists, psychiatrists, specialist mental health nurses, occupational therapists, art, music and drama therapists, and counsellors who have had specific training and supervision in delivering the therapeutic modality they are offering.

PSYCHOTHERAPEUTIC APPROACHES

There are many different approaches to psychotherapy, with research showing efficacy for many different types of psychotherapies for a number of different conditions. This has led to the idea that the success of psychotherapy might be due to certain common therapeutic factors, as opposed to specific theories or techniques. A comprehensive review of psychotherapy research showed that common factors (occurring in any model of therapy) account for 85% of the therapeutic effect, whereas theoretical orientation only accounts for 15%. Common therapeutic factors include client factors (personal strengths, social supports), therapist–client relationship factors (empathy, acceptance, warmth), client expectancy of change and consensus on the goal of the therapy.

> ### HINTS AND TIPS
>
> 'Self-help' is the umbrella term used to describe the process of self-guided improvement. Often, self-help resources utilize psychological techniques (especially cognitive-behavioural therapy and mindfulness) and educational materials. Self-help may involve books, apps, interactive websites and discussion groups (including online forums). Self-help materials may be provided from, and progress followed and reviewed by, healthcare professionals (known as 'facilitated' or 'guided' self-help), and can be incredibly useful for

some people, either in the management of less severe psychological difficulties or as an adjunct to other forms of treatment. Group-based peer support is a form of self-help delivered to groups of patients with shared symptoms, during which experiences can be shared and progress reviewed by a facilitator.

> ### HINTS AND TIPS
>
> The single factor most commonly associated with a good therapeutic outcome is the strength of the client–therapist relationship (therapeutic alliance), regardless of the modality of therapy.

Counselling and supportive psychotherapy

Psychotherapy is usually distinguished from counselling, although they exist on a continuum from counselling and supportive psychotherapy (least complex) to psychodynamic psychotherapy and sophisticated cognitive therapy (more complex and requiring much more specialist training).

Counselling is usually brief in duration and is recommended for patients with less severe mental health or interpersonal difficulties, or for those experiencing stressful circumstances (e.g., grief counselling for bereavement). Counselling helps patients utilize their own strengths, with the therapist being reflective and empathic. The provision of relevant information and advice, which is undertaken by healthcare professionals of all specialties, is also considered to be counselling.

In person-centred counselling, the therapist assumes an empathic and reflective role, allowing patients to discover their own insights using the basic principle that the client ultimately knows best. Problem-solving counselling is more directive and focused, as patients are actively assisted in finding solutions to their problems.

Psychodynamic psychotherapy

Psychoanalysis and psychodynamic therapy have changed substantially since Sigmund Freud introduced psychoanalytic theory in the late 19th century. Fig. 3.1 summarizes some of his ideas regarding personality. The contributions of many other influential theorists (e.g., Melanie Klein, Carl Jung, Alfred Adler, John Bowlby, Donald Winnicott), alongside the expansion of evidence-based practice, have meant the continued evolution of theory and technique. However, the basic assumptions of psychoanalytic theory remain consistent: namely, that it is mainly unconscious thoughts, feelings and fantasies that give rise to distressing symptoms, and that these processes are kept unconscious by *defence mechanisms* (which are employed when anxiety-producing aspects of the self threaten to break through to the conscious mind, potentially giving rise to intolerable feelings – see Table 3.1).

The essential aim of psychoanalysis or psychodynamic psychotherapy is to facilitate conscious recognition of symptom-causing unconscious processes. It is the therapist's role to identify and interpret these processes (of which patients are consciously unaware), and to facilitate their understanding of unconscious processes in the context of a safe, caring relationship. Historically, various methods have been used (free association; hypnosis; interpretation of dreams and fantasy material;

analysis of defence mechanisms – see Table 3.1). However, modern psychodynamic psychotherapy mainly relies on the analysis of *transference* and *counter-transference*:

- Transference is the theoretical process by which the patient unconsciously transfers feelings or attitudes experienced in an earlier significant relationship onto the therapist (e.g., a patient becomes angry with their therapist, whom they see as cold and uncaring, unconsciously reminding them of their mother).
- Counter-transference refers to the feelings that are evoked in the *therapist* during the course of therapy. The therapist pays attention to these feelings, as they may be representative of what the patient is feeling, and so help the therapist to empathize with the patient. Often, therapists have undergone therapy themselves as part of their training – this helps them to separate out which feelings belong to them and which feelings belong to the patient.

Although the terms *psychoanalytic* and *psychodynamic* are often used interchangeably, they differ in the following ways:

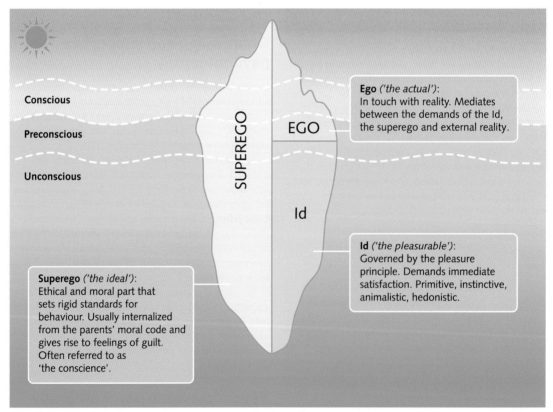

Fig. 3.1 The 'iceberg metaphor', summarizing some of Freud's ideas of personality. The iceberg itself represents the 'structural' model of the mind, while the sea represents the 'topographical model'.

Table 3.1 Some examples of psychoanalytic defence mechanisms

Type	Defence mechanism	Description	Example
Pathological	Denial	Failure to acknowledge the existence of an aspect of reality that is obvious to others.	A person who was badly assaulted reports that it did not happen.
	Projection	Attribution of unconscious feelings to others.	A person who strongly dislikes their neighbour states that their neighbour hates him.
	Splitting	Rigid separation of two extremes.	A person is convinced that their boss is an evil person after they were disciplined at work.
Immature	Fantasy	Use of imagination to avoid acknowledging a difficult or distressing reality.	A school child thinks about killing a bully, rather than taking action to stop the bullying.
	Somatization	The transformation of negative feelings towards others into physical symptoms.	A person stuck in an unhappy marriage develops medically unexplained back pain.
	Regression	Returning to an earlier stage of one's development when facing stressors.	A child begins wetting the bed again after their family migrate to a new country.
Neurotic	Repression	Blocking painful memories from consciousness.	An adult child who has no memory of being beaten by a beloved parent.
	Reaction formation	The switching of unacceptable impulses into opposites.	A person who hates his job works extra hard and performs incredibly well.
	Intellectualization	Concentrating on intellectual aspects to avoid emotional aspects of a difficult situation.	A person diagnosed with terminal cancer develops an intense interest in the classification process of tumour staging.
	Displacement	Shifting the negative feelings towards one person to another.	A person who is angry with their partner shouts at their child instead.
	Withdrawal	Escaping or avoiding situations that may be seen as distressing.	A person avoids going to parties so they don't have to talk to any new people.
Mature	Humour	Using comedy to avoid provoking discomfort in self or others.	A person laughs and mocks themself after arriving at a formal dinner dressed in casual clothes.
	Sublimation	Redirecting energy from unacceptable impulses into socially acceptable activities.	An angry person vigorously works out at the gym.
	Suppression	Consciously avoiding thinking about disturbing problems.	A student cleans the kitchen while waiting on exam results.
	Altruism	Providing a service to others in order to relieve own feeling of anxiety or discomfort	A person who is involved in criminal activity makes a large donation to a local charity.

- Psychoanalysis describes the therapy where clients see their analyst several times per week for a nonspecified period of time. Psychoanalysis is conducted with clients lying on a couch, with the analyst sitting behind them out of view. The analyst may be quieter than in psychodynamic therapy, and there is space for the patient to explore whatever comes into their mind
- Psychodynamic psychotherapy is based on psychoanalytical theory; however, it tends to be more interactive and occurs once weekly for 50 minutes per session, during which time the patient and therapist sit face-to-face. Duration of therapy varies depending on the patient's individual needs, but it can range from a few months to several years. Psychodynamic psychotherapy may be conducted on an individual basis or in a group setting.

Due to the time- and resource-intensive nature (for both the health service and the patient) of classical psychoanalysis, this is very seldom offered within the NHS, with weekly psychodynamic therapy being favoured. However, psychoanalysis is still practised within the private sector.

Mentalization-based therapy is a therapy derived from psychodynamic psychotherapy and is summarized in Table 3.4.

Attachment refers to the bond between an infant and their primary caregiver (see Chapter 33). How a person was treated by their primary caregiver during their early years sets the tone for that person's expectations of the rest of their life: how others are likely to behave towards them, and how they should behave in return. Disrupted attachment during early childhood often contributes to problems with mood, anxiety and self-esteem in adulthood and attachment difficulties (conscious or unconscious) often emerge during encounters with healthcare professionals, particularly during psychological treatment.

COMMUNICATION

Transference and counter-transference are unconscious processes that often occur in settings outside psychodynamic psychotherapy. Patients may react to healthcare professionals as if they were some significant figure from the past. An example is when patients express unwarranted anger towards doctors or nurses when they do not receive immediate attention: this may be considered anger that was initially experienced towards neglectful parents. Similarly, health workers may misplace feelings from their own earlier relationships onto patients.

Behaviour therapy

Behaviour therapy is concerned with changing maladaptive behaviour patterns that have arisen through learning (classical or operant conditioning). The premise is that if a patient changes their behaviour to make it more adaptive, this will have positive effects on how they think about things. Table 3.2 summarizes some of the techniques used in behaviour therapy.

COMMUNICATION

Avoidance increases anxiety. Many of the behavioural techniques used to treat anxiety disorders involve systematic exposure to anxiety-inducing thoughts or situations, supporting the patient to realize that they can tolerate and, in due course, reduce their fear. It can be helpful to explain to patients that they will have to experience some anxiety in order to overcome it.

Cognitive-behavioural therapy

Cognitive-behavioural therapy (CBT) is based on the assumption that the way in which individuals think about things (i.e., their cognitions) subsequently determines how they feel and behave. Likewise, physical or psychological feelings can influence the way in which an individual thinks and behaves.

Automatic thoughts involuntarily enter an individual's mind in response to specific situations (e.g., 'They don't like me'; 'I'm such an idiot'; 'I'm so boring'). *Dysfunctional assumptions* are the faulty 'rules' that individuals live by that are underlying the automatic thoughts which occur. When these rules are broken (as they inevitably are), the result is that the individual experiences psychological distress (e.g., 'If I don't come first, then I am completely useless'; 'If I hurt someone, then I am evil'). The rules themselves may be inherently problematic (e.g., 'If I tell people how I feel, this means I'm weak'). The patient is often encouraged to keep a diary of automatic thoughts, and from this the patient's thinking styles (technically called 'cognitive distortions') can be identified. Some examples are given in Table 3.3.

COMMUNICATION

One way of explaining the process of cognitive-behavioural therapy to patients is that it aims to help them notice and change 'mental bad habits' which we all have to a greater or lesser degree.

The process of therapy draws on the principle that automatic thoughts and dysfunctional assumptions may be challenged (and changed) by *behavioural experiments* (testing dysfunctional thoughts against reality).

Using an example, Fig. 3.2 illustrates the relationship between thoughts, feelings and behaviours; how automatic thoughts and dysfunctional assumptions may affect this relationship; and how challenging these may result in change.

CBT differs from psychodynamic psychotherapy in that: it is time-limited (12–24 sessions); it is goal-oriented and predominantly focuses on present problems (less concerned with the details of how problems developed or unconscious factors); the therapeutic relationship is strongly collaborative (deciding together on the session's agenda and case formulation); it involves patients doing 'homework assignments'. Also, due to its structured format, CBT is more amenable to efficacy studies.

Some other forms of therapy that incorporate elements of CBT are summarized in Table 3.4.

Interpersonal therapy

Interpersonal therapy (IPT) is based on the assumption that problems with interpersonal relationships and social functioning

Table 3.2 Some techniques used in behaviour therapy

Behavioural technique	Clinical uses	Description
Exposure	Phobias and avoidance, post-traumatic stress disorder	Graded exposure: a hierarchy of increasingly threatening situations is created (e.g., spider in another room → spider in the same room → spider near the patient → spider on the patient's hand). Patient exposed to (or imagines) the least threatening situation and stays in the situation until their anxiety reduces towards normal levels. When anxiety relief has been achieved, patients are then exposed to increasingly threatening situations. Flooding: patient instantly exposed to the highest level of their anxiety hierarchy until their anxiety diminishes (e.g., throwing a patient with a fear of water in the deep end of a swimming pool) (flooding by imagination is termed *implosion therapy*).
Exposure with response prevention	Obsessive-compulsive disorder	Patients are encouraged to resist carrying out compulsions until the urge diminishes. They are then exposed to more severe compulsion-evoking situations.
Relaxation	Anxiety	Progressive relaxation of muscle groups; breathing exercises; visualizing relaxing images and situations (*guided imagery*).
Modelling	Phobias and avoidance	Patients observe the therapist being exposed to the phobic stimulus, then attempt the same.
Activity scheduling and target setting	Depression	Patients are encouraged to structure their day with certain activities, as reduced activity can lead to further lowering of mood, due to reduced stimulation and fewer opportunities for positive experiences.

Table 3.3 Some examples of types of cognitive distortion

Cognitive distortion	Description	Example
All-or-nothing thinking	Evaluating experiences using extremes such as 'amazing' or 'awful'.	'If I don't get this job, I'll never work again'.
Mind reading	Assuming a negative response without relevant evidence.	'Because they didn't reply to my text message, they hate me'.
Personalization	Blaming self for an event.	'It's all my fault that the relationship ended'.
Overgeneralization	Drawing negative conclusions on the basis of one event.	'Because I spelt a word wrong in my essay, I'll get a lower grade'.
Fortune telling	Assuming knowledge of the future	'Now I've been told off by my boss, they are going to be on my back forever'.
Emotional reasoning	Confusing feelings with facts.	'I feel so anxious about flying: air travel must be dangerous'.
Labelling	Using unhelpful labels to describe self.	'I'm so horrible'.
Magnification	Blowing things out of proportion.	'I forgot to buy milk: my partner is going to be so angry with me'.

are significant contributors to the development of mental illness, as well as being a consequence of mental illness (particularly depression). IPT attempts to enable patients to evaluate their social interactions and improve their interpersonal skills in all social roles, from close family and friendships to community and work-related roles. One of the following areas is chosen as the main focus: (1) role disputes; (2) role transitions; (3) interpersonal deficits; and (4) loss or grief. IPT tends to focus on current problems and is brief in duration (12–16 sessions).

Dialectical behavioural therapy

Dialectical behavioural therapy (DBT) can be helpful in reducing self-harm and improving functioning in patients with personality disorders with a borderline pattern (see Chapter 30). It uses a combination of cognitive and behavioural therapies, with some relaxation techniques and mindfulness skills. It generally lasts for 2 years, with participants attending one individual and one group therapy session each week. The aim is to equip

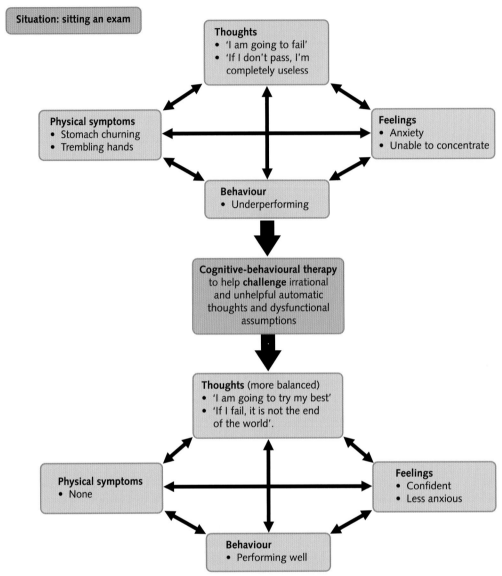

Fig. 3.2 Cognitive-behavioural formulation and the process of therapeutic change.

patients with skills to understand and manage upsetting feelings they may have. Clear, well-boundaried treatment contracts are drawn up regarding missing sessions and self-harming. Patients need to be stabilized (not recently in crisis) before embarking on the treatment course.

Motivational interviewing

Motivational interviewing (MI) is commonly used to help people with substance dependence, but it can be applied to help anyone change their behaviour (e.g., smoking cessation, weight loss). MI aims to strengthen the patient's own motivation and desire to change (making progress along the 'Stages of change' model – see Fig. 20.3). It avoids being directive (telling the patient what to do), as that can provoke the opposite reaction in someone who is ambivalent. Instead, the counsellor takes a curious and collaborative stance, allowing the patient to voice in their own words what their reasons for change might be, what the first steps should be and what they can do to overcome barriers to change. Key skills are asking open questions, offering reflections and summarizing what the patient has said themselves about change.

Table 3.4 Some therapies derived from cognitive-behavioural therapy (CBT) and psychodynamic therapy

Therapy type	Description
Eye movement desensitization and reprocessing	At the same time as giving attention to difficult (usually traumatic) memories, the therapist encourages the patient to attend to another sensory stimulus (e.g., lights or beeps). Eye movements are no longer thought necessary to the therapy. Rather, the gradual exposure to the memory in a relaxed environment seems important.
Mentalization-based therapy	Developed from psychodynamic therapy, this form of therapy focuses on allowing patients to better understand what is going on both in their own minds and in the minds of others. It can utilize both individual and group components. It can involve asking, 'How does my outside appear to other people's insides?'
Cognitive analytic therapy	Cognitive analytic therapy aims to help the patient understand the problematic roles that they repeatedly find themselves and others in, and the (dysfunctional) ways they cope with this. The aim is to increase the patient's flexibility in ways of relating, and to find 'exits' from dysfunctional patterns. The focus is on helping with present circumstances, while understanding from the past how things have arisen.
Mindfulness-based cognitive therapy	Utilizes traditional CBT methods in conjunction with mindfulness and meditation. Mindfulness focuses on becoming aware of thoughts and feelings and accepting them, rather than reacting to them.
Behavioural activation therapy	Behavioural activation is a skill covered as part of CBT, but it can be the basis of a therapy on its own. It works on the basis that low mood and depression prevent people from doing the usual activities that bring them enjoyment in their life. Avoiding these activities causes their mood to become worse however, and it can become a vicious cycle. Behavioural activation helps people restart these activities and assess how their behaviour is influencing their mental state.

Group therapy

Group therapy may be practised according to different theoretical orientations, from supportive, to cognitive-behavioural, to psychodynamic approaches. Most groups meet once weekly for an hour and consist of one or two therapists and about 5 to 10 patients. Therapy can run from months (CBT orientation) to years (psychodynamic orientation). Group therapy allows patients (and therapists) the opportunity to observe and analyse their psychological and behavioural responses to other members of the group in a 'safe' social setting. It is thought that group therapy owes its effectiveness to a number of 'curative factors' (e.g., universality, which describes the process of patients realizing that they are not alone in having particular problems).

Family therapy

Instead of focusing on the individual patient, these forms of therapy treat the family as a whole. It may include just parents and siblings or may also include extended family. It is hoped that improved family communication and conflict resolution will result in an improvement in the patient's symptoms. Similar to group therapy, there are many different orientations, most notably the psychodynamic, structural and systemic approaches. It is the mainstay of treatment in eating disorders in adolescents.

Therapeutic community (milieu therapy)

Therapeutic communities are cohesive residential communities that consist of a group of about 30 patients who are residents

for between 9 and 18 months. During this time, residents are encouraged to take responsibility for themselves and others (e.g., by allowing them to be involved in running the unit). These communities may be useful for patients with personality disorders (especially personality disorders with a borderline pattern) and behavioural problems.

HINTS AND TIPS

Mindfulness is an increasingly common component of a range of psychological therapies. It is also something that many people in the general population choose to explore. In essence, mindfulness is keeping one's attention on the present moment. While trying to do this, it is common for a lot of thoughts and feelings unrelated to the present moment to come into consciousness: mindfulness aims to nonjudgmentally acknowledge these without shifting attention onto them.

INDICATIONS FOR PSYCHOLOGICAL THERAPY

The psychological treatment options for specific conditions have been discussed in each of the relevant chapters on these conditions. The main treatment options with the strongest evidence bases, along with relevant cross-references, are summarized in Table 3.5.

Table 3.5 Main indications for psychological treatments

Psychiatric condition	Main psychological treatment used
Stressful life events, illness, bereavement	**Counselling**
Depression	Guided self-help Cognitive-behavioural therapy Behavioural activation Mindfulness and meditation Interpersonal therapy Counselling Psychodynamic psychotherapy
Anxiety disorders	Cognitive-behavioural therapy Mindfulness-based cognitive therapy Exposure and response prevention (for obsessive-compulsive disorder) Systematic desensitization (for phobias)
Post-traumatic stress disorder	Cognitive-behavioural therapy Eye movement desensitization and reprocessing
Schizophrenia	Cognitive-behavioural therapy Family therapy
Eating disorders	Cognitive-behavioural therapy Focused psychodynamic psychotherapy Interpersonal therapy Family therapy
Personality disorders with a borderline pattern	Dialectical behaviour therapy Mentalization-based therapy Psychodynamic therapy Cognitive-behavioural therapy Cognitive analytic therapy Therapeutic communities
Alcohol dependence	Cognitive-behavioural therapy Group therapy Motivational interviewing

● Chapter Summary

- Psychological therapies are first-line treatments for mild to moderate mood disorders, stress-related disorders, anxiety disorders, eating disorders and personality disorders.
- The therapeutic relationship is more important than the modality of psychological treatment used.
- Self-help is often sufficient for milder problems.
- Counselling is unstructured, allowing the patient to generate their own solutions to problems.
- Psychodynamic psychotherapy aims to facilitate conscious recognition of unconscious processes causing problematic symptoms.
- Cognitive-behavioural therapy aims to help the patient identify and change the links between how they think, feel, sense and behave.

UKMLA Conditions

Anxiety

Anxiety disorder: generalized

Personality disorder

Post-traumatic stress disorder

Depression

OCD

Phobias

UKMLA Presentations

Anxiety

Low mood/affective problems

OCD

Phobias

A fundamental principle of medicine is that patients who are capable of doing so are free to make decisions about their treatment, even if those decisions seem imprudent, and this is no different in psychiatry. However, the very nature of mental disorders can affect some patients' ability to make decisions regarding their care and treatment: in these instances, decisions may need to be made without the informed consent or agreement of the patient. Treatment against patients' wishes is usually only considered when the patient would otherwise be at significant risk to themselves (through self-harm, suicide, self-neglect, exploitation) or may place others at risk. Mental health legislation is therefore in place to protect patients and the public.

Differing legal systems within the United Kingdom mean that there are differences in mental health legislation across the home nations. This book will focus on mental health legislation applicable in England and Wales.

MENTAL HEALTH ACT 1983 AS AMENDED BY THE MENTAL HEALTH ACT 2007

In England and Wales, the Mental Health Act 1983 as amended by the Mental Health Act 2007 (MHA) provides a legal framework for the care and treatment of individuals with mental disorders. The MHA is divided into a number of parts, each of which is divided into 'Sections' (groups of paragraphs).

Part I: Definitions

The term 'mental disorder' is defined as *any disorder or disability of the mind*. However, the Learning Disability Qualification states that *a person with a learning disability* (intellectual disability) *alone can only be detained for treatment or be made subject to Guardianship if that learning disability* (intellectual disability) *is associated with abnormally aggressive or seriously irresponsible conduct*.

The Appropriate Medical Treatment test stipulates that for long-term powers of compulsion (i.e., longer than 28 days) it is not possible for patients to be compulsorily detained or treated unless 'medical treatment' is available and appropriate. Medical treatment includes not only medication but also psychological treatment, nursing and specialist mental health habilitation and rehabilitation.

Certain officials and bodies are designated to carry out specific duties related to implementation of the MHA. Some of these are summarized in Table 4.1.

HINTS AND TIPS

Note that the Mental Health Act 1983 does not regard dependence on alcohol or drugs alone as evidence of a mental disorder. However, mental disorders that arise secondary to substance intoxication or withdrawal (e.g., delirium tremens, drug-induced psychosis) are covered by the MHA.

Part II: Civil sections

Part II of the MHA relates to compulsory assessment and treatment, both in hospital and in the community. Table 4.2 summarizes the most important sections in this part.

Normally, the process starts because concerns are raised about an individual's mental health. Following assessment by the appropriate professionals, the patient may be admitted to hospital under Section 2 or 3 of the MHA.

In an emergency, it may not be possible to arrange a review for consideration of Section 2 or 3. In these cases, there are various options available, depending on circumstances. When any emergency measure is used to detain a patient, this should be reviewed as soon as possible by the appropriate professionals and compulsory measures either revoked, or a Section 2 or 3 granted.

Under Section 135, an Approved Mental Health Professional (AMHP) may apply to a magistrate for a warrant, which allows the police to enter private premises in order to remove someone with a possible mental disorder and take them to a 'place of safety' (usually a police station or hospital) for further assessment. An amendment (2017) also allows the mental health assessment to occur in the private premises if the occupiers consent. Section 136 applies when a police officer has concerns about an individual's mental health in a place that is not the person's dwelling. However, the police officer need not apply for a warrant.

Patients admitted to hospital on an involuntary basis are informed of their detention and their rights. They may apply to have their case reviewed by a Mental Health Review Tribunal or by the Mental Health Act Manager within the hospital, both of whom have the power to remove the detention. Patients may also be discharged from their detention by the Responsible Clinician (RC) or by their nearest relative (unless the right to do this is blocked by the RC).

Table 4.1 Mental Health Act officials

Official or body	Description
Approved Mental Health Professional (AMHP)	A mental health professional (nurse, social worker, occupational therapist, clinical psychologist) with specialist training in mental health assessment and legislation, approved by the local authority. Duties of an AMHP include assessing patients, and (if appropriate) making an application for Mental Health Act 2007 (MHA) detention.
Section 12 approved doctor	A doctor-approved under Section 12 of the Mental Health Act (MHA) as having expertise in the diagnosis and treatment of mental disorders. Section 12 doctors are responsible for the assessment of patients and for recommending MHA detention if appropriate.
Approved Clinician (AC) and Responsible Clinician (RC)	A healthcare professional (usually a doctor, but can also be a nurse, social worker, occupational therapist, clinical psychologist) who has received specialist training and is responsible for the treatment of individuals with mental disorders detained under the MHA. An AC in charge of the care of a specific patient is known as Responsible Clinician for that patient. Their responsibility is to oversee the care and treatment of a patient detained under the MHA and to remain responsible for administrative duties of the MHA pertinent to the patient.
Second Opinion Approved Doctor (SOAD)	Appointed by the Care Quality Commission (CQC – see later), the role of the SOAD is to provide an independent second medical opinion regarding treatment in patients subject to prolonged compulsory treatment who are unable to consent to their treatment, or when a patient refuses electroconvulsive therapy (ECT; not applicable in emergency situations, see Consent to Treatment).
Nearest Relative (NR)	The spouse, child, parent, sibling or other relative of a patient detained under the MHA. This sometimes varies from 'next of kin'. It is the duty of the AMHP to appoint the nearest relative, although this decision can be appealed in court. AMHPs have a duty to inform the NR of the application for MHA detention. NRs can – in some instances – apply for the patient to be discharged from compulsory measures.
Independent Mental Health Advocates (IMHA)	Advocacy is a process of supporting and enabling people to express their views and concerns, access information and services, defend and promote their rights and responsibilities, and explore choices and options. Most patients detained under the MHA have the right to access an independent mental health advocate.
Care Quality Commission	An independent health and social care regulatory body that oversees the use of the MHA and ensures standards are maintained. All NHS and social care providers involved with the care of patients detained under the MHA must be registered with the CQC.
Mental Health Tribunal (MHT)	MHTs hear appeals against detention under the MHA. Their members include a lawyer, a doctor and a layperson. MHTs have the authority to discharge patients from compulsory measures when they determine that the conditions for detention are not met.
Mental Health Act Managers ('hospital managers')	Represent the hospital responsible for a detained patient. Hospital managers will hear appeals from patients against their detention and review renewals of lengthy detentions. Cases are heard in similar settings to those heard by MHRTs, and Mental Health Act Managers have the authority to discharge patients.

For patients liable to be detained under Section 3, it may be appropriate to consider the use of a Community Treatment Order (CTO) under Section 17 of the MHA. This can be useful when treatment in the community is an option (i.e., when the associated risks of the mental disorder do not necessitate ongoing hospital admission). Conditions such as attending appointments may be enforced. However, specific treatment cannot be forcibly given. A CTO allows the RC to recall the patient to hospital should the patient become nonconcordant with treatment or should they become unwell.

HINTS AND TIPS

Note that the term 'informal' applies to hospital patients who are not detained under the Mental Health Act 2007 (i.e., patients who have agreed to voluntary admission).

HINTS AND TIPS

Section 5(2) – doctor's holding power – may be enacted by any hospital doctor provided they are either the Responsible Clinician or another doctor nominated by them (e.g., a specialist registrar or senior house officer). This means that a psychiatrist need not see suspected mentally ill patients on a medical or surgical ward before they can be detained under this section.

Part III: Forensic sections

Part III of the MHA incorporates Sections 35 to 55 and relates to mentally ill patients involved in criminal proceedings or under sentence. Table 4.3 summarizes the most important sections

Table 4.2 Civil sections enabling compulsory admission

Section	Aim	Duration	Application	Recommendation
Section 2 Admission for assessment	Compulsory detention for assessment. Used when diagnosis and response to treatment are unknown. May be converted to a Section 3 if longer admission needed. Medication may be given as part of the assessment process.	28 days	Approved Mental Health Professional (AMHP)	Two doctors (at least one of whom must be Section 12 approved)
Section 3 Admission for treatment	Compulsory detention for treatment. Used when diagnosis and treatment response is established. May be extended.	6 months	AMHP	Two doctors (at least one of whom must be Section 12 approved)
Section 4 Emergency admission for assessment	Emergency admission to hospital for assessment when there is no time to wait for Section 2 procedures in the community.	72 h	AMHP	One doctor, with full GMC registration (usually FY2 or above)
Section 5(2) Doctor's holding power	Detention of a hospital inpatient receiving any form of treatment (not necessarily psychiatric) in order to give time to arrange review for a Section 2 or 3.	72 h	–	Doctor responsible for patient's care or other nominated doctor (with full GMC registration; usually FY2 or above)
Section 5(4) Nurse's holding power	Urgent detention of an inpatient receiving treatment for a mental disorder, to allow for review by doctor.	6 h	–	Registered Mental Health Nurse
Section 17 Community Treatment Order	Allows for supervised treatment in the community in patients liable to detention under Section 3: stipulates that patient must attend appointments. May be recalled to hospital if nonconcordant with treatment or if they become unwell.	6 months	Responsible Clinician (RC)	AMHP and RC
Section 135	Allows police to enter private premises to remove someone with a suspected or known mental disorder to a place of safety for further assessment or to allow an assessment to occur in the private premises if the occupiers agree.	72 h	AMHP	Magistrate
Section 136	Allows a police officer to remove someone with a suspected or known mental disorder from a place that is not their dwelling to a place of safety in their best interests or for the protection of others. If the person is already in a place of safety, a police officer can keep them there or transfer them to another place of safety.	24 h	–	Police officer (following consultation with a mental health professional if practicable)

in this part. It should be noted that patients who are detained under certain forensic Sections and who are not 'restricted' patients (see Table. 4.3) can be considered for supervised community treatment (CTO) if appropriate.

Part IV: Consent to treatment

This part of the MHA clarifies the extent to which treatments can be imposed on patients subject to compulsory measures. Patients detained under Section 3 or 37 (long-term treatment orders) may be treated with standard psychiatric medication for 3 months with or without their consent. However, after 3 months and in other special cases, an extra Section from a Second Opinion Approved Doctor (SOAD) is required for treatment. Such cases include:

- Psychosurgery and surgical implants of hormones to reduce sex drive: these require the informed consent of a patient with capacity to make such a decision, as well as the approval of a SOAD, under Section 57 of the MHA. Neither of these procedures can be carried out on a patient who lacks capacity to make these decisions.
- Administration of medical treatment in a patient who cannot provide, or refuses to provide, informed consent: this requires the approval of a SOAD, under Section 58 of the MHA.
- ECT: if the patient is 'capable of understanding the nature, purpose and likely effects of the treatment' then electroconvulsive therapy (ECT) cannot be given without his consent. If the patient lacks capacity, then ECT must be certified as 'appropriate' by a SOAD, under Section 58A of the MHA.

Table 4.3 Forensic sections

Section	Aim	Duration	Application
Section 35 Remand to hospital for report on mental condition	To prepare a report on the mental condition of an individual who is charged with an offence that could lead to imprisonment	28 days, with option to extend to 12 weeks	Crown or Magistrates' Court, on evidence of one doctor, who must be Section 12 approved
Section 36 Remand to hospital for treatment	To treat an individual who is charged with an offence that could lead to imprisonment	28 days, with option to extend to 12 weeks	Crown Court, on evidence of two medical doctors (one of whom must be Section 12 approved)
Section 37 Hospital order	Detention and treatment of an individual convicted of an imprisonable offence (similar to Section 3)	Initially 6 months, with option to extend	Crown or Magistrates' Court, on evidence of two medical doctors (one of whom must be Section 12 approved)
Section 41 Restriction order	Leave and discharge of Section 37 patients may only be granted with approval of the Home Office (recorded as 37/41) – applied to serious persistent offenders	As for Section 37	Crown Court only, on evidence of one medical doctor (who must be Section 12 approved)

In circumstances where urgent treatment is required to save the patient's life or to prevent serious suffering or deterioration, it may be appropriate to use Section 62 to waive the second opinion requirements of Sections 57 and 58 (e.g., emergency ECT for a patient who is not eating or drinking). Section 62 is only used until a second opinion can be obtained.

> **HINTS AND TIPS**
>
> There is a 'Code of Practice' that accompanies the 1983 Mental Health Act. This provides practical advice to clinicians interacting with the Act, including how to carry out their roles under the Act, and provides statutory guidance around the medical treatment of patients with mental disorders.

> **HINTS AND TIPS**
>
> Unless you choose to specialize in Psychiatry, Section 5(2) of the Mental Health Act 1983 will be the part of the Act you are the most likely to use. It can be used to detain a patient who is already in hospital, to facilitate further assessment and consideration of detention under Section 2 or 3 of the Act. The Responsible Clinician, the Clinician's Deputy or Approved Clinician can examine the patient, and if they are satisfied the grounds for detention are met, they can detain the patient under Section 5(2). The detention lasts for 72 hours.

> **HINTS AND TIPS**
>
> Section 5(2) only applies to patients already admitted to hospital – it cannot be used in an outpatient setting, including in the emergency department.

Reforming the Mental Health Act 1983

In December 2018, the UK Parliament published the findings of an independent review – titled 'Modernising the Mental Health Act'. The goal of the review had been to try and understand why there had been increasing rates of detention under the Mental Health Act in England and Wales, and why there had been disproportionate numbers of people from Black, Asian and minority ethnic groups subject to compulsory measures under the 1983 Act. It also aimed to look at concerns that some processes in place as part of the Mental Health Act 1983 were not compatible with a modern mental health system.

In summary, the review recommended that a new mental health act should make it easier for patients to participate in decisions around their care and treatment, improve patient dignity and increase the recognition of patients' human rights. These recommendations were proposed under four key principles related to the care and treatment of patients. See Table 4.4 for a summary of their recommendations.

Following the publication of 'Modernising the Mental Health Act', the UK government published a white paper titled 'Reforming the Mental Health Act' in January 2021. The government accepted and incorporated most recommendations made by the 'Modernising the Mental Health Act' review into their white paper. Draft legislation in the form of the draft Mental Health

Table 4.4 Key principles underpinning reform of the Mental Health Act 1983

Principle	Recommendations made under this principle
Choice and Autonomy	• Implementation of 'Advance Choice' Documentation – this would allow patients and service users to voice their views about how they would wish their future inpatient care and treatment to be • Right to advocacy • Ability to choose own 'nominated person', rather than a 'nearest relative'
The Use of Least Restriction	• Avoid detention and support people in crisis by improving access to community services and offering opportunities for earlier intervention. • Police cells should not be used as a place of safety for a person with a suspected mental disorder. • Introduction of more detailed care and treatment plans tailored to individuals and shared with them early in their admission. • Improving the ability of a patient or service user to challenge compulsory measures by increasing the role of the tribunal and introducing the right to an early challenge of compulsory treatment. • Reduce the use of community treatment orders.
Therapeutic Benefit	• Investment in the physical environments of mental health wards and improve social interaction and activity for patients and service users who are receiving care and treatment in the wards. • Improved discharge planning • Improve access to long-term support for people with a severe mental illness.
The Person as an Individual	• Value each person as an individual. • Tackle racial disparity by holding organizations to account through the development of a competency framework. • Improve recognition of the ability of young people under 18 to make decisions about their care and treatment and improve safeguards for young people under the age of 18 who may be admitted to wards outside of their local area or into adult wards. • Avoid using the mental health act to compensate for lack of adequate community support and accommodation for people with autism and learning disabilities. • Reduce the time taken to transfer a person with a severe mental illness in prison to a secure hospital environment for their care and treatment.

Bill was introduced to parliament in June 2022. See Box 4.1 for a summary of key amendments to the Mental Health Act 1983 proposed by the bill.

The bill was subject to pre-legislative scrutiny from July to December 2022 by a Joint Committee. They published their report on the bill in January 2023. Overall, the committee was supportive of the reforms proposed, but suggested that the bill had not yet adequately addressed how to reduce rising detention rates or racial inequalities in mental health care and treatment. At the time of publishing, there has not been a confirmed date when the reformed mental health act might come into use in England and Wales, but is expected it could be in law by 2024.

MENTAL HEALTH (CARE & TREATMENT) (SCOTLAND) ACT 2003

Compulsory measures in Scotland are legislated for by the Mental Health (Care & Treatment) (Scotland) Act 2003. They can be used when a patient is suffering (or thought to be suffering) from a mental disorder (mental illness, intellectual disability, personality disorder), by virtue of which the individual's ability to make decisions about treatment of their mental disorder is

BOX 4.1 KEY AMENDMENTS TO THE MENTAL HEALTH ACT 1983 INCLUDED IN THE DRAFT MENTAL HEALTH BILL

• Redefining 'mental disorder' so people with autism and people with a learning disability cannot be treated under Section 3 without a coexisting psychiatric disorder.
• Raising the threshold for detention and reviewing the need for detention more frequently.
• Replacing the Nearest Relative with a Nominated Person, chosen by the patient.
• Expanding access to advocacy services.
• Removing prisons and police cells as places of safety.
• For patients in the criminal justice system, introducing a 'supervised discharge' and a statutory 28-day time limit for transfer from prison to hospital.

From UK Parliament House of Commons Library Research Briefing: 'Reforming the Mental Health Act', Published 31 January 2023.

significantly impaired, when treatment for the mental disorder (including medication, nursing and psychosocial care) is available, and if there would be considerable risk to the health, safety or welfare of the individual, or to the safety of others, without treatment. The use of compulsory powers must be considered necessary and lesser restrictive options must be deemed inappropriate. The use of the Act is overseen by the Mental Welfare Commission for Scotland. Under civil law, the following orders are frequently used:

Emergency Detention Certificate

An Emergency Detention Certificate (EDC) allows an individual with a mental disorder (or suspected mental disorder) to be detained in hospital for up to 72 hours, where hospital admission is required urgently for assessment and when application for a Short-Term Detention Certificate (STDC) would cause undesirable delay. Any doctor (with full GMC registration) can implement an EDC. Wherever possible, the agreement of a mental health officer (MHO – usually a social worker specially trained in mental health) should also be obtained. Patients may not be treated against their will under an EDC, but emergency treatment is possible under common law. It should be reviewed as soon as practical by an Approved Medical Practitioner; a psychiatrist with special training and approval in the use of the Mental Health (Care & Treatment, Scotland, Act 2003) and should either be revoked or converted to an STDC.

Short-Term Detention Certificate

A Short Term Detention Certificate (STDC) allows an individual with a mental disorder (or suspected mental disorder) to be detained in hospital for up to 28 days. It can only be applied by an Approved Medical Practitioner in agreement with an MHO. Patients may be given treatment for their mental disorders under an STDC. Patients have the right to appeal the STDC at any time, with their appeal being heard at a tribunal. The STDC may be revoked before the end of 28 days, or an application for a CTO may be made.

Compulsory treatment order

A Compulsory Treatment Order (CTO) may follow an STDC. An MHO applies to the Mental Health Tribunal for Scotland, asking them to consider granting a CTO. This requires two written medical reports, usually completed by the Responsible Medical Officer (the Approved Medical Practitioner responsible for the care of the patient) and the patient's general practitioner (GP). It also requires a proposed care plan, detailing medical treatment that would be provided if the CTO is granted. The tribunal consists of a lawyer, a doctor and a layperson. They decide whether the application is appropriate before granting the CTO, refusing the CTO, or suggesting an interim order while further information is gathered. A CTO lasts for 6 months initially; however, applications can be made to the Mental Health Tribunal to extend this. Patients have the right of appeal. CTOs can be used to treat patients in the community as well as in hospital.

THE MENTAL CAPACITY ACT (NORTHERN IRELAND, 2016)

The Mental Capacity Act (Northern Ireland, 2016) combines legislation regarding treatment for mental health problems with treatment for those who lack capacity for any reason. When the Act is fully commenced, the Mental Capacity Act (Northern Ireland, 2016) will replace the Mental Health Order (Northern Ireland, 1986). At the time of writing, phase 1 of the Act has been implemented. The most notable change this has brought about is the introduction of 'Deprivation of Liberty Safeguards' (DoLS). DoLS describes the system that ensures a person is only deprived of their liberty (as defined by a person being in place where care or treatment is being provided; they are not free to leave, and they are under continuous supervision and control) when it is right to do so. Safeguards, as defined by the Mental Capacity Act (Northern Ireland, 2016) are summarized in Box 4.2. At the time of writing, it is not clear when the later phases of the Act are due to come into use, and a dual system is in place at present, with both the Mental Health Order (Northern Ireland, 1986) and the Mental Capacity Act (Northern Ireland, 2016) providing legal frameworks around deprivation of liberty. If a person can be detained under the 1986 Order, then the 1986 Order framework must be applied.

CAPACITY TO CONSENT TO TREATMENT

Mental capacity in England and Wales is defined by the Mental Capacity Act 2005 (MCA) as the ability of an individual to make their own decisions. An individual (aged 16 years or older) has the capacity to make a specific decision if they can:
- communicate their decision;
- understand information given to them to make a particular decision;
- retain that information;
- balance or weigh up the information to make the decision.

ETHICS

A significant cause for concern is the higher rates of detention among Black and other ethnic minorities when compared to rates of detention in other ethnic groups. Among the five broad ethnic groups (as defined by NHS Digital), rates of detention for the Black or Black British group were over four times higher in 2021 to 2022 than for the White group. Rates of CTO use for the Black or Black British group was also over 11 times higher than for the White group. The reasons for racial disparities in the use of compulsory measures are likely complex and multifactorial, including institutional racism, higher lifetime prevalence of psychosis in Black people and barriers preventing people from ethnic minorities engaging with general practitioners and community services.

HINTS AND TIPS

Capacity assessment can be remembered by almost the same acronym as the common pneumonia severity assessment: 'CURB' (Communicate, Understand, Retain, Balance).

If an individual is unable to do one or more of the list outline in 'Capacity to consent to treatment' in the ETHICS box left, they lack the capacity to make the particular decision in question.

It should be noted that 'capacity' is not a blanket term and it should be considered according to the decision to be made. For example, a woman with a moderate intellectual disability may have the capacity to decide to buy music by her favourite singer. However, she may lack the capacity to make a decision to take out a mortgage to buy a house.

Under the MCA, an individual:
- Must be assumed to have capacity until it is established that they lack capacity.
- Should not be treated as incapable until all practical steps to help them have been taken without success.
- Must not be treated as incapable merely on the basis of wishing to make an unwise decision.

Any act done or decision made under the MCA:
- Must be in the best interests of the individual.
- Must be undertaken in a manner that is least restrictive to the individual's rights.

BOX 4.2 DEPRIVATION OF LIBERTY SAFEGUARDS, MENTAL CAPACITY ACT (NORTHERN IRELAND, 2016)

If someone wants to deprive an individual of their liberty, they must make sure the following safeguards are in place:
- Believe the person lacks the mental capacity to decide about the deprivation of liberty and this must be written down in a statement of incapacity.
- Believe that the deprivation of liberty will help prevent serious harm coming to the person or serious physical harm to other people.
- Must consult a nominated person.
- Must have authorization for the deprivation of liberty.

Adapted from the Mental Capacity Act Leaflet, available at: https://westerntrust.hscni.net/download/539/new-category/8868/mental-health-capacity-act.pdf

ETHICS

A patient should by default be assumed to have capacity unless it has been demonstrated they do not. Making an unwise decision does not by itself demonstrate incapacity.

HINTS AND TIPS

Capacity is 'decision specific' – this means the principles of assessing capacity need to be applied for each decision an individual makes about their welfare, care and treatment. For example, a person with a learning disability may have the capacity to decide about whether they want to give consent for a simple procedure, e.g., a blood test, but they may not have capacity to decide about a more complex procedure, e.g., a surgical procedure. It is important to try and optimize an individual's capacity by, e.g., providing more accessible information, using communication aids and allowing the individual time and the opportunity to review information given during the decision-making process.

The framework used to assess mental capacity in Scotland is the Adults with Incapacity (Scotland) Act 2000 and in Northern Ireland, the Mental Capacity Act (Northern Ireland) 2016.

With regard to medical treatment, clinicians should provide patients with a clear explanation of the nature and likely benefits of a treatment as well as its potential risks and side effects. An adult who has capacity has the right to refuse treatment, even if this refusal results in death or serious disability. When patients refuse essential treatment, clinicians should ascertain whether they have the capacity to consent to treatment and have made a free decision without coercion.

When making decisions about capacity, you should not hesitate to discuss the case with colleagues, or even a medicolegal defence organization. The process of assessment should be clearly and comprehensively documented in the medical notes.

> **RED FLAG**
>
> An adult who has capacity has the right to refuse treatment, even if this refusal results in death or serious disability. In such cases it is important to document carefully the assessment of capacity and to discuss with senior colleagues.

Deprivation of Liberty Safeguards

The 'Deprivation of Liberty Safeguards' is an amendment to the Mental Capacity Act (2005), which applies only in England and Wales. These safeguards do not apply to someone detained under the Mental Health Act. If a person who lacks capacity in a care home or hospital needs to have their liberty restricted (i.e., they are not free to leave or are subject to continuous supervision and control), then an application to the local authority needs to be made for a 'standard authorization'. Issuing such an authorization ensures that safeguards for the patient are in place (including appointing a patient's representative, the right of appeal and access to advocacy).

Advance Decisions

An Advance Decision (or 'living will') is a statement of an individual's wishes regarding the health care and medical treatment they would wish to have (or not wish to have), if they were to become incapable of making decisions on these matters in the future. The individual must be over the age of 18 years and must have capacity to make the statement. The Advance Decision can become valid when the individual loses capacity to consent to (or refuse) treatment in the future. Advance Decisions are legally enforceable under the MCA in England and Wales.

In Scotland and Northern Ireland, the equivalent of an Advance Decision is called an 'Advance Directive'. Respecting the advance refusal of a competent adult is also a requirement of Articles 5 and 8 of the Human Rights Act 1998. A principle underlying decision-making on behalf of all those without capacity is that the previously known wishes of the individual should be taken into consideration, whether or not they are written down.

Proxy decision-making

A Power of Attorney is a legal document that enables an individual (who has capacity and is over the age of 18 years) to nominate another person ('Attorney') to make decisions on their behalf in the event that they become incapable of doing so in the future. The type of decisions may be specified and may include health care, welfare and financial matters. If the individual lacks capacity and has not made a Power of Attorney, it is possible for the courts to appoint these powers to individuals. Laws regarding Power of Attorney vary between England and Wales, Scotland and Northern Ireland.

> **ETHICS**
>
> Having a serious mental illness does not preclude a patient from having the capacity to consent to physical treatment, as long as their illness does not interfere with their understanding of relevant information and the decision-making process.

> **COMMON PITFALLS**
>
> The Mental Health Acts make provision for the compulsory treatment of mental disorders only, not for the compulsory treatment of physical disorders. Therefore a patient can never be detained under the Mental Health Act 2007 to treat a physical disorder, and patients can refuse physical treatment unless they are assessed as lacking capacity. Patients who require urgent physical treatment, but who do not have capacity, may be treated without their consent (but in their best interests) under the Mental Capacity Act 2005.

COMMON LAW

Common law refers to law that is based on previous court decisions (case law), rather than laws made in Parliament (statute law). The Mental Health Act is an example of statutory law, whereas providing immediate life-saving treatment to an unconscious patient (unable to consent) is justified under common law. The common law *doctrine of necessity* allows for treatment in emergency situations of physical or mental disorders in adults who are unable to consent. Treatment must be in the best interests of the individual and must be necessary to sustain life, to prevent serious deterioration or to alleviate severe pain or suffering. The doctrine of necessity is applicable only in emergency situations, and – if necessary – treatment should be continued under statute law (e.g., MHA, MCA) as soon as practically possible.

Many doctors and nurses who are not familiar with mental health legislation are often concerned about infringing patients' rights and may not act at all (e.g., a man with a life-threatening alcohol withdrawal delirium is allowed to leave the ward with no one attempting to stop him). When considering an action under common law, always ask yourself whether your actions would be defensible in court. Your actions should be consistent with what most individuals with your level of training would do in the same situation. Choosing not to act when you should is indefensible and would be construed as negligent.

COMMON PITFALLS

It is permissible under common law to restrain and medicate patients who are mentally disordered and who present an imminent danger to themselves or others. However, it is not legal to impose psychiatric medication repeatedly on informal patients. Anyone who has required emergency restraint and treatment under common law should be promptly assessed by a senior doctor for treatment under the appropriate Section of the Mental Health Act.

HUMAN RIGHTS LEGISLATION

Human rights are commonly understood as 'inalienable fundamental rights to which a person is inherently entitled simply because she or he is a human being'. The Universal Declaration of Human Rights was established in 1948 and subsequently the European Convention on Human Rights (ECHR) in 1953. These are considered to be international law. The United Kingdom has introduced its own statute law, the Human Rights Act 1998 (HRA).

There are some fundamental incompatibilities between the Human Rights Act 1998 and mental health legislation. The Mental Health Act 2007 has gone some way to address these. However, it is still important to be aware of some important aspects of human rights legislation and to interpret mental health legislation in a way compatible with the Human Rights Act as far as possible.

Article 3 of the ECHR states that 'no one shall be subjected to torture or to inhuman or degrading treatment or punishment'.

This is an absolute right and is always applicable. When a patient is in hospital (whether detained or not), practices that could be considered to be 'inhuman or degrading' may include the use of excessive force during restraint, maintaining high levels of sedation to compensate for staff shortages, a lack of privacy or adequate sanitation, or treatment without consent in cases where it is not medically necessary (under common law or under the MHA). Public authorities have a duty under the HRA to protect the human rights of patients in their care.

Article 8 of the ECHR protects the right to respect for private and family life, home and correspondence. It also sets out, in general terms, circumstances when an interference (also known as a restriction) with this right is acceptable. However, interference must be lawful, necessary and proportionate. Under mental health legislation, seclusion (keeping and supervising a patient alone in a room that may be locked) can occasionally be used. However, if this is not justified as being lawful, necessary and proportionate, it may be a violation of the human rights of the patient.

Article 5 of the ECHR protects the right to liberty. However, it also sets out specific circumstances in which this can be limited. Inappropriate use of the MHA (including undue delays in tribunal or appeal processes) can result in an unlawful restriction of liberty, which may be in violation of Article 5 of the ECHR.

There are also instances when failure to use mental health legislation appropriately may be considered to be in violation of an individual's human rights. Article 2 of the ECHR is an absolute right to life, and professionals or authorities who fail to protect life may be considered to be in violation of the law (e.g., failing to detain a severely depressed and suicidal patient who later committed suicide was considered by the UK Supreme Court to be a violation of Article 2 of the ECHR).

The interface between mental health legislation and human rights legislation is incredibly complex and beyond the scope of this book to discuss in detail. However, it is important to be mindful of human rights law and these potential difficulties and to seek advice from an expert if in doubt.

FITNESS TO DRIVE

Driving is a complex skill requiring good sensory abilities (vision, hearing), good motor control (power, coordination, reaction time), good memory and good executive function (attention and concentration, judgement, planning and organization, ability to self-monitor). It follows that many mental illnesses and psychiatric medications can impair fitness to drive. Clinicians should be aware of the following legal provisions:

- It is the responsibility of the Driver and Vehicle Licensing Agency (DVLA) to make the decision as to whether an individual is fit to continue driving.

- It is the driver's responsibility to inform the DVLA of any condition that may impair driving ability.
- A patient with a condition requiring notification should not drive until they hear back from the DVLA and must not drive during an acute illness.
- It is the doctor's responsibility to advise patients to inform the DVLA of any condition that may interfere with their driving (e.g., psychotic episode, manic episode, dementia). Table 4.5. Doctors may be contacted by the DVLA for further clinical information or may be invited to prepare a medical report
- Medications that can influence safety to drive are those that impair alertness, concentration or coordination. Many medications used in psychiatry are sedating (e.g., tricyclic antidepressants) and/or can affect motor control (e.g., antipsychotics) and patients should be advised not to drive immediately after starting or increasing the dose of such a medication. Those who are not adversely affected can continue to drive. This is particularly important for professional drivers.
- Doctors have a duty to breach confidentiality considerations and contact the DVLA medical advisor themselves if patients fail to take this advice and the potential impairment is serious. The same applies to patients who, due to their illness (e.g., dementia, psychosis), are unable or unlikely, to contact the DVLA.

ETHICS

In order to protect the public, doctors have a duty to break confidentiality and inform the Driver and Vehicle Licensing Agency if they become aware that a patient is continuing to drive or is likely to continue to drive, against medical advice.

Table 4.5 Common mental health conditions about which the DVLA should be notified

Condition	Likely licencing outcome[a]
Anxiety or depression, mild–moderate (without suicidal thoughts, agitation or significant memory or concentration problems)	Can continue to drive, no notification required.
Depression or anxiety, severe (causing significant memory or concentration problems, agitation or suicidal thoughts)	Licence revoked until a period of stability has been achieved (typically 3 months).
Acute psychotic episode	Licence revoked until stable with good insight for 3 months.
Hypomania or mania	Licence revoked until stable with good insight for 3 months.
Schizophrenia	Must not drive during acute illness. After 3 months of stability, licencing can be considered even if continuing symptoms, as long as these are unlikely to affect concentration, memory or cause distraction while at wheel.
Neurodevelopmental disorders (e.g., ADHD)	May be able to drive but must notify DVLA.
Dementia	May be able to drive but must notify DVLA. Early dementia may be licenced with annual review. Impairment in short-term memory, disorientation or lack of insight suggests unfit to drive.
Learning disability	Mild: may be able to drive but must notify DVLA (a driving assessment may be required). Moderate–severe: should not drive.
Personality disorders with severe behavioural disturbance	May be able to drive but must notify DVLA.
Persistent harmful use of alcohol or alcohol dependence	Licence revoked until a minimum of 6 months or 1 year free of alcohol problems (depending on severity of use).
Persistent harmful use of substances or dependence	Licence revoked until a minimum of 6 months or 1 year free of substance use, depending on substance. If multiple substances used, unlikely to be licenced. Methadone or buprenorphine use can be compatible with driving.
Any other psychiatric condition that impairs concentration or awareness, increases distractibility or in any other way is likely to affect safe driving of the vehicle	Case specific, likely that a period of stability required.

[a]Note, although the DVLA provides examples of likely outcomes, each case is assessed individually and may differ from the above. The licencing outcome is not decided by the doctor treating the patient, but by DVLA medical advisors. Standards are much stricter for those with licences to drive buses or lorries.
DVLA, Driver and Vehicle Licensing Agency.

Chapter Summary

- Patients who have capacity are free to make good or bad decisions about their health care.
- Patients who lack capacity may need decisions to be made for them in their best interests. Legislation exists to ensure this is done only when necessary and in a way that protects patients' rights.
- Mental health legislation in the United Kingdom allows people with significantly impaired decision-making ability to be detained in hospital for assessment and to be given treatment for a mental disorder against their will.
- Mental capacity legislation in the United Kingdom allows people who lack capacity to be given treatment for physical disorders and to be accommodated against their will.
- Common law allows immediate treatment to be given to people who cannot consent in emergency situations in order to prevent serious deterioration, severe pain or death.
- Severe mental health problems often impair driving and require the Driver and Vehicle Licensing Agency to be notified; a licence is often returned after a period of stability.

UKMLA Conditions
Driving advice
Mental capacity concerns

UKMLA Presentations
Dementia
Schizophrenia
Anxiety disorder: generalised
Anxiety disorder: post-traumatic stress disorder
Anxiety, phobias, OCD
Bipolar affective disorder
Depression
Substance use disorder

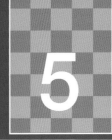

HISTORY

Until the 18th century, the mentally ill in the United Kingdom received no formal psychiatric care and those who were not looked after by their families were kept in workhouses and private institutions. Conditions in such institutions were often poor, with frequent use of physical restraints such as manacles, bars and straightjackets. In 1845, the Lunatics Act led to the building of an asylum in every county so that those patients with severe mental illness could be cared for in large licenced remote communities. Asylum reformers emphasized 'moral treatment' of patients, focusing on treating patients like ordinary people and emphasizing 'rational behaviours'. Since the introduction in the 1950s of chlorpromazine, the first effective medication for schizophrenia, there has been a significant decline in the number of patients in psychiatric hospitals. The attempts to reduce the cost of inpatient care, as well as the criticism levelled at asylums regarding the 'institutionalization' of patients and the loss of patient autonomy, led to the closure of the large asylums and the rise of community care. Today, most patients with mental illness are assessed and managed in the community, and hospital admission, when indicated, is ideally only brief in duration.

PRIMARY CARE

Up to 95% of mental illness is seen and managed exclusively in primary care by general practitioners (GPs), with mild to moderate mood and anxiety disorders and alcohol misuse being the most common conditions. Depression, which is the most commonly treated mental illness, is frequently associated with symptoms of anxiety and physical complaints.

It is important to note that up to half of all patients with mental illnesses go undetected in primary care. This is because many of these patients present with physical, rather than psychological, symptoms. Also, some patients are reluctant to discuss emotional issues with their doctor, due to feelings of embarrassment or uncertainty about how they will be received.

Some GPs have the option of referring patients with mild symptoms or those going through a life crisis (e.g., bereavement) to a practice counsellor (see Chapter 3). Practice and district nurses may be helpful in screening for, and educating patients about, mental illness.

Primary care liaison teams exist in many areas. These act as a single point of contact for GPs to refer. Referrals are allocated

to psychiatrists, psychologists, community psychiatric nurses (CPNs) or occupational therapists as appropriate. This means the GP does not have to work out which professional is best placed to help the patient before referring; the team can discuss this among themselves. Some patients will continue to receive intervention at a primary care level and others will require secondary care. The following box lists the common reasons for referral from primary to secondary mental health care.

REASONS FOR REFERRAL TO SECONDARY MENTAL HEALTH SERVICES

- Moderate to severe mental illness (e.g., schizophrenia, bipolar disorder, severe depression or anxiety disorder)
- Patients who pose a serious risk for harm to self, others or property
- Uncertainty regarding diagnosis
- Poor response to standard treatment, despite adequate dose and concordance
- Specialist assessment required (e.g., dementia, autism, ADHD)
- Specialist treatment required (e.g., psychological therapy, specialist medication regimens)

SECONDARY CARE

Community mental health teams

In the United Kingdom, specialist psychiatric care in the community is mostly coordinated by regional community mental health teams (CMHTs), which consist of a multidisciplinary team of psychiatrists, CPNs, social workers, psychologists, occupational therapists, support workers and pharmacists. Team members usually operate from a base that is easily accessible to the community they serve, and often local GP surgeries are used as venues to meet patients. Patients who are unable to come to the CMHT location are often seen at home. Some subspecialities have specialized community teams, such as Community Learning Disability Teams.

Care programme approach

The approach taken by some secondary care psychiatric services is called the care programme approach (CPA), introduced by the Department of Health in 1991. This approach applies to all patients under specialist psychiatric care and includes patients based in the community, in hospitals and in prisons. The key components of the CPA are:

- The systematic assessment of patients' health and social care needs.
- The formation of an agreed care plan that addresses these identified needs.
- The allocation of a *care coordinator* (previously called 'key worker') to keep in touch with the patient to monitor and to coordinate the care of these needs. This is usually a CPN, social worker or psychiatrist.
- Regular review meetings, which include all relevant professionals, patients and their carers, to adjust the care plan, if necessary.
- Patients may be placed on a *standard* or an *enhanced* CPA according to the severity of their needs.

HINTS AND TIPS

The diverse and multiple needs of patients with mental health problems make a multidisciplinary approach indispensable in psychiatry. A multidisciplinary team consists of members with medical, psychological, social and occupational therapy expertise.

Outpatient clinics

Psychiatric outpatient clinics take place in CMHT centres, GP surgeries, hospitals, and in some cases may be done remotely by video call. Types of clinics include psychiatrists' clinics for new referrals and follow-up patients and special purpose clinics (e.g., depot antipsychotic injection clinics, clozapine monitoring clinics). Some areas offer regional assessment services for neurodevelopmental disorders.

Liaison psychiatry

Liaison psychiatrists work in general hospitals. They provide psychiatric assessment and treatment for people who attend a general hospital with physical health problems, with or without a preexisting mental health problem. Common referrals are for assessment following self-harm, advice on management of delirium, and distinguishing depression from symptoms of physical health disorders. People with intellectual disability can find hospital admissions particularly challenging and therefore some hospitals provide an intellectual disability liaison service who can advise on strategies to manage distress and challenging behaviour.

Day hospitals

Day hospitals are nonresidential units that patients attend during the day. They are an alternative to inpatient care for patients who, although needing intensive support, are able to go home in the evening and at weekends. Having a supportive family is helpful in such cases. They may also be used for patients who have just been discharged from hospital, but who still need a high level of support, as a form of 'partial hospitalization.' They are now mainly used for older adults.

Assertive outreach teams

These are like CMHTs and involve a multidisciplinary team but provide a more intensive service, providing more flexible and frequent patient contact. They are targeted at patients who have not engaged well with mainstream mental health services in the past. Patients who use this service often have histories of severe and enduring mental illness, significant social problems and complex needs, and are usually considered relatively high risk in some regard (e.g., self-harm or suicide, violence to others, self-neglect, or vulnerable). The nature of their illness requires more focused and intensive input.

Home treatment teams

There is increasing emphasis on treating patients at home, thus avoiding expensive and disruptive inpatient admissions. A hospital admission can be very challenging for anyone, particularly someone with an acute mental illness. Treatment at home also allows practical problems with housing and activities of daily living to be better identified and addressed. Most regions now have home treatment teams (sometimes also called crisis teams) who can provide short periods of support (from a few days to weeks) to people who might otherwise have to be admitted to hospital. They can also facilitate earlier discharge from inpatient care than would otherwise be possible. Such teams include similar professionals to a CMHT but generally are available out of hours and can visit patients more often (e.g., multiple times per day, if required). Different home treatment teams will have access to different resources; however, medication, practical help and psychological therapy can often be offered.

Early intervention in psychosis teams

There is some evidence that the longer a psychotic episode goes untreated, the poorer the prognosis, suggesting that early treatment is preferable. However, not all mild or vague symptoms of possible psychosis become a definite psychotic episode, meaning it can be hard to know when to start treatment (e.g., a person who is suspicious of others, but not holding a certain belief of persecution). Specialist teams exist in many regions to manage such cases, offering assessment, medication, psychological strategies and education for patients and families. Teams are open to psychosis secondary to any diagnosis (e.g., schizophrenia, bipolar disorder, substance-induced), and generally accept people aged 14 to 35 years.

Inpatient units

Occasionally, community care is not possible and hospital admission is necessary. Reasons for admission include the following:

- To provide a safe environment when there is: (1) high risk for harm to self or others or (2) grossly disturbed behaviour.
- A period of inpatient assessment is needed (e.g., in response to treatment or when the diagnosis is uncertain).
- It is necessary to initiate treatment in hospital (e.g., electroconvulsive therapy, clozapine therapy – although both of these can be initiated as outpatients if the patient is at low risk for complications).

There are various types of inpatient units. These range from a general adult acute ward for uncomplicated admissions to psychiatric intensive care units (PICUs) for severely disturbed patients who cannot be adequately looked after on an open ward. High-security hospitals (also called 'special hospitals' e.g., Broadmoor, Rampton, Carstairs) are for mentally disordered offenders who pose a significant risk to others. Mother and baby units provide care to women who are in late pregnancy or have a young baby, and eating disorder units provide care to those with severe physical complications resulting from anorexia nervosa. Children are usually admitted to specialized CAMHS units, and hospitals may have specific wards for older adult patients and patients with learning disabilities.

HINTS AND TIPS

Not all psychiatric inpatients are treated in hospital under the Mental Health Act (see Chapter 4). Patients may also not be physically in hospital for their whole admission: time off the ward and visits to the patient's own home are an important part of discharge planning.

Rehabilitation units

These units aim to reintegrate patients whose social and living skills have been severely handicapped by the effects of severe mental illness and institutionalization into the community. Admissions are often for months or even years. The approach taken is holistic and uses the 'Recovery Model' (i.e., learning to live well with ongoing symptoms, rather than aim for complete remission of symptoms).

Accommodation

Certain patients, who are unable to live independently due to severe and enduring mental illness, may need *supported accommodation*. Types of supported accommodation range from warden-controlled property to residential homes with trained staff on hand 24 hours a day.

● Chapter Summary

- Most mental health conditions are managed in primary care.
- Patients with severe and enduring mental illness can benefit from input from a community mental health team.
- Many services exist to manage acutely unwell patients at home.
- High-risk patients are likely to need hospital admission.

● Case summary

The duty psychiatrist is asked for their opinion on Mr SA, a 28-year-old unemployed, recently divorced man, who was brought in by his landlord. The landlord had called round to discuss payment arrears, only to find the door unlocked and Mr SA asleep on his bed with an empty box of paracetamol tablets and several empty cans of lager littered around the floor. He also found a hastily scribbled suicide note on the bedside table, addressed to Mr SA's children. Mr SA was easily roused but was upset to have been found and initially refused the landlord's pleas that they go to the hospital. Only when he was violently sick did Mr SA finally agree. The doctor in the accident and emergency (A&E) department reports that, other than the smell of alcohol on his breath, Mr SA's medical examination was normal. Blood tests revealed raised paracetamol levels, but these were not sufficiently high to require medical treatment. The A&E doctor is concerned because Mr SA is ambivalent about further acts of self-harm or suicide, saying that his 'life is a failure' and that 'there is nothing worth living for'. Before coming to see the patient, the duty psychiatrist checks Mr SA's past medical and psychiatric history.

For a discussion of the case study, see the end of the chapter.

While many psychiatric illnesses can be associated with self-harm or suicidal intent (both as a presenting feature and a chronic symptom), many patients who self-harm or attempt suicide are not previously known to mental health services. Initial assessments of these patients are often made by nonpsychiatric staff, so it is vital that all doctors are able to detect and manage any underlying mental illness, and have a sound approach to assessing and managing risk.

(e.g., cutting, burning, hitting, ingesting foreign bodies). The motives for self-harm are vast and include emotional relief, self-punishment, care elicitation, and can even be a form of self-help (albeit maladaptive) by way of channelling an intolerable emotional experience into a discrete physical sensation, drawing focus to the pain present in the 'here and now'. *Suicide* is the act of intentionally and successfully ending one's own life. *Attempted suicide* refers to an unsuccessful attempt to complete suicide.

COMMUNICATION

The psychosocial assessment can be a therapeutic intervention. Patients who present following self-harm report most valuing having the time to talk and be listened to by a skilled, empathic, competent and nonjudgemental clinician who treats them as individuals, validates their distress and offers hope.

HINTS AND TIPS

Self-harm is one of the top five reasons for acute medical admissions for both men and women in the United Kingdom. Further, it is estimated that a large number of people do not attend hospital following self-harm.

COMMUNICATION

Be curious as to why a person has self-harmed and work collaboratively with the patient to reach a shared understanding of what outcome they were hoping for. You might ask whether it was to stop bad feelings, show other people how bad you are feeling or potentially to end your life.

DEFINITIONS AND CLINICAL FEATURES

Self-harm is a blanket term used to describe any intentional act done with the knowledge that it is potentially harmful. It can take the form of self-poisoning (e.g., overdosing) or self-injury

ASSESSMENT OF PATIENTS WHO HAVE INFLICTED HARM UPON THEMSELVES

Compared with the general population, which has an annual suicide rate of 0.01%, patients who present with self-harm have a 50- to 100-fold greater chance of completing suicide in the following year confusing phrasing, percentages already make clear emphasizing the need for comprehensive risk assessment. It is incredibly difficult to predict suicide reliably, but numerous studies have shown that certain epidemiological and clinical variables are more prevalent among those who have completed suicide (Box 6.1) and it is important to bear these in mind when assessing risk. No patient questionnaire or suicide risk-scoring system has been shown to be more effective at predicting risk of suicide than thorough clinical assessment.

The key areas to assess are:

1. Suicide risk factors
2. Suicidal intent (including circumstances surrounding the act)
3. Mental state examination
4. Current social supports

BOX 6.1 RISK FACTORS FOR SUICIDE

Epidemiological factors:

Male of any age (younger females are more likely to self-harm but less likely to complete suicide)

Being lesbian, gay, bisexual, transgender, queer or intersex (particularly younger people)

Prisoners (especially those on remand)

Being unmarried (single, widowed, divorced)

Unemployment

Working in certain occupations (Women: nurses, primary school teachers, culture/media/sport; care workers. Men: construction workers; care workers)

Low socioeconomic status

Living alone, social isolation

Clinical factors:

Psychiatric illness or personality disorder (see Table 6.1)

Previous self-harm

Alcohol dependence

Physical illness (especially debilitating, chronically painful or terminal conditions)

Family history of depression, alcohol dependence or suicide

Recent adverse life events (especially bereavement)

SUICIDE RISK FACTORS

Box 6.1 summarizes the most important epidemiological and clinical risk factors for suicide.

Psychiatric illness

About 90% of patients who complete suicide have a diagnosed or retrospectively diagnosable mental disorder; however, only around a quarter of these patients have contact with mental health services in the year before completing suicide. Patients recently released from inpatient psychiatric care are at a significantly elevated risk for suicide, particularly during the first couple of weeks after discharge. Table 6.1 summarizes the most important psychiatric conditions associated with suicide.

COMMUNICATION

Every patient with suicidal ideas should be asked about alcohol or substance misuse, no matter how unlikely it seems. Taking a nonjudgemental stance is likely to enhance the therapeutic relationship and help the patient feel understood.

Physical illness

Many disabling or unpleasant medical conditions can be associated with self-harm and suicide. Often, a patient may have comorbid depression that will respond to treatment. However, a minority of patients have no mental illness and make a capacitous decision to die. The most common examples of illnesses associated with suicide are:

- Chronic illnesses which cause a lot of functional impairment or pain (e.g., chronic obstructive pulmonary disease, asthma, stroke, epilepsy).
- Life-limiting illnesses (e.g., cancer, Huntington disease, multiple sclerosis).

Recent adverse life events

Stressful life events are more common in the 6 months prior to a suicide attempt, and include relationship break-ups, health problems, legal/financial difficulties or problems at home or within the family.

Suicidal intent

Suicidal intent, which is commonly defined as the seriousness or intensity of the wish of a patient to terminate their life, is suggested by the following.

The attempt was planned in advance

A lethal suicide attempt typically involves days or weeks of planning. It is rarely an impulsive, spur-of-the-moment idea (the exception is the psychotic patient who impulsively responds to hallucinations or delusions). Planning is strongly suggested by the evidence of final acts. These include the writing of a will or suicide note.

Precautions were taken to avoid discovery or rescue

For example, a patient might check into a hotel room in a distant town or ensure that no friends or family will be visiting over the ensuing hours or days

A dangerous method was used

Violent methods (hanging, jumping from heights, firearm use) are suggestive of lethal intent. That said, use of an apparently ineffective method (e.g., taking six paracetamol tablets) might reflect lack of knowledge of the lethal dose needed, rather than a lack of intent to die. Therefore, it should be ascertained whether the method used was seen as dangerous from the patient's perspective; this is particularly important to clarify in younger patients or patients with learning disabilities.

No help was sought after the act

Patients who immediately regret their action and seek help are less at risk than those who do not seek help and wait to die.

Mental state examination

This should ideally be conducted in a calm, quiet and confidential setting, preferably when the patient has had a chance to rest and is not under the influence of drugs or alcohol. Check specifically for:

- Current mood state: does the patient appear to be suffering from a depressive illness? Assess for features of hopelessness, worthlessness or agitation (all of which are associated with a higher risk for completed suicide).

Table 6.1 Association between psychiatric disorders and suicide

Psychiatric disorder	Risk relative to general population	Comments
Personality disorders	45-fold in borderline pattern, lower but still elevated with other traits[b]	Often have comorbid depression or substance misuse.
Unipolar depression	20-fold[a]	Risk greatest in patients with anxiety/agitation or severe insomnia and higher in patients having received inpatient treatment in the past. Risk greatest in first 3 months of diagnosis.
Substance use	Cocaine dependence 17-fold Alcohol dependence 10-fold Opioid dependence 7-fold Amphetamine dependence 5-fold[a]	Highest risk when comorbid depression.
Schizophrenia	13-fold[a]	Highest risk is young, intelligent, unemployed males with good insight and recurrent illness.
Bipolar affective disorder	6[a]–17[b]-fold	More common in depressive phase but can also happen in manic or mixed affective episodes.
Eating disorders	Anorexia nervosa 8-fold[a] Bulimia lower risk than anorexia	Mortality in anorexia nervosa is also increased due to complications of malnutrition.
Anxiety disorders	3-fold[a]	Increased risk in GAD, panic disorder and PTSD even without comorbid depression. OCD not associated with increased risk.

[a]Ferrari et al. The Burden Attributable to Mental and Substance Use Disorders as Risk Factors for Suicide: Findings from the Global Burden of Disease Study 2010. PLoS One. 2014 Apr 2;9(4):e91936.
[b]Chesney E, Goodwin GM, Fazel S. Risks of all-cause and suicide mortality in mental disorders: a meta-review. World Psychiatry. 2014 Jun;13(2):153–160.
GAD, Generalized anxiety disorder; OCD, obsessive-compulsive disorder; PTSD, posttraumatic stress disorder.

- Other psychiatric illness: does the patient appear to be preoccupied, delusional or responding to hallucinations? Is there evidence of eating disorder, substance abuse or cognitive impairment?
- Current suicidality: is the act now regretted, or is there strong intent to die? What does the patient plan to do if discharged?
- Protective factors: what aspects of the patient's life (family, children and dependents) would guard against further acts? Lack of protective factors, or dismissal of their importance, is a worrying sign.

The following questions might be helpful when asking about suicidal ideation:

- Have you been feeling that life isn't worth living?
- Do you sometimes feel like you would like to end it all?
- Have you given some thought as to how you might do it?
- How close are you to going through with your plans?
- Is there anything that might stop you from attempting suicide?

HINTS AND TIPS

Patients who are tired, emotionally upset or intoxicated may appear to be at greater risk for imminent self-harm. Allowing some time to sober up and reflect can be of great therapeutic value. However, this will always be a matter of clinical judgment.

COMMUNICATION

Often it can be difficult for people to remember or discuss how they sought help after they have attempted to end their life. It can be useful to ask people what happened between the act and arriving in hospital, as sometimes this can prompt people to talk about who they contacted or how they were discovered. Another useful source of information can be the notes taken by the paramedics who have attended to the person, or a collateral history from a family or friend.

PATIENT MANAGEMENT FOLLOWING SELF-HARM OR ATTEMPTED SUICIDE

After taking a thorough history including assessment of risk factors, and conducting a mental state examination; it is then important to consider how best to manage the patient moving forward. It is important to remember that self-harm and suicidality are not discrete illnesses; instead they are symptoms reflecting a complex interplay of mental disorders, personality types and social circumstances. Rather than taking the form of a prescribed care pathway, management of the suicidal or self-harming patient requires clinical judgement, taking into consideration the needs of the individual patient and the availability of local resources. This can often be anxiety-provoking for healthcare workers.

Formulation of a management plan should be made after a thorough review of any available past history, including care programmes or crisis plans if relevant. It is always desirable to obtain a collateral history from a family member or close friend. A good plan should include both short- and long-term management strategies.

Immediate management considerations include the following:

- Is the patient in need of inpatient psychiatric care to ensure their safety? If so, can this be achieved on a voluntary basis, or is the use of mental health legislation required?
- Would the patient benefit from the input of home treatment, outreach or crisis teams (see Chapter 5)?
- Does the patient have existing social supports that could be called upon, e.g., staying with a supportive friend or family member?
- Reducing access to means of self-harm: does the patient have a collection of tablets or rope remaining in their home they could dispose of? Should their prescription medication be dispensed weekly (or more frequently)?
- Is the patient looking after any vulnerable people, e.g., children or older relatives? Were children exposed to the risk of finding the patient during or after their self-harm or suicide attempt? If so, discuss with a senior clinician and contact social work, who will assess what protection the children need and they may be able to offer the patient additional support in their role as a parent or carer.

Longer-term management involves the modification of factors that could increase the risk for further acts of self-harm or suicidality, and may include:

- Treatment of psychiatric illness (medication, self-help, psychological therapies, community mental health team, outpatient appointments, GP follow-up).
- Avoidance of substance use (highlighting association with suicide to patient, encouraging patient to attend third sector organizations and/or addictions services).
- Optimizing social functioning (social work, Citizens Advice Bureau, community groups and activities, encouragement of family support, voluntary support agencies, food banks).
- Crisis planning (relaxation or distraction techniques, telephone counselling services, information on accessing emergency psychiatric services).

DISCUSSION OF CASE STUDY

Self-harm risk assessment

Mr SA's epidemiological risk factors are that he is a young man, recently divorced, unemployed and lives alone in social isolation. His clinical risk factors are that he may have alcohol problems and has recently experienced adverse life events (divorce, financial difficulties). The evidence of final acts (suicide note) and the failure of Mr SA to seek help after the act suggest strong suicide intent. The fact that he would not have been discovered but for the landlord's timely arrival indicates a degree of forward planning, although his leaving the door unlocked and his willingness to go to hospital after vomiting suggest some ambivalence. Mr SA had consumed a significant quantity of alcohol at the time of the overdose, which could have clouded his judgement and increased his impulsivity. On mental state examination, Mr SA has ongoing suicidal ideation and cognitive features of worthlessness and hopelessness, which are associated with suicide.

Further management

The duty psychiatrist should ask about all the epidemiological and clinical risk factors, specifically about: past or current mental illness (is Mr SA known to mental health services?); previous episodes of self-harm; alcohol or substance dependence; physical illness; family history of depression, alcohol dependence or suicide; and recent adverse life events. The duty psychiatrist will also be interested in Mr SA's current social support in order to try and help him formulate the most appropriate management plan.

As this is a complex risk assessment, the duty psychiatrist will probably have to reassess the patient themselves especially as regards detecting mental illness on mental state examination. The psychiatrist might ask the A&E doctor to keep Mr SA overnight, so that a mental state examination can be performed in the morning when he is refreshed and no longer under the influence of alcohol. A hospital admission or follow-up by a high-intensity support mental health team (e.g., crisis team) seems to be the most likely outcome.

● Chapter Summary

Self-harm is a very common presentation with many different causes.
Self-harm increases the risk for completed suicide, but the vast majority of people who self-harm will not die by suicide.
Assess risk for suicide in all those who have self-harmed, by identifying:
- risk factors for suicide (epidemiological and clinical);
- degree of suicidal intent;
- evidence of mental disorder;
- use of alcohol or other substances;
- social support and protective factors.
Management is very specific to the individual but should include crisis planning for all.

UKMLA Conditions
Self-harm

UKMLA Presentations
Self-harm
Suicidal thoughts

Psychiatric emergencies

You will come across situations in multiple specialties that require urgent intervention and a knowledge of psychiatry. This chapter covers management of acute behavioural disturbance and some adverse effects of psychotropic medications and medications commonly taken in overdose. Several other urgent scenarios are covered elsewhere in the book (see Table 7.1).

ACUTE BEHAVIOURAL DISTURBANCE

Acute behavioural disturbance describes a range of behaviours which puts the patient or others at risk. Common examples are patients shouting, pacing, breaking furniture, deliberately hurting themselves, being verbally or physically threatening to others, assaulting others or being very sexually disinhibited.

Patients may present with acute behavioural disturbance for many reasons, including psychosis, mania, delirium, dementia and substance intoxication/withdrawal. Potential exacerbating factors include personality factors, the people around them and their environment. Some people's behaviour is not driven by illness, in which case the police may need to be involved to remove and/or charge them. As well as establishing a correct diagnosis so the cause of agitation can be properly managed, the acute situation requires careful consideration to ensure the safety of the patient and those around them. Many regions have local protocols; however, Fig. 7.1 describes the principles of acute management.

Identify the cause

The best way to treat agitation is to find and treat the underlying cause. Someone with a delirium needs their physical health assessed and treated (see Chapter 19). Someone withdrawing from alcohol or other substances needs proactive pharmacological management (see Chapter 17). Someone with psychosis or mania needs their underlying mental health disorder treated (see Chapters 9 and 10, respectively). However, in some cases the underlying cause of the agitation is not identifiable, is hard to manage, or some time is required to allow definitive treatment to take effect. It is therefore often necessary to provide generic management of behavioural disturbance in the interim.

Environmental management

Hospitals can be very stressful places, particularly for patients who are acutely psychiatrically unwell. Additionally patients who are unable to understand why they are in hospital (such

Table 7.1 Urgent psychiatric conditions covered elsewhere in this book

Presentation/condition	Chapter number
A severely unwell patient requiring ECT	2
A patient requiring detention under the Mental Health Act	4
A patient with acute psychosis	9
A catatonic patient	9
A manic patient	10
A patient with dangerously low body weight	16
A patient in alcohol withdrawal	17, 22
A delirious patient	19
A patient at risk of refeeding syndrome	26
A patient with a postpartum psychosis	29
A child who is being abused	33
A patient who has committed violence against others	34
A patient with suicidal ideation	56

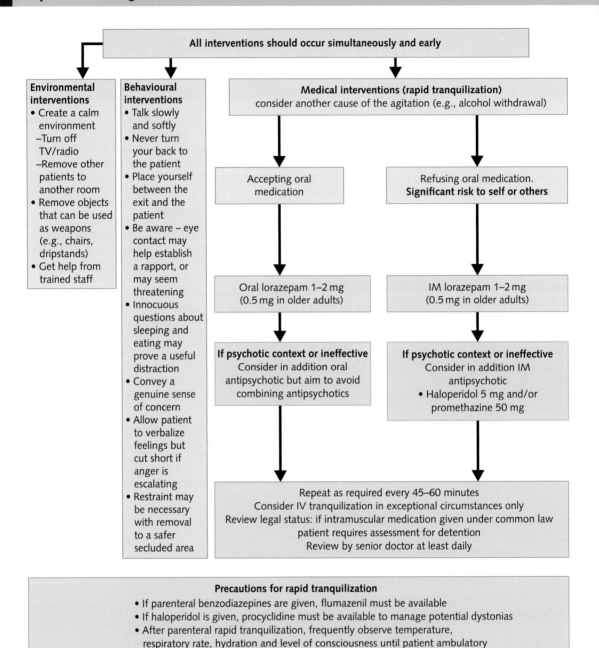

Fig. 7.1 Acute management of the agitated or aggressive patient (NICE, 2015).

as those with dementia or intellectual disability) may be very disstressed by being admitted.

Often simple changes to the environment can be very beneficial in improving agitation. Remove sources of noise (e.g., the television, a beeping IV drip). Directing other patients into different areas, and often reducing the number of people (including staff) in the room where safe to do so can help de-escalate

a situation. Additionally removing potentially dangerous items (e.g., drip stands, throwable chairs) reduces the risk of harm to the patient and others.

In extreme cases it may be that the general ward environment is not suitable to manage the patient's agitation safely. Transfer to more secure settings such as psychiatric intensive care units (PICU) may be considered. If absolutely necessary patients can be placed in seclusion: kept in their rooms or in a special 'safe room' for short periods to reduce the risk of harm.

Behavioural management

Verbal de-escalation includes measures such as speaking softly and quietly to the patient, listening to their concerns in a non-judgemental manner, and giving them the space to feel heard and validated. Patients who are very unwell (such as those with severe thought disorder) may struggle to engage with a conversation, therefore verbal de-escalation may be less successful.

As a last resort the patient may require physical restraint to keep themselves or others safe. This is done by trained staff, and must be done for as short a period as possible to facilitate movement of the patient to a safe area or administration of emergency medication.

> **RED FLAG**
>
> Always be aware of your own safety with an acutely agitated patient. Face the patient, ensure both you and the patient have easy access to an exit (if there is only one, put yourself closest to it), and carry a personal alarm if available (most psychiatric wards will have these). Do not hesitate to remove yourself from the situation if you feel at risk – you can always revisit the interview later if safe to do so.

> **RED FLAG**
>
> Restraints can be dangerous for staff and patients. Never become involved in a restraint unless specifically trained to do so.

Pharmacological management

Many patients in psychiatric wards will have 'as required' or 'PRN' (pro re nata, literally translated from Latin as 'for what arises') medications on their prescription charts for use if they become acutely anxious or agitated. Generally small doses of benzodiazepines (e.g., 1–2 mg of lorazepam) are used as first line. Sometimes, antipsychotics can also be used: if the patient is already prescribed a regular antipsychotic, the same could be used if appropriate to prevent polypharmacy (e.g., a patient on regular olanzapine could be prescribed a small dose of oral olanzapine to be used as required).

Acutely agitated patients may still accept oral medications, and these should always be the first-line option. If a patient is unable or unwilling to accept oral medication, and there is felt to be an imminent threat to themselves or others if they are not

medicated, intramuscular (IM) medication should be considered. Most health boards will have their own policy for this, often referred to as a 'Rapid Tranquilisation' or 'Acute Behavioural Disturbance' policy. Many benzodiazepines and antipsychotics can be given IM as well as orally.

> **RED FLAG**
>
> If parenteral rapid tranquilization is given, frequently observe level of consciousness and respiratory rate until the patient is ambulatory. Check pulse and blood pressure within an hour of administration.

> **RED FLAG**
>
> Withdrawal from alcohol or other substances is a very common cause of acute behavioural disturbance, especially on medical and surgical wards. These require specific pharmacological management (see Chapter 17). In the case of alcohol withdrawal, the core treatments are benzodiazepines and parenteral thiamine. In the case of opioid withdrawal, opioid replacement may be needed.

> **HINTS AND TIPS**
>
> Sometimes patients who are not currently under the Mental Health Act (see Chapter 4) may require medication to be given IM under Common Law if they become acutely agitated. Any informal patient who has been given IM medication should be assessed for consideration of detention under the Mental Health Act.

ADVERSE DRUG REACTIONS

Acute dystonia (antipsychotics)

Dystonia is a sudden spasming of the muscles that leads to an involuntary or abnormal movement. The cause is thought to be linked to dopamine receptor blockade in the nigro-striatal system, which can occur following use of dopamine antagonists such as antipsychotics or the antiemetic metoclopramide. Specific dystonias include oculogyric crises (gaze pulled in a specific direction) and torticollis (twisting of the neck). In severe cases patients are unable to swallow. Dystonias are managed with anticholinergic medications (usually procyclidine), which can be given orally or parentally.

Neuroleptic malignant syndrome (antipsychotics)

Neuroleptic malignant syndrome (NMS) is a rare but life-threatening complication of antipsychotics. It arises in around 1/10,000 patients, generally early in treatment (between 3 and 9 days after starting). It is more likely to occur if doses are very high, rapidly increased, or if the patient has taken an overdose. Mortality rate untreated is around 12% to 20%.

NMS manifests with a triad of neuromuscular hypoactivity (e.g., lead pipe muscle rigidity), altered consciousness level and autonomic dysfunction (e.g., fever, fluctuating blood pressure, and a high heart/breathing rate). Investigations may show a rise in creatinine kinase, and a prolonged QRS/QTc on ECG, increasing the risk of life-threatening arrhythmias. See Table 7.2.

Serotonin syndrome (antidepressants)

Serotonin syndrome arises due to excess serotonin in the central nervous system. It is a highly unpleasant but very rarely fatal condition. It can be caused by high doses of selective serotonin reuptake inhibitors (SSRIs), serotonin and norepinephrine reuptake inhibitors (SNRIs), monoamine oxidase inhibitor (MAOIs), tricyclic antidepressants and tramadol, as well as stimulant drugs of abuse such as cocaine and MDMA. Taking multiple serotonergic medications together is a common cause, e.g., when changing from one antidepressant to another without allowing sufficient washout. The features of serotonin syndrome often increase gradually over a short time after exposure (minutes to hours).

Serotonin syndrome is characterized by a triad of CNS effects (e.g., agitation/delirium or coma), autonomic instability (e.g., pyrexia, tachycardia, and hypertension), and neuromuscular excitability (e.g., clonus/hypertonia, tremors/myoclonus, and raised creatine kinase) Similarly to NMS, ECG may show prolonged QTc and QRS complex.

Management

For both NMS and serotonin syndrome, management is supportive (see Table 7.2). Consider continuous cardiac monitoring if there are abnormalities on ECG. Ensure adequate fluid resuscitation and sedation if necessary. Uncontrolled hyperthermia carries risk of neuronal damage, organ failure and increased permeability of the blood–brain barrier, so cooling methods may be used. Patients may require management in an HDU/ICU setting.

Lithium toxicity

Lithium (most commonly prescribed in bipolar affective disorder, see Chapter 24) requires regular monitoring of levels in the blood to ensure patients do not become lithium toxic. Toxicity can arise in those who take an overdose, due to drug interactions (thiazide diuretics, Nonsteroidal antiinflammatory drugs (NSAIDs)) or who become renally impaired or dehydrated.

Lithium has a narrow therapeutic window between nontherapeutic and toxic blood levels. Therapeutic target ranges vary by indication (see Chapter 2) but should never be much above 1.0 mmol/L. The level is considered toxic if it is above 1.5 mmol/L

Table 7.2 Distinguishing neuroleptic malignant syndrome from serotonin syndrome

	Neuroleptic malignant syndrome	Serotonin syndrome
Defining features	Both conditions characterized by triad of neuromuscular abnormalities, altered consciousness level and autonomic dysfunction (hyperthermia, sweating, tachycardia, unstable blood pressure)	
Neuromuscular abnormalities	*Reduced* activity: severe rigidity ('lead pipe'); stiff pharyngeal and thoracic muscles may lead to dysphagia and dyspnoea; bradyreflexia	*Increased* activity: myoclonus or clonus, hyperreflexia, tremor, muscular rigidity (less severe than neuroleptic malignant syndrome)
Onset	Insidious	Acute
Medication history	Usually occurs within 4–11 days of initiation or dose increase of dopamine antagonist (any antipsychotic, metoclopramide)	Usually occurs after one or two doses of new serotonergic medication; the most common cause is concurrent SSRI and MAOI
Typical blood results	Elevated creatinine kinase, white cell count and hepatic transaminases; metabolic acidosis	
Typical ECG results	Prolonged QRS complex and/or QTc	
General treatment for all patients	Discontinue offending drugs. Cool the patient. Monitor and manage hydration and haemodynamics (e.g., intravenous fluids). Consider intensive care for monitoring and/or ventilation. Monitor for complications (e.g., pneumonia, renal failure). Use benzodiazepines for sedation if agitated	
Specific treatment options to consider (depending on severity of illness)	Bromocriptine (to reverse dopamine blockade) Dantrolene (to reduce muscle spasm) Electroconvulsive therapy	Cyproheptadine (5-HT$_{2A}$ antagonist)
Mortality	20% untreated	Low

MAOI, *Monoamine oxidase inhibitor;* SSRI, *selective serotonin reuptake inhibitor.*

and dangerously toxic above 2 mmol/L. Individual responses vary and older adults may be symptomatic at lower levels than these.

Lithium toxicity (see Table 2.3) predominantly affects the central nervous system, resulting in tremors, blurred vision, muscle weakness, and drowsiness at the mildest end of the spectrum, through to confusion, ataxia, discoordination, and eventually coma. Lithium can also have a cardiotoxic effect resulting in bradycardia, AV conduction (heart) block, and QTc prolongation. ECG and bloods including renal function and lithium level should be carried out in all patients with suspected lithium toxicity.

In mild cases, stopping lithium and monitoring levels may be adequate. More severe cases require management in a medical setting. Ensuring adequate hydration is essential to maintain good renal function and urine output, as well as correcting hypotension. Those with significant neurological features or life-threatening arrythmias should undergo haemodialysis regardless of lithium concentration. Other indications for dialysis include those with renal impairment, or those with very high concentrations. Convulsions can be managed with benzodiazepines.

Opioid toxicity

Consider opioid toxicity in anyone who uses opioids (prescribed or recreational) and presents as physically unwell. Patients may have inadvertently overdosed through a change in preparation or supplier, or they may have lost tolerance after a time away from use. The primary features of opioid toxicity are reduced Glasgow Coma Scale (GCS), depressed respiratory rate and effort, pin-point pupils and cardiovascular collapse.

Treatment is with naloxone, a short-acting opioid receptor antagonist. This will reverse the effect of the opioids very quickly, but has a short half-life, so the patient may require repeat doses or a continuous infusion.

Paracetamol overdose

Paracetamol overdose accounts for 48% of poisoning admissions to hospital, with 235 deaths in 2020 across England and Wales.

Paracetamol is metabolized in the liver. The paracetamol metabolite N-acetyl-p-benzoquinone imine (NAPQI) is incredibly hepatotoxic but is normally conjugated by glutathione into a safe compound. In overdose, the glutathione reserves are depleted leading to a build-up of NAPQI. N-acetylcysteine (NAC), the antidote for paracetamol poisoning, acts to regenerate the depleted glutathione reserves in the liver preventing damage.

Patients may present following an acute overdose (taking all the paracetamol over a period of 1 hour or less) or a staggered overdose (taking the paracetamol over a period greater than 1 hour). Treatment depends on the period over which the overdose was taken.

- If bloods can be taken less than 8 hours after an acute overdose treatment does not need to be started immediately. Bloods (including a paracetamol level) are checked between 4 and 8 hours post overdose, and the level is measured against time since the overdose on a paracetamol nomogram (see Fig. 7.2). Patients who fall above the treatment line will be commenced on NAC, otherwise they do not require treatment.
- If bloods cannot be taken within eight hours of an acute overdose, or the overdose was staggered, NAC is started immediately to minimize harm.

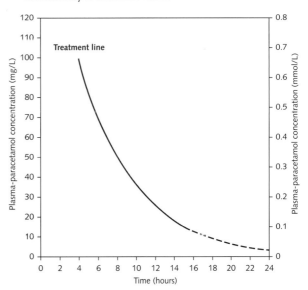

Fig. 7.2 Paracetamol nomogram. Blood paracetamol level is compared to the time since the overdose. Patients who fall over the line will be treated with NAC. (Adapted from Medicines and Healthcare products Regulatory Agency, Treating paracetamol overdose with intravenous acetylcysteine: new guidance. Drug Safety Update September 2012, vol 6, issue 2: A1)

- All patients with paracetamol overdose will require monitoring of liver function tests (LFTs) (particularly alanine transaminase (ALT)) and international normalized ratio (INR). This will determine how long they require NAC treatment.
- In a minority of cases, mostly due to delay in presentation, patients will develop fulminant hepatic failure requiring liver transplantation. These patients should be discussed with liver specialists without delay, and a psychiatric assessment performed promptly to identify any psychiatric contraindications for transplantation.

Other common overdoses

Any drug can be taken in overdose, however some are taken more commonly than others. See Table 7.3 for a description of different drug toxidromes.

Beta-blockers taken in overdose lead to hypotension and bradycardia. Bronchospasm can occur in those with known airway diseases such as asthma or COPD. Bradycardia, and associated cardiogenic shock, is treated with atropine in the first instance. Other treatments include dobutamine, isoprenaline

Table 7.3 Common drug toxidromes

Toxidrome	Example drugs	Clinical signs	Vital signs	Investigations	Management
Opioid	Heroin Methadone Tramadol Prescription opioids	Drowsiness Pin-point pupils	↓Respiratory rate ↓Heart rate/blood pressure ↓GCS	Clinical diagnosis	Naloxone Protect airway +/− oxygen
Serotonin syndrome	SSRIs/SNRIs MAOIs Tricyclic antidepressants Tramadol Stimulant street drugs	Agitated/delirium Sweating Dilated pupils Clonus/hypertonia Tremors	↑Respiratory rate ↑Heart rate/blood pressure ↑Temperature	ECG; ↑QRS ↑QTc ↑Heart rate Bloods; ↑creatinine kinase	IV fluids Benzodiazepines Oxygen (high metabolism) ↑QRS → sodium bicarbonate ↑QTc → magnesium Cyproheptadine (serious cases)
Anticholinergic	Tricyclic antidepressants Antihistamines Antipsychotics Cyclizine Hyoscine Butylbromide	Agitated/delirium Dry skin/mouth Dilated pupils Flushed Tremor Urinary retention Constipation	↑Respiratory rate ↑Heart rate/blood pressure ↑Temperature	ECG; ↑QRS ↑QTc ↑Heart rate Bloods; ↑creatinine kinase	IV fluids Benzodiazepines ↑QRS → sodium bicarbonate ↑QTc → magnesium Oxygen (high metabolism)
Sedative	Benzodiazepine Alcohol GHB Barbiturates	Drowsiness Confused Normal/dilated pupils	↓Respiratory rate ↓Heart rate/blood pressure ↓GCS	Bloods; ↑alcohol level	Protect airway +/− oxygen Benzodiazepines for withdrawal
Neuroleptic malignant syndrome	Antipsychotics Withdrawal of Parkinson's drugs Metoclopramide Prochlorperazine	Sweating Dystonia/rigidity Agitated/delirium Coma/catatonia	↑Respiratory rate ↑/↓Blood pressure ↑Respiratory rate ↑Temperature	ECG; ↑QRS ↑QTc ↑Heart rate Bloods; ↑creatinine kinase Disseminated intravascular coagulation ↑K+ ↑/↓Na+	Discontinue causative drugs IV fluids Benzodiazepines Oxygen (high metabolism) Dopamine agonists Dantrolene ↑QRS → sodium bicarbonate ↑QTc → magnesium
Sympathomimetic	MAOIs Cocaine/MDMA/methamphetamines	Agitated/delirium Sweating Tremor Dilated pupils	↑Respiratory rate ↑Heart rate/blood pressure ↑Temperature	ECG; ↑QRS ↑QTc ↑Heart rate Bloods; ↑creatinine Kinase	IV fluids Benzodiazepines Oxygen (high metabolism) ↑QRS → sodium bicarbonate ↑QTc → magnesium

GCS, *Glasgow Coma Scale;* GHB, *gamma-hydroxy butyrate;* K+, *potassium;* MAOI, *monoamine oxidase inhibitor;* Na+, *sodium;* QRS, *QRS complex;* QTc, *QT interval, corrected;* SNRI, *serotonin and norepinephrine reuptake inhibitor;* SSRI, *selective serotonin reuptake inhibitor.*

and transcutaneous pacing. Fluid resuscitation is first-line management for hypotension; however, in severe cases, IV glucagon and IV high-dose insulin therapy are used.

Insulin can be given in long or short-acting forms, so the duration of toxic symptoms can vary. Hypoglycaemia can lead to symptoms of vomiting, sweating, confusion, drowsiness, convulsions and coma. Due to insulin shifting potassium into cells, life-threatening hypokalaemia can occur.

Management focuses on correcting hypoglycaemia and managing symptoms.

Benzodiazepine overdose results in drowsiness, confusion, respiratory depression and reduced GCS. Street benzodiazepines can be of varying potencies and may be mixed with other drugs such as fentanyl. Management is symptomatic, ensuring the patient's airway and breathing remains uncompromised. Flumazenil, a benzodiazepine antagonist, is rarely used routinely.

● Chapter Summary

- Patients may become acutely agitated to the degree that they are a risk to themselves or others.
- Acutely agitated patients should be managed with a combination of environmental, behavioural and pharmacological measures.
- In extreme cases measures such as physical restraint or IM medications may be needed
- Neuroleptic malignant syndrome is a rare but severe side effect of antipsychotics. Patients are acutely unwell and require management in a medical setting
- Serotonin syndrome is a rare but potentially serious side effect of many antidepressants. Patients are acutely unwell and require management in a medical setting
- Lithium requires careful monitoring, and high levels result in lithium toxicity.
- Opioid overdose requires treatment with naloxone.
- Paracetamol overdose may require no treatment, or require treatment with *N*-acetylcysteine.

UKMLA Conditions
Drug overdose
Self-harm
Substance misuse disorder

UKMLA Presentations
Addiction
Behaviour/personality change
Confusion
Delirium
Overdose
Self-harm
Substance misuse
Suicidal thoughts
Thoughts to harm others

Presenting Complaints

The patient with neurodevelopmental differences

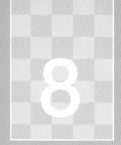

Case summary

JJ, a 9-year-old child, was assessed by the child and adolescent mental health team after their teacher told their parents she thought JJ might have attention deficit hyperactivity disorder (ADHD). She had noticed that JJ was a bright child but made a lot of careless mistakes in their homework, which they often forgot to bring to school. JJ had always been very talkative, which initially endeared them to their peers, but lately they had fallen out with some friends as they said JJ never let them get a word in. They had always been an active child and had been picked for their school football team. However, the coach had dropped them after JJ failed to notice the ball coming in their direction on a number of occasions, seemingly staring off into space. Their high activity levels were becoming increasingly noticeable as they got older and their peers were more able to sit through a class than them. JJ's parents were initially surprised by the suggestion of ADHD but on reflection agreed that JJ often did things without thinking (they broke an arm last year after leaping out of a tree) and they had never considered going to the cinema as a family because they knew JJ would not be able to sit through a film. There were no concerns that they were not looking after JJ well. JJ told the psychiatrist that they generally felt cheerful, had no physical problems and did not have any problems seeing or hearing. In fact, they thought they had extra good hearing because they seemed to notice things other people did not, such as bird calls outside the classroom.

(For a discussion of the case study, see the end of the chapter.)

DEFINITIONS

Neurodevelopmental disorders are common and increasingly identified throughout the lifespan. You will encounter patients with neurodevelopmental disorders in all branches of psychiatry. They are disorders where abnormal development of the central nervous system leads to impairments in brain function resulting in problems acquiring or executing cognitive, motor or social functions. The severest neurodevelopmental disorders tend to present early and are assessed and diagnosed by paediatricians. Disorders that primarily influence subtle aspects of cognition are more likely to present with learning and/or behavioural difficulties in children of school age and are assessed and diagnosed by psychiatry. Because of increasing awareness of neurodevelopmental disorders among both the public and health professionals, as well as changes to diagnostic criteria, some people who had difficulties that were not assessed in childhood and that have persisted into adulthood are now seeking assessment for neurodevelopmental disorders as adults.

The concept of neurodevelopmental disorders is evolving. Recent classification changes have given them increasing precedence, with the DSM-5 and the ICD-11 including them as a diagnostic category in their own right. Some disorders not historically viewed as neurodevelopmental may be categorized as such in due course, for example, brain changes in schizophrenia and bipolar disorder probably occur from a young age, but symptoms only manifest from adolescence or early adulthood. These disorders are covered in Chapters 9 and 10 in this book. Personality disorders also overlap conceptually with neurodevelopmental disorders: both describe dysfunctional patterns of behaviour with onset in childhood causing significant impairment to the patient or others. These are covered in Chapter 18.

This chapter covers the common neurodevelopmental problems that present to psychiatry: difficulties with learning, socializing, paying attention and controlling movements. In defining disorders involving these abilities, it is crucial to recognize that performance in these areas varies normally within the healthy population (see Fig. 8.1). A disorder is only diagnosed if:

1. The person has characteristics that are significantly outside the typical range.
2. These characteristics are associated with functional impairment (i.e., problems in social, occupational or adaptive functioning).

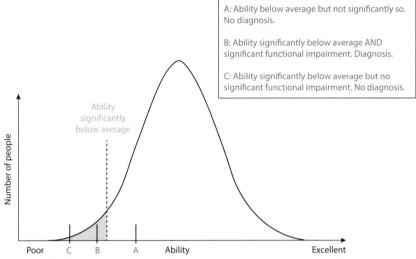

A: Ability below average but not significantly so. No diagnosis.

B: Ability significantly below average AND significant functional impairment. Diagnosis.

C: Ability significantly below average but no significant functional impairment. No diagnosis.

Fig. 8.1 Core criteria for a diagnosis of a neurodevelopmental disorder.

COMMUNICATION

The terms 'intellectual disability', 'learning disability' and 'learning difficulty' are often confused. In the United Kingdom intellectual disability is the preferred medical term; however, learning disability was used more commonly in the past, and is still the preferred name among some self-advocate groups. Broadly, a learning difficulty refers to any condition that impairs learning and is most often not associated with a global reduction in IQ. A specific learning difficulty is impairment in one particular type of learning (e.g., dyslexia, dyscalculia) which ICD-11 terms a 'developmental learning disorder'. An 'intellectual disability' is where there are significant limitations in intellectual functioning across multiple domains and impairments in adaptive functioning.

CLINICAL FEATURES AND DIFFERENTIAL DIAGNOSIS

Problems with learning

Global

A generalized problem with learning new information and skills can arise through physical or mental health problems, sensory impairments or psychosocial adversity. If these are excluded, a diagnosis of intellectual disability should be considered.

Intellectual disability is an umbrella term used to describe diverse difficulties that manifest with all of these three features:

- Significant limitation in intellectual functioning
- Significant impairment in adaptive behaviour functioning
- Have onset during the developmental period

Limitations in *intellectual functioning* are present across multiple domains (e.g., memory, verbal comprehension, processing speed). Limitations in intellectual functioning should be assessed, where possible, using normed standardized tests appropriate for the person's language and culture. ICD-11 recognizes that such tests are not available in all clinical settings and so they are no longer essential for the diagnosis. If testing is available, ICD-11 advises that significant impairment means two or more standard deviations below normal.

In the United Kingdom intellectual functioning is usually defined by the intelligence quotient (IQ). This can be assessed by standardized intelligence tests (e.g., Wechsler Intelligence Scales for Children (WISC)). An IQ of 70 or below, which is two standard deviations below the mean (IQ = 100), represents sub-average intellectual functioning. It is important to remember the limitations of using standardized testing instruments, and they should not be used as the sole evidence for diagnosis. Many standardized tests tend to be aimed at people of (or around) average intelligence and may be unsuitable for patients with more severe difficulties. Also, differences in native language and background, as well as sensory, motor or communication difficulties may lead to patients obtaining falsely low IQ scores. Therefore patients obtaining IQ scores lower than 70 should only be diagnosed as having intellectual disability if there is evidence of significant impairments in adaptive functioning.

Adaptive functioning refers to the conceptual, social and practical skills needed by people in everyday life. Conceptual skills require the application of knowledge (understanding of time, spatial relationships, problem-solving) and communication skills (reading, writing, following instructions, ability to speak). Social skills include managing relationships, social rules, obeying laws and avoiding exploitation. Practical skills include self-care, managing money and maintaining own safety. Adaptive functioning is assessed by a thorough developmental, psychiatric and medical history from the patient's parents and other care providers, particularly occupational therapists who may perform more in-depth assessment of functioning when a diagnosis is unclear.

These issues arise during the developmental period (normally in early childhood but in theory could arise or be identified in adolescence). In practice in the United Kingdom 18 years old is viewed as the upper limit beyond which any new intellectual impairment arising would not be viewed as an intellectual disability. These disorders are generally caused by an interruption in the normal development of the brain resulting from a variety of problems – some genetic, some environmental and some unknown (see Chapter 32). Intellectual disability is a lifelong condition.

Patients may also have clinical features associated with the specific cause of their intellectual disability (e.g., Down syndrome: epicanthic folds with oblique palpebral fissures, broad hands with single transverse palmar crease, flattened occiput, cardiac septal defects). Around 25% of people with intellectual disability have epilepsy, compared to 1% of the general population. People with intellectual disabilities are also more likely to have difficulty with aggression, self-injurious behaviour, repetitive stereotypical motor movements and poor impulse control. Up to a third of people with an intellectual disability have a comorbid psychiatric illness, most commonly schizophrenia which occurs in around 4% of individuals with intellectual disability, higher than the general population.

Intellectual disabilities are classified as mild, moderate, severe and profound, according to the degree of intellectual and adaptive impairment. Table 8.1 summarizes the clinical features of the degrees of intellectual disabilities in adulthood. However, this is simplified and difficulties experienced can vary from person to person. ICD-11 provides detailed tables describing behavioural indicators of adaptive behaviour typically seen with different degrees of intellectual disability during early childhood, later childhood and adolescence and adulthood.

Table 8.1 Degrees of intellectual disability

Degree of intellectual disability	Approximate degree of intellectual limitation	Adaptive functioning expected in adulthood
Mild (85% of cases)	2–3 standard deviations below mean (equivalent to IQ 50–69)	Able to fluently communicate and follow simple three-step instructions Can read or write at about the level of someone who has been at school for 8 years Can apply their abilities in semi-skilled employment, and sometimes skilled employment
Moderate (10% of cases)	3–4 standard deviations below mean (equivalent to IQ 35–49)	Can communicate in short sentences Can follow two-step instructions Can read or write about the level of someone who has been at school for 5 years Some can apply their abilities in semi-skilled employment
Severe (3%–4% of cases)	4 or more standard deviations below mean (equivalent to IQ ≤ 34)	Can use a communication aid to indicate their preferences (e.g., about food) Can follow a one-step instruction Can recognize letters or simple pictures Some can use their abilities in unskilled employment
Profound (1%–2% of cases)	4 or more standard deviations below mean (equivalent to IQ ≤ 34)	Can develop some nonverbal communication strategies Can recognize familiar pictures, and some may recognize familiar places Can perform very simple tasks with support and aids

HINTS AND TIPS

Whereas dementia describes a loss of cognitive ability already acquired, intellectual disability describes the failure to develop a normal level of cognitive functioning. However, individuals with Down syndrome are also at very high risk for developing early-onset Alzheimer disease in later life, with around 2/3 meeting criteria by age 60.

Common intellectual disability syndromes

Foetal alcohol syndrome – Foetal alcohol syndrome is estimated to affect 14 in every 10,000 births, and is a condition caused by maternal ingestion of alcohol during pregnancy. People with foetal alcohol syndrome are often small for their age (<10th percentile for height/weight), have characteristic facial features such as a thin upper lip and a flat philtrum and have an increased incidence of intellectual disability, epilepsy and problems with attention. Due to the risk of foetal alcohol syndrome UK guidance is that women who are pregnant or trying to conceive should not drink alcohol.

Fragile X – Fragile X is an X-linked condition, as such it is more common in males (1/4000 males compared to 1/6000 females). Individuals with Fragile X often have a long face with prominent ears and jaw, and boys with Fragile X typically have macroorchidism. These patients may be very anxious, and girls in particular may present as very shy and withdrawn. There is high comorbidity with autism spectrum disorder (ASD) and ADHD.

22q11.2 Deletion syndrome (DiGeorge syndrome/velocardiofacial syndrome) – DiGeorge syndrome is caused by a deletion at 22q11. Children with DiGeorge syndrome often have congenital cardiac defects, difficulties with speech and hearing (often with a high-pitched voice, and cleft palettes). They may be shorter than average, and are more prone to conditions such as schizophrenia.

Prader–Willi syndrome – Prader–Willi is caused by a loss of genes inherited from the paternal chromosome 15q11-q13 region. Individuals with Prader–Willi have characteristic facial features of a narrow face with almond-shaped eyes, and due to abnormalities of the pituitary gland, experience excessive hunger and weight gain from a young age. Hypogonadism and cryptorchidism are common.

Specific

Some disorders are characterized by the disturbed acquisition of a *specific* cognitive, language or motor function during a child's development (e.g., language, reading, spelling, mathematical ability and motor skills). If other areas of cognitive functioning are normal, a child may have a specific reading disorder (developmental learning disorder with impairment in reading) but be of normal intelligence and have no problem with writing or mathematics. In some children, the consequences of the difficulty (e.g., school problems, bullying) might lead to secondary emotional or behavioural problems. These disorders would normally be assessed and diagnosed by an educational psychologist rather than doctors, so are not discussed in detail here. See Box 8.1 for an overview.

Problems with social interaction and communication

Social interaction is one of the most complex tasks the brain has to negotiate and many factors can influence social ability.

Children

Parents, health visitors or teachers may raise concerns about a child's ability to communicate and interact socially. It is important to exclude an influence of physical or mental health problems, sensory impairments or psychosocial adversity. Intellectual disability reduces social abilities, but if the social impairments are more marked than would be expected for the degree of intellectual disability, they can be diagnosed separately. Clinical features of the neurodevelopmental causes of social difficulty are described in Box 8.1. The differentials are shown in Box 8.2. Selective mutism and reactive attachment disorder are described in Chapter 33.

BOX 8.1 NEURODEVELOPMENTAL DISORDERS INFLUENCING SPECIFIC ABILITIES

Developmental Learning Disorders
- Reading
- Written expression
- Mathematics

Developmental speech or language disorder
- Speech sound
- Speech fluency
- Receptive and expressive language
- Mainly expressive language
- Mainly pragmatic language

BOX 8.2 DIFFERENTIAL DIAGNOSES FOR SOCIAL AND COMMUNICATION DIFFICULTIES IN CHILDREN

Normal for age

Secondary to sensory impairment (e.g., deafness)

Secondary to mental or physical health problem (e.g., depression, childhood schizophrenia, uncontrolled epilepsy)

Secondary to psychosocial adversity (e.g., emotional abuse)

Intellectual disability

Autism spectrum disorder

Rett syndrome

Attention deficit hyperactivity disorder

Reactive attachment disorder

Disruptive behaviour or conduct-dissocial disorder

Selective mutism

Developmental speech or language disorder

Stereotyped movement disorder

Autism spectrum disorder

People with ASD have difficulties with social interaction and communication, and have restricted interests and behaviours. These are clearly atypical or excessive for the person's age and sociocultural context and lead to problems with the person's personal life, their family, their education and their work. The difficulties should be present from a young age, although they may not be noticed until later when social and academic demands exceed the person's capabilities.

The essential diagnostic features of ASD are:

1. Impairment in social interactions and communication. Key domains include:
   - Difficulties imagining and responding to the feelings and emotional **states of others.**
   - Difficulties with **pragmatic language**, i.e., understanding verbal or nonverbal social cues and body language, difficulties integrating spoken language with nonverbal communication (e.g., not making eye contact when speaking to someone).
   - Difficulties forming and sustaining typical **peer relationships**.
2. Restrictive, repetitive and inflexible patterns of behaviours, interests or activities. Key domains include:
   - Difficulty **adapting** to new or unanticipated experiences and circumstances.
   - **Inflexible** adherence to routine and rules (e.g., requiring precise timings for meals).

- **Ritualized behaviours** (e.g., preoccupation with sorting a particular type of object).
- Persistent preoccupation with **special interests** which might include objects or parts of objects (e.g., car tyres).
- **Repetitive stereotyped motor movements** – including whole body (e.g., rocking), atypical gait (e.g., walking on tiptoes) or hands and fingers (e.g., flapping).
- Hypersensitivity or hyposensitivity to **sensory** stimuli (e.g., feel of clothing or food).

In addition to these diagnostic features, individuals may also exhibit behavioural problems such as aggressiveness, impulsivity and self-injurious behaviour. Although children and young people with autism can be of normal intelligence, many have significant intellectual disabilities. Epilepsy develops in about 25% to 30% of people.

Three sets of specifiers are provided for ASD in the ICD-11:

- With or without intellectual impairment
- With or without loss of previously acquired skills
- Level of functional language impairment (none/mild, impaired, complete)

A very small proportion of individuals (more commonly boys) with ASD may present with a loss of previously acquired skills. This regression typically occurs during the second year of life and most often involves language use and social responsiveness. This used to be called Heller Syndrome (or Childhood Disintegrative Disorder) however is now considered part of ASD.

HINTS AND TIPS

You may see reference in notes to Asperger Syndrome (or 'high functioning autism'), and some patients may mention having this diagnosis. This was a subtype of autism where there are no significant abnormalities in language acquisition and ability or in cognitive development and intelligence. It was a diagnosis in the ICD-10, however is not in the ICD-11 or the DSM-5. In ICD-11 it could be specified as ASD without intellectual impairment and with mild or no impairment of functional language.

HINTS AND TIPS

It may be specified that the person has 'co-occurring disorder of intellectual development' if they also have intellectual disability.

You may read notes or hear patients talk about diagnoses that were different in the ICD-10. For neurodevelopmental disorders, differences in the ICD-10 include:

- Mental retardation is now called intellectual disability.
- Pervasive developmental disorder is now classed as ASD.
- Asperger syndrome is no longer a separate diagnosis, it is now classed as a type of ASD.
- Hyperkinetic disorders have been consolidated and renamed as ADHD.

BOX 8.3 DIFFERENTIAL DIAGNOSES FOR SOCIAL AND COMMUNICATION DIFFICULTIES IN ADULTS

Within normal range
Intellectual disability
Autism spectrum disorder
Personality disorder
Disruptive behaviour or conduct-dissocial disorder
Secondary to a psychiatric disorder
- Social anxiety disorder
- Generalized anxiety disorder
- Depression
- Negative symptoms of schizophrenia
Brain injury (e.g., traumatic, cerebrovascular accident, infection, inflammation)
Neurodegeneration (e.g., dementia)

Rett syndrome

Rett syndrome, which has almost only been seen in girls, is caused by mutations in the gene *MECP2* located on the X chromosome and can arise sporadically or from germline mutations. It is initially characterized by an apparently normal antenatal development with a normal head circumference at birth, followed by an apparently normal psychomotor development in the first 5 months after birth. From 6 months to 2 years of age, a progressive and destructive encephalopathy results in a deceleration of head growth; loss or lack of development of language and loss of purposeful hand movements and fine motor skills, with subsequent development of stereotyped hand movements (e.g., midline hand-wringing). After a decade, girls may need to use a wheelchair to mobilize, may have issues with incontinence, muscle wasting and rigidity and significant impairment of language ability.

Adults

In adults presenting with social difficulties, the main differentials are shown in Box 8.3. It is paramount to take a history of the time course of difficulties: have they been present from a young age or only since adulthood? Patients themselves usually struggle to provide an objective account of this, so it is essential to obtain a collateral developmental history from someone who knew the patient well as a child. This can be a parent, a teacher, an older sibling or in written form, for example, school reports. The validity of any diagnosis of this sort in adulthood increases with the number of sources of collateral information available.

If impairments in communication and social abilities have had onset or significantly worsened in adulthood, then it is important to exclude other conditions that could have caused this, for example, a traumatic brain injury, frontotemporal dementia, a depressive episode or schizophrenia.

Anxiety and depression are often comorbid with autism in adults. A primary diagnosis of social anxiety can be distinguished from an ASD in that there should be no associated problems in communication or restricted interests and social abilities should be intact (e.g., able to make normal eye contact). In generalized anxiety disorder, anxiety covers many areas, not just social situations.

Personality disorders can be distinguished from autism by the dominant traits (see Chapter 18), for example, finding little pleasure in anything in those with negative affect personality traits, a desire for perfection in those with anankastic personality traits, feelings of emptiness and frequent self-harm in personality disorders, with a borderline pattern and the ability to read social situations, but to disregard social obligations, in those with dissocial personality traits. People with schizotypal disorder may exhibit magical thinking.

Clinical features of ASDs in adults vs. children are shown in Table 8.2. Because difficulties diagnosed in adulthood are likely to be at the milder end of the spectrum, it is very important to clarify the severity of the person's difficulties and the degree to which they impact their life (e.g., problems in initiating or sustaining employment, education and/or relationships). Your own mental state examination (see Table 8.3) and a collateral history are crucial. People may have difficulties in interacting with others that do not meet criteria for autism or any other psychiatric diagnosis.

Problems with attention

Children

In a child described as paying poor attention, it is important to exclude an influence of physical or mental health problems, sensory impairments or psychosocial adversity. Intellectual disability reduces the ability to pay attention, but if this is more marked than would be expected for the degree of intellectual disability, it can be diagnosed separately. Differentials

Table 8.2 Clinical features of autism spectrum disorder presenting at different ages

Domain	Examples	
	Presenting in childhood	**Presenting in adulthood**
Impaired social interaction and communication	Not interested in peers. Little eye contact. Delayed speech.	Not able to make small talk. Doesn't pick up social cues. Pedantic, overly formal use of language.
Restricted, stereotyped interests and behaviours	Intense interest in physical aspects of objects or numbers (e.g., lining up milk bottle tops). Inflexible adherence to routine. Repetitive movements (e.g., clapping, rocking).	Intense interest in objects or numbers, often enjoyment gained from categorizing or collecting (e.g., listing train timetables). Inflexible adherence to routine. Repetitive movements less common.

Table 8.3 Mental state abnormalities in people with neurodevelopmental disorders

Disorder	Typical findings on mental state examination
Intellectual disability	*Very dependent on severity of disability.* Struggles to understand your questions. Gives short answers with limited vocabulary. Dysarthric.
Autism spectrum disorder (ASD)	Reduced eye contact. Does not pick up on social cues (e.g., when it is the end of the appointment). Speech may have limited intonation, be oddly accented or be unusually formal or pedantic. Talks excessively about topics of particular interest to them, does not take turns as in a normal conversation. Affect unreactive or odd, not able to use facial expression to communicate naturally. May, with effort, be able to mask issues with communication for a brief period.
Attention deficit hyperactivity disorder (ADHD)	Adults may be fidgety. Children may get up from chair, play noisily with toys, run around waiting room, shout. Person may talk at length in a tangential fashion. They may speak over you or finish your sentences. Information may need to be repeated. They may be easily distracted by external noises (e.g., traffic or a distant telephone).
Tourette syndrome	Tics. Features of comorbid attention deficit hyperactivity disorder.

are shown in Box 8.4 and clinical features of the key neurodevelopmental cause of inattention (attention deficit hyperactivity disorder (ADHD)) is described below.

Conduct-dissocial disorder and reactive attachment disorder are described in Chapter 33. They can be distinguished from ADHD in that in conduct-dissocial disorder the child breaks rules deliberately rather than impulsively and resists completing tasks because they do not wish to conform, rather than being unable to sustain attention. In reactive attachment disorder, a child may appear socially disinhibited as with ADHD, but unlike in ADHD will struggle to form sustained relationships.

BOX 8.4 DIFFERENTIAL DIAGNOSES FOR ATTENTION DIFFICULTIES IN CHILDREN

Normal for age
Secondary to sensory impairment (e.g., myopia)
Secondary to mental or physical health problem (e.g., anxiety, restlessness due to pain)
Secondary to psychosocial adversity (e.g., hunger)
Intellectual disability
Attention deficit hyperactivity disorder (ADHD)
Disruptive behaviour or dissocial disorder
Reactive attachment disorder
Tourette syndrome or dyskinesia
Specific learning difficulty

HINTS AND TIPS

Sensory processing abnormalities such as hypersensitivity to sound or touch are common in autism spectrum disorders and attention deficit hyperactivity disorder. The presence of such abnormalities increases the likelihood of a neurodevelopmental diagnosis but is not required for a diagnosis. Their presence is also not diagnostic, you may strongly dislike certain sounds or textures yourself!

Attention deficit hyperactivity disorder

ADHD refers to a pattern of problems with maintaining attention/hyperactivity. This pattern must be persistent (for at least 6 months) and impact multiple areas such as school, work or home life. These should have been present since before age 12, however may not be noticed until later in life. The diagnosis can be of primarily inattentive symptoms, hyperactivity-impulsive symptoms or a mix of both.

1. Inattentive symptoms. Key domains include:
   - Difficulty keeping **focus** on tasks, particularly those which are unstimulating or require sustained mental effort. Not finishing tasks once started. Making careless errors.
   - Easily **distracted.** Appears not to listen when spoken to. Seems to frequently daydream.
   - Difficulty **organizing** day-to-day activities such as arriving on time or homework. Frequently loses things. Forgetful.
2. Hyperactivity-impulsivity symptoms. Key domains include:
   - Struggles to sit still, fidget, feels **restless.**
   - **Talks excessively**/loudly, struggles to participate in quiet activities.
   - Difficulty **taking turns** in games, activities or conversation, blurts out answers, interrupts others.
   - Poor perception of risk, impulsive, **reckless.**

HINTS AND TIPS

When assessing a person's ability to concentrate, remember to take their developmental stage into account. A rule of thumb is that a preschool child would be expected to be able to concentrate for at least 3 minutes, a child at primary school for at least 10 minutes and an adolescent for at least 30 minutes.

Adults

In adults presenting with attentional difficulties, the main differentials are shown in Box 8.5. Even in adults, for a diagnosis of ADHD to be made there must be some evidence of impairment before the age of 12. As with social impairment, it is paramount to take a history of the time course of difficulties with a collateral developmental history from someone who knew the patient well as a child or contemporaneous documentation such as school reports.

If impairments in attention have had onset or significantly worsened in adulthood, then it is important to exclude other conditions that could have caused this, for example, a traumatic brain injury, dementia, a depressive episode or anxiety. Bipolar disorder can present with mood instability similar

---

BOX 8.5 DIFFERENTIAL DIAGNOSES FOR ATTENTION DIFFICULTIES IN ADULTS

Within normal range
Secondary to substance abuse
Intellectual disability
Attention deficit hyperactivity disorder
Personality disorder
 - Borderline pattern
 - Dissocial traits
Disruptive behaviour or dissocial disorder
Secondary to other psychiatric disorder
 - Bipolar disorder
 - Generalized anxiety disorder
 - Depression
Brain injury (e.g., traumatic, cerebrovascular accident, infection, inflammation)
Neurodegeneration (e.g., dementia)

(but more severe) than that seen in ADHD. The use of substances, particularly amphetamines, must be excluded.

Borderline pattern personality traits overlap with ADHD in terms of impulsivity and rapid emotional variation. However, ADHD is not associated with feelings of emptiness or self-harm. Dissocial personality traits overlap with ADHD in that both are associated with lawbreaking and often found in prison populations. However, in ADHD the offences tend to be committed impulsively, whereas in those with dissocial personality traits there is more likely to be premeditation.

HINTS AND TIPS

The symptoms of neurodevelopmental disorders overlap with the symptoms of many other psychiatric disorders and it is important to be aware of the possibility of a missed neurodevelopmental diagnosis. This applies particularly to patients with atypical patterns of symptoms or response (e.g., rapid cycling bipolar, treatment-resistant depression) and to patients with several diagnoses, none of which quite seem to fit.

Clinical features of ADHD in adults vs. children are shown in Table 8.4. In adults presenting for the first time with a possible diagnosis of ADHD, impairments tend to be milder than in those diagnosed in childhood. Because difficulties are likely to be at the milder end of the spectrum, it is very important to clarify the severity of the person's difficulties and the degree to which they impact their life. Mental state examination (see Table 8.3) and a collateral history are crucial.

Problems with controlling movements

Abnormal movements can result from a diverse range of problems, for example, orthopaedic, rheumatological, neurological or nutritional problems. Those covered here are those that are thought to be due to a problem with cortical processing of the coordination of movement (see Table 8.5), rather than a problem with the mechanics of a movement.

Developmental motor coordination disorder

This disorder is characterized by significantly impaired gross and fine motor skills out of keeping with the person's general intellectual ability, sufficient to cause marked functional impairment. For example, gross motor impairment such as being very slow or inaccurate when catching a ball, walking or riding a bike, or fine motor impairment such as issues using scissors, cutlery, zippers or pens.

Stereotyped movement disorder

This disorder is when people persistently show voluntary, repetitive stereotypes (see Table 18.5). It is commonly seen in people with ASD and intellectual disability.

> **HINTS AND TIPS**
>
> Tic disorders were included under 'Mental and Behavioural Disorders' in the ICD-10; however, in ICD-11 they are classified as 'Diseases of the nervous system'. They are often comorbid with neurodevelopmental conditions, so have been left in this chapter for reference.

Tourette syndrome

Tics are sudden, rapid, repetitive, nonrhythmic motor movements or vocalizations (see Table 8.5). They are usually preceded by a premonitory feeling of discomfort. They are involuntary; however, they can be voluntarily suppressed

Table 8.4 Clinical features of attention deficit hyperactivity disorder presenting at different ages

Domain	Examples	
	Presenting in childhood	**Presenting in adulthood**
Inattention	Poor self-organization (e.g., loses school jumper). Needs instructions repeated. Careless mistakes in schoolwork.	Frequently loses important items (e.g., keys, wallet, phone). Struggles to complete administrative tasks.
Impulsivity-hyperactivity	Shouts out answers to questions. Difficulty waiting turn. Easily led. Risk taker. Moves around inappropriately. Excessively talkative, goes off on tangents.	Makes reckless decisions. Completes others' sentences. Avoids queuing. May avoid situations where sitting still is expected (e.g., cinema, theatre). Overtalkative with tangential conversation.

Table 8.5 Types of motor abnormality

Abnormality	Description	Examples
Tic	Quick, sudden, movement arising unpredictably, generally occurring for a brief time. Often stereotyped (i.e., the same movement) and recurrent, but not rhythmic. Suppressible and suggestible. Usually occurs at age 5–7 years.	Eye-blinking, mouth twitching, grunting (simple) or shouting out words, squatting, twirling while walking, making obscene gestures (complex).
Stereotypy	Identical, nonfunctional movement repeated many times. Arises in a fixed, predictable manner. Person can be distracted from movement but cannot voluntarily suppress. Usually occurs by age 2 years.	Hand flapping, twisting, rocking, head banging, grimacing, humming, grunting.
Mannerism	Goal-directed movement that individual performs frequently in a way unique to them. Under voluntary control. May be bizarre if in response to delusional idea.	Twirling hair, rolling eyes, clearing throat (common, part of personality). Jerking head, twiddling finger movements (rarer, bizarre).

(although this can be very difficult, like trying to suppress the urge to sneeze). They are also often suggestible (i.e., can be provoked by discussing them or by observing others' tics) and become more prominent during times of stress. Tics are divided into:

- Simple motor tics (e.g., eye-blinking, neck-jerking, facial grimacing).
- Simple vocal tics (e.g., grunting, coughing, barking, sniffing).
- Complex motor tics (e.g., jumping, touching self, copropraxia (use of obscene gestures)).
- Complex vocal tics (senseless repetition of words, coprolalia (use of obscene words or phrases)).
- Tourette syndrome is characterized by the presence of both motor and vocal tics for more than 1 year, arising during the developmental period. The motor tics usually present by age 7 years, although tics can present as early as 2 years of age. Obsessive-compulsive disorder and ADHD are common comorbidities.

ASSESSMENT

See Fig. 8.2 for an overall approach to assessing neurodevelopmental conditions.

History

The following are the type of questions that may be helpful in screening for the disorders below:

Learning difficulty (see Box 8.6 for communication tips)
- Do you have problems with reading? Or writing? Or maths?

Intellectual disability
- Do you have problems filling in forms?
- Did you need extra help in school?

Autism spectrum disorder
- What does a friend mean to you?
- What are your hobbies?
- How would you know if someone was sad?
- What would you do if someone was sad?
- Can you make small talk?

ADHD
- Do you often make careless mistakes?
- Have you been told you do not listen?
- Are you distracted easily by background noises?
- Are you fidgety?
- What is it like inside your head?
- Have you ever lost anything important such as your bank card/ phone/ keys

Tourette syndrome
- Do you find yourself making pointless movements or sounds?
- Do you get an urge beforehand?
- Can you suppress the urge? (Like with a sneeze or an itch?)
- What happens if you suppress it?

Examination

- Assess for physical signs suggestive of a syndromic intellectual disability, for example, large ears in Fragile X (more typically performed by paediatric services)
- Assess for physical disorders that could cause the presenting complaint.
- Complete a mental state examination focusing on behaviours suggestive of the neurodevelopmental disorder you are assessing for (see Table 8.3).

Investigations

No specific investigations are required to make a diagnosis of a neurodevelopmental disorder. Genetic testing is increasingly used in identifying the cause of intellectual disability, but it is not required for the diagnosis. Some investigations may be useful in excluding differentials or in identifying suspected comorbidities, for example, an EEG in someone with repetitive movements to exclude epilepsy, thyroid function in someone who has become restless and lost weight to exclude hyperthyroidism.

BOX 8.6 COMMUNICATION CONSIDERATIONS IN INTELLECTUAL DISABILITY

Allow extra time

Consider involvement from speech and language therapy

Speak first to the person with the intellectual disability, not their carer

Assess their understanding early and involve them as much as possible

Ask short, simple questions

Use literal, direct language, not abstract or medical terms (e.g., 'Does it hurt when you pee?' rather than 'How are your waterworks?' or 'Do you experience dysuria?')

Consider alternative methods of communication, such as with pictures, using Makaton, or in a written 'Easy Read' format

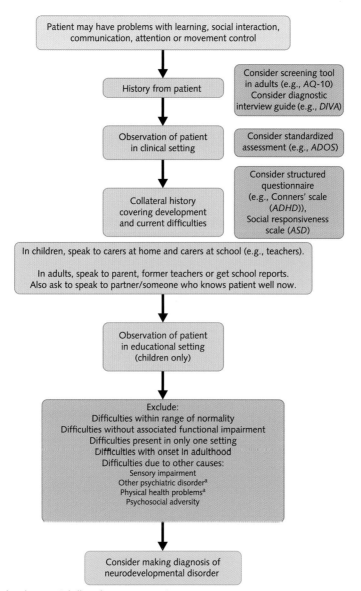

Fig. 8.2 Approach to neurodevelopmental disorder assessment.
[a]Note, Comorbid conditions are very common in neurodevelopmental disorders so do not preclude the diagnosis – but do not diagnose a neurodevelopmental disorder if difficulties are better explained by an alternative disorder.
ADHD, *Attention deficit hyperactivity disorder;* ADOS, *Autism Diagnostic Observation Schedule;* ASD, *autism spectrum disorder;* AQ-10, *autism-spectrum quotient - 10 items;* DIVA, *diagnostic interview guide for ADHD in adults.*

DISCUSSION OF CASE STUDY

JJ is likely to meet criteria for ADHD, although a school observation needs to be arranged. They have problems maintaining attention (e.g., completing schoolwork, remembering homework, on the football pitch), impulse control (e.g., talking over friends, jumping out of trees) and hyperactivity (e.g., not able to sit through a class or a film) that are more severe than those seen in their peers. They may also have sensory hypersensitivity to noise. Their difficulties occur in multiple settings. These problems are causing them functional impairment in educational attainment, socializing and risks to their person. There is no evidence of intellectual disability, sensory impairment, psychosocial adversity or physical or mental health problems.

Now read Chapter 31 about intellectual disability and Chapter 32 about neurodevelopmental disorders and their management.

● Chapter Summary

- Neurodevelopmental disorders are disorders where abnormal development of the central nervous system leads to impairments in brain function.
- To be classed as a disorder, an impairment in brain function should also cause an impairment in social, occupational or adaptive function.
- Intellectual disability refers to a heterogenous group of disorders with both significant limitations in multiple cognitive domains and impairment in adaptive functioning. Developmental learning disorders are specific limitations in learning academic skills when compared to same-age peers (reading, mathematics, written expression).
- Autism spectrum disorders cause impairments in social interaction and communication and restricted or repetitive behaviours.
- Attention deficit hyperactivity disorder causes impairments in attention, impulsivity and hyperactivity.

UKMLA Conditions
Attention deficit hyperactivity disorder
Autism spectrum disorder
Down syndrome
Epilepsy
Fits/seizures
Learning disability
Speech and language problems

UKMLA Presentations
Abnormal development/developmental delay
Behavioural difficulties in childhood
Congenital abnormalities
Dementias
Dysmorphic child
Epilepsy
Fits/seizures
Learning disability
Speech and language problems

The patient with psychotic symptoms

9

CASE SUMMARY

PP, aged 23 years, was assessed by their general practitioner (GP) because their family had become concerned about their behaviour. Over the last 6 months their college attendance had been uncharacteristically poor and they had terminated their part-time work. They had also become increasingly reclusive, spending more time alone in their flat, refusing to answer the door or see their friends. For the last 2 months PP had been expressing ideas their family found odd. After some inappropriate suspiciousness, they allowed their GP into their flat and then disclosed that government scientists had started to perform experiments on them over the last year. These involved the insertion of an electrode into their brain that detected gamma rays transmitted from government headquarters, which issued them with commands and 'planted' strange ideas in their head. When the GP asked how they knew this, they replied that they heard the 'men's voices as clear as day' and that they continually commented on what PP was thinking. They explained that their suspicion that 'all was not right' was confirmed when they heard the neighbour's dog barking in the middle of the night; at that point they knew 'for certain' that they were being interfered with. Prompted by the GP, PP also mentioned that a man in their local pub had sent them a 'covert signal' by conversing about the dangers of nuclear experiments. They also admitted to 'receiving coded information' from the radio whenever it was turned on. PP found these experiences very disturbing and had been considering suicide to escape the situation. The GP found no evidence of abnormal mood, incoherence of speech or disturbed motor function. PP denied use of recreational drugs and appeared physically well. After the GP discussed the case with a psychiatrist, PP was admitted to a psychiatric hospital for a period of assessment and to manage their risk to themselves. PP agreed to a voluntary admission, as they were now afraid of staying alone at home.

For a discussion of the case study, see the end of the chapter.

The patient with psychotic symptoms can present in many varied ways. It is often very difficult to elicit and describe specific symptoms when a patient is speaking or behaving in a grossly disorganized fashion. Therefore it is important to approach the assessment in a logical and systematic fashion as well as to have a good understanding of the psychopathology involved.

DEFINITIONS AND CLINICAL FEATURES

The term 'psychosis' refers to a mental state in which reality is grossly distorted, resulting in symptoms such as delusions, hallucinations and thought disorder. However, patients with schizophrenia and other psychotic disorders often have other symptoms too such as psychomotor abnormalities, mood/affect disturbance, cognitive deficits and disorganized behaviour.

There are many classifications that attempt to describe all the symptoms seen in schizophrenia and psychosis, but it is useful to approach psychotic psychopathology using five somewhat interrelated parameters:

1. Perception
2. Abnormal beliefs
3. Thought disorder
4. Negative symptoms
5. Psychomotor function

Perceptual disturbance

Perception is the process of making sense of the physical information we receive from our sensory modalities (e.g. hearing, vision, smell, taste, touch).

Hallucinations are perceptions occurring in the absence of an external physical stimulus, which have the following important characteristics:

- To the patient, the nature of a hallucination is the same as a normal sensory experience (i.e., it appears real). Therefore patients often have little insight into their abnormal experience.
- They are experienced as external sensations from any one of the sensory modalities and should be distinguished from ideas, thoughts, images or fantasies which originate in the patient's own mind.
- They occur without an external stimulus and are not merely distortions of an existing physical stimulus (see Illusions).

According to which sense organ they appear to arise from, hallucinations are classified as auditory, visual, olfactory, gustatory or somatic. There are special forms of hallucinations which will be discussed in this chapter. See Fig. 9.1 for an outline of the classification of hallucinations.

Illusions are misperceptions of real external stimuli (e.g., in a dark room, a dressing gown hanging on a bedroom wall is perceived as a person). Illusions often occur in healthy people

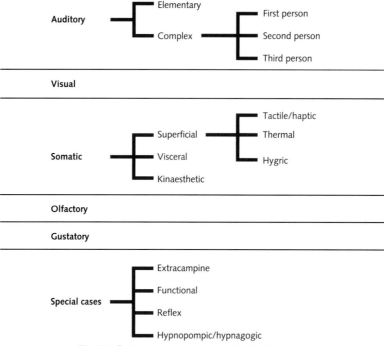

Fig. 9.1 Outline of classification of hallucinations.

and are usually associated with inattention or intense emotional state (e.g., situational anxiety).

A *pseudohallucination* is a perceptual experience which differs from a hallucination in that it appears to arise in the subjective inner space of the mind, not through one of the external sensory organs. Although experienced in internal space pseudohallucinations are not under conscious control (e.g., someone hearing a voice inside their own head telling them to harm themselves or someone experiencing distressing flashbacks in post-traumatic stress disorder). Note that some psychiatrists define pseudohallucinations to mean hallucinations that patients recognize as false perceptions (i.e., they have insight into the fact that they are hallucinating). The former definition is probably more widely used.

COMMUNICATION

One way to identify psuedohallucinations is that the patient is by determining if the source of a hallucination is 'internal' or 'external'. A way to find this out can be by asking something like 'do you hear the voice coming from inside your head, or do you hear it like you're hearing me speak now?'. A voice heard and recognized as being inside the patient's head would be more likely to be called a psuedohallucination.

Auditory hallucinations

These are hallucinations of the hearing modality and are the most common type of hallucinations in clinical psychiatry. Elementary hallucinations are simple, unstructured sounds (e.g., whirring, buzzing, whistling or single words); this type of hallucination occurs most commonly in acute organic states (e.g., epilepsy, migraine, delirium). Complex hallucinations occur as spoken phrases, sentences or even dialogue that are classified as:

- Audible thoughts (first person): patients hear their own thoughts spoken out loud as they think them. When patients experience their thoughts as echoed by a voice after they have thought them, it is termed thought echo.
- Second person auditory hallucinations: patients hear a voice or voices talking directly to them. Second person hallucinations can be persecutory, highly critical, complimentary or can issue commands to the patient (command hallucinations). Second person hallucinations are often associated with mood disorders with psychotic symptoms and are often 'mood congruent' so will be critical or persecutory in a depressed patient or complimentary in a manic patient.
- Third person auditory hallucinations: patients hear a voice or voices speaking about them, referring to them in the third person. This may take the form of two or more voices arguing or discussing the patient among themselves or one or more voices giving a running commentary on the patient's thoughts or actions.

HINTS AND TIPS

Particular types of auditory hallucination are highly suggestive of schizophrenia and known as 'first-rank symptoms'. See Box 9.1 for a list of Schneider's first rank symptoms.

Visual hallucinations

These are hallucinations of the visual modality. They occur most commonly in organic brain disturbances (delirium, occipital lobe tumours, epilepsy, dementia) and in the context of psychoactive substance use (lysergic acid diethylamide, mescaline, petrol/glue-sniffing, alcoholic hallucinosis). An autoscopic hallucination is the experience of seeing an image of oneself in external space. Charles Bonnet syndrome describes the condition where patients experience complex visual hallucinations associated with no other psychiatric symptoms or impairment in consciousness; it usually occurs in older adults and is associated with loss of vision. Lilliputian hallucinations are hallucinations of miniature people or animals and are usually associated with alcohol withdrawal.

Somatic hallucinations

These are hallucinations of bodily sensation and include superficial, visceral and kinaesthetic hallucinations.

Superficial hallucinations describe sensations on or just below the skin and may be:

- Tactile (haptic): experience of the skin being touched, pricked or pinched. Formication is the unpleasant sensation of insects crawling on or just below the skin; it is commonly

associated with long-term cocaine use (cocaine bugs) and alcohol withdrawal.

- Thermal: false perception of heat or cold.
- Hygric: false perception of a fluid (e.g., 'I can feel water sloshing in my brain').

Visceral hallucinations describe false perceptions of the internal organs. Patients may be distressed by deep sensations of their organs throbbing, stretching, distending or vibrating.

Kinaesthetic hallucinations are false perceptions of joint or muscle sense. Patients may describe their limbs vibrating or being twisted. The fleeting but distressing sensation of free falling just as one is about to fall asleep is an example that most people have experienced (see hypnagogic hallucinations later in this chapter).

Olfactory and gustatory hallucinations

These are the false perceptions of smell and taste. They commonly occur together because the two senses are closely related. A classic example is mood-congruent hallucinations of rotting flesh or burning in depression. However, in patients with new olfactory or gustatory hallucinations, it is important to rule out epilepsy (especially of the temporal lobe) and other organic brain diseases.

RED FLAG

If a patient presents with visual, olfactory or elementary hallucinations, consider the possibility of brain disorders such as delirium, migraine, epilepsy or cancer before attributing these symptoms to a primary psychiatric disorder.

Special forms of hallucination

Hypnagogic hallucinations are false perceptions in any modality (usually auditory or visual) that occur as a person goes to sleep; whereas *hypnopompic hallucinations* occur as a person awakens. These occur commonly and do not indicate mental disorder.

Extracampine hallucinations are false perceptions that occur outside the limits of a person's normal sensory field (e.g., a patient describes hearing voices from 100 miles away). Patients often give delusional explanations for this phenomenon.

A *functional hallucination* occurs when a normal sensory stimulus is required to precipitate a hallucination in that same sensory modality (e.g., voices that are only heard when the doorbell rings).

A *reflex hallucination* occurs when a normal sensory stimulus in one modality precipitates a hallucination in another (e.g., voices that are only heard whenever the lights are switched on).

Abnormal beliefs

Abnormal beliefs include primary and secondary delusions and overvalued ideas.

Delusions

A delusion is an unshakeable false belief that is not accepted by other members of the patient's culture. It is important to understand the following characteristics of delusional thinking:

- To the patient, there is no difference between a delusional belief and a true belief; they are the same experience. Therefore only an external observer can diagnose a delusion. A delusion is to ideation what a hallucination is to perception: both have the quality of reality to the person experiencing them.
- The delusion is false because of faulty reasoning. A man's delusional belief that his wife is having an affair may actually be true (she may indeed be unfaithful), but it remains a delusion because the reason he gives for this belief is undoubtedly false (e.g., she 'must' be having an affair because she is part of a top-secret sexual conspiracy to prove that he is a homosexual).
- A delusion is out of keeping with the patient's social and cultural background. It is crucial to establish that the belief is not one likely to be held by that person's subcultural group (e.g., a belief in the imminent second coming of Christ may be appropriate for a member of a religious group, but not for an atheist).

It is diagnostically significant to classify delusions as:

- Primary or secondary
- Mood congruent or mood incongruent
- Bizarre or nonbizarre
- According to the content of the delusion

Primary delusions (autochthonous delusions) do not occur in response to any previous psychopathological state; their genesis is not understandable. They may be preceded by a delusional atmosphere (mood) where patients have a sense that the world around them has been subtly altered, often in a sinister or threatening way. In this state a fully formed delusion has not yet developed and patients appear perplexed and apprehensive. Note that when a delusion occurs after a delusional atmosphere it is still regarded as primary; the delusional atmosphere is probably a precursor to the fully developed primary delusion. A delusional perception is also a primary delusion and occurs when a delusional meaning is attached to a normal perception (e.g., a patient believed he was a terrorist target because he heard an aeroplane flying in the distance). Primary delusions occur typically in schizophrenia and other primary psychotic disorders. *Secondary delusions* are the consequences of preexisting psychopathological states, usually mood disorders

(see Chapters 10 and 11). Many interrelated delusions that are centred on a common theme are termed systematized delusions.

In mood-congruent delusions, the contents of the delusions are appropriate to the patient's mood and are commonly seen in depression or mania with psychotic features.

Bizarre delusions are those which are extremely implausible (e.g., the belief that aliens have planted radioactive detonators in the patient's brain). They are considered to be characteristic of schizophrenia.

Apophenia is when patients make delusional connections between unrelated things.

Table 9.1 lists the classification of delusions by their content. It is important that you can label a delusion according to its content, so take some time to familiarize yourself with this table.

Finally, beliefs that were previously held with delusional intensity but then become held with less conviction are termed partial delusions. This occurs when patients are recovering.

HINTS AND TIPS

Note that the term 'paranoid' refers to any delusions or ideas that are unduly self-referent, typically feelings of persecution, grandeur or reference. It should not be used synonymously with the term 'persecutory' (i.e., when a patient has a false belief that people are trying to harm him, describing him as having a persecutory delusion is more specific than saying he is paranoid).

COMMUNICATION

Direct questioning about perceptual experience may alienate a nonpsychotic patient and raise undue suspicion in a psychotic patient. To maintain rapport with patients, begin these questions with a primer such as: 'I am now going to ask you some questions which may seem a little strange, but are routine questions which I ask all patients'.

Overvalued ideas

An overvalued idea is a plausible belief that a patient becomes preoccupied with to an unreasonable extent. The key feature is that the pursuit of this idea causes considerable distress to the patient or those living around them (i.e., it is overvalued). Patients who hold overvalued ideas have usually had them for many years and typically have abnormalities of personality. They are distinguished from delusions by the lack of a gross abnormality in reasoning; these patients can often give fairly

Table 9.1 Classification of delusions by content

Classification	Content
Persecutory delusions	False belief that one is being harmed, threatened, cheated, harassed or is a victim of a conspiracy
Grandiose delusions	False belief that one is exceptionally powerful (including having 'mystical powers'), talented or important
Delusions of reference	False belief that certain objects, people or events have intense personal significance and refer specifically to oneself (e.g., believing that a television newsreader is talking directly about one)
Religious delusions	False belief pertaining to a religious theme, often grandiose in nature (e.g., believing that one is a special messenger from God)
Delusions of love (erotomania)	False belief that another person is in love with one (commoner in women). In one form, termed 'de Clérambault syndrome', a woman (usually) believes that a man, frequently older and of higher status, is in love with her
Delusion of infidelity (morbid jealousy, pathological jealousy Othello syndrome)	False belief that one's lover has been unfaithful. Note that morbid jealousy may also take the form of an overvalued idea, that is, nonpsychotic jealousy
Delusions of misidentification	Capgras syndrome: belief that a familiar person has been replaced by an exact double – an impostor Fregoli syndrome: belief that a complete stranger is actually a familiar person already known to one
Nihilistic delusions (see Cotard syndrome, Chapter 11)	False belief that oneself, others or the world is nonexistent or about to end. In severe cases, negation is carried to the extreme with patients claiming that nothing, including themselves, exists
Somatic delusions	False belief concerning one's body and its functioning (e.g., that one's bowels are rotting). Also called 'hypochondriacal delusions' (to be distinguished from the overvalued ideas seen in hypochondriacal disorder)
Delusions of infestation (Ekbom syndrome)	False belief that one is infested with small but visible organisms. May also occur secondary to tactile hallucinations (e.g., formication; see Chapter 17)
Delusions of control (passivity or 'made' experiences) Note: these are all first-rank symptoms of schizophrenia	False belief that one's thoughts, feelings, actions or impulses are controlled or 'made' by an external agency (e.g., believing that one was 'made' to break a window by demons) Delusions of thought control include: 'Thought insertion': belief that thoughts or ideas are being implanted in one's head by an external agency 'Thought withdrawal': belief that one's thoughts or ideas are being extracted from one's head by an external agency 'Thought broadcasting': belief that one's thoughts are being diffused or broadcast to others such that they know what one is thinking

logical reasons for their beliefs. They differ from obsessions in that they are not experienced as recurrent intrusive thoughts. However, one will frequently encounter beliefs that span definitions. Typical disorders that feature overvalued ideas are anorexia nervosa, hypochondriacal disorder, dysmorphophobia and morbid jealousy (this can also take the form of a delusion). See Table 13.1 for tips on how to distinguish different types of abnormal thoughts.

Thought disorder

Thought disorder is when someone's speech is so disorganized that it is difficult to follow what is meant. Many patients with delusions are able to communicate in a clear and coherent manner; although their beliefs may be false, their speech is organized (thus delusions are an abnormality of thought content, not thought form). However, there is a subgroup of psychotic patients who speak in such a disorganized way that it becomes difficult to understand what they are saying. The coherency of patients with disorganized thinking varies from being mostly understandable in patients exhibiting circumstantial thinking to being completely incomprehensible in patients with a word salad phenomenon (see Fig. 9.2).

Describing the disturbance of a patient's thought form can be very challenging. This problem is compounded by two factors: it is impossible to know what patients are actually thinking (i.e., thought form has to be inferred from their speech and behaviour); the unfortunate situation has arisen where various authors in psychiatry have described a different conceptual view of thought disorder, which has resulted in conflicting and confusing classification systems. It is not essential to be able to identify

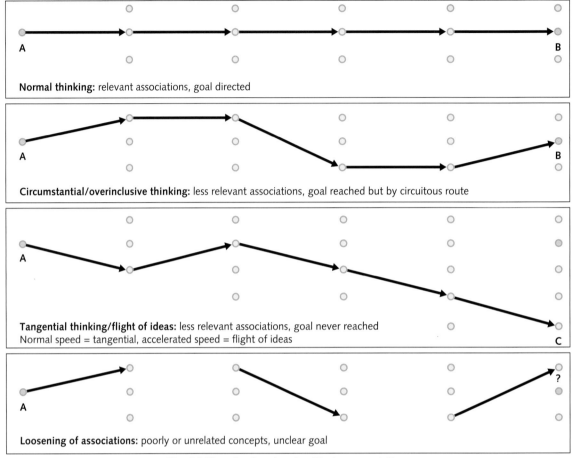

Fig. 9.2 Thought disorder: simplified representation.

all the subgroups of thought disorder, but it is important that you are able to say when thought form is or is not disordered. To describe the nature of the thought disorder you should have a clear understanding of the individual definitions you intend to use. To help describe thought disorder, it is particularly helpful if you document and are able to cite examples of the patient's speech in their own words.

HINTS AND TIPS

Many people have mildly disordered communication styles, particularly when tired or stressed. Perhaps you can think of someone you know who is often circumstantial in their storytelling. To count as thought disorder, the patient's thinking style should significantly impair effective communication.

The following are important signs of disorganized thinking:

Circumstantial and tangential thinking
See Chapter 10.

Flight of ideas
See Chapter 10.

Loosening of association (derailment/knight's move thinking)
This is when the patient's train of thought shifts suddenly from one very loosely or unrelated idea to the next. In its worst form, speech becomes a mixture of incoherent words and phrases and is termed 'word salad'. Loosening of association is characteristic of schizophrenia. Note that some psychiatrists, but not all, use the term 'formal thought disorder' synonymously with loosening of association.

Special forms of thought disorder

Thought blocking occurs when patients experience a sudden cessation to their flow of thought, often in mid-sentence (observed as sudden breaks in speech). Patients have no recall of what they were saying or thinking and thus continue talking about a different topic.

Neologisms are new words created by the patient, often combining syllables of other known words. Patients can also use recognized words idiosyncratically by attributing them with an unrecognized but related meaning (*metonyms*).

Perseveration is when an initially correct response is inappropriately repeated (e.g., unnecessarily repeating a previously expressed word or phrase). Palilalia describes the repetition of the last word of a sentence; logoclonia describes the repetition of the last syllable of the last word. Perseveration is highly suggestive of organic brain disease.

Echolalia is when patients senselessly repeat words or phrases spoken around them by others (i.e., like a parrot).

Irrelevant answers is when patients give answers that are completely unrelated to the original question.

Negative symptoms

Positive symptoms are those that are present when they should not be and include delusions, hallucinations and thought disorder. In contrast, negative symptoms are abilities that are absent when they should be present and include marked apathy, poverty of thought and speech, blunting of affect, reduced engagement and anhedonia. Patients can have positive and negative symptoms simultaneously or, as often happens, develop a negative presentation after initially presenting with predominantly positive symptoms. Remember that patients with a depressed mood or those experiencing significant side effects from psychotropic medication may also present with what appear to be negative symptoms, which often presents a diagnostic challenge.

Psychomotor function

Although a relatively rare phenomenon in high-income countries, some patients with psychosis will present with abnormalities of motor function. Motor system dysfunction in schizophrenia is usually due to the extrapyramidal side effects of neuroleptic medication (see Chapter 2). However, patients with psychosis can occasionally present with striking motor signs that are not caused by psychiatric medication or a known organic brain disease. Although undoubtedly associated with the patient's abnormal mental state, the cause of this psychomotor dysfunction is far from clarified. The term 'catatonia' literally means extreme muscular tone or rigidity; however, it commonly describes any excessive or decreased motor activity that is apparently purposeless and includes abnormalities of movement, tone or position. Table 9.2 describes the symptoms of catatonia. Note that catatonic symptoms are not diagnostic of schizophrenia; they may also be caused by brain diseases (e.g., encephalitis), metabolic abnormalities (e.g., diabetic ketoacidosis) or psychoactive substances, and can also occur in mood disorders and neurodevelopmental disorders, particularly autism spectrum disorders.

Table 9.2 Symptoms of catatonia

Decreased psychomotor activity	
Catatonic stupor	A presentation of 'akinesis' (lack of voluntary movement), 'mutism' and 'extreme unresponsiveness' in an otherwise alert patient
Catatonic negativism	A seemingly motiveless resistance to all instructions or attempts to be moved; patients may do the opposite of what is asked
Increased psychomotor activity	
Catatonic excitement	Agitated, excited and seemingly purposeless motor activity, not influenced by external stimuli
Abnormal motor activity	
Catatonic posturing	Adopting an unusual or bizarre position that is then maintained for some time
Catatonic rigidity	Maintaining a fixed position and rigidly resisting all attempts to be moved
Catatonic waxy flexibility (cerea flexibilitas)	Patients can be 'moulded' like wax into a position that is then maintained
Echopraxia	Patients senselessly repeat or imitate the actions of those around them. Associated with 'echolalia'; also occurs in patients with frontal lobe damage
Mannerisms	Apparently goal-directed movements (e.g., waving, saluting) that are performed repeatedly or at socially inappropriate times
Stereotypies	A complex, identically repeated movement that does not appear to be goal-directed (e.g., rocking to and fro, gyrating)

BOX 9.2 DIFFERENTIAL DIAGNOSES OF PSYCHOSIS

Psychotic disorders
- Schizophrenia
- Schizoaffective disorder
- Schizotypal disorder
- Acute and transient psychotic disorder
- Delusional disorder

Mood disorders
- Manic episode with psychotic features
- Depressive episode with psychotic features

Secondary to a general medical condition

Secondary to psychoactive substance use
- Intoxication
- Withdrawal
- Substance-induced psychotic episode

Dementia/delirium

Personality disorder

Neurodevelopmental disorder (autistic spectrum)

Obsessive-compulsive disorder

BOX 9.3 ICD-11 DIAGNOSTIC GUIDELINES FOR SCHIZOPHRENIA

Two or more of the following symptoms, with at least one from (a) to (d)
a. Persistent delusions
b. Persistent hallucinations
c. Formal thought disorder
d. Experiences of influence, passivity or control
e. Negative symptoms
f. Disorganized behaviour that stops goal-directed activity
g. Psychomotor disturbance such as posturing, waxy flexibility or stupor

Symptoms should be present for most of the time during at least 1 month

Schizophrenia should not be diagnosed in the presence of brain disease or during drug intoxication or withdrawal

BOX 9.4 ICD11 SPECIFIERS FOR SCHIZOPHRENIA

Specifiers based on symptoms (can be mild, moderate or severe):
1. Positive symptoms
2. Negative symptoms
3. Depressive mood symptoms
4. Manic mood symptoms
5. Psychomotor symptoms
6. Cognitive symptoms

Specifiers based on illness course:
1. First episode
2. Multiple episodes
3. Continuous
4. Currently symptomatic
5. In partial remission
6. In full remission

DIFFERENTIAL DIAGNOSES

Psychotic symptoms are nonspecific and are associated with many primary psychiatric illnesses. They can also present secondary to a general medical condition or psychoactive substance use. See Box 9.2 for the differential diagnoses for psychotic symptoms.

Psychotic disorders

Schizophrenia

There are no pathognomonic or singularly defining symptoms of schizophrenia; it is a syndrome characterized by a heterogeneous cluster of symptoms and signs. The ICD-11 has set out diagnostic guidelines based on the most commonly occurring symptom groups, which have been discussed in the preceding section (Box 9.3). It is also important to establish that there has been a clear and marked deterioration in the patient's social and work functioning.

In the past, psychiatrists used Schneider's first-rank symptoms to make the diagnosis of schizophrenia. Kurt Schneider suggested that the presence of one or more first-rank symptoms in the absence of organic disease was of pragmatic value in making the diagnosis of schizophrenia. First-rank symptoms are still referred to, so you should familiarize yourself with them; they are presented in Box 9.1.

The diagnosis of schizophrenia can have specifiers added to it to denote the presence of specific symptoms, and can be divided into mild, moderate or severe (see Box 9.4).

Positive symptoms: hallucinations, delusions.

Negative symptoms: blunted affect, poverty of speech, anhedonia.

Depressive symptoms: feeling down, low or sad.

Manic mood symptoms: elevated mood, increased energy and activity.

Psychomotor symptoms: psychomotor agitation, psychomotor retardation, catatonic symptoms.

Cognitive symptoms: reduced processing speed, impaired attention/concentration, disorientation.

Specifiers can also be added to denote the course of the illness and the presence of symptoms:

First episode: the current episode is the first one the patient has experienced.

Multiple episodes: the patient has experienced at least two episodes with a minimum 2 months gap.

Continuous: the symptoms have been present for at least a year with no significant gaps.

Currently symptomatic: the patient is currently experiencing schizophrenia symptoms and meets criteria for the diagnosis.

In partial remission: the patient is experiencing some schizophrenia symptoms but does not meet criteria for a diagnosis.

In full remission: the patient is not experiencing any significant symptoms.

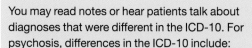

HINTS AND TIPS

You may read notes or hear patients talk about diagnoses that were different in the ICD-10. For psychosis, differences in the ICD-10 include:

- Schizophrenia was separated into subtypes. The commonest subtype, paranoid schizophrenia, was predominantly characterized by positive symptoms (delusions and hallucinations).
- Fewer but more specific symptoms were required to diagnose schizophrenia.
- Delusional disorder had subtypes (infrequently used).
- Acute and transient psychotic disorder was a broader category.
- Schizoaffective disorder was viewed as a lifelong disorder, whereas now schizophrenia or bipolar disorder can also be used as diagnoses, depending on the current presentation.

Schizoaffective disorder

Schizoaffective disorder describes the presentation of both schizophrenic and mood (depressed or manic) symptoms that present in the same episode of illness, either simultaneously or within a few days of each other. The mood symptoms should meet criteria for either a manic episode or a moderate to severe depressive episode.

HINTS AND TIPS

When psychiatrists talk about the typical symptoms of schizophrenia, they are generally referring to points (a) to (d) of the ICD-11 criteria for schizophrenia (or Schneider's first-rank symptoms, e.g., delusions of control, running commentary hallucinations, etc.).

Schizotypal disorder

In general, schizophrenia presents with a clear change in behaviour and functioning, sometimes with a prodrome, whereas patients with schizotypal disorder have often never achieved a normal baseline.

Schizotypal disorder is characterized by eccentric behaviour and peculiarities of thinking and appearance in someone who has never met criteria for diagnosis of schizophrenia/schizoaffective/delusional disorder. These symptoms must have been present to some degree for at least 2 years, and cause some level of distress or impairment of function. Although there are no clear psychotic symptoms evident and its course resembles that of a personality disorder, the ICD-11 includes schizotypal disorder in the chapter on psychotic disorders. This is because it is more prevalent among relatives of patients with schizophrenia and, occasionally, it progresses to overt schizophrenia.

Acute and transient psychotic disorders

Some psychotic episodes have fluctuating and polymorphic positive symptoms, an abrupt onset (without a prodromal phase), and a short duration of symptoms (usually less than one month, maximum 3 months). Premorbid functioning is usually regained. Symptoms may follow an acute stress but this is not required for the diagnosis. The ICD-11 codes these as acute and transient psychotic disorders. Not all psychotic episodes of brief duration are diagnosed as acute and transient psychotic disorder: if negative symptoms are present, there was a clear prodrome, or there is no rapid fluctuation in symptoms then 'Other Primary Psychotic Disorder' should be diagnosed instead. Sometimes these diagnoses are superseded by a later diagnosis of schizophrenia as the clinical picture evolves.

Delusional disorder

In this disorder, the development of a single or set of delusions for the period of usually at least 3 months is the most prominent or only symptom. It usually has onset in middle age and may persist throughout the patient's life. Delusions can be persecutory, grandiose and/or hypochondriacal. The diagnosis is excluded by persistent hallucinations unrelated to the delusion, thought disorder, negative symptoms or delusions of thought control or passivity. Brief depressive symptoms may be evident. Affect, speech and behaviour are all normal and these patients usually have well-preserved personal and social skills. Rarely, patients may present with an induced delusional disorder (*folie à deux*), which occurs when a nonpsychotic patient with close emotional ties to another person suffering from delusions (usually a dominant figure) begins to share those delusional ideas themselves. The delusions in the nonpsychotic patient tend to resolve when the two are separated.

Mood (affective) disorders

Manic episode with psychotic features
See Chapter 10.

Depressive episode with psychotic features
See Chapter 11.

Secondary to a general medical condition

Psychotic episodes secondary to a general medical condition are termed 'Secondary Psychotic Disorders', and these possible causes should always be sought for and ruled out. Box 9.5 lists the medical and substance-related causes of psychotic episodes. The medical condition should predate the development of the psychosis and symptoms should resolve with treatment of the condition. Absence of previous psychotic episodes and absence of a family history of schizophrenia also supports this diagnosis.

Substance-related psychosis

There are three main ways in which substances can cause psychotic symptoms:

- Intoxication (e.g., with hallucinogens).
- Withdrawal (e.g., in alcohol withdrawal with perceptual disturbances).
- Substance-induced psychotic disorder (e.g., alcohol-induced psychotic disorder with hallucinations-sometimes called alcoholic hallucinosis).

For a substance-induced psychotic disorder to be diagnosed, the symptoms must either persist beyond the timeframe of intoxication or withdrawal from the substance (e.g., cannabis triggering an enduring psychosis) and/or be substantially in excess of symptoms which are characteristically seen during intoxication or withdrawal from a substance. Usually, symptoms

---

BOX 9.5 MEDICAL AND SUBSTANCE-RELATED CAUSES OF PSYCHOTIC SYMPTOMS

Medical Conditions:

Cerebral neoplasm, infarcts, trauma, infection, inflammation (including HIV, CJD, neurosyphilis, herpes encephalitis)
Endocrinological (thyroid, parathyroid, adrenal disorders)
Epilepsy (especially temporal lobe epilepsy)
Delirium
Huntington disease
Systemic lupus erythematosus
Vitamin B_{12}, niacin (pellagra) and thiamine deficiency (Wernicke encephalopathy)
Acute intermittent porphyria

Substances:

Alcohol
Cannabis
Novel psychoactive substances
Amphetamines
Cocaine
Hallucinogens
Inhalants/solvents

Prescribed:

Antiparkinsonian drugs
Corticosteroids
Anticholinergics

CJD, *Creutzfeldt–Jakob disease*; HIV, *human immunodeficiency virus*.

---

resolve with abstinence from the substance, but sometimes a major mental illness can be precipitated and persist.

Delirium and dementia

Visual hallucinations and delusions are common in delirium and may also occur in dementia, particularly diffuse Lewy body dementia (see Chapter 20).

Personality disorder

Patients with personality disorder (particularly borderline pattern) may describe psuedohallucinatory experiences that they are able to recognise as not being real.

Neurodevelopmental disorder

Social difficulties and rigid thinking are found in both autistic spectrum disorders and schizophrenia. Patients with intellectual disabilities can also sometimes make unusual connections that can be interpreted as psychotic (see Chapter 8).

Obsessive-compulsive disorder

Patients with obsessive-compulsive disorder often believe there will be negative consequences if they don't complete certain rituals, even if these things are seemingly unrelated. This is not a delusion, but is known as magical thinking (see Chapter 13).

ALGORITHM FOR THE DIAGNOSIS OF PSYCHOTIC DISORDERS

See Fig. 9.3.

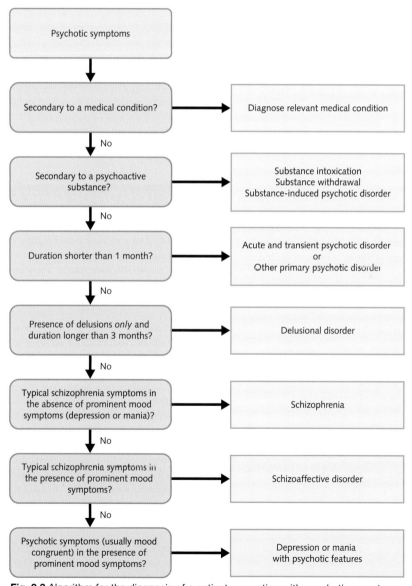

Fig. 9.3 Algorithm for the diagnosis of a patient presenting with psychotic symptoms.

ASSESSMENT

History

The following questions may be helpful in eliciting psychotic phenomena on mental state examination:

Hallucinations

- Do you ever hear strange noises or voices when there is no one else about?
- Do you ever hear your own thoughts spoken aloud such that someone standing next to you might possibly hear them? (audible thoughts; first person auditory hallucinations)
- Do you ever hear your thoughts echoed just after you have thought them? (thought echo)
- Do these voices talk directly to you or give you commands? (second person auditory hallucinations)
- Do these voices ever talk about you with each other or make comments about what you are doing? (third person auditory hallucinations/running commentary)
- Do these voices seem to be coming from inside or outside your head? (pseudohallucinations)

Delusions

- Are you afraid that someone is trying to harm or poison you? (persecutory delusions)
- Have you noticed that people are doing or saying things that have a special meaning for you? (delusions of reference)
- Do you have any special abilities or powers? (grandiose delusions)
- Does it seem as though you are being controlled or influenced by some external force? (delusions of control)
- Are thoughts that do not belong to you being put into your head? (thought insertion)

It is important to obtain collateral information from the patient's GP, family and any other mental health professionals involved in their care to establish premorbid personality and functioning, as well as pattern of deterioration.

Examination

A basic physical examination including a thorough neurological and endocrine system examination should be performed on all patients with psychotic symptoms.

Investigations

Blood investigations are performed to:

- Exclude possible medical or substance-related causes of psychosis.

- Establish baseline values before administering antipsychotics and other psychotropic drugs.
- Assess renal and liver functioning which may affect elimination of drugs that are likely to be taken long term and possibly in depot form.
- If the patient presents with a first episode of psychosis, a good basic screen comprises full blood count, erythrocyte sedimentation rate, urea and electrolytes, thyroid function, liver function tests, glucose, lipids, serum calcium and serology for any suspected infections.
- An oral/urine drug screen should always be done because recreational drugs both cause and exacerbate psychosis.
- An electrocardiogram should be done in patients with cardiac problems as many antipsychotics prolong the QT interval and have the potential to cause lethal ventricular arrhythmia.
- The use of a routine electroencephalogram, computed tomography (CT) or magnetic resonance imaging brain scan to help exclude an organic psychosis (e.g., temporal lobe epilepsy, brain tumour) varies between psychiatric units; they should always be considered in atypical cases, cases with treatment resistance or if there are cognitive or neurological abnormalities.

DISCUSSION OF CASE STUDY

PP meets the ICD-11 criteria for schizophrenia, first episode. They have had a marked deterioration in their social and work functioning. They have delusions of persecution (believing they were a victim of government experiments), thought control (believing that ideas were being planted in their head – thought insertion) and reference (believing that the man in the pub was referring specifically to them). Their statement that they knew these things after hearing the neighbour's dog bark suggests delusional perception. They also report second person command hallucinations and third person running commentary hallucinations. 'Receiving coded information' from the radio might be a hallucination or a delusion of reference depending on how PP described this experience in detail. PP's description that 'all was not right' could indicate the presence of a delusional atmosphere, prior to the development of the full-blown delusions.

It is imperative that a substance-induced psychotic disorder or psychotic disorder secondary to a medical condition is excluded. It would be important to ascertain the duration of PP's psychotic symptoms. It is important to rule out a mood disorder with psychotic features. The presence of a mood episode associated with simultaneous schizophrenic symptoms would suggest a schizoaffective episode. Prominent hallucinations exclude a diagnosis of delusional disorder.

Now go on to Chapter 23 to read more about the psychotic disorders and their management.

Chapter Summary

- Psychosis is when the experience of reality is grossly distorted.
- Psychotic symptoms comprise delusions, hallucinations and thought disorder.
- A delusion is a fixed, false belief which arises through faulty reasoning, is not altered by evidence to the contrary, and is outside cultural norms.
- A hallucination is a perception in the absence of a stimulus.
- Thought disorder is speech so disorganized that communication is impaired.
  When assessing someone with psychotic symptoms, explore:
- the nature and content of their abnormal experiences (their signs and symptoms);
- how these symptoms are affecting them, and their current and past social circumstances (functional impact);
- their physical health and use of recreational substances;
- obtain a collateral history from someone who knows them well (as lack of insight can prevent the patient giving a full history).

The key differentials for someone presenting with psychotic symptoms are: schizophrenia, mania with psychotic symptoms, drug-induced psychosis and psychosis secondary to a general medical condition.

MLA Conditions	MLA Presentations
Anxiety	Anxiety
Autistic spectrum disorder	Auditory hallucinations
Bipolar affective disorder	Behaviour/personality change
Delirium	Elation/elated mood
Dementias	Fixed abnormal beliefs
Depression	Learning disability
OCD	Low mood/affective problems
Personality disorders	OCD
Phobias	Phobias
Schizophrenia	Pressure of speech
Substance use disorder	Visual hallucinations

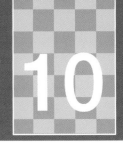
Just as spells of feeling sad and miserable are quite normal to the human experience, so too are periods where we feel elated, excited and full of energy. Although an irritable or elevated mood is not in itself pathological, it can be when grossly and persistently so, and when associated with another psychopathology.

DEFINITIONS AND CLINICAL FEATURES

In Chapter 11 we will observe how a disturbance in mood in addition to various other cognitive, biological and psychotic symptoms, all contribute to the recognition of a depressive episode. A similar approach is taken to hypomanic and manic episodes; these occur on the opposite pole of the mood disorder spectrum to depression.

Core symptoms

The ICD-11 classification system requires evidence of both of the following for a diagnosis of a manic or hypomanic episode:

- Sustained elated, irritable or expansive mood
- Excessive activity or feelings of energy

For a diagnosis of a manic episode these symptoms must have been present for at least a week, however for a hypomanic episode several days is enough for a diagnosis. When manic and depressive symptoms rapidly alternate (e.g., within the same day), this is termed a *mixed affective episode*.

Mood

The hallmark of a hypomanic or manic episode is an elevated or irritable mood. Patients often enjoy the experience of elevated mood and might describe themselves as feeling: 'high', 'on top of the world', 'fantastic' or 'euphoric'. This mood has an infectious quality, although those who know the patient well clearly see it as a deviation from normal. However, some patients tend to become extremely irritable or suspicious when manic and do not enjoy the experience at all. They have a low frustration tolerance and any thwarting of their plans can lead to a rapid escalation in anger or even delusions of persecution.

Increased energy

This initially results in an increase in goal-directed activity and, when coupled with impaired judgement, can have disastrous consequences (e.g., patients may instigate numerous risky business ventures, go on excessive spending sprees or engage in reckless promiscuity that is unusual for them). However, in severe episodes actions can become repetitive, stereotyped and apparently purposeless, even progressing to a *manic stupor* in the extremely unwell. If left untreated, excessive overactivity can lead to physical exhaustion, dehydration and sometimes even death. On mental state examination, increased energy can be seen as *psychomotor excitation*: the patient is unable to sit still, frequently standing up, pacing around the room and gesticulating expansively.

Biological symptoms

Decreased need for sleep

This is a very important early warning sign of mania or hypomania. Sleep disturbance can range from only needing a few hours of sleep a night to a manic patient going for days on end with no sleep at all. Crucially, it is not associated with fatigue.

Increased sexual drive

Manic or hypomanic patients may experience an increase in their sex drive, or may engage in more risky sexual behaviours.

Cognitive symptoms

Elevated sense of self-esteem or grandiosity

Hypomanic patients may overestimate their abilities and social or financial status. In severe cases, manic patients may have delusions of grandeur where they believe themselves to be abnormally powerful or important.

Poor concentration

Manic patients may find it difficult to maintain their focus on any one thing as they struggle to filter out irrelevant external stimuli (background noise, other objects or people in the room), making them, as a consequence, highly distractible.

Accelerated thinking and speech

Manic patients may subjectively experience their thoughts or ideas racing even faster than they can articulate them. When patients have an irrepressible need to express these thoughts verbally, making them difficult to interrupt, it is termed *pressure of speech*. When thoughts are rapidly associating in this way in a stream of connected (but not always relevant) concepts it is termed *flight of ideas*. Some hypomanic patients express themselves by incessant letter writing, poetry, doodling or artwork.

Impaired judgement and insight

This is typical of manic illness and sometimes results in costly indiscretions that patients may later regret. Lack of insight into their illness can be a difficult barrier to overcome when trying to engage patients in essential treatment.

Psychotic symptoms

Psychotic symptoms are far more common in manic than in depressive episodes and include disorders of *thought form, thought content* and *perception*. The presence of psychotic symptoms indicates that an episode is manic rather than hypomanic.

Disordered thought form

Disordered thought form (see Chapter 9 and Fig. 9.2) commonly occurs in schizophrenia but is regularly seen in manic episodes with psychotic features and to a lesser degree in psychotic forms of unipolar depression. The most common thought form disorders in mania are circumstantiality, tangentiality and flight of ideas. However, signs of thought disorder most typical for schizophrenia can also be seen in manic episodes (e.g., loosening of association, neologisms and thought blocking).

Circumstantiality and tangentiality

Circumstantial (over-inclusive) speech means speech that is delayed in reaching its final goal because of the over-inclusion of details and unnecessary asides and diversions; however, the speaker, if allowed to finish, does eventually connect the original starting point to the desired destination. Circumstantiality need not be pathological – most families have at least one person who takes forever to finish a story! Tangential speech, on the other hand, is more indicative of psychopathology and sees the speaker diverting from the initial train of thought but never returning to the original point, jumping tangentially from one topic to the next.

Flight of ideas

As described earlier, flight of ideas occurs when thinking is markedly accelerated, resulting in a stream of connected concepts. The link between concepts can be as in normal communication where one idea follows directly on from the next or can be links that are not relevant to an overall goal. For example, links made through wordplay such as a pun or clang association; or through some vague idea which is not part of the original goal of speech (e.g., 'I need to go to bed now. Have you ever smelt my bed of roses? Ah, but a rose by any other name would smell just as sweet!'). Even though manic patients may appear to be talking gibberish, a written transcript of their speech will usually reveal that their ideas are related in some, albeit obscure, way.

As patients become increasingly manic, their associations tend to loosen as they find it increasingly difficult to link their thoughts. Eventually they approach the incoherent thought disorder sometimes seen in schizophrenia (see Chapter 9).

Abnormal beliefs

Patients with elated mood will typically present with *grandiose delusions* in which they believe they have special importance or unusual powers. *Persecutory delusions* are also common, especially in patients with an irritable mood, and often feature them believing that others are trying to take advantage of their exalted status. When the content of delusions matches the mood of the patient, the delusions are termed *mood-congruent*. Very often, patients with elevated mood may have overvalued ideas as opposed to true delusions, which are important to distinguish, as the former are not regarded as psychotic in nature (see Chapter 9).

Perceptual disturbance

Some hypomanic patients may describe subtle distortions of perception. These are not psychotic symptoms and mainly include altered intensity of perception such that sounds seem louder (hyperacusis) or colours seem brighter and more vivid (visual hyperaesthesia). Psychotic perceptual features develop when manic patients experience hallucinations. This is usually in the form of voices encouraging or exciting them.

HINTS AND TIPS

Always screen for psychotic symptoms in patients suffering from a manic episode. The prevalence is very high – two-thirds report experiencing psychotic symptoms during such an episode. Interestingly, only one-third report psychotic symptoms during a depressive episode.

DIFFERENTIAL DIAGNOSIS

Like depression, an elevated or irritable mood can be secondary to a medical condition, psychoactive substance use or other psychiatric disorder. These will have to be excluded before a primary mood disorder can be diagnosed. Box 10.1 shows the differential diagnosis for patients presenting with elevated or irritable mood.

Mood (affective) disorders

Hypomanic, manic and mixed affective episodes

The ICD-11 specifies three degrees of severity of a manic episode: *hypomania*, *mania without psychotic symptoms* and *mania with psychotic symptoms*. All of these share the above-mentioned general characteristics, most notably: an elevated or irritable mood and an increase in the quantity and speed of mental and physical activity. If psychotic symptoms are present, the episode is by definition mania. In those without psychotic symptoms, the distinction between mania and hypomania can be hard to judge and hinges on the degree of

---

BOX 10.1 DIFFERENTIAL DIAGNOSIS FOR PATIENT PRESENTING WITH ELEVATED OR IRRITABLE MOOD

Mood disorders

- Hypomania, mania, mixed affective episode (isolated episode or part of bipolar affective disorder or cyclothymia)
- Cyclothymia
- Depression (may present with irritable mood)
- Secondary to a general medical condition
- Secondary to psychoactive substance use
  - Intoxication
  - Withdrawal
  - Substance-induced mood episode

Psychotic disorders

- Schizoaffective disorder (may be similar to mania with psychotic features)
- Schizophrenia
- Personality disorder (with prominent traits of disinhibition, negative affect or dissocial features)
- Neurodevelopmental disorder (attention deficit hyperactivity disorder)
- Delirium/dementia

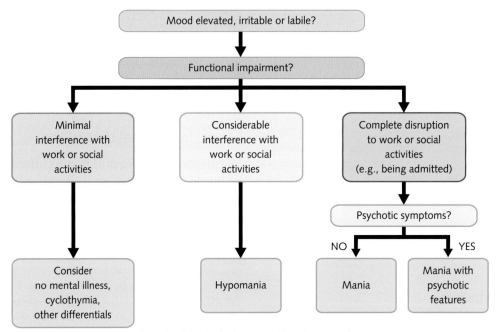

Fig. 10.1 Distinguishing mania from hypomania.

functional impairment (Fig. 10.1). If the person is experiencing rapidly alternating (e.g., within a few hours of each other) manic and depressive symptoms they are diagnosed with a *mixed affective episode*. The symptoms should last for at least a week to be diagnosed as mania (unless a treatment intervention has been given) and for at least several days to be diagnosed as hypomania.

Bipolar disorder

Most patients who present with a hypomanic, manic or mixed affective episode will have experienced a previous episode of mood disturbance (depression, hypomania, mania or mixed). In this case they should be diagnosed with bipolar disorder. Most patients who experience hypomanic or manic episodes also experience depressive episodes, hence, the commonly used term: 'manic-depression'. However, patients who only suffer from manic episodes with no intervening depressive episodes are also classified as having bipolar disorder, even though their mood does not swing to the depressive pole. It is good practice to record the nature of the current episode in a patient with bipolar disorder (e.g., '*bipolar disorder, current episode manic without psychotic features*').

Bipolar disorder type I is diagnosed if a patient has ever had a manic or mixed episode. Bipolar disorder type II is diagnosed if a patient has had at least one hypomanic episode and at least one depressive episode, but has never had a manic episode.

BOX 10.2 SPECIFIERS THAT CAN BE ADDED TO A DIAGNOSIS OF BIPOLAR DISORDER IN THE ICD-11

- With prominent anxiety
- With seasonal pattern
- With rapid cycling
- With melancholia

ICD-11 provides optional specifiers for bipolar disorder including 'rapid cycling' (≥4 episodes in last 12 months, with or without periods of euthymia) (see Box 10.2).

Cyclothymic disorder

Cyclothymic disorder (or cyclothymia) is analogous to dysthymia (see Chapter 11) in that it usually begins in early adulthood and follows a chronic course with intermittent periods of wellness in between. Mood symptoms are present more of the time than not. It is characterized by an instability of mood over at least 2 years resulting in alternating periods of mild elation and mild depression. The low mood should not be sufficiently severe or long enough to meet the criteria for a depressive episode but the elation can meet criteria for hypomania. Symptoms should result in significant distress or functional impairment.

Depression

There are three common scenarios where a patient with a primary depressive disorder may present with an elevated or irritable mood. An 'agitated depression' can present with a prominent irritable mood, which, when coupled with psychomotor agitation, can be difficult to distinguish from a manic episode; depressed patients who are responding to antidepressants or electroconvulsive therapy may experience a transient period of elevated mood; and a patient with a recently resolved depressive disorder might misidentify euthymia for hypomania.

Manic episodes secondary to a general medical condition or psychoactive substance use

A medical or psychoactive substance cause of mania should always be sought for and ruled out. Box 10.3 lists the medical and substance-related causes of mania. The medical condition or substance use should predate the development of the mood disorder and symptoms should resolve with treatment of the condition or abstinence from the offending substance. Absence of previous manic episodes and lack of a family history of bipolar

---

BOX 10.3 MEDICAL AND SUBSTANCE CAUSES OF MANIA

Medical conditions
- Cerebral neoplasms, infarcts, trauma, infection (including HIV), autoimmune encephalitis
- Cushing disease
- Huntington disease
- Hyperthyroidism
- Multiple sclerosis
- Renal failure
- Systemic lupus erythematosus
- Temporal lobe epilepsy
- Vitamin B_{12} and niacin (pellagra) deficiency

Substances
- Amphetamines
- Cocaine
- Hallucinogens
- Novel psychoactive substances

Prescribed
- Anabolic steroids
- Antidepressants
- Corticosteroids
- Dopaminergic agents (e.g., L-DOPA, selegiline, bromocriptine)

---

disorder also supports this diagnosis. Note that antidepressant use does not necessarily exclude the diagnosis of a manic or hypomanic episode, e.g., if a patient has been taking the antidepressant for some time before their elated mood begins.

Schizophreniform disorders

Schizoaffective disorder

See Chapter 9. This can be very difficult to distinguish from a manic episode with psychotic features.

Schizophrenia

Patients with schizophrenia can present with an excited, suspicious or agitated mood and therefore can be difficult to distinguish from manic patients with psychotic symptoms. Table 10.1 compares relevant features that might act as clues to the correct diagnosis.

Personality/neurodevelopmental disorders

Patients with disorders of personality or neurodevelopment often report features similar to hypomania, e.g., impulsivity, irritability and lability of mood in personality disorder with prominent features of negative affect, disinhibition, borderline or dissocial features or in attention deficit hyperactivity disorder. However, personality and neurodevelopmental disorders involve stable and enduring behaviour patterns, unlike the more discrete episodes of bipolar disorder, which are characterised by a distinct, demarcated deterioration in psychosocial functioning. Further, mood instability in personality disorder or neurodevelopmental disorder tends to fluctuate more rapidly (e.g., from hour to hour) (see Chapters 8 and 18). It is possible for bipolar affective disorder to be comorbid with personality disorder or a neurodevelopmental disorder.

Delirium/dementia

Insomnia, agitation and psychotic symptoms in an older adult can be a presentation of hyperactive delirium or of stress and distress in dementia (see Chapter 20).

HINTS AND TIPS

You may read notes or hear patients talk about diagnoses that were different in the ICD-10. For bipolar and related disorders, differences in the ICD-10 include:
- Bipolar Type I and Type II disorders were combined in a single "Bipolar affective disorder" diagnosis.
- Antidepressant use excluded diagnosis of mania or hypomania
- In cyclothymia, elated mood did not meet severity of hypomania

---

Table 10.1 Psychopathological distinctions between mania and schizophrenia (these are guidelines only; typically schizophrenic symptoms can occur in mania and vice versa)

Psychopathology	Mania	Schizophrenia
Thought form	Circumstantiality, tangentiality, flight of ideas	Loosening of association, neologisms, thought blocking
Delusions	Most often mood-congruent (grandiose delusions or persecutory delusions)	Delusions unrelated to mood, bizarre delusions, delusions of passivity (e.g., thought insertion, withdrawal, broadcast)
Speech	Pressured speech, difficult to interrupt	Speech is often hesitant or halting
Biological symptoms	Significantly reduced need for sleep, increased physical and mental energy	Sleep less disturbed, less hyperactive
Psychomotor function	Agitation	Agitation, catatonic symptoms or negative symptoms

ASSESSMENT

History

The following questions might be helpful in eliciting the key symptoms of mania/hypomania:

- Have you been feeling particularly happy or 'on top of the world' lately?
- Do you sometimes feel as though you have too much energy compared with people around you?
- Do you find yourself needing less sleep but not getting tired?
- Have you had any new interests or exciting ideas lately?
- Have you noticed your thoughts racing in your head?
- Do you have any special abilities or powers?

HINTS AND TIPS

Pay attention to countertransference (the way the patient makes you feel). Manic moods can be very infectious, and you may find your own mood becoming elated when speaking to these patients.

Examination

A basic physical examination, including a thorough neurological and endocrine system examination, should be performed on all patients with elevated mood.

Investigations

As for the depressive disorders (see Chapter 11), social, psychological and physical investigations are normally performed on manic patients to establish the diagnosis and to rule out an organic or substance-related cause (see Box 10.2). A urine drug

screen is essential in anyone presenting with a first episode of elated mood.

ALGORITHM FOR THE DIAGNOSIS OF MOOD DISORDERS

See Fig. 10.2.

DISCUSSION OF CASE STUDY

EM appears to be suffering from a *manic episode with psychotic features*. They have an elated mood and have developed the grandiose delusion that they are a world expert (mood-congruent psychotic symptom); note also the rapid switch to irritable mood when confronted. Biological symptoms include the reduced need for sleep and increased mental and physical energy with overactivity. Cognitive symptoms include elevated sense of self-importance, poor concentration, accelerated thinking with pressure of speech and impaired judgement and insight. The episode is classified as manic because of the severe impairment in social and probably work functioning, and because of the psychotic features.

Although EM denied using drugs or alcohol, intoxication with substances (e.g., a novel psychoactive substance) is an important differential. A urine drug screen could exclude amphetamines and a collateral history might help to identify any existing pattern of substance use. However, the long duration of symptoms (2 weeks) is less suggestive of substance-induced manic symptoms, which would typically resolve over a few days.

In this case the diagnosis is: *bipolar type I disorder, current episode manic with psychotic symptoms*. Previous psychotic episodes would add schizoaffective disorder and schizophrenia to the differential diagnosis. Now go on to Chapter 24 to read about the mood disorders and their management.

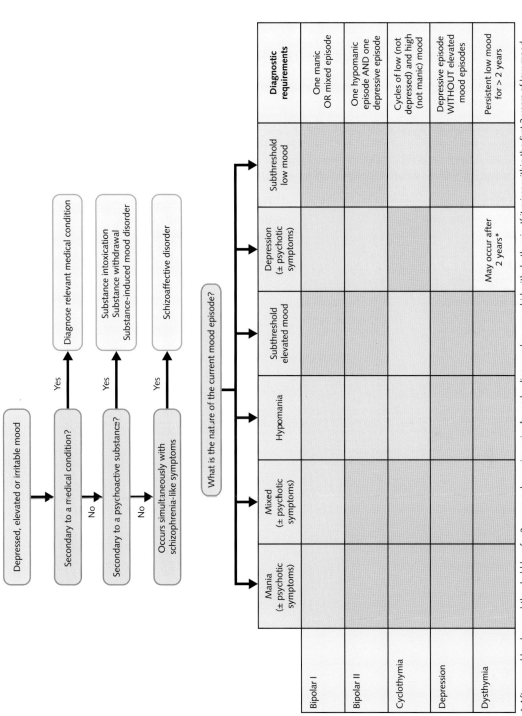

Fig. 10.2 Algorithm for the diagnosis of mood disorders.

* After mood has been subthreshold low for 2 years, a depressive episode can be diagnosed as comorbid with dysthymia. If it arises within the first 2 years of low mood, the diagnosis is simply depression.

Chapter Summary

- A manic episode is a sustained period (at least a week, unless shortened by treatment) of extremely elated or irritable mood associated with increased activity and energy.
- A hypomanic episode has the same symptoms as a manic episode but without marked impairment in functioning and no psychotic symptoms.
- A mixed affective episode is the rapid alternation between symptoms of mania and depression over a sustained period (at least 2 weeks).
- Psychotic symptoms can occur in mania, and are generally mood-congruent.
- The key differential diagnoses for an episode of elated mood are a substance use disorder or psychotic disorder.
- When assessing someone with elated mood, ask about the four domains of: core symptoms, biological symptoms, cognitive symptoms and psychotic symptoms.

UKMLA Conditions
Bipolar affective disorder
Delirium
Dementia
Depression
Personality disorder
Schizophrenia

UKMLA Presentations
Behaviour/personality change
Elation/elevated mood
Low mood/affective problems
Pressure of speech
Substance misuse

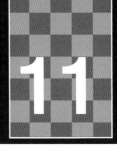

The patient with low mood

Case summary

LM, a 32-year-old married dentist with two young children presented to their general practitioner stating that they were persistently unhappy and had been crying repeatedly over the past few weeks. They had no previous psychiatric history or significant medical history and their only regular medication was oral contraception. They had moved to the area 3 years earlier when their spouse was promoted and, at first, appeared to have integrated well into the neighbourhood by involving themselves in the organization of a toddlers' group. Unfortunately, the group had dissolved a few months ago when their co-organizer and only close confidante had moved away. Deprived of their most important social outlet, LM found themselves increasingly dominated by their young children. Although usually an outgoing person, they noticed that their motivation to keep in touch with other parents from the group had started to dwindle. At the same time, they started feeling persistently weary even though their work schedule had not increased, and often awakened 2 to 3 hours early in the morning. Although their appetite had not increased, they had turned to food for 'comfort' and had gained over 5kg in weight. LM also admitted that they were drinking more alcohol than usual, although this began after their mood lowered. They described feeling incompetent because they were always miserable and had become too tired to look after the children. They felt guilty for burdening their spouse and started crying when talking about their loss of interest in sex and their feelings of unattractiveness. LM maintained that no aspect of their life gave them pleasure and when asked specifically by their doctor, admitted that they had started to wonder whether their family would be better off if they weren't around.

(For a discussion of the case study, see the end of the chapter.)

Feeling sad or upset is a normal part of the human condition; thus a patient presenting with emotional suffering does not necessarily warrant a psychiatric diagnosis or require treatment. However, psychiatrists agree that when patients present with a certain number of key depressive features, they are probably suffering from some form of psychopathology that will require, and usually respond to, specific kinds of treatment.

DEFINITIONS AND CLINICAL FEATURES

The ICD-11 divides depression into three core 'clusters' of ten symptoms in total (see Fig. 11.1). At least five of these symptoms must be present for a diagnosis, plus significant distress or functional impairment. The symptoms should have been present for at least 2 weeks.

Affective cluster

Depressed mood

Whereas feelings describe a short-lived emotional experience, mood refers to a patient's sustained, subjectively experienced emotional state over a period of time. Patients may describe a depressed mood in a number of ways, such as feeling sad, dejected, despondent, 'down in the dumps', 'miserable' 'low in spirits' or 'heavy-hearted'. They are unable to lift themselves out of this mood and its severity is often out of proportion to the stressors in their surrounding social environment. Mood which is consistently worse in the morning and improves as the day goes on ('diurnal variation') is strongly indicative of depression. When meeting a patient, in addition to hearing their account of their mood, you also assess their mood and affect as part of the mental state exam (see Chapter 1). People with depression often have a reduced range of affect, with a monotonous voice and minimal facial expression.

Anhedonia

Anhedonia refers to a markedly reduced interest or pleasure from usual activities, particularly those the person usually enjoys. For example, a patient who is a member of a local drama group may stop attending rehearsals or reading scripts. You could differentiate this from a lack of motivation by asking the patient if they still enjoy rehearsals if they make themselves attend.

HINTS AND TIPS

Remember the distinction between the terms 'mood' and 'affect'; they are not the same. One way to remember the difference is that mood is like the climate and affect like the weather.

Does this patient have depression?

Affective cluster

- ❏ Low mood
- ❏ Anhedonia

1 or 2 of these symptoms

Cognitive-behavioural cluster

- ❏ Poor concentration/indecisiveness
- ❏ Low self-worth/excessive guilt
- ❏ Hopelessness
- ❏ Recurrent thoughts of death/suicide

Neurovegetative cluster

- ❏ Sleep changes
- ❏ Appetite changes
- ❏ Psychomotor retardation/agitation
- ❏ Fatigue

Plus at least 3 or 4 of these symptoms

(total of 5/10 minimum)

Most of the day, nearly every day

Duration ≥ 2 weeks

Marked functional impairment or significant distress

Other diagnostic requirements met

Not better accounted for by another mental, behavioural or neurodevelopmental disorder

Not secondary to a medical condition or substance use/withdrawal

Differentials reviewed

Likely diagnosis of depression

Fig. 11.1 Diagnostic criteria for depression.

Cognitive-behavioural cluster

Cognition has two meanings in psychiatry: it refers broadly to brain processing functions (e.g., concentrating, learning, making decisions) and also more specifically to the thoughts patients have about themselves and the world, which are conclusions arrived at by cognition (e.g., I failed my maths exam, therefore I will fail all exams, see Chapter 3). The latter meaning is used here.

Problems with concentration or attention

Depressed patients report difficulty in sustaining attention while doing previously manageable tasks. They often appear easily distracted and may complain of memory difficulties. They may feel indecisive. As a result depression is an important differential in those presenting with memory impairment.

COMMUNICATION

Questions about concentration can include asking if they can follow their favourite TV programme, read a novel or follow conversations.

Beliefs of low self-worth or excessive guilt

Self-worth includes the interrelated concepts of personal efficacy and personal worth. Depressed patients may have thoughts that they are no longer competent to meet life's challenges and that they are no longer worthy of happiness and the healthy assertion of their needs.

Depressed patients also often have guilty preoccupations about minor past failings. This guilt is often inappropriate and out of proportion to the original 'offence'. Patients often have guilty thoughts about the very act of developing the depressed mood itself.

Hopelessness

Depressed patients can have bleak and pessimistic views of the future, believing that there is no way out of their current situation. They may also have beliefs that their mood will never improve and treatment will not work.

Recurrent thoughts of death or suicide

Depressed patients frequently have thoughts of death and harming themselves. In severe cases suicidal ideation may lead to an actual suicide attempt. At these times, patients may believe that they are faced with insurmountable difficulties or are trying to escape a relentlessly painful emotional state. Self-harm and suicide are discussed fully in Chapter 6.

RED FLAG

Risk needs to be assessed in every patient. During an assessment, the subject can initially be broached by saying that it is common for people who are depressed to feel that life is not worth living and asking the patient if this has occurred to them. Phrases such as 'doing something stupid' are unclear and best avoided. Suicidality can then be formally assessed as discussed in Chapter 6.

Neurovegetative cluster

In the past, psychiatrists distinguished between 'endogenous' or 'reactive' depression. 'Endogenous' depression (also called somatic, melancholic, vital or biological depression) was assumed to occur in the absence of an external environmental cause and have a 'biological' clinical picture. This is opposed to so-called 'reactive' or 'neurotic' depression where it is assumed that the patient is, to some degree, understandably depressed, reacting to adverse psychosocial circumstances. However, most depression is a mixture of the two, and an 'understandable depression' does not require any less treatment than a 'spontaneous depression'. 'Neurovegetative' symptoms (previously called 'biological symptoms' or 'somatic symptoms') are still important to enquire about as, if present, they suggest a more severe depression; however, they are no longer viewed as providing information on aetiology.

Sleep disturbance

Although patients may get off to sleep at their normal time, they wake earlier than they would usually, and then find it difficult to get back to sleep again. Further disturbances of sleep in depression include: difficulty falling asleep (initial insomnia), frequent awakening during the night, early morning wakening (wakening at least 2 hours before the desired wake-up time) and excessive sleeping (hypersomnia).

Changes in appetite or weight

Although some depressed patients have an increased appetite and turn to 'comfort eating', only a dramatic reduction in appetite with weight loss (5% of body weight in last month) is regarded as a biological symptom. Note that the reversed neurovegetative features of overeating and oversleeping are sometimes referred to as 'atypical' depressive symptoms.

Psychomotor retardation or agitation

The term 'psychomotor' is used to describe a patient's motor activity as a consequence of their concurrent mental processes. Psychomotor changes in depression can include retardation (slow, monotonous speech, long pauses before answering questions, or muteness; leaden body movements and limited facial expression (i.e., blunted affect)) or conversely, agitation (inability to sit still; fidgeting, pacing or hand-wringing; rubbing or scratching skin or clothes). Note that psychomotor changes must be severe enough to be observable by others, not just the subjective experience of the patient.

Fatigue or reduced energy

Patients with depression often report feeling tired, low in energy, exhausted or lethargic. This is out of proportion to the demands upon the patient and persists despite rest.

Psychotic symptoms

While not part of the three core clusters, in moderate or severe depressive episodes patients may suffer from delusions, hallucinations or a depressive stupor; these are termed psychotic symptoms (see Chapter 9). Delusions and hallucinations can be classified as 'mood congruent' or 'mood incongruent', which describes whether the content of the psychotic symptoms is consistent with the patient's mood. Delusions and hallucinations in depression are generally mood congruent and so may involve an irrational conviction of guilt or sin or the belief that parts of the body are dead or wasting away. Hallucinations may take the form of accusatory or defamatory voices criticizing the patient in the second person (auditory hallucination) or the smell of rotting flesh (olfactory hallucination).

In severe episodes, psychomotor retardation may progress to the point of unresponsiveness, lack of voluntary movement (akinesis) and near or total mutism. Severe motor symptoms are probably more common in schizophrenia and bipolar affective disorder, but they can and do occur in unipolar depression.

Melancholy

Melancholia is a particularly severe form of depression with biological symptoms and a distinct quality of low mood characterized by a profound sense of despair. Symptoms include anhedonia, early morning wakening, diurnal variation with mood worse in morning, psychomotor retardation/agitation and marked loss of appetite or weight loss. 'With melancholia' can be added as a specifier to the diagnosis of depression in ICD-11.

DIFFERENTIAL DIAGNOSIS

Careful history taking and examination should reveal whether the patient presenting with low mood is suffering from a primary mood disorder, or whether their depression is secondary to a medical condition, psychoactive substance or other psychiatric condition. Box 11.1 presents the differential diagnosis. The most important differential to exclude is bipolar affective disorder as treatment with antidepressants alone may precipitate an episode of elated mood. An algorithm for the diagnosis of mood disorders is presented in Chapter 10.

BOX 11.1 DIFFERENTIAL DIAGNOSIS OF LOW MOOD

Mood disorders
- Depressive episode
- Recurrent depressive disorder
- Dysthymia
- Bipolar affective disorder
- Cyclothymia

Schizoaffective disorder

Secondary to a general medical condition

Secondary to psychoactive substance use (especially alcohol)
- Intoxication
- Withdrawal
- Substance-induced mood episode

Secondary to other psychiatric disorders
- Psychotic disorders
- Anxiety disorders
- Adjustment disorder (including bereavement)
- Eating disorders
- Personality disorders
- Neurodevelopmental disorders (autism or attention deficit hyperactivity disorder)
- Delirium/dementia

Mood (affective) disorders

Depressive episode

The ICD-11 has set out certain diagnostic guidelines for diagnosing a depressive episode (see Fig. 11.1). The minimum duration of the episode is 2 weeks and at least 5 of the 10 symptoms with at least one symptom from the 'affective' cluster must be present. If a patient is experiencing a first depressive episode, the diagnosis is of a 'single episode depressive disorder'.

Depressive episode specifiers

There are a number of specifiers that can be added to a diagnosis of a depressive episode to denote the severity or specific features.

The severity can be mild, moderate or severe.

Mild: there are enough symptoms present to meet criteria for a depressive episode, but none of them are intense. There is some impairment in at least one area of the person's life (e.g., school, work, social life). There are no psychotic symptoms.

Moderate: symptoms are present to a more significant degree and there is impairment in more than one area of the person's life.

Severe: most symptoms are present to a significant degree, and the person has significant difficulty functioning.

There is an additional specifier to denote if the patient is experiencing any psychotic symptoms, which could be either delusions or hallucinations. The presence of psychotic symptoms means the episode is at least 'moderate'. Sometimes it can be hard to differentiate between a delusion and a highly preoccupying anxious rumination with some basis in fact, e.g., a patient believes they are facing extreme financial difficulties and they do indeed have some financial challenges. This might be coded as a depressive episode of moderate severity with psychotic symptoms. However, the majority of cases of depression with psychotic symptoms will be viewed as severe.

ICD-11 also allows depressive episodes to be specified with other features such as 'with prominent anxiety symptoms', 'with panic attacks', 'with seasonal pattern' or 'with melancholia'.

Recurrent depressive disorder

Around 80% of patients who have an episode of depression will go on to have more episodes (the lifetime average is 5). Recurrent depressive disorder is diagnosed when a patient has another depressive episode after their first, and there has been at least a several month gap between the episodes.

Dysthymia

This is a chronically depressed mood (lasting at least 2 years) that usually has its onset in early adulthood and may remain throughout the patient's life, with variable periods of wellness in between. There should be no symptom-free periods lasting longer than 2 months. Within the first 2 years the patient's symptoms should not meet criteria for depressive episodes. Subsequent to this, the patient can be diagnosed with both conditions: a depressive episode on a baseline mood of dysthymia (so-called 'double depression'). Sometimes dysthymia has its onset in later adult life, often after a discrete depressive episode, and is associated with bereavement or some other serious stress.

Bipolar affective disorder/cyclothymia

Unipolar depression means that the patient's mood varies between depressed and normal. When patients suffer from episodes of either depressed or elated mood (often, but not always, punctuated by periods of normal mood), the disorder is termed bipolar, as the mood is considered to deviate from normal to either a depressed or elated (manic) pole. When this instability of mood involves mild elation/hypomania and low mood insufficiently severe to meet criteria for depression it is termed cyclothymia. Bipolar illness and cyclothymia are discussed in Chapter 10.

Schizoaffective disorder

A diagnosis of schizoaffective disorder can be made when patients present with both mood (depression or mania) symptoms and schizophrenic symptoms within the same episode of illness. It is important that these symptoms occur simultaneously, or at least within a few days of each other.

> **COMMON PITFALLS**
>
> Schizoaffective disorder is a difficult diagnosis to establish, as it is not uncommon to have psychotic symptoms in a severe episode of depression; likewise, depressive symptoms often occur in patients with schizophrenia. Schizoaffective disorder is discussed in more detail in Chapter 9.

Anxiety disorders

Many anxiety disorders are often associated with a degree of low mood, because of their unpleasant and pervasive effects. If the low mood is severe enough to meet criteria for depression, this should be diagnosed and treated first (see Chapter 12).

Adjustment disorder

Low mood may be one of several symptoms that appear when a patient has had to adapt to a significant change in life (e.g., divorce, retirement, bereavement). If the symptoms are not severe enough to be diagnosed as depression but are clearly

related to the patient being preoccupied with a stressful life event, an adjustment disorder can be diagnosed (see Chapter 14).

> **HINTS AND TIPS**
>
> A depressive episode can be differentiated from a bereavement by several factors (see Chapter 14). Factors include if the symptoms are unusually prolonged, feelings of low self-worth or guilt that are not related to the death, psychotic symptoms or psychomotor retardation.

Eating disorder

Eating disorders where nutrition is inadequate to maintain body weight are often associated with symptoms of starvation such as low mood, low energy and poor concentration (see Chapter 16).

Personality/neurodevelopmental disorders

Patients with disorders of personality (see Chapter 18) or neurodevelopment (see Chapter 8) often report features similar to depression (e.g., low self-esteem in autism spectrum disorders, feelings of hopelessness and thoughts of self-harm and suicide in borderline pattern personality disorders). However, personality and neurodevelopmental disorders involve stable and enduring behaviour patterns, unlike the more discrete episodes of a depressive disorder, which are characterized by a distinct, demarcated deterioration in psychosocial functioning. It is possible and in fact common for depression to be comorbid with personality and neurodevelopmental disorders.

Delirium/dementia

Low mood, apathy and hypersomnia in an older adult can be a presentation of hypoactive delirium. Depression can cause marked cognitive impairment, but if it persists for more than a few months beyond the remission of low mood, dementia may be the underlying diagnosis (see Chapter 7).

Depression secondary to general medical disorders, or to psychoactive substances

Many general medical conditions are associated with an increased risk for depression (Table 11.1). In some cases, this may be due to a direct depressant effect on the brain. However, any condition that causes prolonged suffering is a risk factor for depression (e.g., chronic pain).

Both prescribed (Table 11.2) and illicit drugs can be aetiologically responsible for symptoms of depression, during intoxication or withdrawal. Alcohol is the psychoactive substance that is probably most associated with substance-induced depression. Chronic use of benzodiazepines and withdrawal from stimulants are also associated with depressed mood.

HINTS AND TIPS

You may read notes or hear patients talk about diagnoses that were different in the ICD-10. For depression, differences in the ICD-10 include:

- Depressive symptoms were grouped into different clusters and there were more of them.
- Psychotic symptoms always indicated a severe episode.
- There were no specifiers.
- Comorbid diagnosis of dysthymia with depression requirements were less well defined.

ASSESSMENT

History

The following questions might be helpful in eliciting the key symptoms of depression:

Affective cluster

- Have you been cheerful or quite low in mood or spirits lately?
- Do you find that you no longer enjoy things the way you used to?

Cognitive-behavioural cluster

- Are you able to concentrate on your favourite TV programme?
- Can you follow lectures at university?
- Are you finding it harder than usual to make decisions?
- Do you feel guilty about things that people say aren't your fault?
- Do you feel like things can get better?
- Do you ever feel that life's not worth living?
- Do you ever have thoughts of hurting yourself or ending your life?

Neurovegetative cluster

- What time did you wake up before your mood became low? What time do you wake up now?
- Do you wake up before your alarm goes off?
- Has your weight changed?
- Has anyone mentioned you seem slowed up or restless?
- Do you find yourself often feeling very tired or worn out?

Psychotic symptoms

- Do you hear people say bad things about you when there's no one there?

Table 11.1 General medical conditions associated with low mood

Neurological	Endocrine	Infections	Others
Multiple sclerosis	Cushing disease	Hepatitis	Malignancies (especially pancreatic cancer)
Parkinson disease	Addison disease	Infectious mononucleosis	Chronic pain states
Huntington disease	Thyroid disorders (especially hypothyroidism)	Herpes simplex	Systemic lupus erythematosus
Spinal cord injury	Parathyroid disorders	Brucellosis	Rheumatoid arthritis
Stroke (especially left anterior infarcts)	Menstrual cycle-related	Typhoid	Renal failure
Head injury		HIV/AIDS	Porphyria
Cerebral tumours		Syphilis	Vitamin deficiencies (e.g., niacin, vitamin D)
			Ischaemic heart disease

Table 11.2 Prescribed drugs causing low mood

Antihypertensives	Steroids	Neurological drugs	Analgesics	Other
β-blockers	Corticosteroids	L-DOPA	Opiates	Antipsychotics
Methyldopa	Oral contraceptives	Carbamazepine	Indometacin	Interferon (alpha and beta)

- Have you ever seen things that you can't explain or you think might not have been real?
- Do you smell anything unpleasant which is hard to explain?
- Do you feel your body is healthy?

A collateral history from the patient's family, partner, carer, community psychiatric nurse or general practitioner (GP) is often helpful.

Examination

A basic physical examination, including a thorough neurological and endocrine system examination, should be performed on all patients with depression.

Investigations

Investigations are performed to: (1) exclude possible medical or substance-related causes of depression; (2) establish baseline values before administering treatment that may alter blood chemistry (e.g., antidepressants may cause hyponatraemia, lithium may cause hypothyroidism); (3) assess renal and liver functioning, which may affect the elimination of medication; and (4) screen for the physical consequences of neglect, such as malnutrition.

- Full blood count: check for anaemia (low haemoglobin), infection (raised white count) and a high mean cell volume (a marker of high alcohol intake).
- Urea and electrolytes (hyponatraemia, renal function).
- Liver function tests and γ-glutamyltranspeptidase (also a marker for high alcohol intake).
- Thyroid function tests (hyperthyroidism or hypothyroidism) and calcium (hypercalcaemia).

If indicated:

- C reactive protein or erythrocyte sedimentation rate (if infection or inflammatory disease is suspected).
- Vitamin D, Vitamin B_{12} and folate (if deficiencies suspected).
- Urine drug screen (if drug use is suspected).
- Electrocardiogram should be done in patients with cardiac problems as tricyclic antidepressants and lithium may prolong the QT interval and have the potential to cause lethal ventricular arrhythmia.

- Electroencephalogram (if epileptic focus or other intracranial pathology is suspected).
- Computed tomography brain scan (if evidence of neurological or cognitive deficit).

DISCUSSION OF CASE STUDY

LM meets the criteria for a depressive episode, at least moderate in severity. They have had both affective symptoms of depression for longer than 2 weeks: depressed mood and loss of interest. They also have neurovegetative symptoms of fatigability and sleep change (with early morning awakening). The GP has also elicited cognitive-behavioural symptoms of feelings of incompetence (reduced self-worth), guilt and possible thoughts of self-harm. As this is a first episode, the diagnosis of recurrent depressive disorder is not appropriate. Dysthymia is not a suitable diagnosis as the period of low mood is far too short, the severity of the present episode too great and the deterioration in functioning too marked. There appear to be no instances of elated mood or increased energy, excluding a diagnosis of bipolar affective disorder or cyclothymia. In order to grade the severity of the depression it would be useful to enquire about all the affective, cognitive-behavioural and neurovegetative symptoms of depression, and to ask about functional impairment. Assessing LM's ability to care for their young children is crucial and is likely to require a collateral history from their partner, with consideration of referral to social work if there are significant concerns. In all cases of suspected depression it is imperative to enquire about thoughts and/or plans of suicide or self-harm (see Chapter 6 for a full discussion). It is also important to rule out secondary causes of depression; these include general medical conditions (Table 11.1), psychoactive substance use (Table 11.2) and other psychiatric conditions. LM admitted to using increased quantities of alcohol subsequent to the onset of their low mood: advising them to abstain from alcohol is an important first step in managing their mood. Patients often use alcohol as a form of self-medication to alleviate feelings of dysphoria; however, alcohol can aggravate and in many cases cause depressive symptoms. LM's use of oral contraception long before the onset of their depressive symptoms suggests that it is unlikely that this prescribed drug is causing their depression.

Chapter Summary

- A depressive episode is a sustained period of low mood (at least 2 weeks) associated with a number of other symptoms, and functional impairment.
- A depressive episode can be associated with impaired cognition and/or psychotic symptoms.
- The key differential diagnoses for a depressive episode are a substance use disorder, anxiety disorder or personality disorder.
- When assessing someone for depression, ask about the three clusters of: affective symptoms, cognitive-behavioural symptoms and neurovegetative symptoms.
- When assessing someone for depression, *always* ask about suicidal thoughts.

UKMLA Conditions
Anxiety disorder: generalized,
Substance use disorder
Bipolar affective disorder
Dementias
Depression
Personality disorders
Self-harm

UKMLA Presentations
Abnormal eating or exercise behaviour
Auditory hallucinations
Behaviour/personality change
Decreased appetite
Elation/elated mood
Fatigue
Loss of libido
Low mood/affective problems
Self-harm
Sleep problems
Substance misuse
Suicidal thoughts
Visual hallucinations
Weight gain
Weight loss

The patient with anxiety, fear or avoidance 12

Case Summary

PA, a 32-year-old divorced interior designer, was referred to a primary care psychologist by their family doctor because of a 6-month history of sudden, dramatic anxiety attacks accompanied by heart palpitations, profuse sweating, dizziness, a choking sensation and a fear that they were going to die. There appeared to be no logical reason for the attacks and PA described them as coming on 'out of the blue'. They reached their maximum intensity within 2 minutes and seldom lasted longer than 15 minutes, occurring two to three times a week. Because of these attacks, which occurred in any situation and at any time of day, PA had stopped going into shops or crowded public places for fear of having an attack and not being able to escape to a safe place and appearing like a 'blubbering fool'. They have started relying on their mother to accompany them on 'absolutely necessary' household excursions 'just in case' they have another attack. Their general practitioner (GP) had signed them off work for the past 3 months, as they were too frightened to visit their potential clients' houses in the event that they had another attack. PA told the psychologist that they had almost become housebound and felt that they were 'losing their mind'. A full physical examination, routine blood tests including: full blood count, urea and electrolytes, fasting glucose, liver function, thyroid function and calcium concentration as well as an electrocardiogram revealed no abnormalities.

For a discussion of the case study, see the end of the chapter.

Feelings of anxiety or fear are both common and essential to the human experience. It is the very uncomfortable nature of this experience that makes anxiety such an effective alerting, and therefore harm avoiding, device. However, for the same reasons, when anxiety is excessive and unchecked, it can create an extremely debilitating condition. To distinguish between normal and pathological anxiety it is important to observe the patient's level of functioning. The Yerkes–Dodson law (Fig. 12.1) states that the relationship between performance and anxiety has the shape of an inverted U: mild to moderate levels of anxiety improve performance, but high levels impair it.

DEFINITIONS AND CLINICAL FEATURES

Both anxiety and fear are alerting signals that occur in response to a potential threat, either known or unknown.

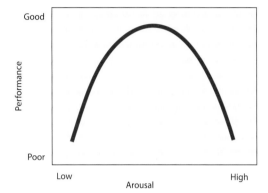

Fig. 12.1 Yerkes–Dodson law (1908).

The experience of anxiety consists of two interrelated components: (1) thoughts of being apprehensive, nervous or frightened; (2) the awareness of a physical reaction to anxiety (autonomic or peripheral anxiety). Box 12.1 summarizes the physical signs of anxiety. The experience of anxiety may lead to a change in behaviour, particularly an avoidance of the real or imagined threat.

There are two patterns of pathological anxiety:

1. Generalized (free-floating) anxiety does not occur in discrete episodes and tends to last for hours, days or even longer and is of mild to moderate severity. It is not associated with a specific external threat or situation (i.e., free-floating), it is excessive worry or apprehension about many normal life events (e.g., job security, relationships and responsibilities).

2. Paroxysmal anxiety has an abrupt onset, occurs in discrete episodes and tends to be quite severe. In its severest form, paroxysmal anxiety presents as panic attacks. These are discrete episodes of short-lived (usually less than 1 hour), intense anxiety. They have an abrupt onset and rapidly build up to a peak level of anxiety. They are accompanied by strong autonomic symptoms (see Box 12.1), which may lead patients to believe that they are dying, having a heart attack, or going mad. This increases their anxiety level and produces further physical symptoms, thereby creating a vicious cycle.

See Fig. 12.2 for a comparison of panic attacks and free-floating (generalized) anxiety. Quite often the two co-occur: someone with a background moderately elevated anxiety level can also have superimposed panic attacks.

Paroxysmal anxiety can further be subdivided into episodes of anxiety that occur seemingly spontaneously, without a specific imagined or external threat (see Panic Disorder, later in this chapter) and those episodes that occur in response to a specific imagined or external threat (the 'focus of apprehension'). Phobic disorders are the most common cause of paroxysmal anxiety in response to a perceived threat.

A phobia is an intense, irrational fear of an object, activity or situation (e.g., flying, heights, animals, blood, public speaking). Although patients may recognize that their fear is irrational, people characteristically avoid the phobic stimulus or endure it with extreme distress. It is the degree of fear that is irrational in that the feared objects or situations are not inevitably dangerous and do not cause such severe anxiety in most other people. In severe cases, phobic anxiety may progress to frank panic attacks.

BOX 12.1 PHYSICAL SIGNS OF ANXIETY

Tachycardia
Palpitations (abnormal awareness of the heart beating)
Hypertension
Shortness of breath/rapid breathing
Chest pain or discomfort
Choking sensation
Tremors, shaking
Muscle tension
Dry mouth
Sweating
Cold skin
Nausea or vomiting
Diarrhoea
Abdominal discomfort ('butterflies')
Dizziness, light-headedness, syncope
Mydriasis (pupil dilatation)

DIFFERENTIAL DIAGNOSIS

When considering the differential diagnosis of anxiety you should determine:

- The rate of onset, severity and duration of the anxiety (i.e., is the anxiety generalized or paroxysmal? Is it lifelong or acquired?)
- Whether the anxiety is in response to a specific threat/thought or arises spontaneously (unprovoked).
- Whether the anxiety only occurs in the context of a pre-existing psychiatric, substance use or medical condition.

Box 12.2 presents the differential diagnosis for patients presenting with anxiety and Fig. 12.3 gives a diagnostic algorithm.

Anxiety disorders

It is useful to consider the primary anxiety disorders under the headings 'Phobic Disorders' and 'Nonsituational Anxiety Disorders'. They are closely related to disorders associated with stress and obsessive-compulsive or related disorders.

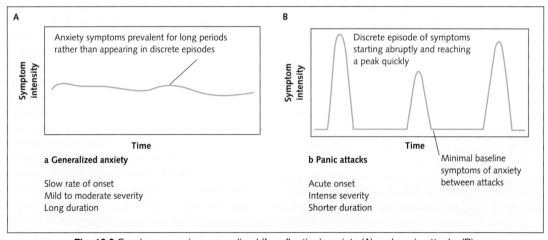

Fig. 12.2 Graphs comparing generalized (free-floating) anxiety (A) and panic attacks (B).

Anxiety disorders (with or without panic attacks):
- Phobic disorders
  - Agoraphobia
  - Specific phobia
- Social anxiety disorder
- Nonsituational anxiety disorders
  - Generalized anxiety disorder
  - Panic disorder

Reaction to stress
- Acute stress reaction
- Adjustment disorder
- Post-traumatic stress disorder
- Complex post-traumatic stress disorder
- Obsessive-compulsive disorder
- Body dysmorphic disorder
- Hypochondriasis
- Bodily distress disorder

Secondary to (any) other psychiatric disorder
- Depression
- Psychosis
- Personality disorder
- Neurodevelopmental disorder
- Other

Secondary to a general medical condition

Secondary to psychoactive substance use (especially alcohol use)

Phobic disorders

Remember that:

- Phobic disorders are associated with a prominent avoidance of the feared situation.
- The situationally induced anxiety may be so severe as to take the form of a panic attack.

Agoraphobia

Agoraphobia literally means 'fear of the marketplace' (i.e., fear of public places). In psychiatry today, it has a wider meaning that also includes a fear of entering crowded spaces (shops, trains, buses, elevators) where an immediate escape is difficult or in which help might not be available in the event of having a panic attack. At the worst extreme, patients may become housebound or refuse to leave the house unless accompanied by a close friend or relative. Sometimes, patients are still able to endure these situations, but it causes them significant distress. If this is the case, a diagnosis of agoraphobia remains appropriate.

There is a close relationship between agoraphobia and panic disorder that occurs when patients develop a fear of being in a place from where escape would be difficult in the event of having a panic attack. In fact, studies have shown that in a clinical setting, up to 95% of patients presenting with agoraphobia have a current or past diagnosis of panic disorder. In the ICD-11, if a patient experiences panic attacks only in situations that trigger their agoraphobia, a diagnosis of 'agoraphobia with panic attacks' can be given. If they also experience panic attacks outside of agoraphobic situations, both agoraphobia and panic disorder can be diagnosed.

Specific phobia

Specific (simple) phobias are restricted to clearly specific and discernible objects or situations (other than those covered in agoraphobia and social anxiety disorder). Examples from adult psychiatric samples in order of decreasing prevalence include:

- Situational: specific situations (e.g., public transportation, flying, driving, tunnels, bridges, elevators).
- Natural environment: heights, storms, water, darkness.
- Blood-injection-injury: seeing blood or an injury, fear of needles or an invasive medical procedure.
- Animal: animals or insects (e.g., spiders, dogs, mice).
- Other: fear of choking or vomiting, contracting an illness (e.g., HIV), children's fear of costumed characters.

HINTS AND TIPS

A diagnosis of a specific phobia should only be made if the fear of the object or situation results in significant functional impairment and/or distress. The patient must also either actively avoid the object or situation, or experience intense fear or anxiety while enduring the situation/presence of the object.

Social anxiety disorder

Patients with social anxiety disorder experience significant fear or anxiety in social situations. For some patients, the fear or anxiety can be experienced in day-to-day social interactions, such as making conversation, or in a situation where they might be observed undertaking an activity (e.g., eating). Situations where an individual is expected to perform in front of others, such as when giving a speech, may also trigger anxiety symptoms. The fear or anxiety can be isolated to one specific area for some patients, whereas for other patients, the fear may involve all social activities outside of the home. The focus of apprehension for individuals with social anxiety disorder is them acting in a way, or displaying anxiety symptoms in a way that might be judged negatively by others. This means that the person starts consistently avoiding social situations, and if they cannot do this, then they endure the situation while experiencing intense anxiety or fear.

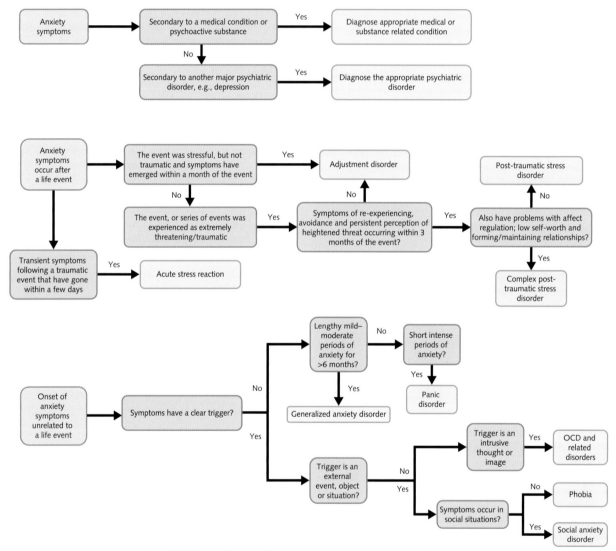

Fig. 12.3 Diagnostic algorithm for anxiety and stress-related disorders.

OCD, Obsessive-compulsive disorder.

Nonsituational anxiety disorders

These disorders, unlike the phobic disorders, are characterized by primary anxiety symptoms that are not restricted to any specific situation or circumstance.

Generalized anxiety disorder

The ICD-11 defines the essential features of generalized anxiety disorder as:

1. Long-standing, free-floating anxiety. Patients describe experiencing excessive worry about everyday events and should be apprehensive on most days for at least several months.
2. One or more additional characteristic symptoms such as tension or restlessness, physical symptoms of anxiety, e.g., palpitations and sweating (see Box 12.1), difficulty maintaining concentration, irritability or sleep disturbance.

Panic disorder

Panic disorder is characterised by the presence of panic attacks that occur unpredictably and are not restricted to any particular situation (indicating a phobic disorder) or objective danger.

A panic attack is a distinct episode of intense fear or apprehension, accompanied by the rapid and simultaneous onset of particular, predictable symptoms. These symptoms include:

1. Palpitations or increased heart rate
2. Sweating
3. Trembling
4. Shortness of breath
5. Chest pain
6. Dizziness or light-headedness
7. Chills or hot flushes
8. Fear of imminent death

Panic attacks are so distressing that patients commonly develop a fear of having further attacks; this is known as anticipatory anxiety. Anticipatory anxiety apart, patients are relatively free from anxiety symptoms between attacks.

Table 12.1 Examples of psychiatric problems commonly associated with anxiety

Focus of anxiety	Psychiatric problem
Gaining weight	Eating disorder (see Chapter 16)
Having many physical complaints	Bodily distress disorder (see Chapter 15)
Having a serious illness	Hypochondriasis (see Chapter 13)
Fear of being poisoned or killed	Delusional beliefs in psychosis (see Chapter 9)
Ruminative thoughts of guilt or worthlessness	Depression (see Chapter 11)
When having an obsessional thought or resisting a compulsion	Obsessive-compulsive disorder (see Chapter 13)
Separation or abandonment	Personality disorders with the borderline pattern specifier (see Chapter 18)
Being rejected or inadequate	Personality disorder with prominent features of negative affectivity with or without the borderline pattern specifier (see Chapter 18)
Not being perfect	Personality disorder with prominent features of anankastia (see Chapter 18)
Feeling restless, unable to concentrate	Attention deficit hyperactivity disorder (see Chapter 32)
Not understanding others	Autism spectrum disorder (see Chapter 32)
Not understanding what is going on	Delirium or dementia (see Chapter 20)

Disorders associated with stress, obsessive-compulsive or related disorders, bodily distress disorder

The disorders associated with stress, obsessive-compulsive or related disorders and bodily distress disorder are discussed in Chapters 14, 13 and 15, respectively.

Other psychiatric conditions

Anxiety is a nonspecific symptom and can occur secondary to other psychiatric conditions. See Table 12.1 for examples of psychiatric problems commonly associated with anxiety.

Note that depression and anxiety are closely intertwined. Not only can anxiety occur secondary to a depressive disorder and vice versa, but some authors have also suggested that the two disorders are aetiologically related. About 65% of patients with anxiety also have depressive symptoms; therefore, when making a diagnosis, it is essential to decide which symptoms came first or were predominant and which were secondary. If symptoms of anxiety occur only in the context of a depressive episode then depression takes precedence and should be diagnosed alone.

Generalized anxiety disorder and personality disorders may both have symptoms from childhood onwards, a chronic course and cause significant distress and functional impairment. They can be distinguished by the focus of the anxiety and by the presence or absence of other traits in personality disorder. For example, someone with a personality disorder with prominent features of anankastia will worry specifically about not doing tasks well enough, and/or about lack of orderliness and control. They are also likely to have a rigid view of appropriate behaviour and find it difficult to deviate from their principles. In contrast, someone with generalized anxiety disorder may well worry about not doing tasks well enough, but they will also worry about many other things (e.g., appearance, finances, personal safety) and they are no more likely than average to have a particularly fixed moral code.

Anxiety secondary to a general medical condition or psychoactive substance use

A medical or psychoactive substance cause of anxiety should always be actively sought and ruled out. The ICD-11 allows for the diagnosis of 'substance-induced anxiety disorder' in the case of most substances, with the exception of nicotine. Table 12.2 lists the medical and Table 12.3 the substance-related causes of anxiety. The medical condition or substance use should predate the development of the anxiety and symptoms should resolve with treatment of the condition or abstinence from the offending substance. Anxiety during alcohol withdrawal is particularly important to exclude (see Chapter 17). Absence of previous anxiety or absence of a family history of anxiety disorder also supports this diagnosis. Often symptoms can arise from a combination of a general medical condition and anxiety, as each predisposes to the other. For example, if someone is having an acute asthma attack they will naturally feel anxious and breathe even faster. Helping them to calm down may be an important intervention.

Table 12.2 Medical conditions and prescribed drugs that are associated with anxiety

Medical conditions	Side effects of prescribed drugs
Causing dyspnoea Congestive cardiac failure Pulmonary embolism Chronic obstructive pulmonary disease Asthma	**Antidepressants** (e.g., SSRIs and tricyclics in first 2 weeks of use or following rapid discontinuation (particularly of paroxetine or venlafaxine)) **Corticosteroids** **Sympathomimetics**
Causing increased sympathetic outflow Hypoglycaemia Pheochromocytoma	**Thyroid hormones** **Compound analgesics containing caffeine** **Anticholinergics** **Antipsychotics (akathisia)**
Causing pain Malignancies	
Other Cerebral trauma Cushing disease Hyperthyroidism Temporal lope epilepsy Vitamin deficiencies	

SSRI, *Selective serotonin reuptake inhibitor.*

Table 12.3 Substances associated with anxiety

Intoxication	Withdrawal	Substance-induced anxiety disorder
Alcohol	Alcohol	Alcohol
Amphetamines	Benzodiazepines	Sedatives
Caffeine	Caffeine	Opioids
Cannabis	Cocaine	Amphetamines
Cocaine	Gamma-hydroxybutyrate/gamma-	Caffeine
Hallucinogens	butyrolactone (GHB/GBL)	Cannabis
Inhalants	Nicotine	Cocaine
Ketamine	Other sedatives and hypnotics	Hallucinogens
Novel psychoactive substances	Opioids	Inhalants
Dissociative drugs		MDMA
		Dissociative drugs

ASSESSMENT

History

The following questions may be helpful in eliciting anxiety symptoms:

- Do you sometimes wake up feeling anxious and dreading the day ahead? (any form of anxiety)
- Do you worry excessively about minor matters on most days of the week? (generalized anxiety)
- Have you ever been so frightened that your heart was pounding and you thought you might die? (panic attack)
- Do you avoid leaving the house alone because you are afraid of having a panic attack or being in situations (like being in a crowded shop or on a train) from which escape will be difficult or embarrassing? (agoraphobia)
- Do you get anxious in social situations, like speaking in front of people or making conversation? (social anxiety disorder)
- Do some things or situations make you very scared? Do you avoid them? (specific phobia)

Examination

A basic physical examination, including a thorough neurological and endocrine system examination, should be performed on all patients with symptoms of anxiety.

Investigations

Anxiety disorders can only be diagnosed when the symptoms are not due to the direct effect of a substance or medical condition. It is impractical to test for each of the large number of drugs and physical health conditions capable of producing anxiety symptoms (see Tables 12.2 and 12.3). It is, however, important to exclude any disease or substance that may be implicated through any clues in the history (e.g., past medical history and drug history) and physical examination. For example, a patient with a rapid pulse and heat intolerance should have thyroid function tests in case thyrotoxicosis is causing the anxiety symptoms. The possibility of withdrawal syndromes (e.g., alcohol, benzodiazepines, opiates) causing anxiety symptoms should always be considered.

DISCUSSION OF CASE STUDY

Repeated, unexpected episodes of short-lived intense anxiety of abrupt onset and rapidly building up to a peak level of anxiety associated with palpitations, sweating, dizziness, a choking sensation and thoughts of being about to die, with no medical cause, suggests a diagnosis of panic disorder.

As is common in many patients with panic disorder, agoraphobia has developed as a super-added problem as evidenced by a fear of going into situations from which escape might be difficult or humiliating. PA is showing the important sign of avoidance of the feared situation by refusing to go out unless it is essential and only when accompanied by their mother. Note that fear of having another panic attack indicates anticipatory anxiety; fear of having a panic attack in a situation from which escape will be difficult or humiliating, thus resulting in avoidance of those situations indicates agoraphobia – PA has both.

It is important to rule out depression or other psychiatric conditions as well as medical conditions and psychoactive substance use.

Now go on to Chapter 25 to read about the anxiety disorders and their management.

Chapter Summary

- Anxiety has two main components: fearful thoughts, and physical symptoms of autonomic arousal.
- Anxiety can be free floating or paroxysmal.
- The main anxiety disorders are phobias, panic disorder, social anxiety disorder and generalized anxiety disorder.
- Many other psychiatric disorders can present with or cause anxiety.
- When assessing anxiety disorders it is important to exclude substance use, particularly alcohol withdrawal, and general medical conditions such as hyperthyroidism.

UKMLA Conditions
Anxiety disorder (generalized)
Anxiety
OCD
Phobias

UKMLA Presentations
Anxiety
Behaviour/personality
change
Chronic abdominal pain
OCD
Phobias

Case summary

OC is a 22-year-old medical student and has recently moved into their own flat. They describe a 5-month history of recurrent thoughts that they have behaved in a sexually inappropriate way towards their mother. They say that even though on one level they know that this is impossible, they are unable to push these thoughts away despite trying 'rigorous mental gymnastics'. The only way they can relieve the distress they experience is to actually contact their mother for reassurance that their fears are not true. On most days, they physically have to go and see their mother, and will spend up to 2 hours analysing their behaviour with her until they feel reassured. Whenever they try to stop themselves from seeking reassurance, they feel a rapid escalation in anxiety, thinking that not contacting their mother is evidence that their thoughts 'might be true'. They shudder in horror when asked whether they have had any sexual feelings for their mother but admit that these distressing thoughts are 'obviously' their own. They are heterosexual and have recently become engaged. They are embarrassed and were eventually persuaded to see their general practitioner by their mother and fiancée when they started falling behind with their studies. They say that the whole thing is starting to affect their mood and that they have lost weight.

(For a discussion of the case study, see the end of the chapter.)

Obsessions or compulsions are terms that are often used in everyday language (e.g., 'she has an obsession with shoes' or 'he is a compulsive liar'). Psychiatrists, however, use these terms in a very specific way and it is important to accurately elicit, recognise and understand obsessive-compulsive psychopathology.

DEFINITIONS AND CLINICAL FEATURES

Obsessions and compulsions

Obsessions are involuntary thoughts, images or impulses which have the following important characteristics:

- They are *recurrent* and *intrusive* and are experienced as *unpleasant* or *distressing*.
- They enter the mind against conscious resistance. Patients *try to resist* but are unable to do so.
- Patients recognise obsessions as being the *product of their own mind* (not from without as in thought insertion - see Chapter 9 and Table 13.1) even though they are involuntary and often repugnant.

Obsessions are not merely excessive concerns about normal life problems, and patients generally retain insight into the fact that their thoughts are irrational. In fact, patients often see their obsessions as foreign to, or against, their 'essence' (ego-dystonic or ego-alien; e.g., a religious man has recurrent thoughts that he has betrayed God). While for some people, obsessive thoughts will remain consistent for the duration of their illness, for others the thoughts can shift and change over time.

COMMUNICATION

If a patient tells you they are suffering from obsessional thinking, always clarify what they mean by 'obsession' (a recurrent, intrusive, unpleasant, resisted thought from within their own mind). This is because, like many psychiatric terms, 'obsession' has other, less specific meanings.

Compulsions are repetitive mental operations (counting, praying or repeating a mantra silently) or physical acts (checking, seeking reassurance, handwashing, strict rituals) that have the following unique characteristics:

- Patients feel forced to perform them in response to their own obsessions (see case study) or irrationally defined 'rules' (e.g., 'I must count to 10,000 four times before falling asleep').
- They are performed to reduce anxiety through the belief that they will prevent a 'dreaded event' from occurring, even though they are not realistically connected to the event (e.g., compulsive counting each night to prevent 'family catastrophe') or are ridiculously excessive (e.g., spending hours handwashing in response to an obsessive fear of contamination).

Compulsions are experienced as unpleasant and serve no realistically useful purpose despite their tension-relieving

Table 13.1 Differentiating types of repetitive or intrusive thoughts or images

Term	Description
Obsession	Unpleasant, recurrent, intrusive thought, image or impulse. Patient attributes origin within self. Involuntary and resisted (ego-dystonic).
Hallucination	Involuntary perception occurring in the absence of a stimulus experienced as indistinguishable from a normal perception.
Pseudohallucination	Involuntary perception in the absence of stimulus experienced in internal space. Experienced vividly, as opposed to an obsessional image which may lack detail or completeness. Not usually resisted.
Flashback	Vivid reexperiencing of memory. Usually visual. Associated with strong affect. Patient recognizes as memory, with origin from within self. Involuntary. Usually unpleasant and resisted.
Rumination	Repeatedly thinking about the causes and experience of previous distress and difficulties. Voluntary, not resisted.
Thought insertion	Intrusive thought, image or impulse. Patient attributes origin outside self. May or may not be resisted.
Over-valued idea	Plausible belief arrived at logically but held with undue importance. Not resisted or viewed as abnormal.
Delusion	Fixed belief arrived at illogically and not amenable to reason. Not culturally normal. May or may not be plausible. Not resisted.

properties. Similar to obsessions, patients resist carrying out compulsions. Resisting compulsions, however, causes increased anxiety.

Obsessions and compulsions are often closely linked, as the desire to resist or neutralise an obsession produces a compulsive act (see Table 13.2 for examples of the most commonly occurring obsessions and compulsions). It can be difficult enquiring about obsessions and compulsions, especially when patients do not offer them as a presenting complaint. Box 13.1 suggests some useful questions in eliciting these symptoms.

Obsessive-compulsive disorder related disorders

The International Statistical Classification of Diseases and Related Health Problems, 11th edition (ICD-11) has listed a group of related disorders in the same section as obsessive-compulsive disorder (OCD). These disorders have similar clinical features, neuroimaging findings, genetics and treatments. They are divided into disorders that feature prominent cognitive components of obsessive thoughts and those which feature prominent compulsive behaviours.

Body dysmorphic disorder

An individual with body dysmorphic disorder (BDD) is persistently preoccupied with a perceived defect or flaw in their personal appearance. The perceived flaw is usually unnoticeable, or only slightly noticeable to other people. This perceived flaw means that the individual is self-conscious, and can feel as though others are talking about or judging them in relation to it.

Table 13.2 Examples of the most commonly occurring obsessions and their associated compulsions in descending order

Obsession	Compulsion
Fear of contamination (feared object is usually impossible to avoid, e.g., faeces, urine, germs)	Excessive washing and cleaning. Avoidance of contaminated object
Pathological doubt ('Have I turned the stove off?' 'Did I lock the door?')	Exhaustive checking of the possible omission
Shameful, blasphemous or sexual thoughts, images or impulses (e.g., impulse to stab husband, having thoughts that one might be a paedophile)[a]	Act of 'redemption' (e.g., repeating 'Forgive me, I have sinned' 15 times) or seeking reassurance (see case study)
Need for symmetry or precision	Repeatedly arranging objects to obtain perfect symmetry

[a]Patients.

In addition, the individual may also engage in repetitive behaviours around the perceived flaw, e.g., repeatedly examining the body part in a mirror, making excessive attempts to camouflage the flaw (e.g., through makeup or cosmetic procedures) or they may avoid social situations that increase their distress (e.g., avoiding the gym due to communal changing rooms). They often have little insight into the accuracy of their beliefs about the flaw.

BOX 13.1 QUESTIONS USED TO ELICIT OBSESSIONS AND COMPULSIONS

1. Do you worry about contamination with dirt even when you have already washed?
2. Do you have intrusive or distressing thoughts entering your mind despite trying hard to keep them out?
3. Do you repeatedly have to check things that you have already done (stoves, lights, taps, etc.)?
4. Do you find that you have to arrange, touch or count things many times over?

RED FLAG

Body dysmorphic disorder is associated with an increased risk of suicide, and rarely, with self-mutilation (in an attempt to correct the perceived flaw). Ensure that you complete a thorough risk assessment for all patients with BDD.

Olfactory reference disorder

Olfactory reference disorder is a new addition to the ICD-11. It involves the individual being preoccupied with the belief that they have offensive body odour, resulting in excessive self-consciousness and concern that others around them are talking about it. They engage in repetitive behaviours to attempt to compensate for their perceived malodour, including checking for odour, seeking reassurance from others about their body odour or making excessive attempts to cover up their body odour.

Hypochondriasis (health anxiety disorder)

Individuals with hypochondriasis have a persistent preoccupation with worries about having one or more serious or life-threatening illnesses. They will engage in behaviours that have a focus on confirming or disproving the diagnosis. Behaviours can include repeated examination of their body, researching the illness or seeking reassurance from medical professionals. They may also display maladaptive behaviours, which include avoiding medical appointments or avoiding situations that trigger thoughts of the illness they are worried about.

HINTS AND TIPS

Individuals with hypochondriasis will often be reassured by negative medical findings, whereas individuals with bodily distress disorder (see Chapter 15) can be frustrated by a lack of findings from any investigations ordered.

Hoarding disorder

Hoarding disorder is a new addition to the ICD-11. It is characterized by the accumulation of possessions because of repetitive urges to acquire items. As a result of the accumulation of possessions, the individual's living space becomes cluttered and ultimately compromises their safety, e.g., due to fire risks. To an outsider looking in, the items accumulated may not look like they hold much value, but to the individual, they can hold emotional significance or they might be viewed as having the potential to be useful in the future. If somebody externally tries to remove the items from the individual's house, it can cause them significant distress and anxiety. Individuals frequently have little insight into the problems caused by the accumulation of their possessions. Hoarding disorder can also be associated with other mental disorders, including depression.

Body-focused repetitive behaviour disorders

These disorders do not have a clear cognitive component, and the repetitive behaviours are directed at the skin (excoriation disorder) or hair (trichotillomania). See Table 13.3 for a summary.

HINTS AND TIPS

The addition of the 'insight specifier' – either 'poor to absent insight', or 'fair to good insight', is new for the ICD-11. It can be applied to all obsessive-compulsive-related disorders, e.g., hoarding disorder with poor to absent insight, or olfactory reference disorder with fair to good insight.

HINTS AND TIPS

A key differential for an obsession is a delusion. They can be distinguished by checking whether the patient knows the thought is false and a product of their own mind (an obsession) or believes it to be true and represents external reality (a delusion).

Table 13.3

Disorders with a prominent cognitive component-associated with obsessive thoughts and compulsive, repetitive behavours	Body-focused repetitive behaviour disorders
Obsessive-compulsive disorder	Trichotillomania (hair-pulling disorder)
Body dysmorphic disorder	Excoriation (skin-picking) disorder
Olfactory reference disorder	
Hypochondriasis (health anxiety disorder)	
Hoarding disorder	

HINTS AND TIPS

When looking at notes documenting the ICD-10 diagnoses, it is good to know:

1. OCD previously had subtypes based on symptoms. Now subtypes reflect degree of insight.
2. Depression used to take priority as a diagnosis over OCD, and a descriptive diagnosis such as 'depression with obsessional symptoms' might be made. Now, if symptoms for both are present, both can be diagnosed.

DIFFERENTIAL DIAGNOSIS

Obsessions and compulsions may occur as a primary illness as in OCD or related disorders or may be clinical features of other psychiatric conditions. If patients have genuine obsessions or compulsions without other psychiatric symptoms, then the diagnosis is simply OCD. ICD-11 diagnostic guidelines are shown in Box 13.2.

Many other psychiatric conditions may also present with repetitive or intrusive thoughts, impulses, images or behaviours (see Table 13.4). However, it is usually possible to differentiate them from OCD by applying the strict definition of obsessions and compulsions. Also, when repetitive thoughts occur in the context of other mental disorders, the contents of these thoughts are limited exclusively to the type of disorder concerned (e.g., morbid fear of fatness in anorexia nervosa, ruminative thoughts of worthlessness in depression, fear of dreaded objects in phobias). Table 13.4 lists the differential

BOX 13.2 THE ICD-11 DIAGNOSTIC GUIDELINES FOR OBSESSIVE-COMPULSIVE DISORDER

Essential features

- Presence of persistent obsessions or compulsions, or most commonly both
  - Obsessions are repetitive and persistent thoughts, images or impulses/urges that are intrusive, unwanted and commonly associated with anxiety. The individual attempts to ignore or suppress the obsessions or neutralise them by performing compulsions. Examples of obsessions include thoughts of contamination or thoughts of a violent or sexual nature.
  - Compulsions are repetitive behaviours that the person feels driven to complete as a response to an obsessive thought. Examples include repetitive cleaning or washing, performing mental acts, e.g., repeating phrases a certain number of times or ordering objects.
- The obsessions and compulsions are time consuming and/or result in significant distress or functional impairment. If function is maintained, it is only through significant effort on the part of the individual.
- The symptoms and behaviours are not due to, or part of another medical condition.

Insight specifiers

- Fair to good insight – the individual can entertain the possibility that their disorder-specific beliefs may not be true and they can accept an alternative explanation.
- Poor to absent insight – most or all of the time, the individual is convinced that their disorder-specific beliefs are true and they cannot accept an alternative explanation.

diagnoses and key distinguishing features of patients presenting with obsessive-compulsive symptomatology. OCD can also be comorbid with other psychiatric conditions, particularly depression and, less commonly, schizophrenia. See Fig. 12.3 for an algorithm to help distinguish OCD from other psychiatric conditions.

Table 13.4 Differential diagnosis for patients presenting with obsessions or compulsions

Diagnosis	Diagnostic features
Obsessive-compulsive or related disorders	
Obsessive-compulsive disorder (OCD)	Persistent, genuine, obsessions and compulsions, which result in significant distress and/or functional impairment (see Box 13.2).
Body dysmorphic disorder (BDD)	Persistent preoccupation with a perceived flaw in personal appearance. Repetitive actions including checking the perceived flaw and avoiding situations where they might need to expose the flawed area.
Hoarding disorder	Persistent and repetitive urges to accumulate items or possessions resulting in an excessive and unmanageable volume of possessions.
Hypochondriasis	Persistent preoccupation with worries about having one or more serious or life-threatening illnesses. Will engage in repetitive behaviours including self-examination and seeking medical reassurance as result of worries.
Olfactory reference disorder	Persistent preoccupation about emitting a foul body odour, with individuals being excessively self-conscious about it.
Body-focused repetitive behaviour disorders (trichotillomania and excoriation disorder)	Repetitive hair pulling or skin picking which is associated with emotional regulation, reduction of tension and sometimes pleasure.
Other mental disorders	
Eating disorders[a] (see Chapter 16)	Morbid fear of fatness (over-valued idea) Thoughts and actions are not recognized by patient as excessive or unreasonable and are not resisted (ego-syntonic). Thoughts do not necessarily provoke, nor do actions reduce, distress.
Personality disorder with prominent features of anankastia (see Chapter 18)	Enduring behaviour pattern of: 1. Perfectionism, which can manifest as hyperscheduling, emphasis on neatness and a focus on following social rules. 2. Emotional and behavioural constraint. This includes stubbornness and inflexibility, risk avoidance and tightly controlling emotional expression. No true obsessions or compulsions, and the behaviours noted are ego-syntonic (i.e., acceptable to the individual).
Autism spectrum disorder (see Chapter 8)	Restricted, stereotyped interests, typically related to physical aspects of objects or to classification and collecting. Pleasurable, not viewed as unreasonable, not resisted. Repetitive behaviours (e.g., rocking or hand-flapping) are performed to gain or reduce sensory input, not to reduce anxiety following an obsessional thought. Associated features are impairments in communication and social understanding.
Depressive disorder (see Chapter 11)	Obsessive-compulsive symptoms occur simultaneously with, or after the onset of, depression and resolve with treatment. Obsessions are mood-congruent (e.g., ruminative thoughts of worthlessness).
Other anxiety disorders (see Chapter 12)	Phobias: provoking stimulus comes from external object or situation rather than patient's own mind. Generalized anxiety disorder: excessive concerns about real-life circumstances. Absence of genuine obsessions or compulsions.
Schizophrenia (see Chapter 9)	Thought insertion: patients believe that thoughts are not from their own mind. Delusion: patients to do not attempt to resist thought. Presence of other schizophrenic symptoms Lack of insight.
Impulse-control disorders, e.g., gambling disorder, kleptomania, pyromania (see Chapter 22)	Repetitious impulses and behaviour (gambling, stealing, setting fires) with no other unrelated obsessions/compulsions. Concordant with the patient's own wishes (therefore ego-syntonic).
Tourette syndrome (see Chapter 8)[b]	Motor and vocal tics, echolalia, coprolalia which are nonintentional and not aimed at counteracting obsessions.

[a]There is a higher incidence of true OCD in patients with anorexia nervosa.
[b]35%–50% of patients with Tourette syndrome meet the diagnostic criteria for OCD, whereas only 5%–7% of patients with OCD have Tourette syndrome.

Overlap with depression

You should always consider depression in patients with obsessions or compulsions because:

- Over 20% of depressed patients have obsessive-compulsive symptoms, which occur at or after the onset of depression. They invariably resolve with treatment of the depression.
- Over two-thirds of patients with OCD experience a depressive episode in their lifetime. Obsessions and compulsions are present before and persist after the treatment of depression.
- OCD is a disabling illness and patients often have chronic mild depressive symptoms that do not fully meet the criteria for a depressive episode. These symptoms usually resolve when the OCD is treated and the patient's quality of life improves.

DISCUSSION OF CASE STUDY

OC has genuine obsessions (recurrent, intrusive thoughts that are distressing, resisted and recognized as being from their own mind) and compulsions (repeatedly and excessively seeking reassurance to relieve anxiety caused by obsessions). They also describe symptoms of depression (depressed mood and weight loss).

Their most likely diagnosis is OCD; however, it is important to consider depression. In this case, the depressed mood developed after the obsessive-compulsive symptoms. If OC now also meets the criteria for a depressive episode, then both OCD and depression would be diagnosed.

Now go on to Chapter 25 to read about OCD and its management.

● Chapter Summary

- An obsession is a recurrent, intrusive, unpleasant, resisted thought experienced as arising from within someone's own mind.
- A compulsion is an irrational or excessive mental operation or physical action performed to reduce anxiety triggered by an obsession.
- Body dysmorphic disorder is characterized by a persistent preoccupation with perceived defects or flaws in an individual's own appearance.
- Obsession-like symptoms often arise in other psychiatric disorders: taking a careful history of the nature of the recurrent thought is important.
- Depression is often comorbid with obsessive-compulsive disorder.

UKMLA Conditions
Anxiety
OCD
Phobias

UKMLA Presentations
Anxiety
Medically unexplained symptoms
OCD
Phobias
Somatization

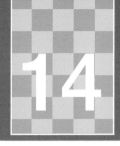

Case summary

28 year old PT was referred to a psychiatrist. They were well and working as a cleaner until 3 months ago when, on their way to work one evening, two men cornered them at a secluded bus shelter. They pushed PT to the ground and attempted to rob them. The men ran off when they heard someone approaching, leaving PT shaken but with only superficial cuts and bruises. They felt low in mood for a few days after the assault but attempted to carry on with their job and forget what had happened. In the month that followed, PT avoided all attempts by their family and friends to talk about the incident. They became socially withdrawn, only leaving the house to go to work. After a month, they started having nightmares about the incident and would wake up drenched in sweat. Their work colleagues noticed that they had become 'jumpy and quick-tempered' and that sudden movements or noises startled them. They had also started avoiding public transportation and refused to watch television for fear that something might remind them of the attack. PT finally sought medical help after their work supervisor found them lying on the floor, seemingly in a trance, screaming 'Leave me alone!' repeatedly. They recounted to their psychiatrist how they 'relived' the attack in their mind and thought they could hear the men threatening them, just like they did during the incident. The psychiatrist noticed that PT could not recall certain important aspects of the assault.

For a discussion of the case study, see the end of the chapter.

It is normal to have some psychological symptoms after a stressful event or bereavement. However, in some cases, these symptoms may be more severe than expected and impact upon everyday functioning. It is important to be able to distinguish what might be a normal reaction to a difficult life event from a specific constellation of symptoms that denote psychopathology requiring clinical attention.

DEFINITIONS AND CLINICAL FEATURES

When assessing someone who may have had a pathological response to a stressful event, it is important to explore two variables: (1) the nature and severity of the life event; and (2) the nature and severity of the person's reaction to the life event.

Nature and severity of the life event

Stress

'Psychosocial stressor' is the term used for any life event, condition or circumstance that places a strain on a person's current coping skills. It is important to remember that what constitutes a 'stressor' is subjective, and dependent on the specific person's ability to adapt or respond to a specific life challenge. For example, one student may breeze through an exam without experiencing any stress, whereas another may feel incredibly strained because of a perceived (or actual) mismatch between their ability and the demands of the situation. Also note that the same person's coping skills vary throughout their developmental life: the death of a distant relative may be far more stressful for a middle-aged man contemplating his own mortality than for an 'invincible' adolescent.

COMMUNICATION

Whenever a patient presents with low mood or anxiety, always check for possible psychosocial stressors and establish how (if at all) they relate to the onset of symptoms. If the stressor seemed insignificant, verify how it was perceived by the patient. Remember, a seemingly innocuous life event may be a significant psychosocial stressor for a vulnerable patient (e.g., a change of accommodation for an elderly widow).

Traumatic stress

A traumatic stressor occurs outside the range of normal human experience, and its magnitude means that it would be experienced as traumatic by most people. This type of stress occurs in situations where a person feels that their own (or a loved one's) physical or psychological integrity is under serious threat. Examples of these situations include natural disasters, physical or sexual assaults, serious road traffic accidents, terrorist attacks, torture and military combat. Bereavement is a special case of traumatic stress that will be discussed later in the chapter.

Nature and severity of patient's reaction

Some people seem to experience few symptoms following a stressful or traumatic life event while others seem more susceptible to developing a pathological response. Depending on the severity of the stressor and the person's underlying vulnerability, a patient may develop: (1) an acute stress reaction; (2) an adjustment disorder; (3) a post-traumatic stress disorder (PTSD); or a complex post-traumatic stress disorder (complex-PTSD) (4) a dissociative disorder; or (5) another major mental illness such as a depressive, anxiety or psychotic disorder. Substance misuse is also common after experiencing a traumatic event.

Acute stress reaction

In the ICD-11 an acute stress reaction is no longer classified as a mental disorder, and has been moved to the subsection of the manual that covers other reasons for clinical encounters that are not related to diseases or disorders. It is felt that an acute stress reaction represents a reaction on the spectrum of 'normal' responses to a significantly stressful life event. The DSM-5 specifies that it should only be diagnosed if the symptoms persist for more than 3 days. The symptoms of an acute stress reaction develop within hours of a traumatic stressor and typically, they subside within a few days. Presentations can vary and people can present with transient symptoms including being in a daze, confusion, reduced or increased activity levels and autonomic symptoms of anxiety. If the symptoms persist for more than 1 month, an alternative diagnosis should be considered.

Adjustment disorder

Feeling unable to cope is common at times of psychosocial stress requiring adjustment or adaptation (such as divorce, moving house, changing job or becoming a parent). However, when preoccupation with the stress is significant enough to cause disturbance to social or occupational functioning, this can be described as an adjustment disorder. For this diagnosis to be made, the emotional and/or behavioural symptoms need to occur within 1 month of the original stressor. It is not the nature of the event that matters but the person's preoccupation with it (in contrast to PTSD, the event does not need to have been of a seriously threatening or horrific nature for a diagnosis of adjustment disorder to be made). The person may present as excessively worried about the event, with recurrent and distressing thoughts about it, or constantly ruminating about it. The person may also experience mood and/or anxiety symptoms, but crucially these symptoms do not meet the threshold for a separate diagnosis of a mood or anxiety disorder. Some people with adjustment disorder can also experience suicidal ideation and there might also be an increase in conduct disturbance, e.g., substance use, particularly in adolescents. In older adults, adjustment disorder is more likely to be characterized by preoccupation with physical health, with the person reporting health anxieties and somatization symptoms. Younger children may also present with somatic symptoms such as headaches and abdominal pain, or alternatively they might present with disruptive behaviours such as tantrums and increased clinginess. Although it is assumed that the disorder would not have arisen without the original stressor, an individual's personality and vulnerability to stress play an important contributing role. Symptoms usually fully resolve within 6 months of onset, and if this is not the case, consideration should be given to a different diagnosis.

> **HINTS AND TIPS**
>
> You should only diagnose an adjustment disorder when patients do not meet the criteria for a more specific diagnosis such as a mood, psychotic or anxiety disorder (including post-traumatic stress disorder), or a normal bereavement reaction.

Post-traumatic stress disorder

The symptoms of PTSD develop in response to an extreme event or stressor and can occur at any point following exposure to the traumatic event. Typically, they occur within 3 months of the traumatic event. The key information required for diagnosis is what the person's subjective experience of the event is (did they perceive their physical or psychological integrity as under serious threat?), and the resulting constellation of symptoms that they experience following it.

There are three core features of PTSD. The presence of all three symptoms is essential to make a diagnosis. The features are as follows:

1. *Re-experiencing the traumatic event in the here and now.* This can take the form of:
   - Vivid, intrusive images and memories of the event (flashbacks).
   - Dreams and nightmares related to the traumatic event.
   - Experiencing intense emotions and physical sensations, that can be overwhelming, e.g., fear or re-experiencing the emotions that occurred at the time of the traumatic event.
2. *Intentional avoidance of things that are reminders of the traumatic event:*

- Avoidance of thoughts or memories associated with the event in the internal space.
- Avoidance of external things that trigger memories or thoughts of the traumatic event, e.g., certain people, places, activities or conversation topics.
- In more extreme presentations, the person might move to a new area, or seek alternative employment in order to avoid reminders of the traumatic event.
3. *Increased arousal or perception of threat:*
    - A heightened startle reaction or hypervigilance.
    - Adopting new behaviours that help the person feel safe, e.g., checking doors and locks repeatedly, never sitting with their back to the door.

The above symptoms must also be severe enough to impact the person's functioning, and often they cause the person significant distress. The biggest risk factor for PTSD is an experience of past trauma, particularly during childhood. It is also more common in females, and females are also more likely to experience symptoms for longer.

Complex post-traumatic stress disorder

Complex post-traumatic stress disorder (complex PTSD) develops in response to an event, or repeated events, that are threatening and horrific in nature. Often, the types of experience that result in the person developing complex PTSD are more severe, or occur for prolonged periods of time, compared to experiences that result in a person developing PTSD. Examples include, but are not limited to, prolonged torture, concentration camps, genocide and repeated childhood physical or sexual abuse. In addition to the three core symptoms of PTSD (re-experiencing, deliberate avoidance and persistent perception of heightened threat), persons with complex PTSD also display severe and sustained difficulties with:

1. *Affect regulation*: the person becomes more reactive to minor stressors and can experience violent outbursts. They can also display self-destructive behaviours, emotional numbing and dissociative symptoms, particularly when under stress.
2. *Developing and sustaining relationships with other people.*
3. *Self-view*: people may have a distorted view of themselves, for example, feeling they are worthless, or they may experience feelings of guilt and/or failure related to the traumatic event.

In addition to the essential features mentioned earlier, complex PTSD is also associated with suicidal ideation, substance use and symptoms of depression and occasionally, psychosis. There is a lot of overlap between the symptoms of complex PTSD and other psychiatric disorders, in particular personality disorders with a borderline pattern (see Chapter 18). Often, people may meet diagnostic criteria for both complex PTSD and personality disorder.

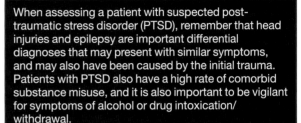

RED FLAG

When assessing a patient with suspected post-traumatic stress disorder (PTSD), remember that head injuries and epilepsy are important differential diagnoses that may present with similar symptoms, and may also have been caused by the initial trauma. Patients with PTSD also have a high rate of comorbid substance misuse, and it is also important to be vigilant for symptoms of alcohol or drug intoxication/withdrawal.

COMMUNICATION

Not everyone who tells you they are 'traumatised' has post-traumatic stress disorder (PTSD): PTSD is only diagnosed following an event which the majority of people would experience as life-threatening or catastrophic to themselves or to their loved ones. For example, domestic violence, rather than a relationship break-up.

Dissociation

In psychiatry, 'dissociation' describes an involuntary disruption in the usually integrated functions of consciousness and cognition. In this phenomenon, memories of the past, awareness of identity, thoughts, emotions, movement, sensation and/or control of behaviour become separated from the rest of an individual's personality and are not under voluntary control. The disruption can be complete or partial and there is a huge variety in the length of the dissociative experience, ranging from hours to years depending on the specific disorder. In contrast to the ICD-10, the ICD-11 does not require a person to have experienced a stressor or trauma prior to developing dissociative symptoms, but it is important to remember that stress and trauma remain important aetiological factors in the development of dissociative symptoms.

HINTS AND TIPS

Depersonalization is feeling yourself to be strange or unreal. Derealization is feeling that external reality is strange or unreal. These can be considered as types of dissociation, and may be caused by psychiatric illness (e.g., depression, anxiety, schizophrenia), physical illness (e.g., epilepsy), psychosocial stress and substance abuse.

Of note, the DSM-5 classifies dissociative memory symptoms with dissociative disorders and dissociative neurological symptoms as somatic disorders. The shifting classification system reflects shifts in understanding of the causes of these syndromes. They are now falling more under the umbrella of 'medically unexplained symptoms' and of 'functional symptoms'.

There are several brain networks that are thought to be associated with the development of dissociative symptoms. Rather than a purely psychological causation, it is now thought that dysfunction in high-level cortical processing of motor and sensory information can lead to symptoms which are genuinely experienced, involuntary and not necessarily related to past or current trauma, even though no structural or physiological abnormality is identified.

Dissociative disorders should not be diagnosed if there is evidence of a physical or psychiatric disorder that plausibly explains the symptoms. In addition to assessing for evidence of known physical disorders, it is also useful to check for positive signs of functional neurological disorder (see Table 14.1). If present, these strengthen the evidence for a functional (dissociative) neurological condition. However, if in doubt it is safest to ask a neurologist for their opinion too.

In the ICD-11, there are several different diagnostic categories of dissociative disorder. These include:

1. Dissociative neurological symptom disorders. In order for a diagnosis of dissociative neurological symptom disorder to be made, there needs to be involuntary disruption to the person's cognitive, motor or sensory functioning for a period of at least several hours. The symptoms must not correspond with known neurological patterns, or anatomic dermatomes (if the symptoms are sensory). The ICD-11 has various symptom specifiers as follows:
   - with visual disturbance
   - with auditory disturbance
   - with vertigo or dizziness
   - with other sensory disturbance
   - with non-epileptic seizures (previously known as "pseudo-seizures" and sometimes called "functional seizures" or "non-epileptic seizures" in clinical practice)
   - with speech disturbance
   - with paresis or weakness
   - with gait disturbance
   - with movement disturbance (this category includes functional tremor).
   - with cognitive symptoms.

2. Dissociative amnesia: this disorder is characterized by the person having the inability to recall autobiographical memories, particularly those related to a recent traumatic event. The person can often be unaware of their memory loss and they cannot voluntarily recall memories of the specific event, although they can still experience dreams and flashbacks to the event. A subtype of dissociative amnesia is a dissociative fugue, where a person experiences a sudden loss of their identity, and is commonly associated with them suddenly travelling away from the area where they work or live. Other cognitive functions are unaffected, e.g., language, problem-solving skills.

3. Trance disorder and possession trance disorder: in these disorders the person enters a trance state and they experience altered consciousness. Trance-possession disorder is associated with the person's personal identity being replaced with a 'possessing' entity. These experiences can occur as part of some peoples' normal religious and cultural practices, so in order to make the diagnosis it must be a distressing, involuntary experience outside of the person's cultural and religious norms.

4. Depersonalization–derealization disorder: depersonalization is where a person experiences themselves as strange or unreal and derealization is where the person experiences the world around them as strange or unreal. Episodes can also be associated with an altered sense of time. A diagnosis is made when a person experiences either or both depersonalization and derealization, and the symptoms have an impact on their functioning.

5. Dissociative identity disorder: the ICD-11 and the DSM-5 both include dissociative identity disorder, previously referred to as multiple personality disorder in the ICD-10. People with dissociative identity disorder experience two or more distinct personalities, with each personality having its own experience of the person's self, body and environment. Each personality takes control of the person's consciousness, and typically there are episodes of amnesia associated with the different personalities.

Table 14.1 Some positive signs of functional neurological disorders

Disorder	Signs
Dissociative neurological symptom disorder, with non-epileptic seizures (functional seizures)	Eyes shut, resisting opening. Ictal or postictal weeping. Long duration. Memory of ictal events (e.g., 'I was shaking all over').
Dissociative neurological symptom disorder, with paresis or weakness	Hoover sign. A 'give way' quality to the weakness. A limb that when left suspended in the air 'hovers' for a moment before falling.
Dissociative neurological symptom disorder, with other sensory disturbance	Nondermatomal pattern of sensory loss (e.g., sensory abnormalities that stop at the groin or shoulder).
Dissociative neurological symptom disorder, with movement disturbance (functional tremor)	Entrainment (i.e., the tremor frequency aligns with that of a voluntary rhythmic movement). Stops with distraction (e.g., mental arithmetic). Worsens when attempts made to immobilize (e.g., if limb held onto by examiner).

Dissociative identity disorder generally occurs in people who have experienced significant trauma, with shifts in personality occurring in response to stressful events, both related and unrelated to the original traumatic event. People with dissociative identity disorder are also at high risk of self-harm and suicidal behaviours.

HINTS AND TIPS

Interviewing someone who knows the patient well, such as friends or family members, can be helpful as part of your clinical assessment of dissociative symptoms, particularly if there is amnesia present.

RED FLAG

Before accepting the diagnosis of a dissociative disorder, a neurological or other psychiatric disorder should be carefully sought for and adequately excluded (see Fig. 15.1).

HINTS AND TIPS

Although dissociative disorders are covered in this chapter, around one in three functional neurological disorders arise in the absence of a stressor.

HINTS AND TIPS

The Hoover sign is weakness of hip extension which returns to normal with contralateral hip flexion against resistance. This can be demonstrated to the patient to reassure them that it is a problem with muscle control, not structure, which is causing their leg weakness.

Precipitation or exacerbation of an existing mental illness

The influence of a patient's environment on their mental health cannot be overemphasised. Almost all forms of mental illness

(e.g., depression, psychotic illness, anxiety) can be precipitated or exacerbated by psychosocial ('life events') or traumatic stressors.

BEREAVEMENT

Bereavement is a unique kind of stress experienced by most people during their life and is a normal human experience. A bereavement reaction usually occurs after the loss of a loved person, but can also result from other losses, like the loss of a national figure or a beloved pet. The normal course of grief after bereavement occurs in five phases (Fig. 14.1), although these should not be regarded as a rigid sequence that is passed through only once. Each response to bereavement is unique to the person, and will vary greatly in severity, duration and content.

HINTS AND TIPS

The length of a bereavement reaction is variable and tends to be longer if the death was sudden and unexpected. There is also significant variety in lengths of bereavement reaction within different cultural groups, so asking a person's family or friends, who are familiar with their culture, whether their reaction is atypical, can be helpful.

Although most people will meet the criteria for a depressive episode at some stage during the grieving process, bereavement reactions are not pathological, so no psychiatric diagnosis should be made. However, patients who have been bereaved are at higher risk for developing a severe depressive illness requiring treatment. The DSM-5 now suggests that bereaved people meeting criteria for a depressive episode should be assessed and treated as normal. Although the shift is away from defining 'normal' or 'abnormal' grief reactions, both the DSM-5 and the ICD-11 do include an option to describe extremely prolonged and intense grief (causing significant functional impairment) as a disorder. Table 14.2 compares symptoms suggested by the DSM-5 that may help to distinguish depression from bereavement.

Prolonged grief disorder

Prolonged grief is where a person continues to experience an intense grief reaction for a longer period of time than would be expected within their culture. It should not be diagnosed within the first 6 months of a bereavement. The person may report feelings of intense emotional pain, including sadness, guilt, anger and longing for the deceased person. These emotional responses

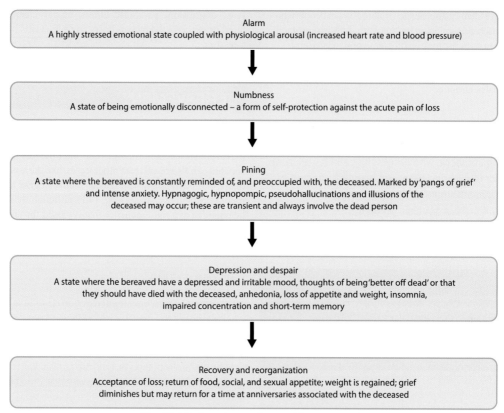

Fig. 14.1 Parkes stages of normal bereavement.

are common within earlier stages of a grief reaction, but usually they start to decrease in intensity as time passes. The person may also become preoccupied with the deceased person, which can take the form of focusing on the circumstances of the deceased persons death, or adopting behaviours focused on preserving possessions of the deceased so they remain unchanged from how they were before their death.

DIFFERENTIAL DIAGNOSIS

Following thorough exploration of the nature and severity of both the life event and patient's reaction, the diagnosis is usually clear (see Box 14.1 and Fig. 12.3 for a diagnostic algorithm). Major mental illnesses are often triggered by major stressors. Even if the onset of symptoms is clearly linked with a stressor, diagnosis of a specific major mental illness (mood disorder, psychotic disorder) should be given if diagnostic criteria are met.

If a patient presents with psychiatric symptoms after a life-threatening event, always screen for features of depression as well as features of PTSD. This is because the risk for developing depression increases sixfold in the 6 months that follow a stressful event.

> **HINTS AND TIPS**
>
> You may read notes or hear patients talk about diagnoses that were different in the ICD-10. For reactions to stress, differences in the ICD-10 include:
>
> - Acute stress reaction was a psychiatric diagnosis.
> - Complex PTSD was not a diagnosis.
> - Prolonged grief disorder was not a diagnosis.

DISCUSSION OF CASE STUDY

PT experienced a traumatic stressor in which they believed that their physical integrity was under immediate threat. The event was outside the range of normal human experience and

Table 14.2 Distinguishing depression from grief

	Depression	Bereavement
Mood symptoms	Pervasively low and anhedonic	Feeling empty and lost, but also able to experience positive emotions
Variation	Diurnal, worse in morning	Triggered by reminders of deceased
Cognitions	Guilt, worthlessness	Self-esteem intact, preoccupied with deceased
Suicidal thoughts	With intent to end a worthless, pointless or unbearable existence	With intent to join the deceased or end the pain of unbearable existence
Psychotic symptoms	Mood-congruent, persistent	Transient hallucinations of the deceased
Motor function	Psychomotor retardation in severe cases	Intact

BOX 14.1 DIFFERENTIAL DIAGNOSIS FOR PATIENTS PRESENTING WITH A REACTION TO STRESS OR TRAUMA

Acute stress reaction

Adjustment disorder

Post-traumatic stress disorder

Complex post-traumatic stress disorder

Normal bereavement reaction

Prolonged grief disorder

Dissociative disorder

Exacerbation or precipitation of other psychiatric illness:

- Mood disorders
- Anxiety disorders
- Psychotic disorders (especially acute and transient psychotic disorders)
- Substance use disorders

Malingering or factitious disorder (see Chapter 15)

would have been experienced as traumatic by most people. They subsequently developed avoidance of stimuli associated with the trauma (avoided talking or thinking about it, avoided public transportation and television), amnesia for aspects of the trauma and social withdrawal. Later on, they showed signs of increased arousal (startle response, being 'jumpy and quick-tempered'). Finally, PT repetitively reexperienced the trauma through nightmares, flashbacks and dissociation (reliving and behaving as though the trauma were occurring at that moment through mental imagery and hallucinations). All of the above suggest a diagnosis of PTSD.

Now go on to Chapter 25 to read about the anxiety- and stress-related disorders and their management.

Chapter Summary

- Unpleasant responses to stressful events such as bereavement are normal and generally not pathological.
- Life-threatening or potentially catastrophic trauma can lead to post-traumatic stress disorder (PTSD) in vulnerable individuals.
- The three core features of PTSD are: reexperiencing, deliberate avoidance and persistent perception of heightened threat. Complex PTSD comprises the core features of PTSD plus additional features of problems with affect regulation, relationships and beliefs about oneself.
- Dissociative disorders are when the normal integration of consciousness with cognition is disrupted.
- Dissociative disorders can disrupt motor, sensory and memory function. A subset is termed 'functional neurological disorders'.
- Bereavement does not exclude the diagnosis of depression.

UKMLA Conditions
Acute stress reaction
Anxiety disorder (post-traumatic stress disorder)
Personality disorder

UKMLA Presentations
Behaviour/personality change
Child abuse
Low mood/affective problems
Memory loss
Sleep problems
Somatization/medically unexplained symptoms
Substance misuse
Suicidal thoughts

FURTHER READING

Good explanation and advice regarding functional neurological symptoms www.neurosymptoms.org.

Description of functional facial weakness: BBC Radio 4 Inside Health 10th Oct 2012 along with a commentary. www.bbc.co.uk/programmes/b01n65zl.

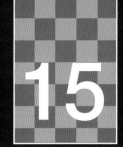
Case summary

Mrs SD, a 32-year-old shop assistant, had consulted her general practitioner (GP) at least once every 2 weeks for the past year. Her GP had known her for just over a year since she moved to the area after an acrimonious divorce. Her medical history, part of which was obtained from her previous GP, was substantial, and her health difficulties had precluded her from employment. At menarche, she was diagnosed with dysfunctional uterine bleeding and dysmenorrhoea. Extensive investigations, including three exploratory laparoscopies, revealed no physical cause for persistent upper abdominal pain with alternating diarrhoea and constipation. Three years ago, Mrs SD presented with urinary frequency and dysuria. Exhaustive investigations including cystoscopy, urodynamic studies and radiography, were all normal. She had also been referred to various specialists including a rheumatologist due to chronic neck pain that she had described as: 'the pain that has ruined my life!' She has not worked for several months due to the pain. Again, physical examination and investigations revealed no abnormalities. Mrs SD was taking up to 30 codeine tablets daily and could not sleep without two different types of sleeping tablets.

For a discussion of the case study, see the end of the chapter.

Medically unexplained symptoms (symptoms where no cause can be found despite adequate investigation) are a common clinical problem, representing around a third of medical outpatient appointments and a large proportion of primary care appointments. Patients with such symptoms are often stigmatized by healthcare providers, with their genuine difficulties being labelled as 'all in the mind' or 'the worried well'. Understanding the psychiatric disorders leading patients to have unusual physical symptoms or an abnormal response to physical symptoms is invaluable for all junior doctors.

COMMUNICATION

Many of the terms used for medically unexplained symptoms are perceived as stigmatizing but the term *functional symptoms* is acceptable to most patients and colleagues. Functional symptoms are those without identifiable structural cause. They can be likened to 'software' rather than 'hardware' problems in the body.

DEFINITIONS AND CLINICAL FEATURES

A structural or physical cause should always be considered in response to reported 'physical symptoms'. However, in certain cases, the reported symptoms are medically unexplained, that is they:

- do not correspond to or are clearly not typical of any known physical condition;
- are associated with an absence of any physical signs or structural abnormalities;
- are associated with an absence of any abnormalities in comprehensive laboratory, imaging and invasive investigations.

Medically unexplained symptoms represent a large and diverse group of symptoms and underlying difficulties:

- It is likely that some disorders for which no medical cause can be found are still secondary to 'physical aetiology' – subtle presentations of a disorder yet to fully manifest or a vanishingly rare genetic disorder, toxin or occult infection which can never be detected.
- Some symptoms are recognized to arise as part of a common syndrome, without associated structural abnormalities, but with unclear aetiology. These are generally now termed 'functional disorders'. For example, fibromyalgia, irritable bowel syndrome or dissociative disorders (see Chapter 14).
- Some symptoms are associated with undue distress, causing a high degree of anxiety and impairment despite reassurance and beyond what would be a normal response to a given symptom. These disorders of bodily experience are the focus of this chapter.

Table 15.1 Functional disorders affecting individual systems

System	Disorder
Cardiovascular	Atypical chest pain
Respiratory	Hyperventilation
Gastrointestinal	Irritable bowel syndrome
Neurological	Dissociative seizures, weakness and sensory symptoms (see Chapter 14)
Rheumatology	Fibromyalgia
Infectious diseases	Chronic fatigue syndrome

It is worth noting that even though no structural or physiological disease has been identified, it does not mean that one does not exist – it may remain thus far undiscovered by medical science. For example: epilepsy, migraine, multiple sclerosis and stomach ulcers were historically considered 'functional' illnesses. See Table 15.1 for a (non-exhaustive) list of what are currently termed functional disorders.

It is also worth noting that many patients with medically unexplained symptoms will be reassured by normal investigations or an explanation that they are functional symptoms which are likely to get better. Those patients who are unable to accept reassurance may have a psychiatric disorder.

Disorders of bodily distress or bodily experience

Bodily distress disorder

Bodily distress disorder has the following diagnostic features in ICD-11:

1. The patient experiences bodily symptoms that are distressing to them (the exact nature of these may vary over time).
2. Patients are persistently preoccupied on these symptoms and what they may mean (often leading to frequent contact with health professionals beyond that which could be considered medically necessary).
3. Neither the severity of the symptoms nor the amount of attention directed towards them is fully explained by an underlying medical condition.
4. Patients remain concerned even when examinations or investigations show no underlying physical cause.
5. Some sort of distressing bodily symptom is present on most days for at least several months (the symptoms may vary).
6. The distressing symptoms are associated with significant functional impact.

It is normal to experience occasional bodily symptoms which are concerning: in bodily distress disorder the degree and persistence of distress is out of proportion to the symptoms. Similarly, patients may have a comorbid physical health condition (e.g.,

mild asthma), but feel unduly preoccupied about the risks of this (e.g., to the point of having regular episodes of hyperventilation or of never wanting to go outside to minimise air pollution exposure). The bodily symptoms are not under voluntary control: they occur unintentionally, as opposed to the intentional feigning or production of symptoms in factitious disorder and malingering.

COMMUNICATION

It is important to acknowledge that even though no physical pathology has been found, the functional impairment and distress caused by bodily distress disorder are genuine and that the symptoms are neither under conscious control nor are they being feigned. Empathic acknowledgement and explanation can be very therapeutic in itself. Dismissing a patient by telling them that their symptoms are 'all in your mind' is unhelpful and potentially harmful.

The most commonly experienced symptoms in bodily distress disorder are pain (e.g., musculoskeletal pain, headaches), fatigue, gastrointestinal symptoms (e.g., abdominal pain, constipation/diarrhoea), cardiovascular (e.g., chest pain) or respiratory symptoms (e.g., hyperventilation).

Bodily distress disorder can be classified as mild, moderate or severe:

- Mild: the patient spends a limited amount of time focusing on symptoms and there is only mild impairment of their usual functioning.
- Moderate: the patient is persistently preoccupied with their symptoms (for at least several hours a day) and there is moderate impairment of functioning. They make frequent visits to healthcare services.
- Severe: focus on symptoms becomes the primary focus of the patient's life and they have extensive contact with health services. There is severe impairment of the patients' usual functioning.

HINTS AND TIPS

Health-seeking behaviours in bodily distress disorder:
- Present in general medical rather than mental health settings
- Reluctant to accept possibility of psychological component to their experience
- Dissatisfaction with previous care
- Change health providers frequently

Body integrity dysphoria

Body integrity dysphoria is a new diagnosis in the ICD-11. It is an extremely rare condition where a patient has an intense and persistent desire to become physically disabled, and may attempt to intentionally make themselves disabled. They may also simulate behaviours associated with the disability such as using crutches or a wheelchair.

HINTS AND TIPS

You may read notes or hear patients talk about diagnoses that were different in the ICD-10. For medically unexplained symptoms, differences in the ICD-10 include:

- Bodily distress disorder has replaced a cluster of 'somatoform disorders' of which the commonest diagnosis was somatization disorder.
- Neurasthenia has now been combined with bodily distress disorder.
- Hypochondriasis was classed as a somatoform disorder, it is now classified as an OCD-related disorder.
- Body dysmorphic disorder did not exist as a disorder.
- Dissociative disorder subtypes were a little different and 'conversion' was included in the diagnosis name.

Obsessive-compulsive disorder-related disorders

Two disorders related to obsessive-compulsive disorder (OCD) can present with medically unexplained symptoms. The psychopathology in both takes the form of intrusive thoughts. They are briefly covered below and also in Chapter 13.

Hypochondriacal disorder

In hypochondriacal disorder, patients misinterpret normal bodily sensations, which lead them to believe that they have a serious and progressive physical disease. These patients tend to ask for investigations to definitively diagnose or confirm their underlying disease. However, despite repeated normal examination and investigations, hypochondriacal patients refuse to accept the reassurance of numerous doctors that they do not suffer from a serious physical illness – although they are often reassured for a short while. This is in contrast to bodily distress disorder, where patients are seeking relief from their symptoms and normal investigations are very rarely reassuring even temporarily.

Body dysmorphic disorder

Body dysmorphic disorder is when someone is persistently preoccupied with a perceived defect or flaw in their personal appearance. Objectively the perceived flaw is absent or very minor. The nose is a common area of preoccupation but any body part can be involved. The preoccupation causes significant distress or functional impairment. Patients may seek surgical procedures to reverse the perceived flaw.

Functional and dissociative disorders

These two types of disorders are closely related, and their classification is evolving rapidly. *Conversion* is a psychoanalytical term that describes the hypothetical process whereby psychic conflict or pain undergoes 'conversion' into somatic or physical form to produce physical symptoms. The DSM-5 uses this term interchangeably with 'functional neurological symptom disorder', although a recent stressor is not required for the diagnosis, whereas ICD-11 considers these to be dissociative disorders and no longer uses the term 'conversion'. This book describes these in Chapter 14. See also Table 15.1. The details of these individual conditions are not covered here.

Factitious disorder

In factitious disorder patients intend to convince medical professionals that they have certain symptoms, either through falsifying symptoms, trying to intentionally induce them or aggravating more mild symptoms. Patients may give convincing histories that fool even experienced clinicians and often manufacture signs (e.g., warfarin may be ingested to simulate bleeding disorders, insulin may be injected to produce hypoglycaemia, urine may be contaminated with blood or faeces, etc.). Certain patients feign psychiatric symptoms such as hallucinations, delusions, depression or dissociation. The central feature of factitious disorder is focus on the primary (internal) gain of assuming the sick role (the aim to be cared for like a patient, usually in hospital). Often patients have a history of studying or working in healthcare-related fields. This is an uncomfortable but important diagnosis to make and collateral history is crucial.

Although symptoms are feigned, it is important to understand that this care-seeking behaviour is usually a manifestation of psychological distress.

There are two different subtypes:
- Factitious disorder imposed on self: the patient is attempting to falsify symptoms in themselves.
- Factitious disorder imposed on another: the patient is attempting to falsify symptoms in another, most commonly a parent trying to create symptoms in a child.

HINTS AND TIPS

Munchausen syndrome is an unofficial diagnostic term often used synonymously and interchangeably with factitious disorder. Strictly, Munchausen syndrome refers to a subgroup of patients with factitious disorder imposed on self who travel between hospitals and care providers (peregrination), often giving different names and details. Munchausen syndrome by proxy (factitious disorder imposed on another) is when the symptoms are imposed on another person under their care, typically a child. The syndrome's name derives from Rudolf Erich Raspe's literary character, Baron Munchausen, a well-known teller of fantastic and implausible stories about his travels and adventures.

HINTS AND TIPS

Clinical features that should prompt consideration of factitious disorder:

- Evidence of feigning/inducing/falsifying symptoms identified (e.g., foreign objects placed in wounds)
- Course of illness does not follow usual natural history (e.g., antibiotics not working)
- Patient eagerly agrees to or requests invasive procedures or operations
- Multiple previous admissions with poor response to treatment
- Multiple consults with different specialties with no relevant cause for symptoms found

Malingering

Malingering patients focus on secondary (external) gain of the secondary consequence of being diagnosed with an illness (avoidance of military service, evading criminal prosecution, obtaining illicit drugs, obtaining benefits or compensation). It is not considered a mental illness.

DIFFERENTIAL DIAGNOSIS

The differential diagnosis for patients presenting with an abnormal response to physical symptoms is shown in Box 15.1.

BOX 15.1 DIFFERENTIAL DIAGNOSIS FOR PATIENTS PRESENTING WITH MEDICALLY UNEXPLAINED SYMPTOMS

- Undiagnosed unknown medical condition
- Undiagnosed known medical condition (e.g., insidious multisystem disease)
- Functional disorders (also known as dissociative disorders or conversion disorders)
- Bodily distress disorder
- OCD-related disorders
  - Hypochondriasis
  - Body dysmorphic disorder
- Factitious disorder
- Malingering
- Other psychiatric conditions
  - Anxiety disorders
  - Mood disorders
  - Psychotic disorders

The flow chart in Fig. 15.1 can help with reaching the correct diagnosis.

An underlying physical condition should be ruled out when patients present with physical symptoms. Bodily distress disorder can resemble insidious multisystem diseases such as systemic lupus erythematosus, multiple sclerosis, acquired immune deficiency syndrome, hyperparathyroidism, occult malignancy and chronic infections.

Physical complaints often occur in the context of other psychiatric conditions. Patients with schizophrenia may have somatic delusions or visceral somatic hallucinations. However, the explanation of these symptoms is often quite odd and there are usually other psychotic symptoms accompanying the physical complaints. Individuals with depressed mood often present with numerous somatic complaints; these tend to be episodic and resolve with the treatment of the depression. Patients with panic disorder have multiple somatic symptoms while having panic attacks, but these resolve when the panic subsides. Patients with generalised anxiety disorder may also have multiple somatic preoccupations, but their anxiety is not limited to physical symptoms. Dissociative disorders (e.g., motor disorders, nonepileptic seizures) can present with neurological symptoms without any evidence of a structural cause. However, these symptoms are usually clearly defined and isolated as opposed to the ill-defined, multiple symptoms in bodily distress disorder.

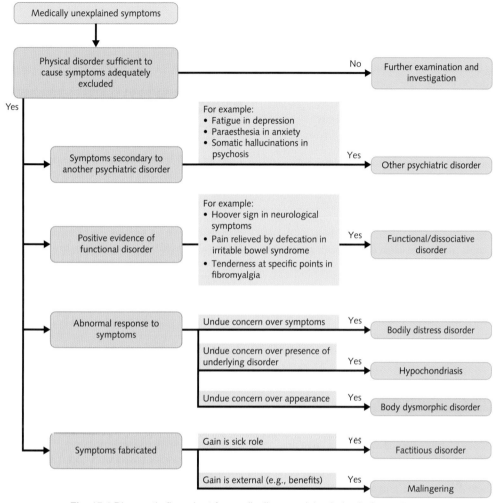

Fig. 15.1 Diagnostic flow chart for medically unexplained physical symptoms.

The difficulty in distinguishing other mental disorders from bodily distress disorder is illustrated by the observation that at least half of patients with bodily distress disorder have another coexisting mental illness.

RED FLAG

Bodily distress disorder usually has its onset in early adult life. The onset of multiple physical symptoms late in life is more likely to be due to a physical illness.

RED FLAG

In patients who present with unusual or unexplained physical symptoms, care should be taken to ensure there are no physical illnesses before a diagnosis such as bodily distress disorder is given. Particularly in those with a psychiatric history, there can be a tendency to blame any physical symptoms on the psychiatric illness, known as 'diagnostic overshadowing'.

ASSESSMENT

History

The following questions may be helpful in screening for bodily distress disorder on mental state examination:

- Do you often worry about your health?
- Are you bothered by many different symptoms?
- Are you concerned you may have a serious illness?
- Are you concerned about your appearance?
- Do you find it hard to believe doctors when they tell you that there is nothing wrong with you?

Examination

A thorough physical examination with special focus on the presenting problem is imperative when dealing with somatoform complaints.

Investigations

Clinicians dealing with patients with a bodily distress disorder need to investigate physical complaints judiciously. It is important to take all symptoms seriously, yet excessive and needless investigations to placate an anxious patient can result in a vicious circle with worsening of symptoms. Invasive investigations can result in iatrogenic harm. See Chapter 25 for guidance on management.

DISCUSSION OF CASE STUDY

Mrs SD has a long history of multiple, recurrent, frequently changing physical symptoms for which no physical causes have been found despite extensive investigation. She is unduly distressed by her symptoms (e.g., describing pain as 'ruining her life'). Her functioning has been impaired, and she is now unable to work. Because she is focused on symptoms, not the idea that she has a serious and progressive illness, Mrs SD has bodily distress disorder as opposed to hypochondriacal disorder. As is typical, Mrs SD has a secondary (possibly iatrogenic) substance misuse problem (codeine and sleeping tablets). It would be important to exclude other mental illness, such as depression and anxiety, as causative factors. If there was evidence that Mrs SD intentionally produced or feigned her symptoms, then factitious disorder or malingering should be considered.

Now go on to Chapter 25 to read about the bodily distress disorder and its management.

Chapter Summary

- Medically unexplained symptoms are common in all fields of medicine.
- In bodily distress disorder, patients have an abnormal response to physical symptoms.
- In functional/dissociative disorders, the normal integration of consciousness with cognition is disrupted, leading to disrupted sensory perception and motor control.
- In factitious disorder and malingering, patients feign physical symptoms.

UKMLA Condition
Somatization

UKMLA Presentations
Child abuse
Chronic abdominal pain
Fatigue
Somatization/medically unexplained physical symptoms

The patient with eating, feeding or weight problems

Case summary

Miss FD, a 19-year-old law student, eventually agreed to see a psychiatrist after much persuasion from her mother and general practitioner (GP). Her weight had fallen from 65 to 41 kg over the previous 6 months and she appeared emaciated. Her GP had measured her height at 1.65 metres and had calculated her body mass index (BMI) to be 15 kg/m^2. The psychiatrist saw Miss FD alone and spent some time putting her at ease. After an initial reluctance, she admitted that she was repulsed by the thought of being fat and felt that she was still overweight and needed to lose 'just a few more pounds'. She had stopped menstruating 4 months ago and had also noted that she was feeling tired and cold all the time and was finding it difficult to concentrate. The psychiatrist elicited that she only ate one small meal a day and was exercising to the point of almost collapsing. She denied binge eating or self-induced vomiting but did admit to using 20 senna tablets daily. She reported symptoms of depression, but no suicidal ideation. Physical examination revealed a pulse rate of 50 beats per minute and fine, downy hair covering her torso.

(For a discussion of the case study, see the end of the chapter.)

Many people are concerned about what they eat and how this affects their body weight and shape. However, some individuals become morbidly concerned with their body image to the point that their life revolves around the relentless pursuit of thinness. This life-threatening psychopathology needs to be distinguished from other physical, psychiatric or substance-associated causes of weight loss.

DEFINITIONS AND CLINICAL FEATURES

An eating disorder is characterised by abnormal eating behaviours, with an associated preoccupation with weight and shape. In feeding disorders, there are also abnormal eating behaviours present, but crucially they are not related to, or as a result of, concerns about weight and shape. It is important to exclude the presence of a medical condition or side effect of a medication (e.g., appetite suppression secondary to stimulant medication) prior to making the diagnosis of a feeding or eating disorder.

It is also important to ensure that the behaviour is considered within the developmental and cultural background of the patient, e.g., periods of fasting as part of religious and cultural practices would not represent abnormal eating behaviour for an individual from that cultural background.

Eating disorders

Anorexia nervosa and *bulimia nervosa* are two psychiatric disorders characterised by conscious and deliberate efforts to reduce body weight. Individuals with anorexia nervosa are significantly underweight, whereas weight in bulimia is generally normal, or slightly above normal. Binge-eating disorder is characterized by frequent and recurrent episodes of binge eating leading to significant functional impairment. Individuals with binge-eating disorder are often overweight or obese.

Anorexia nervosa

There are three key diagnostic features of anorexia nervosa:

1. *Significantly low body weight for the individual's age, height and developmental stage.* There are no absolute weight thresholds required for a diagnosis to be made and clinical judgement can be used for diagnosis. Commonly used thresholds to aid diagnosis applied by the ICD-11 include a body mass index (BMI) <18.5 in adults and <5th percentile in young people under the age of 18. However, if an individual displays rapid weight loss, e.g., >20% weight loss in a 6-month period, or a young person fails to gain weight as expected for their developmental stage and growth trajectory, a diagnosis of anorexia nervosa would still be appropriate.
2. *Persistent pattern of restrictive eating and other behaviours in an effort to establish and maintain low body weight.* Other behaviours can include purging, use of appetite suppressants, diuretics and laxatives and excessive exercise.
3. *Overvaluation and excessive preoccupation with weight and shape.* For individuals with anorexia nervosa, low body weight is overvalued, and having a low body weight becomes central to their sense of self. Individuals can also inaccurately perceive their body weight and shape, believing that they are overweight or a normal weight, when in fact they are underweight. Preoccupation with weight and shape can manifest as checking behaviours, e.g., regular weighing of self and calorie counting. It can also manifest as avoidant behaviours, e.g., covering mirrors and wearing oversized clothes.

BOX 16.1 THE BODY MASS INDEX

The body mass index (BMI) relates weight to height and is used as a crude test to assess nutritional status in patients who are fully grown.

$$BMI = \frac{\text{weight (kilograms)}}{\text{height (metres)}^2}$$

Morbid obesity	greater than 40 kg/m²
Obesity	greater than 30 kg/m²
Normal	20–25 kg/m²
Anorexia nervosa	less than or equal to 18.5 kg/m² (also apply clinical judgement)
High risk for medical complications	less than 13 kg/m²

The ranges of values listed above relate to adults and differ during growth and development. A BMI growth chart should be consulted for younger people.

In order for a diagnosis to be made, the above features need to have been present for at least several months.

Once the core features of anorexia nervosa have been established, there are weight and behaviour pattern specifiers that can be added to give further context to the diagnosis.

Weight specifiers
- Normal body weight (in recovery).
- Significantly low body weight (BMI 14–18.5 kg/m² for adults and 0.3–5th centile for young people under 18).
- Dangerously low body weight (BMI <14 kg/m² for adults and <0.3 centile for young people under 18).

Box 16.1 summarizes how to calculate BMI.

Behaviour pattern specifiers
- Restrictive: low food intake and/or excessive exercising.
- Binge-purge: presence of episodes of binge eating and/or purging.

In addition to the core diagnostic features of anorexia nervosa, individuals with anorexia will also have features of generalised endocrine disturbance of the hypothalamic–pituitary–gonadal axis. This can include amenorrhoea in postmenarcheal women; loss of sexual interest and impotency in men; raised growth hormone and cortisol levels; and reduced T_3. In prepubertal sufferers of anorexia, expected weight gain during the growth period can be impaired and pubertal events (menarche, breast and genital development) may be delayed or arrested.

Bulimia nervosa

In bulimia nervosa, patients usually have a normal or increased body weight. In addition to sharing similar over-valued ideas with anorexia nervosa, bulimia nervosa is characterised by a preoccupation with eating and an irresistible craving for food that results in binge eating. This is associated with a sense of lack of control and is invariably followed by feelings of shame and disgust. To counteract this caloric load, patients not only engage in purging (self-induced vomiting, laxative and diuretic use), fasting or excessive exercise but can also employ a number of ingenious, even dangerous, strategies (e.g., misuse of thyroid drugs, diabetic patients refusing to administer insulin). In order for a diagnosis of bulimia nervosa to be made, an individual must experience episodes of binge eating at least once per week, over a minimum period of 1 month.

HINTS AND TIPS

Some patients with anorexia nervosa may also engage in binge eating and purging behaviour, which is characteristic of bulimia nervosa. This does not preclude the diagnosis of anorexia nervosa: the key diagnostic difference is that patients with anorexia nervosa have a significantly low body weight. The specifier anorexia nervosa with binge-purge pattern can be used for these patients.

Binge-eating disorder

Binge-eating disorder is characterised by frequent and recurrent episodes of binge eating. An episode occurs when a patient experiences a subjective loss of control over what they are eating, in a way that is different from how they feel usually. For the diagnosis to be made, the episodes of binge eating need to occur regularly, i.e., once per week or more for at least 3 months. Unlike bulimia nervosa, the patient does not engage in compensatory behaviours such as purging to offset the calories consumed during the episode of binge eating. Binge eating episodes are typically very distressing for the patient, but they are not preoccupied with body shape or weight. Although patients often become obese, this is not required for the diagnosis.

Feeding disorders

Avoidant restrictive food intake disorder

Avoidant restrictive food intake disorder (AFRID) describes a pattern of eating where someone avoids or restricts their food intake, resulting in an insufficient quantity or variety of food being consumed to meet their nutritional requirements. Crucially, this is not done in attempt to alter weight or appearance. Instead, patients report restricting or avoiding foods due to the foods' sensory properties or perceived adverse consequences of eating (e.g., choking). Patients can experience significant weight loss and nutritional deficiencies and become dependent on oral supplements or tube feeding. ARFID has associations with other mental disorders, in particular neurodevelopmental disorders such as autism spectrum disorder.

Pica

Pica is characterised by the regular consumption of substances without any nutritional value. Examples can include eating raw food ingredients, e.g., flour, salt or nonfood substances, such as chalk, soap and paper. The consumption of these substances must be severe enough to cause either functional impairment or health problems for the individual. It is important to consider a person's developmental stage – for example, it would be inappropriate to diagnose Pica in an individual with an intellectual disability who is unable to distinguish between food stuffs with and without nutritional value. The onset of Pica often occurs in childhood, and is associated with neurodevelopmental disorders and intellectual disability. It is also important to be aware that during pregnancy, it can be normal for women to consume substances with no nutritional value. A diagnosis of Pica would only be appropriate if consuming the substances was causing the woman significant health or functional problems.

Rumination-regurgitation disorder

Individuals intentionally regurgitate food that they have chewed and swallowed back into their mouth, which they then either rechew and reswallow, or spit out. It can only be diagnosed if the individual has reached the developmental stage of a 2-year old. The episodes of regurgitation are frequent and occur over periods of several weeks.

Fig. 16.1 summarizes the ICD-11 criteria for anorexia nervosa, bulimia nervosa, binge-eating disorder and ARFID.

ASSESSMENT

History

It is important to define the extent of the eating disorder, yet at the same time not alienate a patient who might be ambivalent about treatment. Focusing initially on the patient's life history, premorbid personality, social circumstances, family, friendships, relationships and functionality can aid engagement and build rapport. These factors can also be very relevant to the aetiology of the disorder, and useful in determining appropriate treatment (see Chapter 26). Later in the interview, it is important to focus on weight and eating. Remember that direct questions may lead to confrontation and denial, and a technique that can be helpful to avoid alienating the patient is to 'normalize' symptoms for the purposes of the interview. The following questions may be useful:

Anorexic symptoms
- Body weight and shape can be very important to some people. Do you find that you are quite concerned about your weight?

<table>
<tr><td>

Anorexia Nervosa

1. Significantly low body weight for height/age/ developmental stage
2. Persistent pattern of restrictive eating +/- other behaviours to establish and maintain a low body weight
3. Excessive preoccupation and overevaluation of weight and slender body shape

</td><td>

Bulimia Nervosa

1. Frequent and recurrent episodes of binge eating that occur at least once per week over a period of at least 3 months
2. Repeated, inappropriate behaviours to compensate for an episode of binge eating aimed at preventing weight gain
3. Distress about the pattern of binge eating and compensatory behaviours.

</td></tr>
<tr><td>

Binge Eating Disorder

1. Frequent and recurrent episodes of binge eating that occur at least once per week over a period of at least 3 months
2. Binge eating episodes are not accompanied by compensatory behaviours aimed at avoiding weight gain
3. Significant distress associated with the pattern of binge eating

</td><td>

Avoidant Restrictive Food Intake Disorder (ARFID)

1. Avoidance or restriction of food intake, that results in either significant weight loss, nutritional deficiencies, dependence on supplemental feeding, negative physical health consequences or significant impairment in social functioning.
2. The behaviours are not motivated by a preoccupation with weight or shape

</td></tr>
</table>

For all: Symptoms are not better accounted for by another condition or related to the availability of food and are not culturally sanctioned

Fig. 16.1 The ICD-11 diagnostic criteria for anorexia nervosa, bulimia nervosa, binge-eating disorder and avoidant restrictive food intake disorder *(ARFID)*.

- Do you think you are a healthy weight? (This is a key diagnostic question: an underweight person who recognises they are too thin does not have anorexia nervosa.)
- A common way of losing weight is to eat less or to exercise a lot. Are these things that you do?
- Sometimes when women lose weight, their periods can become irregular or stop. Has this happened to you?

Bulimic symptoms

- Often when people try to lose weight, they have episodes when their eating seems excessive or out of control. Has this ever happened to you?
- After eating a lot, some people can feel guilty and uncomfortable and can vomit to make themselves feel better. Is this something that you have ever done?
- Sometimes people might use prescribed or street drugs to help control their weight. Have you ever tried this?

Other psychiatric symptoms

Sufferers of eating disorders may report other psychiatric symptoms. Anxiety classically surrounds eating but may appear more generalised. If symptoms are sufficiently severe to be disorders in their own right, then a comorbid psychiatric illness may be present. Distinguishing depression from anorexia is discussed below (under differential diagnosis).

Physical symptoms

Eating disorders are associated with a number of physical sequelae, and therefore a thorough medical history is required. Physical complications of starvation and vomiting are listed in Boxes 16.2 and 16.3. Important factors to ascertain include a menstrual history, episodes of syncope or presyncope, palpitations, tiredness, muscle weakness and sensitivity to cold. A history of syncope or palpitations is very concerning and places the patient at high physical risk.

Examination

Both anorexia nervosa and bulimia nervosa cause medical sequelae, and a physical examination is essential to accurately assess the physical risk to the patient (see Red Flag box later in this chapter). Patients may be reluctant to be examined; however, this can be facilitated when preceded by a clinical interview in which good rapport is established. Other than measuring height and weight and calculating BMI, important areas to examine are:

- Skin: 'lanugo' hair (fine, downy hair on body); loss of head hair; calluses on knuckles (from self-induced vomiting: Russell sign).
- Dentition: abrasions; tooth decay.
- Cardiovascular: lying and standing blood pressure (postural hypotension may occur if dehydrated); pulse.

BOX 16.2 PHYSICAL COMPLICATIONS OF EATING DISORDERS RELATED TO STARVATION

Signs and symptoms	Laboratory results
• Emaciation	• Normocytic anaemia
• Amenorrhoea; infertility; reproductive system atrophy	• Leucopoenia
	• Acute kidney injury (dehydration)
• Cardiomyopathy	• Raised transaminases
• Constipation; abdominal pain	• Hypoglycaemia
• Cold intolerance; lethargy	• Raised cortisol
• Bradycardia; hypotension; cardiac arrhythmias; heart failure	• Raised growth hormone
• Lanugo: fine, downy hair on trunk; loss of head hair	• Reduced T_3
	• Reduced follicle-stimulating hormone and luteinizing hormone
• Peripheral oedema	
• Proximal myopathy; muscle wasting	• Hypercholesterolaemia
• Osteoporosis; fractures	• Raised ferritin
• Seizures; impaired concentration; depression	

BOX 16.3 PHYSICAL COMPLICATIONS OF EATING DISORDERS RELATED TO VOMITING

Signs and symptoms	Laboratory results
• Permanent erosion of dental enamel; dental cavities	• Hypokalaemic, hypochloraemic alkalosis
• Enlargement of salivary glands (especially parotid)	• Hyponatraemia
	• Hypomagnesaemia
• Calluses on the back of hands from repeated teeth trauma (Russell sign)	• Raised serum amylase (acute pancreatitis)
• Oesophageal tears; gastric rupture	

- Abdomen: constipation.
- Musculoskeletal: muscle wasting; ability to sit up from lying and rise from a squat without using hands (the 'SUSS' test (sit-up, stand-squat test)); pathological fractures.

- Other: core temperature; mucous membranes (dehydration); facial glands (swollen parotid glands may suggest frequent vomiting).

RED FLAG

High-risk examination findings in patients with eating disorders (Red flag items on Medical Emergencies in Eating Disorders (MEED) Guidelines)
- BMI <13 in over 18s or <70% mean BMI/weight for height percentage in under 18s
- Recent weight loss >1 kg/week for 2 weeks in an underweight patient
- HR <40 bpm
- Recurrent syncope with standing BP <90 mmHg systolic and a postural drop of >20 mmHg or increase in heart rate >30
- Fluid refusal or signs of dehydration (decreased urine output, decreased skin turgor, sunken eyes, tachypnoea)
- Unable to sit up from lying flat or get up from squat on SUSS test
- Temperature <35.5°C
- Long QTc or other ECG abnormalities
- Low glucose/sodium/potassium/calcium/phosphate/albumin/white cell count on blood tests
- Acute food refusal – <500 kcal/day for 2 or more days
- >2 hours per day of exercise in the context of malnutrition
- Multiple episodes of purging and/or laxative abuse
- Moderate to high risk of completed suicide
- Staff/carers unable to implement meal plan

Investigations

Numerous biochemical and metabolic changes are associated with being underweight and engaging in excessive purging as summarised in Boxes 16.2 and 16.3. These complications may be associated with long-term consequences or result in sudden death. Investigations should therefore include: electrocardiogram (ECG), urea and electrolytes, full blood count, liver function tests, serum glucose and lipids, thyroid function tests and amylase. Changes in hormone levels (cortisol, insulin, luteinizing hormone, follicle-stimulating hormone, growth hormone) have been described, but these are of limited diagnostic value and are not routinely measured. Bone density (DXA) scanning may be considered for identification of osteopenia and osteoporosis.

Fig. 16.2 shows an algorithm to help establish diagnosis in patients with a suspected eating disorder.

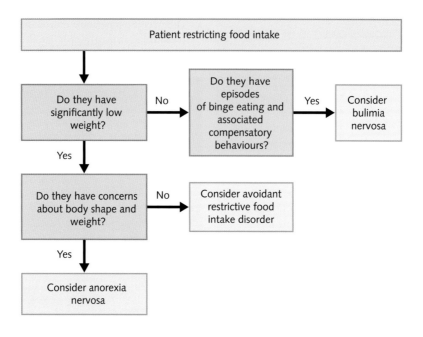

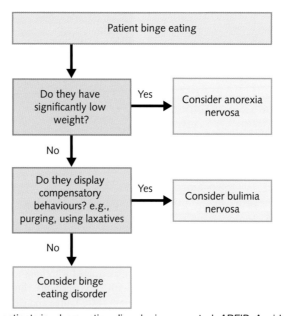

Fig. 16.2 Diagnostic approach for patients in whom eating disorder is suspected. *ARFID*, Avoidant restrictive food intake disorder.

HINTS AND TIPS

When weighing someone with a suspected eating disorder, always ensure they remove their shoes and any outdoor clothing. It is common for patients to attempt to artificially increase their weight by wearing heavy clothing or accessories, and even to drink a lot of water shortly before review.

DIFFERENTIAL DIAGNOSIS OF PATIENTS WITH LOW WEIGHT

Box 16.4 lists the other causes of significant weight loss that should be considered, especially when the onset of illness is later than adolescence or early adulthood.

It is very important to exclude physical causes of weight loss, including malignancies, gastrointestinal disease, endocrine diseases (e.g., diabetes mellitus, hyperthyroidism), chronic infections and chronic inflammatory conditions. Note that rare neurological syndromes associated with gross overeating include the Kleine–Levin, Klüver–Bucy and Prader–Willi syndromes.

Before diagnosing an eating or feeding disorder, consider the age and developmental stage of the patient, as some disorders, e.g., rumination-regurgitation disorder, cannot be diagnosed if the patient's age or developmental age is less than 2 years old. Also note that within certain cultural and religious communities, it can be normal to have periods of prolonged fasting, therefore a diagnosis of a feeding or eating disorder would not be appropriate for behaviours observed during these periods, as it is within cultural norms for that community.

BOX 16.4 DIFFERENTIAL DIAGNOSIS FOR PATIENT PRESENTING WITH WEIGHT LOSS

- Medical causes of low weight
- Alcohol or substance abuse
- Dementia
- Psychotic disorders
- Depression
- Obsessive-compulsive disorder
- Anorexia nervosa
- Bulimia nervosa
- Avoidant restrictive food disorder (ARFID)

Poor nutrition often occurs due to self-neglect in patients with alcohol or substance abuse and dementia. Patients with psychosis may not eat due to delusions about food or hallucinations commanding them not to. The negative symptoms of schizophrenia can also result in substantial weight loss due to self-neglect.

Severe weight loss may occur in depression, but this is usually associated with a marked loss of appetite and interest in food. Patients with anorexia maintain their appetite until late in the disease and remain interested in food-related subjects (e.g., low-calorie recipes). Note that patients with anorexia and bulimia often have comorbid depression and that depressive symptoms may be secondary to the biological consequences of starvation and thus resolve with subsequent weight gain.

Patients with obsessive-compulsive disorder may lose weight when time-consuming compulsions prevent an adequate diet. Also, obsessions of contamination of food might curtail their caloric intake. As with depression, the issue is clouded by the observation that patients with anorexia nervosa have an increased incidence of obsessive-compulsive disorder, which should only be diagnosed when obsessions or compulsions are unrelated to food or body shape.

HINTS AND TIPS

In the differential diagnosis of weight loss, anorexia and bulimia nervosa are associated with the overvalued idea and dread of fatness. Weight loss occurring in depression results from loss of appetite and lack of interest and enjoyment in food.

DISCUSSION OF CASE STUDY

Miss FD's BMI is 15 kg/m^2, which represents a significantly low weight. She admits to a dread of fatness and consequently pursues a target weight significantly below that which is healthy. Her weight loss methods include restrictive eating, excessive exercise and laxative abuse. She displays the core diagnostic features of anorexia nervosa: significantly low body weight, persistent pattern of restrictive eating and a pattern of other behaviours (exercise/laxative abuse) to maintain low body weight. She also displays features of preoccupation with her weight and overvalues thinness. The weight specifier of 'significantly low body weight' and behaviour pattern specifier of 'restrictive pattern' would also be clinically appropriate. The depressive symptoms may signify a comorbid disorder or be secondary to the biological effects of malnutrition. Medical complications include amenorrhoea, lethargy, bradycardia and lanugo (fine, downy hair on torso). Her extremely low BMI, moderate bradycardia and history of almost collapsing while exercising place her at moderate to high physical risk. She requires a complete physical examination, and same day bloods and ECG to assess for any acute life-threatening complications. She will require urgent treatment to stabilise and then increase weight.

Now go on to Chapter 26 to read about the eating disorders and their management.

Chapter Summary

- The key psychopathology in eating disorders is the overvalued idea of being overweight.
- Anorexia nervosa is associated with a significantly reduced body mass index (BMI), bulimia with a normal or high BMI.
- Purging behaviours are common in both disorders, including vomiting and laxative misuse.
- Restrictive behaviours are common in anorexia nervosa, including over-exercise and fasting.
- ARFID is characterised by low body weight with nutritional and physical health consequences, but the weight loss is not associated with a preoccupation with weight or body shape.
- Significant weight loss can be associated with life-threatening physical complications, and it is important to perform a full physical examination (including muscle power), blood tests and electrocardiogram at presentation and frequently during treatment.

UKMLA Conditions
Eating disorders

UKMLA Presentations
Weight loss

The patient with alcohol or substance use problems 17

Case summary

AD, aged 42, presented to their GP smelling of alcohol and complaining of depression, anxiety, relationship difficulties and sexual dysfunction. They admitted to drinking up to a bottle and a half of whisky per day. They reported drinking increasing amounts over the past year as the same amount no longer gave them the same feeling of well-being. Recently, they noticed that they had to drink in order to avoid shaking, sweating, vomiting and feeling 'on edge'. These symptoms meant having to take two glasses of whisky before breakfast, just to feel better. AD admitted that they had neglected their family and work because of their drinking. Whereas in the past, they would vary what and when they drank, they now tended to drink exactly the same thing at the same time each day, irrespective of their mood or the occasion. They found themselves craving alcohol and felt unable to walk home past the pub without going in. They continued to drink although they knew it was harming their liver. They were also concerned about their mental health because, on more than one occasion, they thought they saw a witch, about the same height as the kitchen kettle, walking around the room. They decided to contact their GP after they were charged with drink-driving by the police. AD had no previous psychiatric history or family history of psychiatric illness and was not taking any medication.

For a discussion of the case study, see the end of the chapter.

Psychoactive substances have been used for centuries, and their use is seen in many cultures as entirely acceptable. They have many beneficial effects including relief of pain and distress. However, psychoactive substances may cause symptoms and behaviour changes which are damaging to the individual or those around them, particularly when the substance is used regularly or to excess. Initial use of a substance can lead to a cycle of further use even when the person wishes to stop, as many recreational substances are associated with dependence, and withdrawal can be unpleasant and, with a minority of substances, fatal.

DEFINITIONS AND CLINICAL FEATURES

The term 'psychoactive' refers to any substance that has an effect on the central nervous system. This includes recreational drugs,

alcohol, nicotine, caffeine, prescribed or over-the-counter medication and poisons or toxins.

The ICD-11 describes the use of substances with three axes:

- The nature of the substance used (e.g., alcohol, cocaine)
- The pattern of use over time (hazardous use, harmful use, dependence)
- The effect of the substance at a given point in time (withdrawal, intoxication or mental disorder)

See Fig. 17.1 for an overview.

Nature of substance

The ICD-11 has codes for 14 different classes of psychoactive substances (Box 17.1).

Pattern of use

Hazardous use

Hazardous use is a quantity or pattern of substance use which is sufficient to substantially increase the risk of physical or mental harm to the user or others, but has not yet caused harm or dependence. In the ICD-11 it is defined as a risk factor, not a mental disorder. It warrants attention and advice from health care professionals, but is not yet a disorder. For example, drinking alcohol above the recommended limits (see Fig. 17.2) is hazardous use, whether or not the person feels they have come to any harm.

Harmful use of substance

Harmful use of a substance is defined as a quantity or pattern of substance use that actually causes adverse consequences to the user or others, without dependence. It may result in difficulties within interpersonal relationships (e.g., domestic violence, erectile dysfunction); problems meeting work or educational obligations (e.g., absenteeism); impaired physical health (e.g., alcohol-related liver disease, trauma); worsening of mental health problems (e.g., low mood or anxiety); or legal difficulties (e.g., arrest for disorderly conduct, stealing to fund habit, drink-driving).

The ICD-11 splits harmful use into an *episode* of harmful use and a harmful *pattern* of substance use. The diagnosis of an episode of harmful use can occur where there has only been one episode of harm, or where there is insufficient information to describe the pattern of use, e.g., if someone is unconscious following an opiate overdose and unable to give a history.

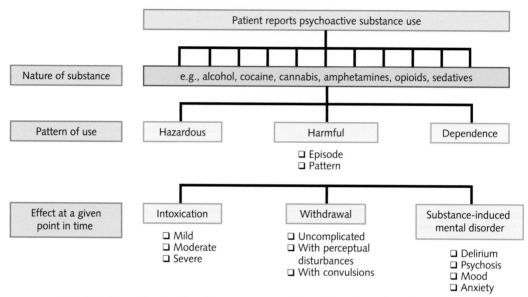

Fig. 17.1 Diagnostic algorithm for a person presenting with psychoactive substance use.

BOX 17.1 PSYCHOACTIVE SUBSTANCE CLASSES IN THE ICD-11

1. Alcohol
2. Cannabis
3. Synthetic cannabinoids
4. Opioids
5. Sedatives, hypnotics and anxiolytics
6. Cocaine
7. Stimulants (e.g., amphetamine)
8. Synthetic cathinones
9. Caffeine
10. Hallucinogens
11. Nicotine
12. Volatile inhalants
13. MDMA and related drugs
14. Dissociative drugs, e.g., ketamine

There are also categories for unknown, other and mixed psychoactive substances, including medications.

COMMUNICATION

Remember the 'Four Ls' (love, livelihood, liver, law) as a framework for assessing harm arising from substance use.

Substance dependence

HINTS AND TIPS

The confusion regarding use of the term 'addiction' led the World Health Organization (1964) to recommend that the term be abandoned in scientific literature in favour of the term 'dependence'.

COMMUNICATION

Substance 'misuse' is a general term used to refer to substance use without legal or medical guidelines. It includes both harmful or dependent use of substances. Substance 'abuse' has the same meaning but is usually avoided because it has negative connotations.

Substance dependence describes a syndrome that incorporates physiological, psychological and behavioural elements. The dependence syndrome has been simplified for the ICD-11 and is now conceptualised as a triad of impaired control, increased priority and physiological features (of tolerance or withdrawal). Changes in two or more of these domains are required for diagnosis (see Box 17.2). Patients can meet the criteria for the dependence syndrome without having developed physiological

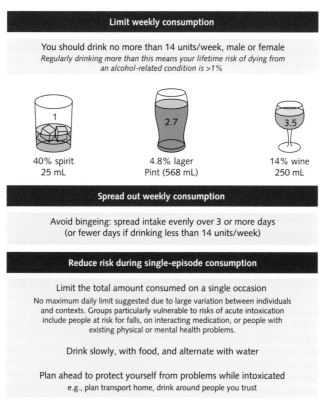

Limit weekly consumption

You should drink no more than 14 units/week, male or female
Regularly drinking more than this means your lifetime risk of dying from an alcohol-related condition is >1%

1

40% spirit
25 mL

2.7

4.8% lager
Pint (568 mL)

3.5

14% wine
250 mL

Spread out weekly consumption

Avoid bingeing: spread intake evenly over 3 or more days
(or fewer days if drinking less than 14 units/week)

Reduce risk during single-episode consumption

Limit the total amount consumed on a single occasion
No maximum daily limit suggested due to large variation between individuals
and contexts. Groups particularly vulnerable to risks of acute intoxication
include people at risk for falls, on interacting medication, or people with
existing physical or mental health problems.

Drink slowly, with food, and alternate with water

Plan ahead to protect yourself from problems while intoxicated
e.g., plan transport home, drink around people you trust

Fig. 17.2 How to keep health risks from drinking alcohol to a low level. (Modified with permission from UK Chief Medical Officers' Low Risk Drinking Guidelines, 2016.)

BOX 17.2 THE ICD-11 FEATURES OF DEPENDENCE ON A SUBSTANCE

1. *Impaired control* over substance use, including how often, how much, and when to stop.
2. *Increasing priority* given to substances, over e.g., relationships, work, school or activities of daily living.
3. *Physiological features* of dependence such as increasing tolerance or withdrawal symptoms.

Typically dependence will require at least 12 months of use to manifest, but if use has been daily (or near daily) the diagnosis can be made after 3 months.

There are a number of specifiers that can be added to a diagnosis of substance dependence, which denote whether or not the patient is actively using substances:

- Current use: the patient meets criteria for substance dependence.
- Sustained partial remission: the patient has managed to reduce their substance use for at least 12 months, and does not meet criteria for substance dependence.
- Early full remission: the patient has not used substances for <12 months.
- Sustained full remission: the patient has not used substances for >12 months.

Effect at a given point in time

Substance intoxication

Substance intoxication describes a transient, substance-specific condition that occurs following the use of a psychoactive substance. Symptoms can include disturbances of consciousness, perception, mood, behaviour and physiological functions. Severity of intoxication is normally proportional to dose or levels, and may be impacted by the

changes, particularly if the substance they are using is not associated with tolerance or withdrawal, e.g., hallucinogens or dissociative drugs. In addition to these requirements patients will often have an urge or a craving to use substances, although this is not required for diagnosis. While substance dependence often leads to harm, proof of harm is not required for a diagnosis.

individual's weight, height and tolerance. Intoxication can be classed as:

- Mild: recognisable disturbances in functions such as coordination or attention, but no change to consciousness.
- Moderate: marked disturbances in functioning with some disturbance to consciousness level.
- Severe: obvious disturbances in functioning with marked impairment of consciousness level. The person may not be able to care for themselves or communicate.

Substance withdrawal

Substance withdrawal describes a substance-specific syndrome that occurs on reduction or cessation of a psychoactive substance that has generally been used repeatedly, in high doses, for a prolonged period. Not all substances (e.g., hallucinogens, dissociative drugs) will cause a withdrawal state. Some substances can cause a withdrawal state with complications, e.g., withdrawal from alcohol or benzodiazepines can be associated with perceptual disturbances or convulsions. If withdrawal is associated with a delirium, this is now classed as substance-induced delirium.

Substance-induced mental disorder

Substance-induced mental disorders are those in which the symptoms resemble those from other diagnostic categories (e.g., psychotic symptoms, anxiety symptoms) but are caused directly by the use of substances. If the symptoms were present prior to the onset of substance use then the diagnoses should not be used. The symptoms should arise during or shortly after intoxication or withdrawal from a substance. The amount and duration of the substance use should be capable of producing the symptoms. The intensity or duration of the symptoms should be significantly in excess of those typically seen during uncomplicated intoxication or withdrawal (if this is not the case, simply diagnose intoxication or withdrawal).

There are six classes of substance-induced mental disorders. Most of the disorders can be caused by multiple different substances, with the exception of the final two:

- Substance-induced delirium
- Substance-induced psychotic disorders
- Substance-induced mood disorders
- Substance-induced anxiety disorders
- Substance-induced obsessive-compulsive disorders*
- Substance-induced impulse control disorders*

---

*Caused only by stimulants (e.g., cocaine, amphetamines, synthetic cathinones).

ALCOHOL-RELATED DISORDERS

Many people who drink alcohol come to no apparent harm. However, drinking even a small amount of alcohol without overt harm at the time increases the risk for many subsequent illnesses (e.g., cancer, stroke, heart disease, liver disease) and also death through accidents (e.g., head injuries, fractures, facial injuries). It has previously been suggested that there are potential health benefits of moderate consumption, in particular a small reduction in risk for ischaemic heart disease in women over 55 years old who drink around five units per week; however, more recent evidence suggests this is not the case. The Chief Medical Officer (2016) advised that 'there is no safe level of alcohol consumption'. However, for many people alcohol is a large part of their social lives and they may feel the benefits of consumption outweigh the risks (similar decisions are made by those who choose to partake in high-risk sports). For those who choose to drink alcohol, a number of steps can be taken to keep the associated harms to a low level: see Fig. 17.2.

HINTS AND TIPS

One unit of alcohol = 8 g (10 mL) of pure alcohol *(note this varies between countries)*

One unit is approximately equivalent to the amount of alcohol metabolized in 1 hour. For example, if you drink a large glass of wine (usually containing around three units) it will typically be at least 3 hours before blood alcohol concentration returns to zero.

Alcohol metabolism follows zero-order kinetics; it cannot be speeded up (e.g., by drinking coffee).

You can calculate units by multiplying alcohol by volume (ABV) in percent by volume in litres: ABV × vol = units (e.g., a pint (568 mL) of 5.3% lager would contain 5.3 × 0.568 = 3 units.

COMMUNICATION

The Chief Medical Officer's advice on alcohol consumption can be summarized as:

- There's no safe level at which to drink alcohol.
- Drinking at most 14 units/week keeps risks low (but some people will be harmed by less).
- Don't drink all 14 units in one night.
- Have several alcohol-free days a week.

Hazardous use of alcohol

Hazardous use is a pattern of consumption which places the individual at harm, but harm has not yet occurred. In the United Kingdom, this is defined as drinking more than 14 units per week, regardless of gender.

Harmful use of alcohol

Harmful use of alcohol is when drinking causes physical, psychological or social harm to the patient or others around them. People who harmfully drink are not dependent on alcohol; if features of dependence are present, the patient has alcohol dependence syndrome (Box 17.1). Box 17.2 lists the adverse physical, psychological and social consequences of drinking.

COMMUNICATION

It is frequently useful to explain that, although a patient may not be suffering from alcohol dependence, they are drinking at harmful levels, and are likely to benefit from support to reduce their consumption.

Alcohol dependence

After a significant time of heavy, regular drinking, users may develop dependence (Box 17.1). Alcohol dependence does not just mean physical dependence (although that is an important part of it), but describes a heterogeneous collection of symptoms, signs and behaviours which are determined by biological, psychological and sociocultural factors. There is a range in the severity of dependence; one dependent drinker may experience a mild tremor and anxiety while at work ('the fear') whereas another may shake so much after waking that they are unable to drink a cup of tea in the morning without spilling it.

Acute intoxication

Ingestion of alcohol results in transient psychological, behavioural and neurological changes, the severity of which is roughly correlated to the alcohol concentration in the blood and brain. Initially, this may produce an enhanced sense of well-being, greater confidence and relief of anxiety, which may lead to individuals becoming disinhibited, talkative and flirtatious. As blood levels increase, some drinkers may exhibit inappropriate sexual or aggressive behaviour whereas others might become sullen and withdrawn, with labile mood and possibly self-injurious behaviour. As levels rise further, drinkers can suffer incoordination, slurred speech, ataxia, amnesia (discussed later in this chapter) and impaired reaction times. Very high concentrations may lead to, a lowered level of consciousness, respiratory depression, coma and death.

HINTS AND TIPS

Extreme alcohol intoxication states can cause impaired concentration, inability to sustain attention, global cognitive impairment, and can meet diagnostic criteria for delirium. However, this should not be confused with delirium tremens, associated with alcohol withdrawal.

RED FLAG

Alcohol intoxication can cause dangerous disinhibition, increasing a person's likelihood of having and acting upon thoughts of self-harm or suicide. Seven out of 10 men who complete suicide are intoxicated.

Alcohol intoxication can be a potentially life-threatening condition due to the risk of respiratory depression, aspiration of vomit, hypoglycaemia, hypothermia and trauma (e.g., head injury, fractures or blood loss following accidents or assaults).

HINTS AND TIPS

Patients may report drinking alcohol in order to sleep better. This is counterproductive. It is true that alcohol reduces sleep latency and leads to increased slow-wave (deep) sleep during the first half of the night. However, alcohol also inhibits the time to onset and duration of REM sleep, causing disruption to sleep architecture during the second half of the night and overall reduced quality sleep.

Alcohol withdrawal (including delirium)

The development of withdrawal symptoms upon discontinuation of substance use is part of the dependence syndrome. Box 17.3 summarises the continuum of clinical features of alcohol withdrawal, from uncomplicated withdrawal to life-threatening delirium tremens ('the DTs'). However, 'uncomplicated' does not mean not serious. All withdrawal states are potentially life-threatening, if they are associated with autonomic hyperactivity or perceptual disturbances which may cause a person to engage in risky behaviour.

BOX 17.3 COMPLICATIONS OF EXCESSIVE ALCOHOL USE

MENTAL HEALTH

- Substance-related disorders (Fig. 17.1)
- Self-harm or suicidal behaviour

SOCIAL

- Absenteeism from, or poor performance at, work or education
- Victim of theft (e.g., wallet, phone, keys)
- Unprotected sex with risk for sexually transmitted disease or unplanned pregnancy
- Legal problems (increased risk for violent crime, drink-driving, alcohol-related disorderly conduct, child abuse)
- Interpersonal problems (arguments with friends or family due to alcohol)
- Financial problems (expense of drinking, unemployment)
- Homelessness

PHYSICAL HEALTH

- *Nervous system*
  Intoxication delirium
  Withdrawal delirium (delirium tremens)
  Withdrawal seizures
  Cerebellar degeneration
  Haemorrhagic stroke
  Peripheral and optic neuropathy
  Wernicke–Korsakoff syndrome
  Alcohol-related cognitive impairment
- *Gastrointestinal system*
  Alcoholic liver disease (fatty liver, alcoholic hepatitis, alcoholic cirrhosis)
  Acute and chronic pancreatitis
  Peptic ulceration and gastritis
  Cancers: oropharynx, larynx, oesophagus, liver, breast, colon and pancreas
- *Cardiovascular system*
  Hypertension
  Arrhythmias
  Ischaemic heart disease (in heavy drinkers)
  Alcoholic cardiomyopathy
- *Immune system*
  Increased risk for infections (especially meningitis and pneumonia)
- *Metabolic and endocrine system*
  Hypoglycaemia
  Hyperlipidaemia/hypertriglyceridemia
  Hyperuricaemia (gout)
  Hypomagnesaemia, hypophosphatemia, hyponatraemia
  Alcohol-induced pseudo–Cushing syndrome
- *Haematological system*
  Red cell macrocytosis
  Anaemia
  Neutropenia
  Thrombocytopenia
- *Musculoskeletal system*
  Acute and chronic myopathy
  Osteoporosis
- *Reproductive system*
  Intrauterine growth retardation
  Foetal alcohol syndrome
  Erectile dysfunction
  Infertility
- *Increased incidence of trauma (fractures, head injury, soft tissue injury following accidents or assaults)*

RED FLAG

Always check whether previous episodes of alcohol withdrawal have been complicated by medical problems (such as delirium tremens or seizures) or psychiatric problems (such as suicidality or hallucinations). These points will be important in determining where detoxification takes place.

Alcohol-related cognitive disorders

Blackouts

Episodes of anterograde amnesia ('blackouts') can occur during acute alcohol intoxication. Memory loss may be patchy, or for a discrete block of time during which nothing can be remembered. Blackouts are common, studies of university students found that approximately half had a blackout at some point in their lives. Blackouts refer to amnesia, not collapsing

BOX 17.4 CLINICAL FEATURES OF ALCOHOL WITHDRAWAL

UNCOMPLICATED ALCOHOL WITHDRAWAL
SYNDROME

- Symptoms develop 4–12 hours after drinking cessation
- Tremulousness ('the shakes')
- Sweating
- Nausea and vomiting
- Mood disturbance (anxiety, depression, 'feeling edgy')
- Sensitivity to sound (hyperacusis)
- Autonomic hyperactivity (tachycardia, hypertension, mydriasis, pyrexia)
- Sleep disturbance
- Psychomotor agitation

WITH PERCEPTUAL DISTURBANCES

- Illusions or hallucinations (typically visual, auditory or tactile)

WITH WITHDRAWAL SEIZURES

- Develop 6–48 hours after drinking cessation
- Occurs in 5%–15% of all alcohol-dependent drinkers
- Generalised and tonic–clonic
- Predisposing factors: previous history of withdrawal fits, concurrent epilepsy, low potassium or magnesium

WITHDRAWAL DELIRIUM (DELIRIUM TREMENS)

- Develops 1–7 days after drinking cessation (mean = 48 hours)

- Altered consciousness and marked cognitive impairment (i.e., delirium; see Chapters 19 and 20)
- Vivid hallucinations and illusions in any sensory modality (Specific hallucinations in withdrawal include Lilliputian visual hallucinations (miniature humans/animals) and fornication (a sensation of insects crawling on the skin). Patients may be able to interact with these hallucinations.)
- Marked tremor
- Autonomic arousal (heavy sweating, raised pulse and blood pressure, fever)
- Paranoid delusions (often associated with intense fear)
- Mortality (5%–15% of people with delirium tremens die from cardiovascular collapse, hypothermia/hyperthermia, infection)
- Predisposing factors such as physical illness (hepatitis, pancreatitis, pneumonia)

WITHDRAWAL OFTEN PRECIPITATES WERNICKE ENCEPHALOPATHY

- Triad of ataxia, ophthalmoplegia and acute cognitive impairment
- Risk for long-term cognitive impairment (Korsakoff syndrome)

or 'passing out' at the end of the night. They are evidence of hazardous use of alcohol as they place an individual at great vulnerability.

Wernicke–Korsakoff syndrome

Both Wernicke encephalopathy and Korsakoff syndrome occur because of thiamine (vitamin B_1) deficiency. Although the two disorders were initially described separately it is now clear they represent a continuum, with Wernicke encephalopathy occurring during acute brain damage due to thiamine deficiency and Korsakoff being the chronic state that emerges later. Any disorder that is associated with low thiamine can cause Wernicke–Korsakoff syndrome, but heavy drinkers are at particular risk. This is because of nutritional deficiency secondary to poor dietary intake and impaired absorption.

Wernicke encephalopathy is characterised by the classical clinical triad of delirium, ophthalmoplegia (mainly nystagmus, sixth nerve palsy or conjugate gaze palsy) and ataxia (which can be impossible to distinguish from intoxication). All three triad components are found in only a minority of cases; the presence of any of them should prompt treatment. Early treatment with parenteral thiamine (Pabrinex) can reduce the likelihood of progression to Korsakoff syndrome. Korsakoff syndrome is characterized by extensive anterograde and retrograde amnesia, frontal lobe dysfunction and psychotic symptoms occurring in the absence of delirium. See Chapter 22 for more details on treatment.

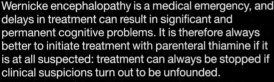

RED FLAG

Wernicke encephalopathy is a medical emergency, and delays in treatment can result in significant and permanent cognitive problems. It is therefore always better to initiate treatment with parenteral thiamine if it is at all suspected: treatment can always be stopped if clinical suspicions turn out to be unfounded.

The classic triad of Wernicke encephalopathy is delirium (82% of cases), ophthalmoplegia (29% of cases) and ataxia (23% of cases). However, all three features are only found in around 1 in 10 patients, and at presentation, 1 in 5 patients have none of these features. In someone who is withdrawing from alcohol, treatment with parental thiamine is required for:

- Anyone who is detoxing as an inpatient
- Anyone who is at high risk for Wernicke encephalopathy (malnutrition, malabsorption)
- The presence of any symptom consistent with Wernicke encephalopathy

Alcohol-related brain damage

Long-term alcohol excess leads to impairment of memory, learning, visuospatial skills and impulse control associated with cortical atrophy and ventricular enlargement (alcohol-related brain damage, sometimes called dementia). If memory is predominantly affected then alcohol-related amnestic disorder can be diagnosed. These changes persist beyond the time of alcohol intoxication or withdrawal. Withdrawal from alcohol is associated with cognitive impairment, which often does not fully recover. Alcohol-dependent people are also at risk for brain damage due to years of poor nutrition, trauma (e.g., head injury) and comorbid physical illness (e.g., alcoholic liver disease). It is therefore important to screen for other causes of cognitive impairment, particularly reversible causes of dementia. Unlike neurodegenerative dementias, subsequent abstinence from alcohol often leads to stabilization or some improvement in cognitive functioning.

HINTS AND TIPS

'Alcohol-related brain damage' (ARBD) is an umbrella term which includes chronic brain damage/dementia due to use of alcohol, Wernicke–Korsakoff syndrome arising following single or repeated withdrawals and amnestic syndrome. Abstinence from alcohol is often associated with some improvement in cognition.

Alcohol-related psychotic disorder

The interplay between alcohol excess and psychotic symptoms is complex, and is not as simple as 'cause and effect'. While both hallucinations and delusions can occur in the context of heavy alcohol consumption, alcohol misuse is also a common comorbidity in many patients who suffer from disorders associated with psychotic symptoms (e.g., schizophrenia, bipolar disorder). Alcohol misuse is also strongly (but rarely) associated with overvalued ideas or delusions of infidelity (morbid jealousy, or 'Othello syndrome'; see Table 9.1). However, drinkers may experience psychotic symptoms that resolve or significantly improve with abstinence from alcohol and can thus be directly attributed to alcohol. These can range from fleeting perceptual disturbances with retained insight, to more persistent auditory or visual hallucinations ('alcoholic hallucinosis'), to persecutory or grandiose delusions. These are distinguished from acute intoxication or alcohol withdrawal delirium by the absence of cognitive impairment and by clarifying when someone last had a drink. Psychotic symptoms directly due to alcohol are far rarer than psychotic symptoms due to a comorbid psychiatric disorder, so always carefully assess for the presence of other psychiatric disorders even if a patient is drinking heavily.

Alcohol-related mood disorder

Again, the relationship between alcohol and depression is complex. Heavy alcohol consumption may cause low mood, and similarly, low mood may cause sufferers to drink heavily to 'escape' their difficulties. This problem is often compounded by the social damage that alcohol can have on a patient's personal life (relationships, marriage, employment, finances, physical ill health, criminality, etc.). Differentiating low mood secondary to alcohol and true depressive disorder is very difficult, and usually starts with abstinence (following detoxification if necessary). Because of the potent psychoactive depressant effects of alcohol, pharmacological treatment of depression with antidepressants in a patient who continues to drink heavily is extremely unlikely to work and potentially dangerous. The first step in treating low mood is abstinence.

Alcohol-related anxiety disorder

Large amounts of alcohol can deplete levels of GABA in the brain, causing increased anxiety and feelings of panic. As in depression, establishing whether alcohol is a cause or a consequence of anxiety disorders is difficult. The anxiolytic properties of alcohol often result in attempts at self-medication in patients with PTSD, agoraphobia and social anxiety disorder, and alcohol withdrawal symptoms can mimic anxiety and panic symptoms. Patients often find it difficult to remember which came first: the alcohol or the anxiety. Whatever the direction of the relationship, reducing alcohol consumption will be of benefit.

RED FLAG

Self-harm and suicide are strongly associated with alcohol misuse. Over 50% of patients who present to hospital after harming themselves have recently consumed alcohol. Alcohol dependence is associated with a 12-fold increase in the risk for completed suicide.

OTHER SUBSTANCE-RELATED DISORDERS

It is beyond the scope of this book to describe in detail the individual psychiatric consequences of every recreational drug. Like alcohol, use can be harmful, dependent or result in psychiatric disorders such as psychosis. The effects of common recreational drugs are described in Table 17.1.

Table 17.1 Effects of common recreational drugs

Drug group[a]	Common examples	Mood and cognition effects	Physical effects	Withdrawal syndrome[b]	Associated psychiatric disorders
Opioids	Heroin, dihydrocodeine (DF118), methadone, buprenorphine (Subutex), fentanyl, oxycodone	Euphoria, drowsiness, apathy, personality change	Miosis, conjunctival injection, nausea, pruritus, constipation, bradycardia, respiratory depression, coma, death	Muscle aches, nausea, piloerection, sweating, mydriasis, lacrimation, rhinorrhoea, tachycardia, tremor, anxiety/irritability (rate using COWS) Short-acting opioids within 12 hours, long-acting within 2 days Lasts around a week	None typical
Sedatives	Temazepam, diazepam (Valium), flunitrazepam (Rohypnol) Gamma-hydroxybutyrate (GHB), gamma-butyrolactone (GBL)	Drowsiness, disinhibition, confusion, poor concentration, reduced anxiety, feeling of well-being	Hypotension, impaired coordination, respiratory depression	Similar to alcohol withdrawal with onset and duration depending on half-life: seizures, hallucinations, sweating, tachycardia, tremor, nausea	Substance-induced cognitive impairment
Stimulants	Amphetamine, cocaine, crack cocaine, MDMA (Ecstasy), mephedrone, novel psychoactive substances (commonly stimulants)[c]	Alertness, hyperactivity, euphoria, irritability, aggression, paranoid ideas, hallucinations (especially cocaine – formication), psychosis	Mydriasis, tremor, hypertension, tachycardia, arrhythmias, perspiration, fever (especially Ecstasy), convulsions, perforated nasal septum (cocaine)	Within a few hours to days of stopping heavy use: dysphoria, fatigue, hyperphagia, nightmares, insomnia or hypersomnia, psychomotor retardation or agitation	Substance-induced psychosis and/or mood disorder Trigger for manic episode in those with bipolar disorder
Hallucinogens	Lysergic acid diethylamide (LSD), magic mushrooms	Marked perceptual disturbances including chronic flashbacks, paranoid ideas, suicidal and homicidal ideas, psychosis	Mydriasis, conjunctival injection, hypertension, tachycardia, perspiration, fever, loss of appetite, weakness, tremors	No specific withdrawal syndrome	Substance-induced psychosis

Continued

157

Table 17.1 Effects of common recreational drugs—cont'd

Drug group[a]	Common examples	Mood and cognition effects	Physical effects	Withdrawal syndrome[b]	Associated psychiatric disorders
Cannabinoids	Cannabis, hashish, hash oil	Euphoria, relaxation, altered time perception, psychosis	Impaired coordination and reaction time, conjunctival injection, nystagmus, dry mouth	Generally mild–moderate symptoms lasting 2–4 weeks Irritability, anxiety, low mood, restlessness, insomnia, tremulousness, headaches	Substance-induced psychosis and/or mood disorder Trigger for schizophrenia
Dissociative anaesthetics	Ketamine, phencyclidine (PCP)	Hallucinations, paranoid ideas, thought disorganization, aggression	Mydriasis, tachycardia, hypertension, ulcerative cystitis	No specific withdrawal syndrome	Substance-induced psychosis
Inhalants	Aerosols, glue, lighter fluid, petrol, toluene	Disinhibition, confusion, euphoria, hallucinations, stupor	Similar to alcohol intoxication: headache, nausea, slurred speech, loss of motor coordination, muscle weakness, nystagmus Also arrhythmia and pneumonitis. Chronic use: damage to brain/liver/kidneys/myocardium	Existence of withdrawal syndrome unclear. Around half of heavy users may experience hypersomnia, low mood and nausea over the first days post-cessation	Substance-induced psychosis

[a]Many drugs affect a person in more than one way so one drug can fit into multiple categories. There are other ways to categorize drugs, for example, as 'empathogens' (drugs which increase empathy). See Fig. 17.3.

[b]Stopping any recreational drug that has been taken long-term is often associated with cravings and anxiety about discontinuation; this is not the same as a specific physiological withdrawal syndrome.

[c]Not all novel psychoactive substances are stimulants, they can occur in all classes (e.g., synthetic cannabis, 'spice').

COWS, Clinical Opiate Withdrawal Scale.

DIFFERENTIAL DIAGNOSIS

Patients using psychoactive substances can present with features similar to primary psychiatric disorders, posing a diagnostic challenge. The relationship between substance use and psychiatric symptoms can be reduced to three diagnostic possibilities:

1. There is a primary psychiatric disorder (e.g., depression or schizophrenia) and the patient is coincidentally using drugs or alcohol (remember that patients suffering from mental illness often use psychoactive substances to obtain relief from their symptoms).
2. The symptoms are entirely due to the direct effect of the substance and no primary psychiatric diagnosis exists.
3. Psychiatric symptoms are due to a combination of the above, as occurs when psychoactive substances are used by those

with a predisposing vulnerability to the development of mental illness.

The following features suggest a substance-related psychiatric disorder:

- The psychiatric symptoms are known to be associated with the specific drug in question (e.g., psychotic symptoms with amphetamine use).
- There is a temporal relationship (hours or days) between the use of the suspected drug and the development of psychiatric symptoms.
- There is a complete recovery from all psychiatric symptoms after termination and metabolic clearance of the suspected drug.
- There is an absence of evidence to suggest an alternative explanation for psychiatric symptoms (e.g., previous history of primary psychiatric illness or family history of psychiatric illness).

The Drugs Wheel
A new model for substance awareness

[NPS/Established version 1.0.4 • 15/04/2022]

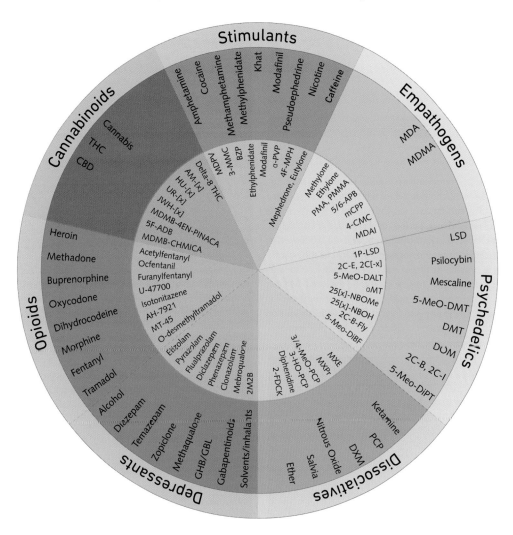

Outer ring: Established psychoactive substances

Inner ring: Newer psychoactive substances

 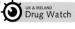

Fig. 17.3 The drugs wheel. (Modified with permission from The Drugs Wheel by Mark Adley.)

COMMUNICATION

You cannot completely exclude the use of substances, or gauge the severity of established misuse, without a collateral history (or in some cases even with one). A urine or oral toxicology screen are useful in establishing recent use of common recreational substances, and essential if considering a treatment such as methadone.

ASSESSMENT

History

The CAGE and AUDIT questionnaires can be helpful in screening for alcohol dependence. A thorough clinical history should pay particular attention to all substances used, the pattern of use, the route of use, features of dependence, periods of abstinence or controlled use, reasons for relapse, previous treatments, and consequences of substance use (relationships, employment, physical health, criminality). History of psychiatric illness and substance misuse, as well as family history of substance misuse should be explored. Mental state examination is important to establish psychiatric comorbidity or sequelae, current suicidality, and insight into current substance misuse (e.g., whether the patient considers it to be a problem and what they would consider to be helpful).

RED FLAG

Taking multiple substances at once is a major risk factor for drug-related death, with recreational, prescribed and over-the-counter drugs all implicated. The commonest drugs involved in fatalities are opiates and benzodiazepines. Always ask about polydrug use, and whether the person has ever unintentionally overdosed. All patients prescribed opioid substitution treatment should be offered a take-home naloxone kit, and training in how to recognise and treat an overdose.

The CAGE questionnaire is a simple tool to screen for alcohol dependence. If patients answer yes to two or more questions, regard the screen as positive and go on to check if they meet criteria for the alcohol dependence syndrome:

1. Have you ever felt you ought to **C**ut down on your drinking?
2. Have people ever **A**nnoyed you by criticizing your drinking?
3. Have you ever felt **G**uilty about your drinking?
4. Have you ever needed an '**E**ye-opener' (a drink first thing in the morning to steady your nerves or get rid of a hangover)?

The Alcohol Use Disorders Identification Test (AUDIT) is a 10-item screening questionnaire for problem drinking developed by the WHO. It takes 3 minutes to complete and score, and is recommended by NICE (2011). Severity of dependence can be rated using the 'Severity of Alcohol Dependence Questionnaire' (SADQ).

RED FLAG

Always ask about driving and the patient's responsibilities for caring for children or vulnerable adults. These are common areas of risk to others caused by alcohol or other substance use.

RED FLAG

Substance use disorders are common among doctors and other healthcare professionals, for whom accessing appropriate treatment is often problematic due to issues with stigma, discretion and confidentiality, not least because the General Medical Council considers these as fitness to practice issues. In an attempt to address these barriers, specialist, dedicated and confidential services have been developed for doctors and other healthcare professionals to access proper treatment for addiction and mental health difficulties. In England, this is via the Practitioner Health Programme, and in Scotland via the Workforce Specialist Service. This applies to medical students as well as qualified doctors and is intended to be supportive rather than punitive, aiming to protect patient safety while facilitating the doctor or student to engage in treatment and recovery. As a medical student, if you are misusing substances, similarly you may be able to access specialist services via your university or seek support via your supervisor/director of studies or your general practitioner. If you suspect a peer or senior colleague is misusing substances in a way which may influence patient care, speak to a senior doctor or your medical school.

Examination

The physical examination requires an awareness of both the acute and chronic effects of alcohol or substance use and should focus on:

- Evidence of acute use or intoxication (e.g., pupil constriction with opioid use; incoordination and slurred speech with alcohol use).

- Signs of withdrawal (e.g., tremulousness, sweating, nausea and vomiting, tachycardia and pupil dilatation with opioid withdrawal).
- Immediate and short-term medical complications of substance use (e.g., head injury following alcohol intoxication; infection caused by intravenous drug use (always inspect injection sites)).
- Long-term medical complications (e.g., alcohol-related liver disease, hepatitis B or C or HIV infection with intravenous drug use).

Investigations

There is no investigation that is absolutely indicative of substance dependence. A urine or saliva drug-screening test is extremely helpful whenever the use of psychoactive substances is suspected. Saliva testing is more dignified than urine testing, and is now most commonly used. Hair testing is occasionally used to get an accurate picture of drug use over longer time periods. However, toxicology testing generally is only set up to detect a limited number of well-known drugs (and testing laboratories will often not yet be set up to detect drugs which are new to the black market). Breath alcohol level (via a breathalyser) only detects recent alcohol use; however, a high reading in the absence of signs of intoxication suggests some degree of tolerance, which is likely to be indicative of chronic heavy drinking.

Investigations are also useful to identify possible longer-term complications of alcohol (see Table 17.1) and include a full blood count (mean corpuscular volume, or MCV, may be elevated), urea and electrolytes, liver function tests (gamma-glutamyl transpeptidase may be raised; elevated aminotransferases (ALT or AST) indicate liver injury and a high AST:ALT ratio suggests alcohol is the cause), clotting screen (prolonged prothrombin time is a sensitive marker of liver function) and electrocardiogram.

HINTS AND TIPS

If a patient is drinking too much alcohol, check their liver function. If a patient has abnormal liver function tests (LFT), take an alcohol history. Alcohol can cause abnormalities in any LFT.

If the patient has injected drugs ensure serology for blood-borne viruses has been performed (hepatitis B and C, HIV)

subsequent to the most recent injection (and consider the need to repeat testing after potential seroconversion). Signpost the patient to a needle exchange where they will also get access to a wide variety of harm-reduction information and education, including sexual health issues.

If the patient is suffering from a withdrawal delirium, brain imaging may be necessary to exclude an alternative cause or additional complication (e.g., infection, head injury, stroke).

HINTS AND TIPS

All patients, especially people presenting for the first time with psychotic symptoms, should have a urine or saliva drug-screening test. It is important to collect the sample as soon as possible because the half-lives (and hence detection windows) of some drugs are short. Urine dip-sticks are the fastest way to get a result.

DISCUSSION OF CASE STUDY

AD has an alcohol dependence syndrome as evidenced by their impaired *control* over their consumption (strong desire to drink alcohol, unable to walk past pub without going in, drinking regardless of context), the high priority they give it (continued drinking despite awareness of harmful consequences, neglecting their family and work in order to drink) and physiological features (tolerance, withdrawal symptoms, relief of withdrawal by drinking). They have physical (sexual, possibly other systems), social (relationship problems, neglect of family and work), legal (drink-driving offence) and mental health (depression, anxiety, hallucinations) complications of alcohol use. The first priority is treating the alcohol dependence. Following detoxification, it is important to reassess their mental health to ensure that their depression, anxiety and hallucinations are not indicative of a primary psychiatric disorder. The visual hallucinations may be suggestive of a withdrawal syndrome or be one of the perceptual disturbances sometimes caused by heavy alcohol use (alcoholic hallucinosis), although the latter is much less likely.

Now go on to Chapter 22 to read about the alcohol and substance disorders and their management.

Chapter Summary

- Problematic substance use can be classified according to three features:
  - nature of the substance used (e.g., alcohol, cocaine)
  - pattern of use over time (hazardous use, harmful episode or pattern of use, dependence)
  - effect of the substance at a given point in time (withdrawal, intoxication or substance-induced mental disorder)
- Substance-induced mental disorders are: delirium, psychotic disorders, mood disorders, anxiety disorders, obsessive-compulsive disorders and impulse control disorders.
- Substance use is often comorbid with primary psychiatric disorders.
- Intoxication by and withdrawal from psychoactive substances can be life-threatening.
- When assessing substance misuse, do not forget to assess for impact on physical health and psychosocial function.

UKMLA Conditions

Alcoholic hepatitis
Anxiety
Delirium
Dementias
Depression
OCD
Overdose
Phobias
Self-harm
Substance use disorder
Wernicke–Korsakoff syndrome

UKMLA Presentations

Addiction
Behaviour/personality change
Confusion
Driving advice
Loss of libido
Low mood/affective problems
Memory loss
Overdose
Sleep problems
Substance misuse
Suicidal thoughts
Threats to harm others
Visual hallucinations
Weight loss

FURTHER READING

Clinical Opiate Withdrawal Scale (COWS). https://www.drugabuse.gov/sites/default/files/files/ClinicalOpiateWithdrawalScale.pdf.

Alcohol Use Disorders Identification Test (AUDIT), https://www.drugabuse.gov/sites/default/files/files/AUDIT.pdf.

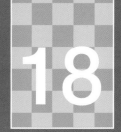
Case summary

The on-call psychiatrist was asked to assess BP, a 27-year-old who had been known to mental health services since they were 17 with symptoms that had been fairly consistent. They have never managed to sustain a job or long-term relationship, and have lived with their mother for most of their adult life. Their mother had contacted services because BP was threatening to jump in front of a bus. BP's father had sexually abused them as a child and they have a long history of self-harm that included cutting and repeated overdoses. Their mother was inclined to challenge their promiscuous behaviour and binge drinking, which led to many heated arguments. At interview, BP told the psychiatrist that they were feeling 'more depressed than ever' because their mother had suggested that they move out. With gentle questioning, it transpired that they were afraid that their mother would stop caring for them if they moved out. They also described chronic feelings of emptiness. The psychiatrist, who had known BP for years, recognised that this behaviour was not unusual for them and was able to help them to see another perspective to their mother's suggestion. BP's mood quickly lifted and their suicidal ideation resolved.

For a discussion of the case study, see the end of the chapter.

The description and management of 'personality disorder' is one of the most controversial subjects in psychiatry. Personality disorders overlap substantially with the concept of neurodevelopmental disorders (see Chapter 32) but are currently considered separately. People use the term 'personality' with varying meanings, even within the psychological and psychiatric specialties. From as early as 3 years old, children begin to exhibit personality traits that gradually become more stable over the course of their lives. Early life experiences, particularly traumatic events, influence the trajectory of how an individual's personality develops. Ways of thinking and feeling which help someone adapt effectively to the environment in which they are growing up may become maladaptive in later life. Personality disorders are important: they are common, associated with significant distress to the sufferer and often with great cost to health care, social services and criminal justice agencies.

DEFINITIONS AND CLINICAL FEATURES

Personality traits are enduring patterns of perceiving, thinking about, and relating to both self and the environment, exhibited in a wide range of social and personal contexts. A *personality disorder* is when an individual has traits that cause persistent disturbance (at least 2 years) in regard to one or both of two key areas:

1. Problems in functioning in aspects of the self: this can present as an unstable sense of identity, low or extremely high and unrealistic sense of self-worth, challenges in making decisions for oneself and inaccuracies in self-view of personal characteristics.
2. Interpersonal dysfunction across a variety of contexts and relationships: this presents as an individual having difficulties making and sustaining close relationships and managing conflict and challenges within the relationships. It can also manifest as an individual being unable to understand other peoples' perspectives, or lacking any consideration for them.

These two general features manifest in specific maladaptive patterns of:

- Cognition, e.g., extreme hopelessness (self) or believing "everyone hates me" (interpersonal).
- Emotional experience, e.g., frequent mood swings (self) or feeling overwhelmed with emotion if others do not act as desired (interpersonal).
- Emotional expression and behaviour, e.g., very limited emotional experience (self) or callousness towards the suffering of others (interpersonal).

The noted disturbance must also be present across different areas of an individual's life, e.g., employment, friendships, romantic relationships and education, and must be causing the person significant distress and impairment.

People with a personality disorder often do not regard their patterns of behaviour as inherently abnormal. Instead, they usually present to healthcare services with a wide range of problems related to or as a consequence of their abnormal personality traits (e.g., self-harm, feelings of depression or anxiety, violence or disorderly conduct, post-traumatic stress disorder, eating disorders, dissociative or bodily distress disorders). Having a major psychiatric illness such as schizophrenia does not preclude patients from also having a personality disorder; however, care should be taken to differentiate symptoms to avoid attribution of aspects of the primary disorder (e.g., negativism, self-harm, impulsivity) to a separate personality disorder.

A diagnosis of personality disorder can be stigmatising, as an individual's personality is essential to their sense of self. It is therefore important to consider whether making the diagnosis is useful, for example if it will direct the patient towards appropriate therapy or direct them away from potential iatrogenic harm. It is also important to hold in mind that the pattern of behaviours and display of emotions observed in individuals with personality disorder are part of the individual's attempt to adapt to the environment in which their personality developed.

CLASSIFICATION

Personality disorders can be classified into two groups according to their aetiology.

The first group includes 'acquired' personality disorders where the disorder clearly develops after, and is directly related to, a recognisable 'insult'. *Secondary personality disorder* results when this 'insult' is some form of brain damage or disease (e.g., a brain tumour or stroke). A common example is seen in patients with frontal lobe lesions, which can be characterised by disinhibition (e.g., stealing, sexual inappropriateness) and abnormalities of emotional expression (e.g., shallow cheerfulness, aggression, apathy). Patients can also develop enduring personality changes after experiencing a catastrophic event (e.g., concentration camp or hostage situation leading to complex post-traumatic stress disorder) or after the development of a severe psychiatric illness, e.g., schizophrenia. In such cases, a mental illness rather than personality disorder should be diagnosed.

The second group includes what is referred to in the ICD-11 as personality disorders and related traits (these are far more prevalent and therefore simply referred to as 'personality disorders'; this is the term that will be used for the rest of this chapter). In this group of personality disorders, it is difficult to find a direct causal relationship between personality traits and any one specific insult, although genetic and environmental factors have been implicated (see Chapter 30). The onset of personality disorders is in adolescence or early adulthood and any change

in symptoms tends to occur very gradually over a long period of time.

The ICD-11

The ICD-11 takes a hybrid categorical/dimensional approach to classifying personality disorder (see Fig. 18.1). If the essential features of a personality disorder are present, they should be categorized by *severity* (categorical). Then there is the option to add *trait domain specifiers*, to comprehensively describe the nature of an individual's personality disturbance *(dimensional)*. There is also an option to assign the *borderline pattern specifier*.

Severity

Severity is categorized as mild, moderate or severe. The degree of severity diagnosed is dependent on the degree and pervasiveness of disruption to the individual's functioning in the following areas:

- Sense of self and relationships
- Intensity and range of emotional, cognitive and behavioural symptoms
- Associated distress or psychosocial impairment
- Associated risk of harm, to self and others

Table 18.1 summarizes the severity descriptors in the ICD-11.

Specifiers

The ICD-11 specifies five personality trait domains which exist on a continuum with typical personality traits: negative affectivity, detachment, dissociality, disinhibition and anankastia (see Table 18.2). Each domain describes different features of an individual's personality that culminate in maladaptive patterns of behaviour and emotional experience. As many of the specifiers can be applied to the personality disorder diagnosis as necessary to accurately describe how an individual's personality is functioning.

In addition to the personality trait domains, the ICD-11 also includes a stand-alone pattern specifier of 'borderline pattern'. Borderline pattern can be described using the personality trait domains of negative affectivity, dissociality and disinhibition but the borderline pattern specifier was included to help identify individuals who may respond to certain psychotherapeutic treatment approaches and to ensure clinical continuity from the ICD-10.

The DSM-5

In contrast to the ICD-11, the DSM-5 uses a *categorical* approach to personality disorders. It assumes there are several

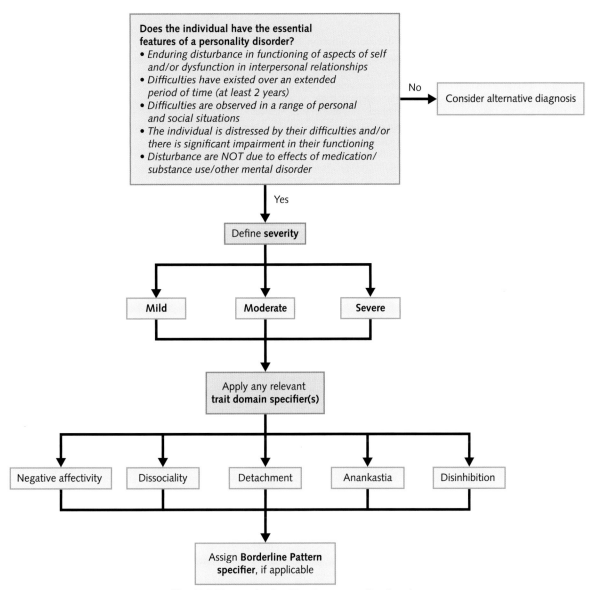

Fig. 18.1 Diagnostic algorithm for personality disorders

different distinct personality types, split into three clusters. Describing odd or eccentric individuals, Cluster A personality disorders include paranoid, schizoid and schizotypal personality disorders. Cluster B personality disorders include borderline, antisocial, histrionic and narcissistic personality disorders. Cluster C personality disorders include avoidant, dependent and obsessive-compulsive personality disorders. The DSM-5 classification systems are no longer commonly used in clinical practice in the United Kingdom, and this information is included for reference and as similar terms were included in the ICD-10. Table 18.3 summarizes the DSM-5 categorical classification of personality disorders.

Table 18.1 Summary of the ICD-11 severity descriptors

Severity	Overall functioning	Cognition, emotion, behaviour examples[a]
Mild	Impairment limited to a narrow range of functioning or many areas of functioning to a lesser degree	Someone who has a somewhat contradictory sense of identity and very low self-esteem but good ability to make decisions Someone who struggles to form intimate relationships but is able to form lasting friendships and get on well with colleagues Typically not associated with self-harm or harming others
Moderate	Noticeable and marked impairment in multiple areas of functioning, but the person may be able to function in some areas	Someone with poor emotion regulation in the face of setbacks but able to cope with challenges at work Someone with major difficulties in the ability to understand the perspective of others, resulting in relationships which are often conflictual or one-sided, but is able to get on well with their grandparents Sometimes associated with self-harm or harming others
Severe	Severe impairment evident in all areas of the person's life	Someone who is unable to experience or report emotions Someone who is unwilling or unable to sustain regular employment Someone who has no relationships with family members Often associated with self-harm or harming others[a]

[a]Note each person will have their own individual pattern of strengths and difficulties; these are just examples.

Table 18.2 Prominent personality traits or patterns in the ICD-11

Personality specifier	Description of diagnostic features
Negative affectivity	Broad range of negative emotions including anger/sadness/fear/guilt/shame, often disproportionate to the situation Difficulties with emotional regulation, including frequent mood shifts and prolonged distress Negative attitudes such as hopelessness Low self-esteem and self-confidence; may become dependent on others Difficulty trusting others
Detachment	Avoidance of social interactions Few/no friends and often a lack of interest in sexual relations Limited emotional expression and experience, aloofness
Dissociality	Self-centredness and a sense of self-entitlement. Over valuation of own qualities and expectation that they should be the subject of admiration Needs of others may not be considered at all Lack of empathy – can manifest as manipulation and exploitation of others May be physically violent and take pleasure in harming others
Disinhibition	Impulsivity and a desire to pursue short-term pleasures, e.g., in sexual relationships, gambling Distractibility, quick to become bored and tired of routine Irresponsibility and unreliability, will often lack a sense that they are accountable for their actions Recklessness and a lack of caution Difficulty planning or focusing beyond the here and now resulting in failure to meet any goals
Anankastia	Perfectionism, focus on rules and strong sense of right and wrong Highly systematic and detail orientated Rigid control over how their own emotions are expressed Inflexible and lack of spontaneity; risk avoidant Can be indecisive if they feel lacking in sufficient information
Borderline pattern	Significant efforts to avoid real or imagined abandonment Sense of self-image and sense of self is unstable Self-damaging behaviour when experiencing negative emotions, e.g., binge eating, promiscuity, binge drinking Recurrent episodes of self-harm Emotional instability, triggered by own thoughts or external factors Chronic feeling of emptiness Difficulties with anger management Can experience transient dissociative or psychotic symptoms in periods of heightened distress

Table 18.3 Categorical classification of personality disorders (DSM-5)

Cluster A: 'odd or eccentric'	
Paranoid personality disorder Schizoid personality disorder Schizotypal personality disorder	Suspects others are exploiting, harming or deceiving them; doubts about spouse's fidelity; bears grudges; tenacious sense of personal rights; litigious Emotional coldness; neither enjoys nor desires close or sexual relationships; prefers solitary activities; takes pleasure in few activities; indifferent to praise or criticism Eccentric behaviour; odd beliefs or magical thinking; unusual perceptual experiences (e.g., 'sensing' another's presence); ideas of reference; suspicious or paranoid ideas; vague or circumstantial thinking; social withdrawal
Cluster B: 'dramatic, emotional, erratic'	
Borderline (emotionally unstable) personality disorder Antisocial (dissocial) personality disorder Histrionic personality disorder Narcissistic personality disorder	Unstable, intense relationships (fluctuating between extremes of idealization and devaluation); unstable self-image; impulsivity (sex, binge eating, substance abuse, spending money); chronic feelings of emptiness; repetitive suicidal or self-harm behaviour; fluctuations in mood; frantic efforts to avoid (real or imagined) abandonment; transient paranoid ideation; pseudohallucinations; dissociation Repeated unlawful or aggressive behaviour; deceitfulness; lying; reckless irresponsibility; lack of remorse or incapacity to experience guilt Dramatic, exaggerated expressions of emotion; attention seeking; seductive behaviour; labile shallow emotions Grandiose sense of self-importance, need for admiration
Cluster C: 'anxious or fearful'	
Dependent personality disorder Avoidant (anxious) personality disorder Obsessive-compulsive (anankastic) personality disorder	Excessive need to be cared for; submissive, clinging behaviour; needs others to assume responsibility for major life areas; fear of separation Hypersensitivity to critical remarks or rejection; inhibited in social situations; fears of inadequacy Preoccupation with orderliness, perfectionism and control; devoted to work at expense of leisure; pedantic, rigid and stubborn; overly cautious

Note that the ICD-10 included all the personality disorders described in the DSM-5 clusters above, except for schizotypal and narcissistic personality disorder. However, schizotypal disorder (similar to the DSM-5's schizotypal personality disorder) is included in the ICD-10 and ICD-11 section on psychotic disorders.

HINTS AND TIPS

You may read notes or hear patients or clinicians talk about diagnoses that were different in the ICD-10. For personality disorder, differences in the ICD-11 include:

- Removal of individual categories of personality disorder (because patients often presented with overlapping traits in multiple disorders).
- Addition of the requirement to classify personality disorder by severity (because this is the best predictor of outcome).
- Addition of trait domain specifiers and borderline pattern specifier.
- 'Emotionally unstable personality disorder' in the ICD-10 would be 'Personality Disorder (of given severity, with applicable personality trait specifier) with borderline pattern'.

The underlying symptoms of personality disorder remain the same: if someone was diagnosed with a personality disorder using the ICD-10 diagnostic criteria, they will also have a personality disorder using the ICD-11 criteria; but the name will be different.

HINTS AND TIPS

Everybody has a personality that, no matter how 'normal', can have dysfunctional traits. These traits often become more prominent at times of psychological stress, such as mental or physical illness, pain and discomfort, work-related stress, and even tiredness and hunger. It is important to remember that personality disorders occur in many settings, remain stable over time and cause significant personal distress or functional impairment – do not assume someone has a personality disorder after meeting them only once during a time of stress.

HINTS AND TIPS

The term 'borderline personality disorder' is derived from the early 20th century psychoanalysts, who described a group of patients who were 'on the borderline' between the neuroses and the psychoses.

ASSESSMENT

History

As with other mental illnesses, giving a patient a label of personality disorder gives those involved with their care only a limited amount of information. Patients with a possible personality disorder often present at times of crisis and distress, and therefore diagnosis at the first interview can be difficult because of the quantity of background and collateral information required and because diagnosis requires the features to persist over time.

A practical approach includes making a comprehensive assessment of:

- Sources of distress (thoughts, emotions, behaviour and relationships) to self and others
- Any comorbid mental illness
- Specific impairments of functioning at work, home or in social circumstances

It is usually possible to establish some idea of a patient's personality by taking a detailed history of their life, focusing on the areas of education, work, criminality, relationships and sexual behaviour. When patients are not able to describe aspects of their personality, it can be useful to ask how those close to them might describe them. It is also useful – with consent – to obtain collateral information from the patient's friends or family and general practitioner, all of whom might be able to provide information to help distinguish between transient and enduring patterns of behaviour.

It is important to recognise that patients with a personality disorder may exhibit strong emotional reactions (transference and countertransference – see Chapter 3) and that they are often perceived as 'difficult patients' because of this. Being aware of your own emotions (often strong feelings of anger or anxiety) and taking a nonjudgmental and empathic stance during assessment can be greatly beneficial, as well as providing insight into the diagnosis itself.

A number of self-rating questionnaires that focus on personality traits are available. These can be helpful in the diagnosis of personality disorder; however, they should not be used as a substitute for a comprehensive clinical history. Structured interviews are also available, although these tend to be used for research purposes and are seldom used clinically.

Examination and investigation

There are no specific physical signs that help in the diagnosis of personality disorders. However, the consequences of associated behaviours may be seen on examination or investigation (e.g., marks from self-inflicted lacerations or burns, musculoskeletal injuries from assaults or accidents, the sequelae of drug or alcohol misuse, and sexually transmitted infections following promiscuity).

DIFFERENTIAL DIAGNOSIS

A personality disorder should not be diagnosed if symptoms are better explained by a physical problem, substance misuse or a mental illness. Almost all the mental illnesses described in this book can

Table 18.4 Important differential diagnoses for the prominent personality traits

Prominent personality trait or pattern	Differentials to consider (also consider 'no psychiatric disorder' in all cases)
Negative affectivity	Complex-PTSD; recurrent depressive disorder; bipolar disorder; dysthymia, cyclothymia; substance use (especially alcohol dependence)
Detachment	Autism spectrum disorder; prodromal or negative symptoms of schizophrenia
Dissociality	Mania
Disinhibition	Mania; ADHD; substance misuse
Anankastia	OCD; anxiety disorders; autism spectrum disorder
Borderline pattern	PTSD; complex PTSD; depression; substance misuse

ADHD, *Attention deficit hyperactivity disorder;* OCD, *obsessive-compulsive disorder;* PTSD, *post-traumatic stress disorder.*

feature some of the behaviours that characterise personality disorders. Examples include social withdrawal, suspiciousness and odd ideas in schizophrenia; self-harm, low mood and poor self-image in depression; aggression, irresponsibility and impulsivity in substance misuse or mania (see Table 18.4). The diagnostic task is also complicated by the observation that many patients with a major mental illness or intellectual disability also have a concurrent personality disorder. A personality disorder should only be diagnosed when the clinical features begin in adolescence or early adulthood, are relatively stable over time and do not only occur during an episode of a major mental illness (e.g., depressive, manic, psychotic episode).

When an individual develops a dramatic personality change after a period of normal personality functioning, consider a personality disorder secondary to a general medical condition, or mental disorder triggered by a catastrophic event, or onset of a severe psychiatric illness.

HINTS AND TIPS

Remember that personality disorders may present with features similar to the psychotic disorders (e.g., suspiciousness, social withdrawal and eccentric beliefs) but are differentiated by the absence of true delusions or hallucinations.

DISCUSSION OF CASE STUDY

BP has a chronic condition that first presented in adolescence and has changed little over time. They have a number of maladaptive and inflexible personality traits that manifest as repeated self-harm, suicidal behaviour, impulsivity (promiscuity, binge drinking), fluctuations in mood, and a marked fear of abandonment by their mother. These characteristics are consistent with a diagnosis of a severe personality disorder, with a borderline pattern. It would be important to exclude another mental illness that may coexist with the personality disorder, such as depression, complex PTSD or harmful use of/dependence on alcohol. Note that there is an association between personality disorders with a borderline pattern and adverse childhood experiences, including physical, emotional and sexual abuse.

Now go on to Chapter 30 which covers personality disorders and their management.

● Chapter Summary

- A personality disorder is when someone has ways of thinking, feeling or behaving in regard to themselves or others that cause considerable personal or social disruption.
- Patterns of emotion and behaviour represent an individual's attempt to adapt effectively to their early life experiences.
- Personality disorder should be classified as mild, moderate or severe, determined by functional impact.
- Trait domain specifiers can be used to describe what aspect of personality is disturbed (negative affectivity, detachment, dissociality, disinhibition, anankastia) or the pattern specifier 'borderline'.
- Many people manifest both a personality disorder and a mental disorder.
- Symptoms should not be diagnosed as a personality disorder if symptoms can be better explained by a physical problem, substance abuse or a mental disorder.

UKMLA Conditions
Personality disorder
Self-harm

UKMLA Presentations
Behaviour/personality
change
Overdose
Self-harm
Substance misuse
Suicidal thoughts
Threats to harm others

The patient with impairment of consciousness or cognition

Case summary

DD, aged 78 years, lived at home with their partner with carers visiting twice daily. Their general practitioner (GP) had referred them to a psychiatrist 6 years earlier, after they started experiencing difficulty remembering things. At first, they would forget things like the social arrangements they had made. Later they started forgetting activities they had engaged in only the day before. Their partner had noticed a gradual change in their personality in that they became increasingly withdrawn and sullen and, at times, verbally aggressive. Their language deteriorated to the point where they would ramble incoherently, even when there was no one else in the room. Despite having smoked for many years, DD seemed unable to recognize their pipe and would stare at it quizzically for hours. They lost the ability to dress themselves or complete simple multistep tasks such as making a cup of coffee.

Their partner contacted their GP when DD was too sleepy to get out of bed one morning. The GP arranged hospital admission for further investigation. Nurses were concerned because their consciousness level was fluctuating from hour to hour. They slept through most of the day, but would wander around the ward at night looking very agitated and appeared to have visual hallucinations. The senior nurse pointed out that they had developed a productive cough.

(For a discussion of the case study, see the end of the chapter.)

Cognitive impairment is common and important, but often underdiagnosed and underinvestigated. It is associated with a high morbidity and mortality, and you are likely to frequently encounter people with cognitive impairment in most specialties of medical practice.

DEFINITIONS AND CLINICAL FEATURES

Consciousness

To be conscious is to be aware, both of the environment and of oneself as a subjective being. It is a global cognitive function. It is a poorly understood, complex phenomenon with multiple vaguely defined terms for its abnormalities. It is best to avoid terms such as 'confused', 'obtunded', 'clouding of consciousness' and 'stupor' as they are not well-defined and mean different things to different specialties. Clinically, the key question is whether someone has a normal or altered conscious level. This is assessed at a practical level by observing arousal level (hyper-aroused or lowered) (Fig. 19.1).

Cognition

This chapter considers 'cognition' in its broadest sense as meaning all the mental activities that allow us to perceive, integrate and conceptualise the world around us. These include the global functions of consciousness, attention and orientation and the specific domains of memory, executive function, language, praxis and perception. The term 'cognition' is also used more narrowly in cognitive psychology and cognitive therapy where individual thoughts or ideas are also referred to as 'cognitions'.

Impairments in cognition can be generalized (multiple domains) or specific (one domain only). An altered level of consciousness is generally associated with a generalized impairment in all aspects of cognition, as it is difficult to concentrate on any tasks when feeling very agitated or drowsy.

A large number of specific cognitive impairments exist (Table 19.1). These can be isolated impairments, for example, if they are developmental or secondary to a small stroke or occur together in disorders of generalized cognitive impairment such as dementia.

Memory

Memory is one of the commonest cognitive domains to be impaired. There are two main ways to categorise memory: the duration of storage (working or long-term) or the type of information stored (implicit or explicit). Explicit memory (sometimes called *declarative memory*) includes all stored material of which the individual is consciously aware and can thus 'declare' to others. Implicit memory (sometimes called *procedural memory*) includes all material that is stored without the individual's conscious awareness (e.g., the ability to speak a language or ride a bicycle).

Explicit memory is the most common type of memory to be disrupted. It can be further subdivided into *semantic* and *episodic* memory. Semantic memory is knowledge of facts (e.g., Edinburgh is the capital of Scotland). Episodic memory is knowledge of autobiographical events (e.g., remembering a trip to Edinburgh when you were 10 years old). See Table 19.2

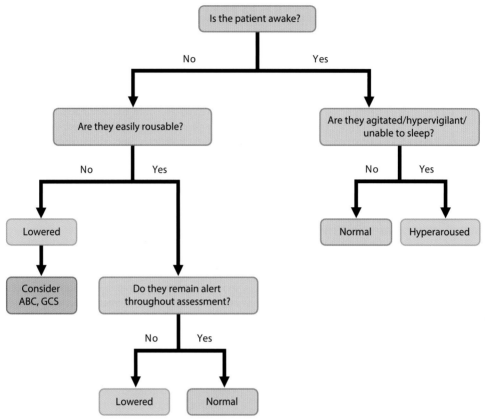

Fig. 19.1 Assessment of conscious level. *ABC,* Airway, breathing, circulation; *GCS,* Glasgow Coma Scale.

Table 19.1 Specific cognitive impairments		
Cognitive domain	**Term(s) for impairment**	**Description**
Language	Dysphasia/aphasia	Loss of language abilities despite intact sensory and motor function (e.g., difficulty in understanding commands or other words [receptive dysphasia] or difficulty using words with correct meaning [expressive dysphasia]). Not being able to name items correctly despite knowing what they are (nominal dysphasia) is a subtype of expressive dysphasia
Praxis	Dyspraxia/apraxia	Loss of ability to carry out skilled motor movements despite intact motor function (e.g., inability to put a letter in an envelope, use a tin opener, button up a shirt)
Perception	Dysgnosia/agnosia	Loss of ability to interpret sensory information despite intact sensory organ function (e.g., not able to recognize faces as familiar)
Memory	Amnesia	Loss of ability to learn or recall new information (e.g., not able to recall time or recent events, not able to learn new skills)
Executive function (umbrella term for many abilities)	Many terms, including: Disinhibition, perseveration, apathy, dysexecutive syndrome	Loss of ability to plan and sequence complex activities, or to manipulate abstract information (e.g., not able to plan the preparation of a meal, not able to return to a task once distracted)

Table 19.2 Explicit memory types, disorders and tests

Explicit memory type	Capacity duration	Key brain regions	Tests
Working/short-term	7 ± 2 items 15–30 s	Frontal cortex	Recall of unrelated words (e.g., 'lemon, key, ball')
Long term (recent)	Unlimited Minutes to months	Hippocampus Mamillary bodies	Anterograde: delayed recall of an address or objects Retrograde: questions about recent events (e.g., what did you have for breakfast?)
Long term (remote)	Unlimited Lifetime	Frontal and temporal cortex	Questions about past important events. Ask about personal events (episodic; e.g., what school did you attend?) and general knowledge (semantic; e.g., which US president was assassinated in the 1960s?)

for the characteristics of different durations of explicit memory and how to test them.

COMMUNICATION

There are different ways of classifying memory, and different terms have similar or overlapping meanings. For example, some clinicians use the term 'short-term memory' to mean recent long-term memory whereas others mean working memory. When speaking to colleagues it can be useful to define the type of memory referred to by the name of the test used to measure it.

Amnesia refers to the loss of the ability to store new memories or retrieve memories that have previously been stored. Anterograde amnesia is when the patient is unable to store new memories (impaired learning of new material), although the ability to retrieve memories stored before the event or onset of disorder may remain unimpaired. Anterograde amnesia usually results from damage to the medial temporal lobes, especially the hippocampal formation.

Retrograde amnesia results in the patient being unable to retrieve memories, although the ability to store new memories may remain unaffected. Retrograde amnesia usually results from damage to the frontal or temporal cortex.

HINTS AND TIPS

Implicit memory (procedural memory) is typically preserved despite severe disruptions to explicit (declarative) memory, probably due to its independent neural location. Implicit memory is associated with basal ganglia circuitry. Explicit memory is associated with the hippocampal, diencephalic and cortical structures.

COMMON COGNITIVE DISORDERS

Delirium

Delirium is a syndrome manifesting as acute or fluctuating cognitive impairment associated with altered consciousness and impaired attention. If someone is newly disorientated and is drowsy or agitated, they are very likely to have delirium. Psychotic symptoms such as hallucinations or persecutory delusions are often present but are not essential to make the diagnosis. Delirium often fluctuates, so a patient may present as alert and attentive on the morning ward round but cognitively impaired and agitated in the evening.

Delirium is a final common pathway of severe injury to the brain or body and is a marker of severity of illness (e.g., the 'C' in the CURB65 score for severity of community-acquired pneumonia stands for 'confusion'). It is usually multifactorial and often arises from illnesses that do not directly affect the brain (Box 19.1). It has a high mortality, with around a third of people with delirium dying during the presentation. It is therefore a medical emergency and the cause should be thoroughly investigated and treated. It is particularly common in those with vulnerable brains, such as a preexisting dementia, where a relatively minor insult (e.g., dehydration or a new medication) can result in delirium. Delirium is also a risk factor for development or worsening of dementia. Delirium usually resolves when the cause is treated, but sometimes can be prolonged for weeks or months. The terms 'acute confusional state' and 'encephalopathy' have roughly the same meaning as delirium. Prominent symptoms of delirium are described further later. There are three main subtypes: hyperactive, hypoactive and mixed.

HINTS AND TIPS

Key risk factors for delirium are an abnormal brain (e.g., dementia, acquired brain injury, alcohol misuse), age (children, adults over 65 years), polypharmacy and sensory impairment.

BOX 19.1 CAUSES OF DELIRIUM (ANYTHING THAT DISRUPTS HOMEOSTASIS)

Environmental change or stress

- Hospital admission, particularly intensive care
- Urinary catheterization
- Use of physical restraint
- Major surgery
- Sleep deprivation

Drugs (use or discontinuation)

Prescribed (plus many more)

- Anticholinergics
- Benzodiazepines
- Opiates
- Antiparkinsonian drugs
- Steroids

Recreational

- Alcohol (delirium tremens, see Chapter 8)
- Opiates
- Cannabis
- Amphetamines

Poisons

- Heavy metals (lead, mercury, manganese)
- Carbon monoxide

Systemic illness

Infections and sepsis

Hypoxia

- Respiratory failure
- Heart failure
- Myocardial infarction

Metabolic and endocrine

- Dehydration
- Electrolyte disturbances
- Renal impairment
- Hepatic encephalopathy
- Porphyria
- Hypoglycaemia
- Hyper- and hypothyroidism
- Hyper- and hypoparathyroidism
- Hyper- and hypoadrenocorticism (Cushing syndrome, Addison disease)
- Hypopituitarism
- Constipation

Nutritional

- Thiamine (Wernicke encephalopathy), vitamin B_{12}, folic acid or niacin deficiency

Trauma

- Any fracture, but frequently hip fracture

Intracranial causes

Space-occupying lesions

- Tumours, cysts, abscesses, haematomas

Head injury (especially concussion)

Infection

- Meningitis
- Encephalitis

Epilepsy

Cerebrovascular disorders

- Transient ischaemic attack
- Cerebral thrombosis or embolism
- Intracerebral or subarachnoid haemorrhage
- Hypertensive encephalopathy
- Vasculitis (e.g., from systemic lupus erythematosus)

HINTS AND TIPS

The four key diagnostic features of delirium are: (1) impaired consciousness, (2) impaired attention and (3) impaired cognition, all with (4) acute or fluctuating onset. Supportive diagnostic features are perceptual and thought disturbance, sleep–wake cycle disturbance and mood disturbance.

RED FLAG

There are two types of delirium. Hypoactive delirium is characterised by drowsiness, inactivity, decreased speech and withdrawal. Hyperactive delirium is characterised by increased activity, restlessness and wandering. Patients with hypoactive delirium can sometimes go unnoticed as they do not draw as much attention on wards.

Impaired consciousness

Patients may have a reduced level of consciousness ranging from drowsiness to coma (hypoactive delirium), or they can be hypervigilant and agitated (hyperactive delirium).

Impaired attention

Ability to sustain attention is reduced and patients are easily distractible. Assess attention using tests such as serial sevens or months of the year backwards.

Impaired cognitive function

Short-term memory and recent memory are impaired with relative preservation of remote memory. Patients with delirium are most commonly disoriented to time, and often disoriented to place. It is uncommon for patients to be disoriented to self, and this would suggest a patient is severely unwell. Language abnormalities such as rambling, incoherent speech and an impaired ability to understand are common.

Perceptual and thought disturbance

Patients may have perceptual disturbances ranging from misinterpretations (e.g., a door slamming is mistaken for an explosion) to illusions (e.g., a crack in the wall is perceived as a snake) to hallucinations (especially visual and, to a lesser extent, auditory). Transient persecutory delusions and delusions of misidentification may occur.

Sleep–wake cycle disturbance

Sleep is characteristically disturbed and can range from daytime drowsiness and night-time hyperactivity to a complete reversal of the normal cycle. Nightmares experienced by patients with delirium may continue as hallucinations after awakening.

Mood disturbance

Emotional disturbances such as depression, euphoria, anxiety, anger, fear and apathy are common.

> **RED FLAG**
>
> A physical illness should always be sought when a patient presents with visual hallucinations in isolation because patients with schizophrenia or psychotic mood disorders more commonly present with auditory hallucinations.

> **RED FLAG**
>
> Delirium is a medical emergency. Around a third of people with delirium die during the episode. Thoroughly assess for and treat the probable cause(s).

> **RED FLAG**
>
> Medication is one of the easiest causes of delirium to reverse. Always check the patient's prescription. The top three drug classes which precipitate delirium are benzodiazepines, anticholinergics and opiates. Benzodiazepines may worsen many deliriums, although they are indicated in patients in GABA-ergic withdrawal deliriums such as alcohol withdrawal, where they are used in treating the underlying cause as opposed to simply being used as a sedative or anxiolytic.

Dementia

Dementia is a syndrome of acquired progressive generalized cognitive impairment associated with functional decline. There should be evidence of impairment in two or more cognitive domains (attention, memory, language, verbal fluency, visuospatial) compared to the patient's baseline. Conscious level is nearly always normal. The following text describes the general categories of impairment in dementia.

Functional impairment

Functional impairment must be present to make a diagnosis of dementia. Functional impairment means difficulties with basic or instrumental activities of daily living (ADL). Basic ADLs refer to self-care tasks such as eating, dressing, washing, toileting, continence and mobility (being able to make crucial movements such as from bed to chair to toilet). Instrumental ADLs refer to tasks which are not crucial to life, but which allow someone to live independently, such as cooking, shopping and housework. As well as being diagnostically important, someone's ability to perform ADLs determines what level of support they need (home carers or 24-hour residential care).

> **RED FLAG**
>
> A diagnosis of dementia does not automatically prevent someone from driving, but must be reported to the DVLA. The decision about driving will then be made by the DVLA based on medical reports, the person's individual cognitive functioning and in some cases a driving assessment.

Memory impairment

Impairment of memory is a common feature of dementia. Recent memory is first affected (e.g., forgetting where objects are placed, conversations and events of the previous day). With disease progression, all aspects of memory are affected, although highly personal information (name, previous occupation, etc.) is usually retained until late in the disease. Note that memory is essential for orientation to person, place and time and this will also be gradually affected (e.g., patients may lose their way in their own house).

Other cognitive symptoms (aphasia, apraxia, agnosia, impaired executive functioning)

See Table 19.1.

Stress and distress in dementia

Stress and distress in dementia, also known as 'behavioural and psychological symptoms of dementia' (BPSD), is an umbrella term for noncognitive symptoms associated with dementia, including changes in behaviour, mood and psychosis. Behavioural symptoms are very common and include pacing, shouting, sexual disinhibition, aggression and apathy. Depression and anxiety may occur in up to 50% of all those with dementia. Delusions, especially persecutory, may occur in up to 40% of patients. Hallucinations in all sensory modalities (visual is more common) occur in up to 30% of patients. Stress and distress symptoms can be similar to symptoms of delirium, but generally have a more gradual onset and conscious level is normal. See Table 19.3 for more ways to differentiate stress and distress in dementia from delirium.

Neurological symptoms

Between 10% and 20% of patients will experience seizures. Primitive reflexes (e.g., grasp, snout, suck) and myoclonic jerks may also be evident.

COMMUNICATION

When seeing a new patient with a likely diagnosis of dementia, always take a collateral history as patients may have poor insight and recall of their difficulties.

Distinguishing the type of dementia

Dementia is an umbrella term that describes a particular set of symptoms. It can be caused by a variety of underlying aetiologies, including neurodegenerative processes, cerebrovascular disease and occasionally, it can be secondary to another medical condition. Prolonged substance use (particularly alcohol, benzodiazepines and inhalants) can also present with severe and disabling cognitive impairment, beyond the period of intoxication/withdrawal. In the ICD-11, this is termed "dementia", but it can also be conceptualised as an acquired brain injury with terms such as 'alcohol-related brain damage' in widespread use. Unlike neurodegenerative dementia, a patient's cognitive

Table 19.3 Factors differentiating delirium from dementia

Feature	Delirium	Dementia
Onset	Acute	Gradual
Duration	Hours to weeks	Months to years
Attention	Impaired	Normal
Course	Fluctuating	Progressive deterioration
Consciousness	Altered	Normal
Context	New illness/ medication	Health unchanged
Perceptual disturbance	Common	Occurs in late stages
Sleep–wake cycle	Disrupted	Usually normal
Orientation	Usually impaired for time and unfamiliar people/places	Impaired in late stages
Speech	Incoherent, rapid or slow	Word finding difficulties
Things you may think	'Why aren't they listening?', 'Why won't they wake up properly?' or 'They need to calm down'	'Why do they keep telling me about the past?', 'Why do they keep asking me the same question?'

functioning generally improves somewhat over the weeks and months after abstinence from the substance. Box 19.2 describes the different diseases that can cause dementia.

HINTS AND TIPS

You may come across the term "early onset dementia"- this is a descriptor given when the onset of dementia has occurred before the age of 65.

By far the most common causes of dementia are neurodegeneration and/or vascular disease. Table 19.4 describes the distinguishing clinical features of the various types of dementias although clinically, it is often difficult to tell what form of dementia is present and definitive diagnosis can normally only be made by postmortem examination. It is important to establish the likely underlying type of dementia because:

- A secondary process causing progressive cognitive impairment (e.g., brain tumour) may be detected and possibly treated.
- The progress of certain types of dementia may be slowed with specific medication (e.g., cholinesterase inhibitors in Alzheimer dementia).

BOX 19.2 POSSIBLE CAUSES OF DEMENTIA

Neurodegenerative
- Alzheimer disease
- Frontotemporal dementia (includes Pick disease)
- Dementia with Lewy bodies (DLB)
- Parkinson disease
- Huntington disease
- Progressive supranuclear palsy

Cerebrovascular disease
- Vascular dementia
- Mixed Alzheimer and vascular dementia

Space-occupying lesions
- Tumours, cysts, abscesses, haematomas

Trauma
- Head injury
- Dementia pugilistica (sometimes called 'punch-drunk syndrome')

Infection
- Creutzfeldt–Jakob disease (including 'new variant CJD')
- HIV-related dementia
- Neurosyphilis
- Viral encephalitis
- Chronic bacterial and fungal meningitides

Metabolic and endocrine
- Chronic renal impairment (also called 'dialysis dementia')
- Liver failure
- Wilson disease
- Hyper- and hypothyroidism
- Hyper- and hypoparathyroidism
- Cushing syndrome and Addison disease

Nutritional
- Thiamine, vitamin B_{12}, folic acid or niacin deficiency (pellagra)

Drugs and toxins
- Alcohol (see Chapter 17), benzodiazepines, barbiturates, solvents

Chronic hypoxia

Inflammatory disorders
- Multiple sclerosis
- Systemic lupus erythematosus
- Normal pressure hydrocephalus

- Certain drugs may be contraindicated in some dementias (e.g., antipsychotics can cause a catastrophic parkinsonian reaction in patients with dementia with Lewy bodies).
- The prognoses of the various dementias differ; this may have practical implications for patients and their families with regards to final arrangements (e.g., wills).
- The patient's relatives may enquire about genetic counselling (e.g., Huntington disease, early-onset Alzheimer dementia).

In a minority of cases the distinction will be obvious, based on other symptoms produced by the disease process (e.g., jerky movements of the face and body [chorea]) and a positive family history would be suggestive of Huntington disease. In the majority of cases, the different dementias may be distinguished to some degree based on a detailed history from the patient and an informant, physical examination, relevant investigations and follow-up over time. However, the definitive diagnosis of a dementia subtype can only be established with absolute certainty on detailed microscopic examination of the brain at autopsy, and even then, a conclusive diagnosis may not be possible. To aid the clinical distinction of dementia, some authors differentiate dementias based on the predominance of cortical or subcortical dysfunction (see Table 19.5 for the features of cortical and subcortical dementias). This is often of limited benefit as there is often a considerable overlap of symptoms in advanced dementia of whatever type. In the ICD-11 there are specifiers that can be added to a dementia diagnosis to note the severity and specific behaviours the patient displays (see Box 19.3).

HINTS AND TIPS

At this point you might find it helpful to read up on the aetiology and neuropathology of the various neurodegenerative dementias in Chapter 20.

DIFFERENTIAL DIAGNOSIS

There are four key questions when a patient presents with possible cognitive impairment:

- Is there objective evidence of cognitive impairment on a standardised test?

Table 19.4 Distinguishing clinical features of the commonest types of dementia

Dementia type	Distinguishing clinical features
Alzheimer dementia (62%)	Gradual onset with progressive cognitive decline Early memory loss
Vascular dementia (multiinfarct dementia) (17%)	Focal neurological signs and symptoms Evidence of cerebrovascular disease or stroke May be uneven or stepwise deterioration in cognitive function
Mixed (10%)	Features of both Alzheimer and vascular dementia
Lewy body dementia (4%)	Core: Day-to-day (or shorter) fluctuations in cognitive performance Recurrent visual hallucinations Motor signs of parkinsonism (rigidity, bradykinesia, tremor) (not drug-induced) Supporting: REM sleep behaviour disorder Recurrent falls and syncope Transient disturbances of consciousness Extreme sensitivity to antipsychotics (induces parkinsonism)
Frontotemporal dementia (including Pick disease) (2%)	Behavioural variant: Early decline in social and personal conduct (disinhibition, tactlessness) Dietary changes (preference for sweet food) Early emotional blunting and loss of insight Primary progressive aphasia (nonfluent and semantic variants): Attenuated speech output, echolalia, perseveration, mutism Loss of semantic knowledge and naming Relative sparing of other cognitive functions
Parkinson disease with dementia (2%)	Diagnosis of Parkinson disease (motor symptoms over a year prior to cognitive symptoms) Dementia features very similar to those of Lewy body dementia

Percentages are prevalence of dementia subtypes in the UK population (Dementia UK report, 2007).

Table 19.5 Features of cortical and subcortical dementias

Characteristic	Cortical dementia	Subcortical dementia
Language	Aphasia early	Normal
Speech	Normal until late	Dysarthric
Praxis	Apraxia	Normal
Agnosia	Present	Usually absent
Calculation	Early impairment	Normal until late
Motor system	Usually normal posture/tone	Stooped or extended posture, increased tone
Extra movements	None (may have myoclonus in Alzheimer disease)	Tremor, chorea, tics

Cortical:
Alzheimer disease and the frontotemporal dementias (including Pick disease)

Subcortical:
Parkinson disease, dementia with Lewy bodies, Huntington disease, progressive supranuclear palsy, Wilson disease, normal pressure hydrocephalus, multiple sclerosis, HIV-related dementia

Mixed:
Vascular dementias, infection-induced dementias (Creutzfeldt–Jakob disease, neurosyphilis and chronic meningitis)

BOX 19.3 ICD-11 SPECIFIERS IN DEMENTIA

Severity specifiers

- Mild: Some impairment in cognitive functions, but may be able to live on their own. Someone meeting them for the first time may not notice any issues.
- Moderate: Require help to function outside of their house and require assistance with ADLs. May behave inappropriately in social situations.
- Severe: Often have severe memory problems and may be disoriented. They require significant help from others for personal care and may struggle to understand what is happening around them.

Behaviour specifiers:

- Psychotic symptoms in dementia
- Mood symptoms in dementia
- Anxiety symptoms in dementia
- Apathy in dementia
- Agitation or aggression in dementia
- Disinhibition in dementia
- Wandering in dementia
- Other specified behavioural or psychological disturbance in dementia
- Behavioural or psychological disturbances in dementia unspecified

- If so, is it acute, chronic or acute-on-chronic? (this may require a collateral history)
- Is the patient's conscious level normal or abnormal?
- What impact is the cognitive impairment having on the patient's functioning?

See Fig. 19.2 for a diagnostic algorithm and Box 19.4 for a summary of differential diagnosis.

Acute, acute-on-chronic or fluctuating cognitive impairment: delirium

See 'Common Cognitive Disorders' section earlier for clinical features of delirium.

Chronic cognitive impairment

Key questions when a patient presents with chronic cognitive impairment:

- Which cognitive domains are impaired? (one or many?)
- Is the impairment stable, fluctuating or progressive?
- Is the cognitive impairment causing functional impairment?
- Are there any other associated symptoms? (e.g., mood change, personality change, perceptual disturbance).

Chronic impairment in multiple cognitive domains is due most often to dementia, mild neurocognitive disorder or depression (see Box 19.4 for more differentials). Sometimes a patient has an isolated impairment (see Table 19.1 for examples), most often due to an acquired brain injury or stroke. Causes of isolated amnesia (amnesic syndrome) are considered in more detail at the end of the section.

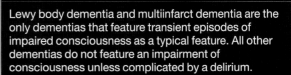

RED FLAG

Lewy body dementia and multiinfarct dementia are the only dementias that feature transient episodes of impaired consciousness as a typical feature. All other dementias do not feature an impairment of consciousness unless complicated by a delirium.

Dementia

See 'Common Cognitive Disorders' section for clinical features.

Older adults presenting with both physical health problems and generalized cognitive impairment are very common, and it is imperative that you understand how to differentiate between dementia and delirium. Table 19.3 summarizes the factors differentiating delirium from dementia – learn it well.

HINTS AND TIPS

Dementia and delirium are by far the most common causes of generalized cognitive impairment. A key question in differentiating them is the duration of impairment: is it acute, chronic or acute-on-chronic? The patient may not be able to tell you, but their notes or a collateral history from a relative or GP can be invaluable.

Mild neurocognitive disorder

Mild neurocognitive disorder (also known as 'mild cognitive impairment') is objective cognitive impairment (confirmed with a standardised test) that does not interfere notably with ADL. Mild neurocognitive impairment is a risk state for dementia, with around 10% to 15% of patients developing dementia each year. However, in some cases the impairment remains stable or even improves. All the processes that cause dementia can also cause mild neurocognitive impairment, so it is normally investigated in the same way.

Subjective cognitive impairment

Subjective cognitive impairment, also known as functional cognitive disorder, is when a patient complains of cognitive problems but scores normally on standardised tests or has normal observed

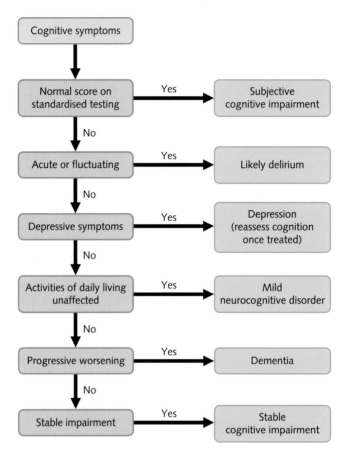

Note: Other differentials of cognitive impairment include intellectual disability, psychotic illness, amnestic disorder, dissociative disorders, factitious disorder and malingering (see Box 19.4).

Fig. 19.2 Diagnostic algorithm for cognitive symptoms.

BOX 19.4 DIFFERENTIAL DIAGNOSIS OF COGNITIVE IMPAIRMENT

Delirium
Dementia
Mild neurocognitive disorder
Subjective cognitive impairment
Stable cognitive impairment post insult (e.g., stroke, hypoxic brain injury, traumatic brain injury)
Depression
Psychotic disorders
Intellectual disability
Dissociative disorders
Factitious disorder and malingering
Amnesic syndrome

cognitive functioning. The cognitive symptoms are inconsistent with a recognised neurodegenerative disease process. It can reflect anxiety or depression, but can also represent early deterioration in a highly educated individual that is unidentifiable using standard tests. People with subjective memory impairment are at increased risk for later developing mild neurocognitive disorder or dementia.

Stable cognitive impairment

Some 'one off' insults to the brain can impair one or more aspects of cognition but not cause progressive deterioration (e.g., following a stroke, hypoxic brain injury, traumatic brain injury or viral encephalitis). Improvement post-insult can occur over several months, so it is important not to make a firm diagnosis of stable chronic impairment too soon. Often someone who has had one cerebrovascular event continues to have further episodes, so an initially stable post stroke cognitive impairment can evolve into vascular dementia.

Depression

Both depression and dementia can be associated with a gradual onset of low mood, anorexia, sleep disturbance and generalized cognitive and functional impairment, and they can be very difficult to distinguish. If there is uncertainty, treatment for depression is trialled and cognition rechecked after mood has improved. Unfortunately, depression presenting with cognitive impairment is a risk factor for later developing dementia.

HINTS AND TIPS

Often patients with dementia do not realise or acknowledge they have issues with their cognition, but depressed patients are typically more aware their memory has changed.

Psychosis

Patients with schizophrenia often have multiple cognitive deficits, particularly relating to memory, but unlike dementia, the age of onset is earlier and psychotic symptoms are present from the start. An acute psychotic state may resemble a delirium due to disturbed behaviour, vivid hallucinations, distractibility and thought disorder. However, patients generally remain orientated and symptoms do not fluctuate to the same degree as in delirium.

Intellectual disability

Patients with intellectual disability have an impaired ability to adapt to their social environment. Unlike dementia, intellectual disability manifests in the developmental period (before age 18 years) and the level of cognitive functioning tends to be stable over time, not progressively deteriorating (see Chapter 31). However, intellectual disability can be comorbid with dementia or delirium: around 50% of people with Down syndrome will develop Alzheimer dementia, often early-onset.

Dissociative disorders

Memory loss and altered conscious levels can also occur in the dissociative disorders such as dissociative amnesia, with or without dissociative fugue, see Chapter 14. These usually occur in younger adults; however, there is no evidence of a physical cause and they are usually precipitated by a psychosocial stressor.

Factitious disorder and malingering

See Chapter 15.

Amnestic disorder

While dementia is the most common cause of chronic memory dysfunction overall, certain brain diseases can cause a severe

BOX 19.5 CAUSES OF AMNESIC SYNDROME

Diencephalic damage
Vitamin B$_1$ (thiamine) deficiency (i.e., Korsakoff syndrome):
   Chronic alcohol abuse
   Gastric carcinoma
   Severe malnutrition
   Hyperemesis gravidarum
   Bilateral thalamic infarction
   Multiple sclerosis
   Post subarachnoid haemorrhage
   Third ventricle tumours/cysts

Hippocampal damage
Bilateral posterior cerebral artery occlusion
Carbon monoxide poisoning
Closed head injury
Herpes simplex virus encephalitis
Transient global amnesia

disruption of memory with minimal or no deterioration in other cognitive functions. This is termed 'amnestic disorder' and usually results from damage to the hypothalamic–diencephalic system or the hippocampal region (see Box 19.5 for the causes of amnestic disorder). Amnestic disorder is characterized by all of the following:

- Anterograde amnesia.
- Often, retrograde amnesia. The impairment of memory for past events is in reverse order of their occurrence (i.e., recent memories are the most affected).
- There is no impairment of attention or consciousness or global intellectual functioning. There is also no defect in working memory as tested by digit span.
- There is strong evidence of a brain disease known to cause amnestic disorder.

Although there is no impairment of global cognitive functioning, patients with amnestic disorder are usually disorientated in time due to their inability to learn new material (anterograde amnesia). Other associated features are confabulation (filling of gaps in memory with details which are fictitious, but often plausible), lack of insight and apathy.

The commonest cause of amnestic disorder is thiamine deficiency resulting in Wernicke encephalopathy, followed by Korsakoff syndrome. See Chapter 17 for details.

HINTS AND TIPS

Due to their unimpaired intellectual functioning, maintained communication and language skills, tendency to confabulate and lack of insight, patients with amnestic disorder can present as problem-free. Therefore, as in dementia, a collateral history is crucial.

ASSESSMENT

History

The following questions may be helpful in eliciting symptoms of cognitive impairment:

To the patient:

- Do you find yourself forgetting familiar people's names?
- Do you get lost more easily than you used to?
- Are you able to handle money confidently?
- Do you feel being forgetful is stopping you from doing anything?

To the informant:

- Are they repetitive in conversation?
- Has their personality changed?
- Are they having difficulty with aspects of their day-to-day life?
- Do you have any concerns about their safety?

Examination

Cognitive examination

The key when assessing cognition is to use a standardised test and avoid vague descriptions such as 'alert and orientated'. Many patients maintain a good social veneer, making it surprisingly easy to miss cognitive impairment if it is not formally assessed. There is a wide range of tests available of varying comprehensiveness, length and generalizability across cultures. The one you choose depends on the time available and degree of concern about a patient's cognition. In the United Kingdom, it is recommended that all hospital inpatients aged more than 65 years have their cognition screened whether or not they appear impaired. Table 19.6 lists the advantages and disadvantages of some widely used screening tests. There are many more cognitive tests which may be useful for specific disorders (e.g., the Wisconsin card test to assess frontal lobe function). Assessment of conscious level is described in Fig. 19.1.

Table 19.6 Standardised tests of cognition: advantages and disadvantages

Test	Acronym	Time to perform (min)	Advantages	Disadvantages
Abbreviated Mental Test	AMT	3	Fast	Not sensitive to mild to moderate impairment
Montreal Cognitive Test	MoCA	10	Tests all cognitive domains Sensitive to mild impairment Different versions available, e.g., MoCA-Blind and MoCA-Basic (for people with literacy problems)	Influenced by premorbid IQ, language and culture Tester needs to practice prior to administration
Addenbrooke's Cognitive Examination – III	ACE-III	20	Tests all cognitive domains Sensitive to mild impairment	Lengthy Influenced by premorbid IQ, language and culture
Frontal Assessment Battery	FAB	5	Fast, can identify frontal lobe impairment in otherwise unimpaired patients	Limited in differentiating frontal lobe impairment from other cognitive impairment
4AT	4AT	3	Fast, easy to learn	Low scores do not exclude cognitive impairment. Does not assess severity.

In the past, the MMSE (mini-mental state exam) was commonly used but is less so now because of both licensing restrictions and availability of more comprehensive tests.

Try to ensure the result of a cognitive assessment reflects cognitive abilities rather than other difficulties as far as possible: check for medications which may be influencing cognition, ensure the patient has their glasses and/or hearing aid, is not hungry, needing the toilet or exhausted. Many tests are available in a range of languages, and there are modified versions for patients with sensory impairment such as blindness or deafness.

Physical examination

A physical examination, including a neurological examination, is important for everyone with cognitive impairment as it may provide evidence of:

- Reversible causes of impairment such as hypothyroidism or a space-occupying lesion.
- Risk factors for dementia (e.g., hypertension or atrial fibrillation).
- Differential diagnosis of dementia (e.g., a hemiparesis or visual field defect suggestive of a stroke and hence increased risk for vascular dementia).
- Complications of impairment such as self-neglect or injuries from falls.
- Factors that may influence future prescribing decisions (e.g., bradycardia should lead to caution with cholinesterase inhibitors).

Investigations

The main aim of investigation in cognitive impairment is to exclude reversible causes (Table 19.7). In delirium, additional investigations for acute illness are likely to be appropriate, including an electrocardiogram (ECG) and a septic screen in the presence of infective symptoms or pyrexia.

Although some types of dementia have characteristic radiological findings (Table 19.8), these differences are not yet robust enough to be diagnostic. In some rarer forms of dementia, genetic testing may be useful (Huntington disease and early onset Alzheimer; see Chapter 20). If the diagnosis is in doubt or atypical, a more detailed cognitive assessment by a neuropsychologist may be of benefit (often accessed via a 'memory clinic').

Table 19.7 Investigations recommended in chronic cognitive impairment

Investigation	Potentially treatable cause
Full blood count, Vitamin B_{12}/folate level	Anaemia, nutrient deficiency/malabsorption
Liver function tests, thyroid function tests, calcium, urea and electrolytes, CRP, ESR, HbA1c	Liver disease, hypothyroidism, hypercalcaemia, Cushing or Addison disease, infection, autoimmune disease, diabetes

The above investigations are recommended by NICE (2022 Clinical Knowledge Summary) for excluding reversible causes of dementia in the United Kingdom. Neuroimaging (CT/MRI head scan) is also commonly used and particularly important if there are any focal neurological signs. Other investigations may also be appropriate depending on features in the history or examination (e.g., HIV or syphilis serology, heavy metal screen, autoantibodies).

CRP, C-reactive protein; CT, computed tomography; ESR, erythrocyte sedimentation rate; MRI, magnetic resonance imaging.

While radiological imaging is not required for diagnosing dementia, it can be useful if the diagnosis is unclear or there is a suspicion there may be a reversible cause.

DISCUSSION OF CASE STUDY

DD first presented with memory loss for recent events. Their personality gradually changed (withdrawn, prone to verbal aggression) and they also developed numerous other cognitive deficits: aphasia (rambling incoherently), agnosia (unable to recognize their pipe), apraxia (unable to dress themselves) and impaired executive functioning (unable to make a cup of coffee). This 6-year deterioration in cognitive and functional abilities associated with a normal level of consciousness suggests the diagnosis of dementia.

DD then developed a delirium as evidenced by the rapid onset of a fluctuating conscious level, disturbed sleep–wake cycle, psychomotor agitation and apparent perceptual disturbances (visual hallucinations). It is crucial that the cause of the delirium is diagnosed and treated. In this case, it could be pneumonia as DD had developed a productive cough.

Now go on to Chapter 20 to read about delirium and dementia and their management.

Table 19.8 Typical CT appearances for the main forms of dementia

Condition	CT appearance
Normal ageing	Progressive cortical atrophy and increasing ventricular size
Alzheimer disease	Generalized cerebral atrophy Widened sulci Dilated ventricles Thinning of the width of the medial temporal lobe (in temporal lobe-oriented CT scans)
Vascular dementia	Single/multiple areas of infarction Cerebral atrophy Dilated ventricles
Frontotemporal dementia (including Pick disease)	Greater relative atrophy of frontal and temporal lobes Knife-blade atrophy (appearance of atrophied gyri)
Huntington disease	Dilated ventricles Atrophy of caudate nuclei (loss of shouldering)
Creutzfeldt–Jakob disease (CJD)	Usually appears normal
nvCJD (new variant CJD)	nvCJD has a characteristic MRI picture: a bilaterally evident high signal in the pulvinar (post thalamic) region

Note that an MRI scan is generally preferable to a CT scan for aiding in the diagnosis of dementia because more detailed images can be obtained. CT findings are provided here because MRI is less commonly available.

CT, *Computed tomography;* MRI, *magnetic resonance imaging.*

Chapter Summary

- Cognitive impairment is common and associated with high morbidity and mortality, but is often under-recognised.
- Delirium is a syndrome of impaired consciousness, impaired attention and impaired cognition, all with acute or fluctuating onset.
- Dementia is a syndrome of acquired, gradually progressive, generalized cognitive impairment associated with functional decline.
- Always assess cognition using a standardised cognitive test.
- A collateral history is often crucial to establish the temporal pattern of cognitive difficulties and degree of functional impairment.
- Always screen for treatable causes of delirium and dementia.

UKMLA Conditions	UKMLA Presentations
Delirium	Auditory hallucinations
Dementias	Behaviour/personality change
Depression	Confusion
	Driving advice
	Memory loss
	Sleep problems
	Speech and language problems
	Struggling to cope at home
	Visual hallucinations

Cause and management

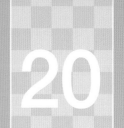

This chapter discusses the most common disorders associated with the complaints described in Chapter 19, which you might find helpful to read first.

DEMENTIA

Epidemiology

The overall prevalence of dementia is approximately 1% of the total UK population, rising sharply with increasing age. Fig. 20.1 illustrates the increasing prevalence of dementia with age. The Alzheimer's Society Dementia UK update, published in 2014 suggested that the prevalence of dementia in people aged 60 to 65 is 0.9%, increasing to 2% to 3% in people between the ages of 65 and 75, 6% to 11% in people ages 75 to 85 and 30% to 40% in people aged 85 or older. Dementia that manifests before the age of 65 years is referred to as early onset. This arbitrary age cut-off is sometimes important when determining which service will treat a patient (see Chapter 21). Alzheimer dementia (AD) is more common in women and vascular dementia is more common in men.

Dementia is a syndrome due to various diseases, most commonly neurodegeneration or vascular damage as below:

- Alzheimer Dementia, 62% of cases
- Vascular dementia, approximately 17%

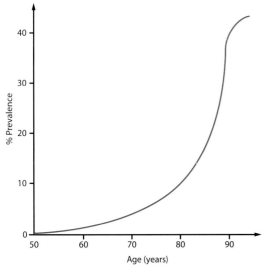

Fig. 20.1 Graph showing increasing prevalence of dementia with age.

- Combined Alzheimer and vascular ('mixed') dementia, approximately 10%
- Dementia with Lewy bodies (DLB), 4%
- Frontotemporal dementia, approximately 2% (20% of early onset dementia)
- Parkinson disease dementia 2%
- Other causes of dementia 3%
  Source: NICE 2022 Dementia Clinical Knowledge Summary.

Aetiopathology

There are many potentially modifiable risk factors for dementia as a whole, which if eliminated could reduce the prevalence of dementia by up to 40%. Many of these factors are vascular, but others include low educational attainment, hearing loss, traumatic brain injury, alcohol consumption of >21 units per week, obesity, depression, social isolation and air pollution. Although many risk factors are shared, the pathology of each type of dementia will now be discussed separately.

Alzheimer dementia

AD is classified as:

- Early onset (onset before age 65 years, usually familial, with relatives also affected before age 65 years).
- Late onset/sporadic (onset after age 65 years, either no family history or relatives affected after age 65 years).

At present, the cause of most cases of AD is unknown. It appears to be a combination of multifactorial genetic risk factors, vascular risk factors and other uncertain environmental factors. The characteristic pathological changes are:

1. Beta-amyloid **plaques** between neurones
2. Neurofibrillary **tangles** of hyperphosphorylated tau inside neurones

It is unclear whether either of these changes are a cause or a consequence of neuronal damage and death. The abnormalities generally begin in the medial temporal lobe (where key structures relating to memory are located) before becoming more diffuse, resulting in generalized cortical atrophy and compensatory ventricular enlargement. Degeneration of cholinergic neurons in the nucleus basalis of Meynert leads to a deficiency of acetylcholine, which can be partially reversed by some antidementia medications (cholinesterase inhibitors). These drugs can temporarily slow the loss of cognitive function, but not reverse or ultimately prevent it.

Genetic factors

Late-onset AD. First-degree relatives of people with AD have a threefold increased risk for developing AD themselves. The most important gene associated with late-onset AD is the gene that codes a protein involved in cholesterol metabolism called apolipoprotein E (ApoE), which is encoded by three different common alleles (ε2, ε3 and ε4). Individuals who inherit one copy of the ApoE ε4 allele are at a roughly three-fold increased risk for developing AD and those with two copies are at a roughly 10-fold increased risk. However, other environmental and genetic factors must be involved because having two ApoE ε4 alleles does not guarantee the development of AD and many patients with AD have no copies of the allele. Genome-wide association studies have identified approximately 40 genes in which polymorphisms contribute a small increase in risk for AD. These genes are involved in amyloid processing, lipid transport and metabolism, endocytosis and immune response.

Early-onset AD. Some forms of early-onset familial AD are inherited in an autosomal dominant fashion. Three genes have been isolated so far:

- Amyloid precursor protein (APP)– chromosome 21
- Presenilin-1 – chromosome 14
- Presenilin-2 – chromosome 1

These genes are all involved in metabolism of the amyloid protein. These autosomal dominant dementias present between the ages of 30 and 60 years, sometimes as early as 28 years of age when there is a mutation at presenilin 1.

Adults with Trisomy 21 (Down syndrome) invariably develop neuropathological changes similar to AD by middle age and many will develop dementia. This has been attributed to triplication and over-expression of the gene for APP.

HINTS AND TIPS

You should be aware of four genes in AD – one in late-onset AD, and three in early-onset autosomal dominant AD:

- In late-onset AD, the ApoE ε4 allele increases an individual's susceptibility to develop AD.
- In early-onset AD, the possession of a mutated version of one of three genes, amyloid precursor protein, presenilin-1 and presenilin-2, is strongly associated with development of AD.

Late-onset sporadic AD accounts for the overwhelming majority of all AD cases.

BOX 20.1 NONGENETIC RISK FACTORS FOR ALZHEIMER AND VASCULAR DEMENTIA

Vascular	Both	Alzheimer
Previous stroke	Smoking	Head injury
Atrial fibrillation	Hypertension	Low educational attainment
	Diabetes	
	Hypercholesterolaemia	
	Previous myocardial infarct	
	Obesity	
	Late-onset depression	
	Air pollution	

Nongenetic factors

The main environmental risk factors for AD are vascular (see Box 20.1). It is unclear whether vascular insufficiency in part causes the plaques and tangles seen in AD or whether vascular damage reduces the brain's reserve, making a given amount of neurodegeneration more likely to manifest clinically. Head injury and low educational attainment are also risk factors.

HINTS AND TIPS

Neurodegeneration seems to be associated with misplaced proteins: Alzheimer disease, dementia with Lewy bodies and frontotemporal dementia all involve the accumulation of degradation-resistant protein aggregates (see Table 20.1 for more detail).

HINTS AND TIPS

The National Institute for Health and Care Excellence (2015) recommends that individuals reduce their risk for dementia in later life by quitting smoking, being more active, reducing alcohol, eating healthily and maintaining a healthy weight.

Vascular dementia

The cause of vascular dementia is presumed to be multiple cortical infarctions or many small subcortical infarctions in white matter (Binswanger disease) resulting from widespread

Table 20.1 Neuropathology of dementia

Dementia type	Abnormal protein(s)	Macroscopic findings	Microscopic findings
Alzheimer dementia	Beta-amyloid Tau	Generalised cerebral atrophy, beginning in medial temporal lobes	Extracellular amyloid plaques Intracellular neurofibrillary tangles containing hyperphosphorylated tau and ubiquitin
Frontotemporal dementia (a heterogeneous collection of dementias including Pick disease and progressive supranuclear palsy)	Tau TDP FUS	Atrophy of frontal and temporal lobes, particularly anteriorly	Intracellular aggregates of tau, TDP or FUS
Dementia with Lewy bodies	α-synuclein	Mild atrophy frontal, parietal, occipital lobes	Lewy bodies (intracellular aggregates of α-synuclein and ubiquitin) in cortex
Parkinson disease (dementia point prevalence of 25%, increasing with duration)	α-synuclein	Atrophy of substantia nigra and locus coeruleus	Lewy bodies in brainstem nuclei
Huntington disease	Huntingtin	Marked atrophy of basal ganglia and often frontal lobes	Intracellular aggregates of huntingtin and ubiquitin
Creutzfeldt–Jakob disease	Prion protein	Spongiform changes throughout cortex and subcortical nuclei	Extracellular prion protein plaques, particularly in cerebellum
Vascular dementia	None identified (in most cases)	Infarction – multiple small infarcts, or single large or strategic infarct	Infarcted grey and or white matter

FUS, *Fused-in-sarcoma protein;* TDP, *TAR DNA-binding protein with molecular weight 43 kDa.*

cerebrovascular disease. On occasions, vascular dementia can arise from a single infarct in a strategic area. As with both AD and cerebrovascular disease, vascular dementia is closely associated with increasing age. In rare cases, the disease is linked to *NOTCH3*, a gene on chromosome 19 involved in vascular smooth muscle cells response to injury (cerebral autosomal dominant arteriopathy with subcortical infarcts and leukoencephalopathy (CADASIL). The risk factors for developing vascular dementia are the same as for cerebrovascular disease in general (Box 20.1).

HINTS AND TIPS

A diagnosis of mixed dementia refers to the presence of features of both vascular dementia and Alzheimer dementia. It is important to establish whether Alzheimer disease is also present, as this can dictate future treatment options, as discussed later in this chapter.

Lewy body dementias

Dementia with Lewy bodies and Parkinson disease dementia are now viewed as part of a continuum with the umbrella term Lewy body dementias (LBD). They have the same pathogenesis and as both diseases progress they become increasingly similar. Both are associated with the deposition of Lewy bodies: neuronal inclusions composed of abnormally phosphorylated neurofilament proteins aggregated with ubiquitin and α-synuclein. The initial distribution of Lewy bodies probably determines which symptoms occur first and hence which diagnosis is given initially. Early deposition in the brain stem is thought to underlie the rapid eye movement (REM) sleep behaviour disorder that often precedes the onset of LBD by several years (see Chapter 27). Deposition in the substantia nigra, with associated neuronal death, results in parkinsonism. Deposition in the cortex results in cognitive impairment and hallucinations.

Familial cases of dementia with Lewy bodies are rare but can be caused by mutations in the genes coding for α-synuclein (*SNCA*), an intracellular signaling protein (LRRK2) and lysosomal processing. Fifteen percent of people with Parkinson disease have a family history of the disorder, associated with mutations in the same genes as dementia with Lewy body and with mutations in genes coding for proteins involved in the ubiquitin-proteasome system (e.g., parkin).

The syndrome of parkinsonism (as opposed to the specific disorder of idiopathic Parkinson disease) can be due to any injury to the basal ganglia: cerebrovascular disease, head injury, carbon monoxide poisoning, dopamine antagonists (including antipsychotic medication) or other neurodegenerative disorders (e.g., Parkinson-plus syndromes such as progressive supranuclear palsy).

HINTS AND TIPS

If dementia occurs at the same time or within a year of onset of parkinsonism, dementia with Lewy bodies is diagnosed. If dementia occurs more than a year after well-established Parkinson disease, Parkinson disease with dementia is diagnosed. The umbrella term Lewy body dementia describes both disorders.

RED FLAG

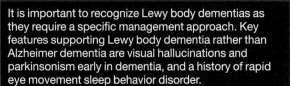

It is important to recognize Lewy body dementias as they require a specific management approach. Key features supporting Lewy body dementia rather than Alzheimer dementia are visual hallucinations and parkinsonism early in dementia, and a history of rapid eye movement sleep behavior disorder.

Frontotemporal dementia

Frontotemporal dementias are a heterogeneous group of neurodegenerative disorders associated with degeneration of the anterior part of the brain. Their pathology and presentation overlap with motor neurone disease. There are 3 main variants of frontotemporal dementia, identified on the basis of presenting symptoms. These include:

- *Behavioural variant*
- *Primary progressive aphasia:* this is further subdivided into nonfluent and semantic subtypes.
- *Motoric variant:* this includes progressive supranuclear palsy, corticobasal degeneration and amyotrophic lateral sclerosis (ALS). Typically the motoric variant presents with progressive impairment in motor functioning, but progressive neurocognitive impairment can occur simultaneously.

See Table 19.4 for further details. Macroscopically, they are associated with bilateral atrophy of the frontal and anterior temporal lobes (atrophied paper-thin gyri known as 'knife-blade atrophy') and degeneration of the striatum. Microscopically, three main types of intracellular inclusion body have been identified, containing mainly tau (e.g., Pick bodies; 30%–50% cases) the TAR DNA-binding protein (50% of cases) or the fused-in-sarcoma protein (10% of cases). Mutations in genes encoding three proteins account for around 60% of familial frontotemporal dementia: tau (microtubule stabilization), C9orf72 (endosomal trafficking) and progranulin (a protein involved in neuronal repair and lysosomal degradation).

COMMUNICATION

Pick disease is strictly a neuropathological diagnosis requiring the presence of Pick bodies at postmortem, but previously it was used to mean the clinical diagnosis of any type of frontotemporal dementia.

Huntington disease

Huntington disease has autosomal dominant inheritance with complete penetrance. It is caused by an excessive number of trinucleotide (CAG) repeat sequences, usually more than 40, in the gene encoding the protein 'huntingtin'. The length of the abnormal trinucleotide repeat sequence is inversely correlated to the age of onset of the disease. This abnormal protein is associated with neuronal death, particularly in the basal ganglia, giving rise to the distressing motor signs of the disease.

Creutzfeldt–Jakob disease and other prion-related diseases

A prion is an infectious protein. All the prion-related dementias result in a spongiform degeneration of the brain in the absence of an inflammatory immune response, associated with the deposition of the prion protein (PrP) in the form of beta-pleated sheets.

A number of prion diseases exist: kuru (prion transmitted by cannibalism of neural tissue, described in the highland tribes of New Guinea), Gerstmann–Sträussler syndrome (autosomal dominant condition caused by mutation of PrP gene on chromosome 20), scrapie in sheep and BSE (bovine spongiform encephalopathy) in cattle.

Most cases of Creutzfeldt–Jakob disease (CJD) appear to be sporadic, affecting people aged in their 50s, although it can be transmitted iatrogenically (e.g., via infected corneal transplants and surgical instruments). It presents with a rapidly progressing dementia with cerebellar ataxia and myoclonic jerks over 6 to 8 months. The electroencephalogram (EEG) characteristically shows stereotyped sharp wave complexes. Often patients present with visual symptoms first due to the effect on the occipital lobe, and as such may initially present to optician or TIA clinic.

New variant CJD (nvCJD) is thought to be secondary to the ingestion of BSE-infected beef products. It typically presents in young adults with mild psychiatric symptoms such as depression and anxiety preceding the development of ataxia, dementia and finally death over a period of 18 months. There are no characteristic EEG changes, although nvCJD may have a characteristic magnetic resonance imaging (MRI) picture: a bilaterally evident high signal in the pulvinar (postthalamic) region. As a result of public health measures, the incidence of this rare disorder has declined further, only affecting one or two people per year in the United Kingdom since 2012.

HIV-related dementia

Infection with the human immunodeficiency virus (HIV) is thought to cause direct damage to the brain in addition to the complications of HIV infection, such as opportunistic infections (cerebral cytomegalovirus infection, cryptococcosis, toxoplasmosis, tuberculosis, syphilis) and cerebral lymphoma. HIV encephalopathy presents clinically as a subcortical dementia and neuropathological examination shows diffuse multifocal destruction of the white matter and subcortical structures.

Assessment, clinical features, investigations and differential diagnosis

Discussed in Chapter 19.

Management

There is no cure for any of the neurodegenerative forms of dementia. Although the prognosis is invariably continued deterioration, considerable improvements in the quality of patients' lives are possible through a variety of psychosocial and pharmaceutical approaches. The principles of management are:

- Treating the underlying cause if possible (e.g., hypothyroidism, modifying vascular risk factors).
- Slowing down the rate of cognitive decline using antidementia drugs if indicated.
- Managing associated disorders or complications (e.g., aggression, depression, psychotic symptoms).
- Addressing resulting functional problems (e.g., kitchen skills, financial management, social isolation).
- Advising on driving.
- Providing advice and support for carers.
- Advising on legal measures to prepare for loss of capacity (e.g., Power of Attorney, Advance Statements).

Specific management strategies
Maintaining cognitive functioning

Alzheimer dementia:

- The cholinesterase inhibitors, donepezil, rivastigmine and galantamine, are recommended by National Institute for Health and Care Excellence (NICE; 2018) for patients with mild-moderate AD. Up to half the patients given these drugs will show a slower rate of cognitive decline and possible improvement in behavioural and psychological symptoms.
- Memantine is recommended by NICE (2018) for those with moderate to severe AD or for those who cannot tolerate cholinesterase inhibitors. It is an N-methyl-D-aspartate (NMDA) receptor channel blocker, thought to reduce excitotoxic damage by reducing the influx of calcium.

- A current area of research focus is on the development of monoclonal antibody treatments for Alzheimer dementia. Examples of drugs in this category includes aducanumab, lecanemab and donanemab. At the time of publishing, none of these medications are licensed for use in the UK.

Vascular dementia: Cholinesterase inhibitors are not recommended (NICE 2018). The cornerstone of treatment is optimally managing vascular risk factors. In mixed Alzheimer/vascular dementia, cholinesterase inhibitors can be prescribed.

Lewy body dementias: Cholinesterase inhibitors are recommended. Rivastigmine has the most evidence of benefit in both LBD and dementia associated with Parkinson disease.

Frontotemporal dementias: Cholinesterase inhibitors can worsen behavioural abnormalities and are not usually recommended.

Promoting cognition, independence and wellbeing

NICE (2018) recommend the following interventions for people with dementia:

- Cognitive stimulation therapy groups: patients take part in activities designed to help promote communication, memory, confidence and wellbeing.
- Group reminiscence therapy: this helps patients revisit events from their past by discussing past experiences with the help of prompts, e.g., photographs, films, sound recordings.
- Occupational therapy or cognitive rehabilitation to help support the functional abilities of patients with dementia.

Reducing symptoms of stress and distress in dementia

- Symptoms of stress and distress in dementia (also known as behavioural and psychological symptoms of dementia or BPSD) are the noncognitive symptoms of dementia, including anxiety, agitation, delusions, hallucinations, aggression, wandering and sexual disinhibition (see Chapter 19).
- If a patient develops stress and distress symptoms, the first course of action should be carefully assessing for a change in the patient's physical health, including pain, constipation and infection. People with dementia may find it very difficult to communicate discomfort. Consider medication side effects. Assess for depression. Consider also a change in the person's environment – are they troubled by noise, extremes of temperature, other people's behaviour?
- NICE (2018) recommends offering 'a range of activities to promote wellbeing that are tailored to the person's preferences'. They also recommend cognitive stimulation therapy, cognitive rehabilitation or group reminiscence therapy for people with mild to moderate dementia.

Pharmacological treatment can be considered for disturbed behaviour such as aggression or agitation that does not respond to nonpharmacological strategies and is causing significant distress or risk. Anxiolytic medication such as trazodone can be useful. Benzodiazepines should be avoided if at all possible because they worsen cognition, predispose to delirium, increase falls risk and may paradoxically disinhibit and agitate those with dementia.

- Psychotic symptoms do not require treatment if they are not distressing to the patient or causing risk to others. If there is felt to be significant distress, a trial of an antipsychotic can be considered. Consider, discuss and document the increased risk for cerebrovascular events. Review every 6 weeks. Discontinue if there is no benefit within 12 weeks.
- Depression in dementia is managed similarly to depression in older adults but with even more care taken to avoid anticholinergic drugs, which can worsen cognition.

HINTS AND TIPS

Most medications should be prescribed at lower doses in older adults. In general, prescribe according to the rule 'start low and go slow'. This is particularly true when prescribing psychotropic medications for those with vulnerable brains (e.g., dementia) where doses a tenth of what would be used in a younger adult can be sufficient.

RED FLAG

Antipsychotics prescribed to patients with dementia increase the risk of a cerebrovascular event, with studies showing a threefold increased risk compared to placebo. They are also associated with increased all-cause mortality of 1% to 2%. It is important to discuss these risks alongside potential benefits when prescribing antipsychotics, regularly review the prescription and stop the medication if there is no clear benefit.

Legal issues

- People with dementia are likely, at some point in the course of their illness, to lose the capacity to be able to make decisions about their welfare and financial affairs. It is advisable to arrange Power of Attorney as early as possible, before the person loses capacity to authorise this. They may also wish to consider an Advance Statement.
- People with dementia may lose the ability to drive safely and they and their carers should be advised to notify the Driver and Vehicle Licensing Agency (DVLA) and their insurer of their diagnosis.

RED FLAG

- Benzodiazepines should be avoided if at all possible in most patients with dementia, as they are particularly vulnerable to their adverse effects such as sedation, falls and delirium.
- Remember that 50% of patients with dementia with Lewy bodies will have a catastrophic reaction to antipsychotics (even atypicals), precipitating potentially irreversible parkinsonism, impaired consciousness, severe autonomic symptoms and a two- to threefold increase in mortality. Benzodiazepines and cholinesterase inhibitors are safer in this group of patients. This exemplifies the need to exercise caution when prescribing antipsychotics and the importance of differentiating the various types of dementia.

Course and prognosis

The course of dementia is invariably progressive. Around a third of people with dementia live in residential care. Dementia is a life-shortening illness directly and indirectly, because it reduces the ability to communicate and tolerate management of physical problems. A diagnosis of dementia roughly halves a person's remaining life expectancy. The average duration of survival from the time of diagnosis of a late-onset dementia is 4 years, although there is a wide range.

DELIRIUM

Epidemiology

Most research into the epidemiology of delirium concentrates on older adults, who, along with infants and young children, are more vulnerable to this disorder. The prevalence in hospitalised, medically unwell patients ranges from 10% to 30%. Between 10% and 35% of patients over the age of 65 years are delirious on admission and a further 10% to 40% develop a delirium during hospitalisation, with incidence increasing up to 87% in those admitted to intensive care. Patients with dementia are at an increased risk for developing a delirium; up to two-thirds of cases of delirium occur in patients with dementia.

Aetiology

Delirium is a final common pathway of disrupted homeostasis. It is nearly always multifactorial. In healthy individuals, multiple severe insults are required to cause it (e.g., head injury followed by sedative medication followed by surgery). In those with already vulnerable brains (e.g., dementia, acquired brain injury), a minor insult is sufficient (e.g., constipation, or a urinary tract infection). The commonest causes are medication (most commonly anticholinergics, opiates or benzodiazepines) or systemic illness, particularly infection. See Box 19.1 for a fuller list. Often, no cause is found – this does not preclude the diagnosis. Around a third of cases are viewed as preventable.

The pathophysiological mechanism remains unclear and may vary with cause. Suggested mechanisms include: aberrant stress response (neurotoxic effects of excess glucocorticoids), disrupted blood–brain barrier (allowing entry of toxins and cytokines to the brain) and impaired cholinergic neurotransmission.

HINTS AND TIPS

The cause of delirium is almost always multifactorial. This means prevention and management should address multiple factors too.

RED FLAG

Delirium is not just a condition of older adults – consider it as a diagnosis in patients of any age presenting with acute and fluctuating consciousness, disturbed cognition, attention and perception

Assessment, clinical features, investigations and differential diagnosis

Discussed in Chapter 19.

Management

Delirium can be highly distressing for patients and anxiety-provoking for medical ward staff who are not experienced in dealing with agitated patients. It can also be very distressing for the families and friends of the patient. Fortunately, it is treatable if managed appropriately and urgently. See Fig. 20.2 for a management algorithm incorporating recommendations by NICE (2010). General principles of management are as follows:

- Hospitalization is essential: delirium is a medical emergency (unless prior ceiling-of-care discussions have concluded that this is not appropriate).
- Vigorously investigate and treat any underlying medical condition.
- Always assess medication use, including over-the-counter treatments: this is a high-yield intervention.
- To limit confusion and foster trust, try to ensure that the patient is nursed by the same staff consistently.
- Merely the physical presence of a reassuring person is often enough to calm a distressed patient.
- Maximize visual acuity (e.g., glasses, appropriately lit environment) and hearing ability (e.g., hearing aid, quiet environment) to avoid misinterpretation of stimuli.
- Encourage a friend or family member to remain with the patient to help comfort and orientate them.
- Clocks, calendars and familiar objects may be helpful with orientation.
- Avoid tranquilizing medication unless the patient's agitation is causing them extreme distress, posing a significant risk to themselves or others or preventing them from receiving essential medical investigations or treatment. If medication is required:
  - Antipsychotics, especially low-dose haloperidol, are generally effective in treating delirious symptoms, in part due to their sedative qualities, but perhaps also due to their effects on the dopamine–acetylcholine balance.
  - Olanzapine can be given if haloperidol is ineffective or contraindicated (e.g., history of dystonia, long QTc). Low doses should be given initially (e.g., 2.5 mg).
  - Avoid benzodiazepines unless the patient is at high risk and has not responded to haloperidol, as they tend to prolong delirium. The exception is delirium relating to GABA-ergic (e.g., alcohol) withdrawal, in which they are highly effective because they are treating the underlying cause.

The specific management of delirium tremens is outlined in Chapter 22.

RED FLAG

Remember that delirium indicates the presence of a medical condition that should be managed on a medical, not a psychiatric, ward. Remember this when making referrals.

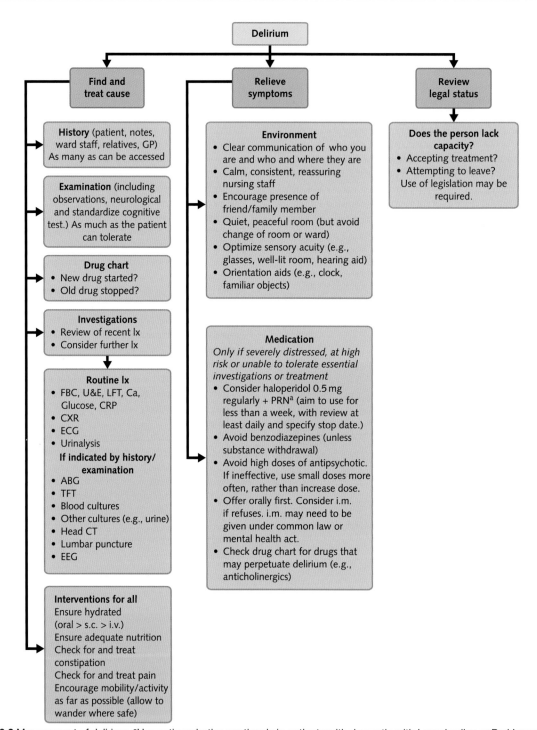

Fig. 20.2 Management of delirium. [a]Use antipsychotics cautiously in patients with dementia with Lewy bodies or Parkinson disease (see earlier) or with a prolonged QTc. Use benzodiazepines instead. ABG, *Arterial blood gas;* Ca, *calcium;* CRP, *C-reactive protein;* CT, *computed tomography;* CXR, *chest X-ray;* ECG, *electrocardiogram;* EEG, *electroencephalogram;* FBC, *full blood count;* GP, *general practitioner;* i.m., *intramuscular;* i.v., *intravenously;* LFT, *liver function test;* PRN, *when necessary;* s.c., *subcutaneous;* TFT, *thyroid function test;* U&E, *urea and electrolytes.*

Course and prognosis

The average duration of a delirium is 7 days, but delirium can be prolonged for weeks or months, even after the initial insult is treated. Some studies suggest that symptoms of disorientation, inattention and memory impairment might persist for up to 12 months. Inpatients who develop delirium have an increased mortality, with around a third dying during that admission. This is unsurprising given that delirium is often a sign of severe systemic illness. Those who survive have an increased duration of admission, are at increased risk for complications such as pressure sores and falls and are more likely to be discharged to institutional care. An episode of delirium increases the risk for developing dementia sixfold and, in those with preexisting dementia, delirium can accelerate cognitive decline. Factors that worsen prognosis following an episode of delirium include the patient having a preexisting dementia or cognitive impairment, older age, frailty, hypoxic illness (e.g., severe pneumonia), visual impairment, hypoactive delirium and prolonged duration of delirium.

● Chapter Summary

- Dementia is very common, affecting around 7% of those aged over 65 years and increasing with age.
- The four commonest types of dementia in older adults are: Alzheimer > vascular > Lewy body > frontotemporal.
- Neurodegenerative dementia arises due to abnormally folded proteins, vascular dementia due to one or many infarcts.
- Dementia cannot be cured, but some of the commonest forms can be slowed using cholinesterase inhibitors.
- Stress and distress symptoms in dementia should be managed nonpharmacologically wherever possible.
- Delirium is very common in hospitalised older adults, particularly those with preexisting cognitive impairment, sensory impairment, polypharmacy or who are severely unwell. Think delirium!
- Delirium is a medical emergency that requires prompt assessment and treatment of causes.
- Management of the symptoms of delirium requires environmental approaches for all and medication for a minority.

UKMLA Conditions
Delirium
Dementia

UKMLA Presentations
Behaviour/personality change
Concerns
Confusion
Driving advice
Memory loss
Mental capacity
Struggling to cope at home

Ageing is associated with an increased prevalence of both mental and physical health problems. Older adults may also face new social challenges such as coming to terms with retirement; income reduction; living alone or being separated from family; death of spouse, siblings and peers and coping with deteriorating physical health and mobility.

The most common psychiatric disorders in older adults are dementia and delirium (see Chapter 20). This chapter considers other psychiatric disorders in older adults.

Patients used to arbitrarily come under the care of older adult psychiatrists at the age of 65 years. However, concerns were raised that an automatic transfer to older adult services at a given age resulted in age-based discrimination. Instead, a 'needs-based' approach is now being taken in the majority of areas, whereby patients with problems that older adult services are expert in are transferred, with everyone else remaining under the care of general adult services, whatever their age. This also has the advantage of maintaining continuity of care. Examples of patients that older adult services are best placed to manage are:

- People with dementia of any age.
- People with a mental disorder and significant physical problems or frailty which cause or complicate the management of their mental illness (e.g., someone with both schizophrenia and chronic obstructive pulmonary disease requiring nursing home care).

Regardless of which services care for them, the number of people aged over 65 years is set to increase substantially over coming decades. Currently, around one in five of the UK population is over 65 years of age but by 2040 one in four people is projected to be aged over 65 years. The number of 'very old' people (aged over 85 years) is also continuing to increase.

MENTAL ILLNESS IN OLDER ADULTS

Epidemiology

The prevalence of all mental illnesses tends to increase with age and tends to be higher in residential homes. Fig. 21.1 summarizes the prevalence of the individual psychiatric disorders in older adults.

Depression

Depression in older adults presents similarly to that in younger people, but a slightly different symptom set needs to be focused

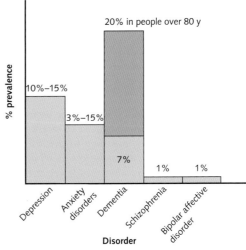

Fig. 21.1 Prevalence of mental illness in people over the age of 65 years.

on. Symptoms such as fatigue, insomnia and anorexia are more likely to arise in older adults for reasons other than depression and so are less specific in supporting the diagnosis. Similarly, poor concentration and memory are very common in older adult depression but could also reflect a cognitive disorder (see Chapter 19). Instead, negative cognitions such as guilt, hopelessness and suicidality are given more diagnostic weight. There are also certain features of depression that are more common in older adults:

- Severe psychomotor agitation or retardation.
- Cognitive impairment
- Poor concentration.
- Generalized anxiety.
- Excessive concerns about physical health (hypochondriasis).
- When psychotic, older adults are particularly likely to have hypochondriacal delusions, delusions of poverty and nihilistic delusions (see Table 9.1).

Depression is often underdiagnosed in older adults, so a high index of suspicion is needed. Older adults are also less likely to be referred to mental health services regarding depression. This may reflect a perception that low mood is part of normal ageing: it is not. Effective management of depression is important not least because older adults are at high risk for completed suicide, even though the prevalence of self-harm in this group is lower than in younger adults.

RED FLAG

Always think about depression in an older adult presenting with abnormal illness behaviour: hypochondriasis is a common presenting symptom.

RED FLAG

Self-harm in an older adult should be considered to be with suicidal intent until proven otherwise.

The principles of treatment are the same as for younger adults, taking a stepwise approach guided by severity of illness. In addition, it is particularly important to check for physical problems or medication that can cause low mood as the likelihood of these is higher in older adults (see Tables 11.1 and 11.2).

Mild depression and subthreshold symptoms may respond well to psychosocial interventions alone (e.g., befriending, assistance in accessing community supports such as lunch clubs, structured exercise programmes).

Psychological therapies for depression (mainly cognitive-behavioral therapy) are just as effective in older adults as in younger adults and are recommended in those with moderate-to-severe depression. Psychological therapies are particularly useful for patients whose comorbidities place them at high risk of side-effects from medications.

The National Institute for Health and Care Excellence (NICE) also recommends antidepressant medication for those with moderate-to-severe depression, although medication should be introduced cautiously as older adults have an increased risk of developing adverse side effects and generally need lower doses. Selective serotonin reuptake inhibitors are first line. Tricyclic antidepressants should be avoided if possible as postural hypotension and cognitive impairment are very common side effects in older adults, due to the burden of anticholinergic side effects. Response to antidepressants is often slower in older adults, with benefits taking 6 to 8 weeks to emerge. Lithium augmentation may be used in treatment-resistant cases, although the dose is generally lower than that used in younger adults.

HINTS AND TIPS

Some selective serotonin reuptake inhibitors side effects are more likely to occur in older adults than younger adults: hyponatraemia (consider monitoring sodium), gastrointestinal bleeding (consider proton pump inhibitor) and drug interactions (least likely with citalopram and sertraline).

Electroconvulsive therapy (ECT) is a very effective treatment for severe depression in older adults and should be considered for severe symptoms of psychosis, suicidality or life-threatening food and fluid refusal. Dementia is not a contraindication.

Poor prognostic factors include comorbid physical illness, severity of illness and poor concordance with antidepressant medication. The median duration of an episode is 18 months, longer than in younger adults. Having depression reduces life expectancy in older adults by on average 3 years, even when physical illness is taken into account. It also doubles the person's risk of developing dementia.

HINTS AND TIPS

Cotard syndrome describes the presence of nihilistic and hypochondriacal delusions as part of a depressive psychosis and is typically seen in older adults.

HINTS AND TIPS

A common triad in older adults is depressive symptoms, cognitive impairment and functional impairment. It is often difficult to tease out whether someone is experiencing depression manifesting with cognitive impairment or an early dementia leading to comorbid depression. Ideally, depression is treated first, then cognition reassessed once mood is euthymic.

Anxiety disorders

Studies that have assessed prevalence of anxiety disorders in older adults alongside younger adults have found that anxiety disorders reduce with age. Generalized anxiety disorder is the commonest specific anxiety disorder in those aged over 65 years (affecting 2%–7%), specific phobias affect around 3% and social phobia, obsessive-compulsive disorder and panic disorder are all uncommon, each occurring in less than 1%. It is rare for anxiety disorders to arise for the first time in older adults. Importantly, anxiety (particularly health related) is a common presenting symptom of depression in older adults, so anyone presenting for the first time with anxiety in later life should be carefully assessed for depression.

Treatment of anxiety disorders in older adults is broadly similar to that in younger adults, with evidence supporting benefits from both medication and psychological therapies (although psychological therapies appear to be not as beneficial as in younger adults). Benzodiazepines should be avoided where at all possible because of the risks of cognitive impairment and falls in older adults.

Mania

Unlike depression, the incidence of bipolar disorder does not increase with age, although late-onset cases seem to be less influenced by genetic factors (fewer of these patients have positive family histories for mood disorders). In a fifth of cases, mania is precipitated by an acute medical condition (e.g., stroke or myocardial infarction), making it particularly important to screen for physical or medication causes (see Box 10.1). Hyperactive delirium is an important differential. The presentation and treatment are similar to those of younger adults.

Late-onset schizophrenia

Older adult psychiatrists in the United Kingdom use the term *late-onset schizophrenia* to denote a group of patients who develop their first psychotic symptoms late in life, usually over the age of 60 years. Late-onset schizophrenia is characterized predominantly by delusional thinking, usually of a persecutory or grandiose nature. These delusions tend not to be as bizarre as they sometimes are in earlier-onset schizophrenia (e.g., rather than believing that secret agents are monitoring them by satellite, a patient with late-onset schizophrenia may assert that the neighbours have been poisoning their water supply). They are also more likely to experience 'partition delusions', which is the belief that people or objects can pass through an impermeable barrier. Hallucinations may occur, but disorganized thinking, inappropriate affect and catatonic features are rarer than in younger adults. The key differentials are dementia, delirium or medication-induced psychotic symptoms.

The aetiology of late-onset schizophrenia seems different to early onset schizophrenia in that affected patients are less likely to have a family history of schizophrenia. In addition, late-onset schizophrenia is far more common in women than men – unlike early-onset schizophrenia, which is slightly more likely to arise in men. Sensory deprivation, particularly hearing loss, and social isolation are also implicated in its aetiology.

The treatment is with antipsychotics, but some work is needed in building up a therapeutic relationship as these patients are often difficult to engage and poor concordance is associated with a poor treatment response. Note that although late-onset schizophrenia does seem to be a distinct entity, it is not a term used by the ICD-11 or the DSM-5; here, these patients would be classified simply as having schizophrenia or delusional disorder.

HINTS AND TIPS

Diogenes syndrome is the term used to describe a self-isolated person who lives in a state of significant self-neglect, which may include hoarding and squalid living conditions. This is purely a descriptive term and may occur in individuals who misuse alcohol or have frontal lobe dysfunction, personality disorder and chronic psychotic illness. It may also occur at a younger age.

ASSESSMENT CONSIDERATIONS IN OLDER ADULTS

- Home assessments are a very important part of older adult psychiatry. Patients can be assessed in their normal environment and collateral information can be obtained from family members. It is important to ascertain whether the patient can be managed at home (i.e., risk of harm to self and others; ability to carry out activities of daily living, drive, manage financial affairs), or whether additional community support or hospitalisation is needed.
- Collateral information from the patient's general practitioner (GP), family and carers is an important part of history taking.
- Ensure the patient has any aids they require to optimize their communication (e.g., glasses, hearing aids, dentures).
- Mental state examination follows the same format as for all adults, although extra consideration should be given to the assessment of cognitive functioning and it is advisable to always do a standardized test (see Table 19.6 for examples).
- A thorough physical assessment is very important – this may be best done by the patient's GP. Do not forget to consider hearing and vision as well as tremors and involuntary movements.
- Routine investigations in newly diagnosed or hospitalised older adults include: full blood count, urea and electrolytes, liver function tests, thyroid function tests, calcium, glucose, urinalysis (with midstream urine microscopy and culture if indicated), chest X-ray, electrocardiogram and consideration of serum magnesium, phosphate, vitamin B_{12} and folate and a computed tomography or magnetic resonance imaging scan of the head. Remember that the chances of a physical illness causing or aggravating a mental disorder are significant in older adults.
- It is also important to be aware of the possibility of elder abuse. Abuse can happen in many locations, including a person's own home or within a residential care setting. Older

people who physically or mentally depend on others for help with activities of daily living are more vulnerable to abuse. Abuse can be physical, emotional, financial or sexual, or may take the form of neglect. Consider elder abuse in any older adult presenting with unexplained physical injuries, physical signs, e.g., bed sores that are associated with neglect, who looks unkempt with unwashed clothes or hair, who becomes more withdrawn or who has unpaid living expenses where someone else has access to or has responsibility for managing their finances.

HINTS AND TIPS

Patients' homes can give assessing clinicians important information about their mental state. It can also give an indication of their level of functioning and whether they are coping at home. This can help inform decisions about the most appropriate place for ongoing care.

TREATMENT CONSIDERATIONS IN OLDER ADULTS

Physiological changes with ageing

There are a number of physiological changes that occur with ageing, which may affect the way the body handles certain drugs. Table 21.1 describes the most important changes and their effects. The net result of these changes is that the tissue

concentration of a drug may be increased by over 50%, especially in malnourished, dehydrated and debilitated patients. Therefore, the adage, 'start low and go slow' applies especially to the use of psychotropic drugs in the older adult.

Polypharmacy

It is estimated that around 1 in 10 people over the age of 65 take at least seven prescribed medications, and that 1 in 5 hospital admissions are caused by adverse effects of medicines. Polypharmacy increases the risk of adverse reactions, drug interactions and poor concordance. Therefore, prescribing psychotropic drugs for common, self-terminating symptoms such as insomnia and headache should be avoided wherever possible. When psychotropic drugs are recommended, follow-up arrangements should include a timely assessment of response and discontinuation of any ineffective treatments. Medication should not be a substitute for adequate social care, the lack of which often underlies many nonspecific symptoms.

Concordance

Concordance is often a problem in older adults, especially with those who are visually impaired, cognitively impaired, take numerous drugs, and live alone. This may be improved by simplifying medication regimens, taking time to explain dosing schedules, using large font prescription labels or concordance aids such as dosette boxes. Organizing supervision of medication by a relative, friend or support worker may be necessary.

Psychosocial interventions

Psychological treatments, such as cognitive-behavioural therapy, can be used with success in older adults as with younger adults. Reality orientation and reminiscence therapies have

Table 21.1 Age-related changes in drug handling and effects: in general lower doses are needed in older adults

Physiological changes	Effects
Reduction in renal clearance (glomerular filtration rate and tubular function)	Drugs excreted by filtration (e.g., lithium) need lower doses. Drug concentrations may rise rapidly with dehydration, heart failure, etc.
Decreased lean body mass and total body water and increased body fat	Volume of distribution increases for lipid-soluble drugs (most psychotropic drugs), and reduces for water-soluble drugs (e.g., lithium). Half-life of lipid-soluble drugs prolonged (e.g., diazepam half-life doubled).
Decreased plasma albumin	Reduced drug binding resulting in increased physiologically active unbound fraction.
Reduced hepatic metabolism and first-pass metabolism	May increase the bioavailability and elimination of some drugs.
Increased sensitivity to central nervous system drugs	Sedating drugs may result in drowsiness, confusion, falls and delirium. Tricyclics are more likely to be associated with anticholinergic and postural hypotensive effects. Antipsychotics are more likely to be associated with parkinsonism and increased risk of cerebrovascular accident.
Decreased total body mass	Lower doses of drugs needed (think in terms of milligram/kilogram as opposed to standard dose for all).

been used to reduce disorientation and stimulate remote memories in patients with dementia. Practical psychosocial interventions such as memory aids (e.g., notebooks, calendars) and assistance with mobility and daily activities by a support worker should not be underestimated. Occupational therapy assessment of activities of daily living, which assess skills such as washing, dressing, eating, and shopping, give carers an indication of patients' strengths and weaknesses and enable a care package to be tailored that caters specifically to these.

● Chapter Summary

- Mental illness in older adults is overall similar in presentation and management to younger adults.
- Depressive episodes in older adults often have prominent features of cognitive impairment, agitation and health-related anxiety.
- Self-harm in an older adult should be considered to be with suicidal intent until proven otherwise.
- New-onset mood, anxiety and psychotic illnesses are rare but do occur.
- Be cautious with psychotropic medication use in older adults.
- Psychological interventions are effective in older adults.

UKMLA Conditions
Depression
Schizophrenia
Anxiety Disorder: Generalized

UKMLA Presentations
Confusion
Elation/elated mood
Elder abuse
Fixed abnormal beliefs
Suicidal thoughts
Anxiety, Phobias, OCD

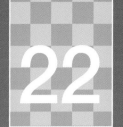

Alcohol and substance disorders · 22

This chapter discusses the disorders associated with the complaints described in Chapter 17, which you might find helpful to read first. Alcohol-related disorders will be presented first, followed by other psychoactive substances. Disorders due to addictive behaviours will be discussed briefly at the end of the chapter.

ALCOHOL DISORDERS

Epidemiology

Alcohol use is declining in the United Kingdom but is still associated with high morbidity and mortality and overall is the most harmful psychoactive substance in common use (see Fig. 22.1).

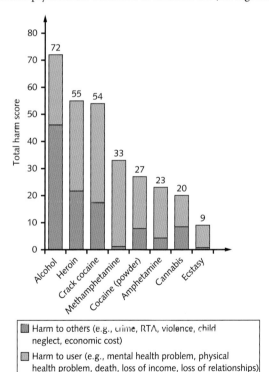

Fig. 22.1 Relative harmfulness of commonly used psychoactive substances. Alcohol causes the most harm to others with heroin and crack cocaine causing the most harm to users. When scores are combined, alcohol is the most harmful substance. *RTA, Road traffic accidents.* (Modified from Nutt, DJ, et al. Drug harms in the UK: a multicriteria decision analysis. *Lancet* 2010; 376(9752): 1558–1565.)

In England, among people aged 15 to 49 years, alcohol is the leading cause of ill-health, disability and death. Rates of alcohol use were impacted by the COVID-19 pandemic, in general, lighter drinkers drank less than usual during the pandemic, and heavier drinkers drank more. Middle-aged people are the most likely to drink dependently and to die of complications from alcohol abuse. Men are more likely to drink excessively than women (see Table 22.1).

Aetiology

The causes of alcohol dependence are multifactorial and are determined by biological, psychological and sociocultural factors.

Genetic and biochemical factors

Strong evidence shows a genetic component to alcohol dependence. Family studies show an increased risk for dependence among relatives of dependent individuals. Twin studies indicate that monozygotic twins have a higher concordance rate than

Table 22.1 Epidemiology of alcohol use[a]

	Prevalence	Association with gender and age
Alcohol use	57% drank any alcohol within the last week (*this proportion is gradually reducing*). 20% reported not drinking at all.[b]	62% men, 52% women Age 16–24 years least likely to drink[b]
Hazardous use (>14 units/week)	24% regularly exceed guidelines[b]	25% of men, 11% of women[b]
Hospital admissions related to alcohol	6% of all hospital admissions (814,595)[c]	72% male, 28% female[c]
Deaths related to alcohol	1.5% of all deaths (8974)[d]	Male-to-female ratio 2:1. Highest percentage in Scotland and Northern Ireland[d]

[a]These are self-report values; alcohol sales figures show actual consumption is higher.
[b]*Office of National Statistics Adult Drinking Habits in Great Britain (2017).*
[c]*Local Alcohol Profile England (2021).*
[d]*Office of National Statistics, Alcohol Specific Deaths in the UK (2021).*

dizygotic twins and adoption studies indicate a heritable component. The nature of this influence is unclear. It may operate at the level of heritable personality characteristics or it might relate to the body's inherited biochemical susceptibility to alcohol and its consequences. For example, 50% of East Asians have a deficiency in mitochondrial aldehyde dehydrogenase, leading to flushing and palpitations after small quantities of alcohol; this may explain reduced rates of consumption and dependence in these cultures.

From a biochemical perspective, chronic alcohol consumption influences a range of receptors and intracellular signalling proteins to cause long-term changes in plasticity in reward pathways, and to cause epigenetic changes. Some of the systems implicated are decreasing activity (downregulation) of γ-aminobutyric acid (GABA) systems and increasing activity (upregulation) of glutamate (mainly N-methyl-D-aspartate, or NMDA) systems.

Psychological factors

Behavioural models explain dependence in terms of operant conditioning where:

- Positive reinforcement occurs when the pleasant effects of alcohol consumption reinforce drinking behaviour (despite adverse social and medical consequences).
- Negative reinforcement occurs when continued drinking behaviour is reinforced by the desire to avoid the negative effects of alcohol withdrawal symptoms.

An alternative behavioural explanation is the observational learning theory (modelling), which suggests that patterns of drinking are modelled on the drinking behaviour of relatives or peers. Family studies support the idea that drinking habits follow those of older relatives.

The presence of psychiatric (anxiety, bipolar disorder, depression, schizophrenia) or physical illness appears to increase the risk for alcohol abuse and dependence, although differentiating cause and effect can be difficult (see Chapter 17). There is also evidence linking alcohol dependence with dissocial and borderline personality traits. Possible explanations for this could include any of the following: attempts to self-medicate to relieve symptoms, the use of alcohol as a (maladaptive) coping mechanism, the lack of a supportive environment, impulsivity or the lack of insight into the risks associated with excessive alcohol.

Social and environmental factors

The cultural attitude towards alcohol affects the prevalence of alcohol-related problems (e.g., lower rates in Jewish societies as opposed to Mediterranean countries). Enormous cross-cultural variation in the way that people behave when drinking alcohol has been noted (e.g., alcohol consumption in the United Kingdom, United States and Australia is associated with antisocial behaviour and violence, while in Mediterranean countries it is generally more peaceful), suggesting that the effect that alcohol has on behaviour is linked to social and cultural factors rather than solely to the chemical effects of ethanol. Alcohol consumption is greatly affected by price; strong evidence exists to suggest that the more affordable alcohol is, the more is consumed and the more harm results (see

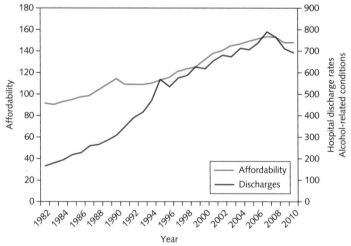

Fig. 22.2 Increasing alcohol affordability is associated with increasing alcohol-related harm. Alcohol has become around 45% more affordable in the United Kingdom since 1980, and alcohol-related hospital admissions have quadrupled. As the affordability of alcohol has increased, so has the number of hospital discharges for alcohol-related conditions (rates shown here are per 100,000 people in the population of Scotland). This is the rationale for minimum unit pricing which has been introduced in Scotland. The impact is due to be assessed in 2023. (Modified from Scottish Government (2012). Framework for Action: Changing Scotland's Relationship With Alcohol. Available at: https://www.gov.scot/Publications/2009/03/04144703/14.)

Fig. 22.2). Since May 2018, every alcoholic drink sold in Scotland has cost a minimum amount per unit, reducing alcohol sales by 3% by 2022. Data from the first 3 years after the policy was introduced shows it has so far resulted in a 13.4% reduction in deaths wholly attributable to alcohol and a 4.1% reduction in admissions wholly attributable to alcohol.

There is an association between certain occupations and deaths from alcoholic liver disease. The highest-risk professions are members of leisure and catering trades (publicans especially), doctors, journalists and those involved with shipping and travel. Furthermore, higher rates of dependence are noted in unskilled workers and the unemployed compared with those with higher incomes. This may be partly explained by the 'social drift' caused by alcohol dependence (see Box 17.3).

The frequency of significant life events increases the risk for harmful drinking. Although the anxiolytic properties of alcohol are often used as a means of coping with stress, the social and physical complications of heavy drinking often lead to further stress.

Assessment, clinical features, investigations and differential diagnosis

Discussed in Chapter 17.

Management

The management of alcohol-related problems varies markedly depending on the pattern of use. Advice about reducing intake may be sufficient for hazardous drinkers and can be delivered by general practitioners (GPs) or any healthcare professional. See the box (FRAMES) for guidance on how to deliver a brief alcohol intervention. Up to a third of people with alcohol problems manage to abstain from alcohol without any formal treatment or self-help programme. NICE CKS (2022) recommends that all people who are seeking help for alcohol misuse are directed to community support networks such as Alcoholics Anonymous. Those with mild dependence should be offered referral for a psychological intervention (e.g., CBT or behavioural therapy focused on alcohol-related thoughts and actions). Those who are moderately severely dependent should be referred to specialist alcohol services. NICE CKS (2022) also recommends that GPs offer oral thiamine to patients who are harmful/dependent drinkers who are malnourished or have decompensated liver disease. Management of alcohol dependence can be considered as having two overlapping objectives: the treatment of alcohol withdrawal and the longer-term maintenance of abstinence: these are considered further below.

HINTS AND TIPS

COMPONENTS OF A BRIEF ALCOHOL INTERVENTION (FRAMES)

Research has shown that the features below contribute to the effectiveness of a brief alcohol intervention. Remember the acronym FRAMES:

F – Feedback: after taking a history or using a screening tool, point out the patient's alcohol problem and/or how alcohol may have contributed to their presenting complaint.

R – Responsibility: the decision whether or not to change is the patient's responsibility. Emphasizing this is less likely to trigger resistance.

A – Advice: clearly state that cutting down or stopping alcohol will reduce the patient's risk for future health problems.

M – Menu: provide a range of options the patient can use for change (e.g., a substance diary, alternative activities to drinking, identifying and avoiding high-risk situations, attending mutual aid groups). Encourage the patient to select one or two to begin with.

E – Empathy: be warm, reflective and understanding

S – Self-efficacy: help the patient to feel confident they can make the proposed changes. Encourage the patient to describe their ability to make the change in their own words, for example; 'Do you think this is a change you'll be able to make?'.

Treatment of alcohol withdrawal

All clinicians need to be able to recognize alcohol withdrawal because of its high mortality and morbidity. The treatment of the alcohol withdrawal syndrome is commonly termed 'detoxification'. The following points are important:

- For the majority of patients, an outpatient or community-based detoxification will be safe and effective.
- Contraindications to detoxification in the community include severe dependence, a history of withdrawal seizures or delirium tremens, an unsupportive home environment, significant physical or psychiatric comorbidity, advanced age, pregnancy, cognitive impairment or learning disability or a previous failed community detoxification. In these cases, inpatient detoxification is advised.
- Unplanned, short-notice detoxification should only be undertaken if absolutely necessary (e.g., if a patient has to be an inpatient for another reason). In general, detoxification works best when it is planned in advance to allow the

perpetuating factors for dependence to be addressed alongside detoxification.

- In order to relieve severe symptoms and reduce the risk for developing seizures or delirium tremens, a drug with similar neurochemical effects to alcohol is prescribed, usually a benzodiazepine (such as chlordiazepoxide, diazepam or lorazepam). This may be given in a reducing regime (where high doses are given and then gradually reduced over 5–7 days) or a symptom-triggered regime (where doses are only given if the patient exhibits withdrawal symptoms).
- Medication may not be necessary if the patient has been drinking less than 15 units/day (men) or 10 units/day (women) and has no current or previous withdrawal symptoms.
- Alcohol withdrawal is a high-risk time for precipitating Wernicke encephalopathy (brain damage due to thiamine deficiency). Thiamine is therefore given prophylactically to those undergoing alcohol withdrawal. If a patient is well nourished and otherwise physically well, oral supplements are recommended. However, parenteral thiamine (Pabrinex) is needed if there is any suspicion of the onset of Wernicke, if someone is acutely physically unwell for any reason, if they are admitted to hospital, if they are malnourished or if they have decompensated liver disease.
- Every time the brain withdraws from alcohol, it is at risk for delirium with persistent cognitive impairment. However, continuing alcohol also places the individual at risk for brain damage. If a person relapses after detox, it is usually recommended to wait for at least 6 months before initiating a further detox, to balance the risk of brain damage from withdrawal with the risk of brain damage from ongoing alcohol use.
- Acamprosate is given in some centres because of its potential neuroprotective effect during alcohol withdrawal.

The box below summarizes the management of delirium tremens and Wernicke encephalopathy.

MANAGEMENT OF DELIRIUM TREMENS

Emergency hospitalization essential

Physical examination and investigations:

Thorough search for alternative cause of delirium associated with alcohol use, for example

- Infection
- Head injury
- Liver failure
- Gastrointestinal haemorrhage

Assess for signs of:

- Wernicke encephalopathy

Medication:

Control withdrawal symptoms and reduce risk for seizures

- Large doses of a drug with similar neurochemical actions to alcohol (e.g., benzodiazepines. Intravenous therapy seldom needed). Also prevents and controls seizures.
- Follow local guidelines regarding dosage and choice of benzodiazepine: in general, dosage is symptom driven (e.g., using CIWA) or follows a reducing regime.
- Only use antipsychotics (e.g., haloperidol) for severe psychotic symptoms (risk for lowering seizure threshold).

Prophylaxis against or treatment of Wernicke encephalopathy

- Large dosages of parenteral (intramuscular or slow intravenous) thiamine (Pabrinex). Oral thiamine is not adequate in delirium tremens.

Monitoring of temperature, fluid, electrolytes and glucose:

Risk for hyperthermia, dehydration, hypoglycaemia, hypokalaemia, hypomagnesaemia

General principles for managing delirium:

See Chapter 20.

COMMUNICATION

Some patients think that 'detoxification' refers to the treatment of alcohol dependence. However, it only refers to the management of physical and psychiatric symptoms of withdrawal. Treating alcohol dependence involves addressing biological, psychological and social factors that may have precipitated and perpetuated its development.

RED FLAG

Delirium tremens is a medical emergency that is common on medical and surgical wards. Despite appropriate care and treatment, it is associated with a mortality of 5% to 15% (estimated to be as high as 35% if untreated), emphasizing the need for prompt recognition and appropriate treatment. Make sure that you know the symptoms (Chapter 17) and management well.

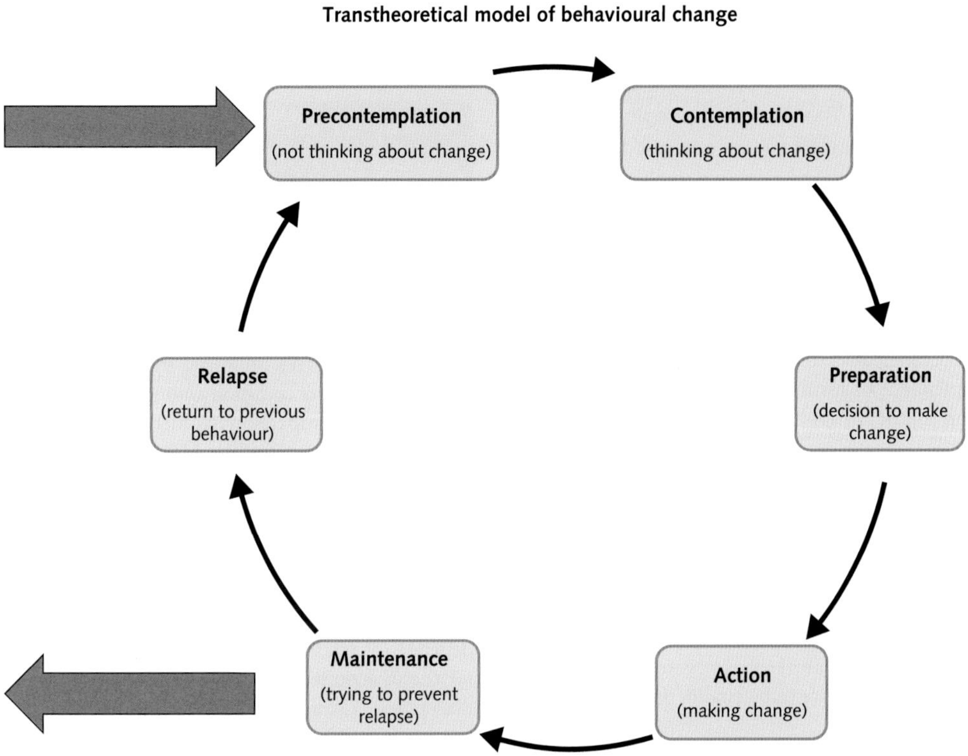

Transtheoretical model of behavioural change

Fig. 22.3 Prochaska and DiClemente stages of change. (Adapted with permission from Prochaska JO, et al. In search of how people change; applications to addictive behaviours. *American Psychologist*. 1992; 47: 1102–1114.)

Maintenance after detoxification

Remaining abstinent from alcohol is not as simple as a successful detoxification. Often the period post detoxification highlights psychosocial issues to the patient that intoxication had previously allowed them to ignore. This may include the reasons they started to drink to excess in the first place and the psychological/ social impacts on themselves and others subsequent to becoming dependent. For this reason, psychosocial interventions are crucial in allowing the patient to process emotional distress and to develop a new network of friends with similar experiences who are now sober. Recovery can be a transformational process, with changes far wider reaching than simply achieving abstinence.

Psychosocial interventions

Not all interventions are suited to all patients, but the huge range available means there will be something that meets the needs of everyone. Many interventions include assessing where a patient's motivation for change is using Prochaska and DiClemente's stages of change model (Fig. 22.3).

The various forms of psychosocial intervention that have been shown to be effective in managing alcohol problems include:

- Motivational interviewing (see Chapter 3).
- Cognitive behavioural therapy (CBT): focusing on cue exposure, relapse prevention work, behavioural contracting, dealing with trauma symptoms.
- Mutual aid organizations.
- 12-step fellowship organizations (e.g., Alcoholics Anonymous): based around a 12-step programme of spiritual and personal development.
- SMART recovery uses CBT to facilitate group self-help.
- Social support: social workers, probation officers and citizens' advice agencies may be able to help with homelessness, criminal charges and debt.
- Residential rehabilitation communities: these can provide intensive periods of structured holistic support (e.g., 12 weeks or longer) in the difficult period immediately following detoxification.
- Peer support.

HINTS AND TIPS

For every person who drinks to excess, multiple others are adversely affected. The families of people who misuse alcohol or other substances can also benefit from mutual aid through organizations such as Al-Anon. Support for families can also indirectly help the user.

Pharmacological therapy

Various pharmacological strategies have been shown to be useful in the maintenance of abstinence from alcohol. They should be offered as an adjunct to appropriate psychosocial measures:

- Disulfiram (Antabuse): blocks the aldehyde dehydrogenase enzyme, causing an accumulation of acetaldehyde if alcohol is consumed or makes contact with the skin (such as a body spray). This causes unpleasant symptoms of anxiety, flushing, palpitations, headache and nausea very soon after alcohol consumption. It is contraindicated in patients with heart failure, stroke or coronary heart disease and caution is advised in people with hypertension, severe liver disease, renal impairment, cognitive impairment, psychosis and personality disorder.
- Acamprosate (Campral): enhances GABA transmission and inhibits glutamate transmission via NMDA receptors and appears to reduce the likelihood of relapse after detoxification by reducing craving. It is safe to use while drinking.
- Naltrexone (Nalorex) and nalmefene (Selincro): block opioid receptors, and appear to both reduce cravings for alcohol, and – when taken in conjunction with normal drinking – reduce the pleasant effect of alcohol, therefore decreasing the desire to drink and the amount consumed.
- The use of antidepressants and benzodiazepines is not recommended as pharmacological means for the maintenance treatment of abstinence from alcohol.

Course and prognosis

Alcohol dependence has a variable course and is often associated with numerous relapses. However, the prognosis is not as poor as is often thought, with around 50% to 60% of people with alcohol dependence showing abstinence or significant functional improvement 1 year after treatment. Good prognostic indicators include being in a stable relationship, employment, having stable living conditions with good social supports, lack of cognitive impairment and having good insight and motivation. People with any alcohol use disorder have an increased risk for death compared to age-matched controls (threefold in men, fivefold in women). Alcohol dependence is associated with a 12-fold increase in the risk for completed suicide, with deaths through accidents, cancer and cardiovascular disease also common.

OTHER PSYCHOACTIVE SUBSTANCES

Epidemiology

According to the Office of National Statistics, in 2022, 35% of 16- to 59-year-olds in England and Wales had tried an illicit substance in their lifetime. The most commonly used substance was cannabis (31%), followed by cocaine (11%) and ecstasy (10%). Use is more common among young people. Opioid use is rare (0.7%) in comparison to other drug use, but has the highest morbidity and mortality. See Fig. 22.1 and Table 22.2.

Aetiology

Occasional or experimental use of recreational substances is not the same as drug dependence. However, ongoing use of recreational substances over a period of time can lead to development of a dependence syndrome, particularly drugs with a strong potential for the development of dependence (namely opioids and benzodiazepines). Using opioids for as little as seven consecutive days can result in dependence. Dependence on any drug is associated with stimulation of the brain's 'reward system' (by increasing dopamine release in the mesolimbic pathway). Aetiological factors for recreational drug dependence are not well understood, although they appear to be related to a mixture of biopsychosocial factors. The operant conditioning model described in the alcohol section also applies to other psychoactive substances. Similarly, price, availability and cultural attitudes appear to be key factors influencing

Table 22.2 Epidemiology of substance use

Lifetime prevalence within adults in England and Wales in 2022	
In their lifetime, 16- to 59-year-olds report:	
Any recreational drug use	35.3%
Cannabis use	31.2%
Cocaine use	11.3%
Ecstasy use	9.9%
Hallucinogen use	8.7%
Amphetamine use	8.7%
Ketamine use	4.1%
Novel psychoactive substance use	3.1%
Opioid use	0.7%

Office of National Statistics, Drug Misuse in England and Wales: year ending June 2022

the use of recreational substances. In addition, social deprivation, childhood adversity, a family environment of substance abuse, conduct disorder in childhood, personality disorder with prominent features of dissociality and severe mental illness all increase the likelihood of substance misuse problems.

Assessment, clinical features, drug classification and differential diagnosis

Discussed in Chapter 17.

Management

Management of recreational drug dependence involves

- Harm-reduction of continued use
- Physical detoxification (if a withdrawal syndrome exists)
- Maintenance of abstinence if patient wishes to stop using

A detailed description of management strategies regarding the use of all recreational substances is beyond the scope of this book. Patients should be directed to local substance use services (run by National Health Service or third sector staff) who will be able to direct patients towards appropriate resources. There is a great deal of information on harm reduction techniques online (e.g., Know the Score, CREW). Patients who are dependent on opioids tend to be seen by NHS teams because prescriptions are often involved in management. However, for many drugs there is no medication-based treatment (cannabis, cocaine, amphetamines, novel psychoactive substances). People who wish to receive help in reducing use of such substances are likely to be able to find suitable support via third sector organizations and mutual aid (e.g., fellowship organizations such as Narcotics Anonymous or Cocaine Anonymous). Key points on the treatment of opioid and benzodiazepine use are described later.

Opioids

Opioid use is associated with high rates of drug-related death, and other health complications such as blood-borne viruses, infective endocarditis and abscesses. It is also associated with a high cost to society through unemployment, crime and child neglect. One of the primary aims, when someone is opioid dependent, is to minimize the harms associated with chaotic drug use. This can be achieved through a period of stabilization with long-acting opioid substitution therapy, removing the patient's need to purchase illicit opioids (often funded by criminal activities, prostitution or neglect of other aspects of their lives) to manage cravings and withdrawal. Table 22.3 compares the two forms of opioid substitution therapy recommended by NICE: methadone and buprenorphine. If they are felt equally suitable, methadone should be prescribed. However,

management of opioid dependence is more than just a prescription (see Table 22.4 for the key areas to address). Establishing a therapeutic alliance with the patient where they feel in control of their management is important.

> ### HINTS AND TIPS
>
> Buvidal is a relatively new treatment, and is a prolonged-release version of buprenorphine, given via a monthly subcutaneous injection. Patients do not need to regularly visit a pharmacy, reducing the impact on their work or education. It can also be used where there is concern about opioid replacement medications being diverted, or if there are concerns about the patient having medications in their home.

> ### RED FLAG
>
> Drug-related deaths via unintentional overdose are increasing in the United Kingdom, with opioids, alcohol, benzodiazepines, antidepressants, antipsychotics and gabapentinoids frequently implicated. Always provide a take-home naloxone kit to someone who uses opioids and offer training on how to use it to the patient and those who are in close contact with them.

> ### RED FLAG
>
> Patients can provide inaccurate information. When a patient is admitted to hospital, always confirm opioid replacement and benzodiazepine doses with the dispensing pharmacy as soon as possible. Also confirm with the pharmacy when the patient last picked their prescription up, and whether usage has been supervised, as if they have not been using it they may need retitration. Prescribing doses higher than the patient has actually been taking can result in death.

Benzodiazepines

Benzodiazepine dependence often arises iatrogenically when patients are prescribed benzodiazepines every day for longer than 2 to 4 weeks. It can also arise when patients purchase benzodiazepines illicitly. If someone is dependent on illicit benzodiazepines, they can be offered a detoxification prescription if they are truly committed to abstinence, but they should not be offered a maintenance prescription (unlike with opioids, there is no evidence that this reduces harm).

Table 22.3 Opioid substitute prescribing: comparison of methadone and buprenorphine

	Methadone	Buprenorphine
Mechanism	Long-acting mu-opioid receptor agonist	Long-acting mu-opioid receptor partial agonist
Side effects	As all opioids: constipation, sedation, euphoria, nausea At doses above 100 mg/day, electrocardiogram to check for QTc prolongation recommended	Less sedating, less euphoric than methadone
Overdose risk	Prolonged action increases risk for overdose if other depressants used on top	Lower risk as partial agonist
Withdrawal symptoms	A few days to weeks	A few days
Precipitated withdrawal	Does not occur	Can occur if taken by a person with opioid dependency and circulating opioids
Methods to prevent diversion	Supervised consumption	Give as intramuscular injection. Supervised consumption or combination with naloxone (opioid antagonist which is inactive if taken orally but blocks receptors if injected (Suboxone))
Ceiling effects	None	Cannot satisfy very strong cravings as partial agonist (less suitable for people using large amounts of heroin)
Starting daily dose (oral)	10–40 mg	4–8 mg
Maintenance daily dose (oral)	Typically 60–120 mL	Typically 12–16 mg
Formulations available	Oral	Oral, orodispersable, long-acting intramuscular injection (Buvidal)

Table 22.4 Biopsychosocial management of different stages of opioid dependence

Domain	Key actions
Harm reduction	Psychoeducation Offer substitute prescribing Consider child protection and give advice on minimizing harm to children from drug use Offer • take-home naloxone kit • needle exchange • contraception advice/condoms • blood-borne virus screening (hepatitis B and C, HIV)
Psychosocial intervention	Encourage attendance at mutual aid groups (fellowships or SMART Recovery) Signpost to extra support if needed with housing, benefits, food, debts Signpost to training and vocational opportunities Consider: • Motivational interviewing • Trauma-specific psychoeducation or CBT • Behavioural couples therapy • Family interventions • Contingency management • Residential rehabilitation
Substitute prescribing	Before initiation, confirm dependent use via toxicology screens and attendance in withdrawal (see Table 17.1) Consider methadone or buprenorphine (see Table 22.3) Initiate under supervised consumption Regular review for dose titration to be sufficient to remove cravings but not to cause intoxication Long-term aim can be stability on maintenance prescription or abstinence

Table 22.4 Biopsychosocial management of different stages of opioid dependence—cont'd

Domain	Key actions
Detoxification	Minimize withdrawal symptoms by providing gradual reduction in opioid substitution therapy (e.g., 5 mg methadone/fortnight) Opioid withdrawal is uncomfortable and distressing, although it is not life-threatening. If required, offer symptomatic relief: • A range of symptoms: lofexidine (alpha-2 adrenoreceptor agonist) • Diarrhoea: loperamide • Nausea: metoclopramide or prochlorperazine • Stomach cramps: mebeverine or hyoscine butylbromide • Pain: paracetamol or ibuprofen • Anxiety/agitation/insomnia: propranolol or diazepam (short term only)
Abstinence	Encourage ongoing attendance at mutual aid meetings. Encourage participation in recovery community activities (e.g., cafes, sports groups). Naltrexone (an opioid antagonist) can be used to block the euphoriant effects of future opioid use. It induces withdrawal if the patient has circulating opioids. Develop a crisis plan. Ensure patient is aware of how to regain rapid access to services should relapse occur.

CBT, *Cognitive-behavioural therapy.*

Caution must be exercised when attempting withdrawal from benzodiazepines as it can be fatal (albeit rarely). The benzodiazepine withdrawal syndrome may include hallucinations, convulsions and delirium. Symptoms can emerge within hours to days, depending on the half-life of the benzodiazepine. Management of benzodiazepine withdrawal involves initially converting drugs with a shorter half-life (e.g., lorazepam) to drugs with a longer half-life (usually diazepam). Doses are then reduced very slowly by around an eighth every fortnight, depending on patient response. If withdrawal symptoms emerge, the rate of reduction can be slowed, but increasing the dose should be avoided if at all possible.

HINTS AND TIPS

Sudden discontinuation of a patient's long-term sleeping tablet when they are admitted to hospital can lead to a withdrawal syndrome: only consider this if the patient's condition means benzodiazepines must be avoided and ideally reduce the dose gradually.

Course and prognosis

Drug-related deaths are increasing in the United Kingdom, with 4589 registered in 2021 in England and Wales, 6.2% higher than the previous year. Mortality in heroin users is 12-fold that of the general population. A longitudinal study in the United States found that after two decades, 28% of male heroin users had died, 18% were in prison, 23% were still using and 29% were abstinent. The median duration of opioid use is 10 years. As with alcohol, relapse rates following detoxification are high and are most likely to succeed with psychosocial support in place. A quarter to a third of people entering treatment achieve and maintain long-term abstinence.

ADDICTIVE DISORDERS

ICD-11 introduced the category of 'addictive disorders' which have features of dependence which overlap with those seen in substance use, but arise due to repetitive rewarding behaviours. The dependence features of loss of control and undue priority are seen, but not physiological features of dependence. The behaviours should also be causing distress or interference with functioning, and should be present over at least 12 months. The symptoms should not be better explained by another condition such as autism spectrum disorder or obsessive compulsive disorder. The diagnoses specifically exclude sexual behaviours.

Gambling disorder

Persistent or recurrent gambling leading to distress and negative consequences for the patient, such as financial losses or an impact on personal relationships. There is some evidence that naltrexone may have a role in treatment, but it is not currently licensed for this use. CBT and programs such as Gambler's Anonymous may be of benefit. People can register for websites such as GamStop which will prevent them accessing gambling sites.

Gaming disorder

Persistent pattern of uncontrolled gaming behaviour (whether online or offline) for a period of greater than 12 months. While gaming is a hobby enjoyed by many, if someone cannot control their gaming behaviour or persistently gives gaming priority over other aspects of their life or health, they may meet criteria for gaming disorder. Some countries have taken measures to curb the impact of excessive gaming, in South Korea until 2021, children under 16 were not able to play online video games between midnight and 6 am, and in China, children are limited in how long they can play online games every week.

● **Chapter Summary**

- Alcohol is the most harmful psychoactive substance in common use.
- Alcohol and substance problems are more common in men.
- Alcohol withdrawal is a potentially fatal condition that requires treatment with benzodiazepines and thiamine.
- Management of all alcohol and substance use disorders requires psychosocial interventions.
- Mutual aid is a key component of maintaining abstinence for many people dependent on substances.
- Harm from opioids is reduced by opioid substitute therapy.
- Harm can also be caused by addictive behaviours such as gambling or gaming.

UKMLA Conditions
Drug overdose
Substance use disorder
Wernicke encephalopathy

UKMLA Presentations
Addiction
Substance misuse

The psychotic disorders | 23

The main types of psychotic disorder are schizophrenia, schizoaffective disorder, delusional disorder and acute and transient psychoses.

SCHIZOPHRENIA

History

Ideas about the disorder we now term 'schizophrenia' crystallized towards the end of the 19th century. The concept of this disorder has evolved during the 20th century. Important landmarks in the definition of this disorder are:

- 1893: Emil Kraepelin separated affective psychoses (e.g., mania) from nonaffective psychoses; he gave the term 'dementia praecox' to clinical conditions resembling the main forms of schizophrenia.
- 1911: Eugen Bleuler coined the term 'schizophrenia' (splitting of the mind); his description placed more emphasis on thought disorder and negative symptoms than on positive symptoms.
- 1959: Kurt Schneider defined first-rank symptoms, which are still relevant to diagnosis now (see Box 9.1).
- 1970 to the present: the main international classification systems, the ICD-11 and the DSM-5, have further clarified the diagnostic criteria.

Epidemiology

- The incidence is approximately 15/100,000 individuals per year.
- The prevalence varies geographically but is approximately 1% in most settings.
- The lifetime risk is approximately 1% (see also Table 23.1).
- The age of onset is typically between late teens and mid-30s. Women have a later age of onset. Men: 18 to 25 years; women: 25 to 35 years.
- Women also have a second peak of onset in late middle age.
- Men have a higher incidence than women (ratio of 1.4:1) but equal prevalence (possibly due to a higher rate of mortality among male sufferers).

- There is an increased prevalence in lower socioeconomic classes (classes IV and V). This is more likely to be due to social drift (impairment of functioning caused by schizophrenia results in a 'drift' down the social scale) rather than social causation (poor socioeconomic conditions contribute to the development of schizophrenia).
- There is an increased incidence in urban (inner city) compared with rural areas.
- The incidence and prevalence are higher in migrants.

Aetiology

The aetiology of schizophrenia involves a complex interaction of biological and environmental factors.

Genetic

There is a strong tendency for schizophrenia to run in families. Table 23.1 shows the lifetime risk for developing schizophrenia if relatives have schizophrenia. Twin studies show a higher concordance rate for monozygotic twins (50%) than for dizygotic twins (10%), although this also shows that environmental factors are important, as monozygotic concordance is not 100%. Adoption studies provide further evidence for a genetic factor: babies adopted away from parents with schizophrenia to parents without retain their increased risk, whereas the risk is not increased when babies are adopted to parents with schizophrenia from biological parents without. Genome-wide association studies have found that there are over 200 genes implicated in schizophrenia, mainly in genes implicated in neurodevelopment, immune function, glutamatergic and dopaminergic neurotransmission, and calcium signalling. Rare high-penetrance genetic variations also exist, for example, deletion of a region of chromosome 22 is associated with a 30% risk for schizophrenia. The overall risk is

Table 23.1 Lifetime risk for developing schizophrenia if relatives have schizophrenia

No relatives with schizophrenia	1%
Sibling and dizygotic twin	10%
One parent	13%
Both parents	50%
Monozygotic twins	50%

likely to result from a complex interaction of a large number of genes and their interaction with environmental factors.

COMMUNICATION

Schizophrenia is not purely genetic in aetiology – environment is also important. You may want to bear this in mind when discussing the diagnosis with patients and their families: parents may find a genetic description accusational, while for the patient it will have ramifications about having children themselves.

Developmental factors

Schizophrenia is associated with complications during pregnancy and birth. In addition, the observation that more people with schizophrenia are born in late winter or spring has led to the theory that schizophrenia is linked to second-trimester influenza infection. Prenatal malnutrition may also increase risk: maternal starvation early in gestation doubles the risk for schizophrenia in offspring.

Brain abnormalities

Structural and functional brain abnormalities are associated with schizophrenia, even in those with first-episode psychosis who have never received treatment. Structural imaging is not yet diagnostic, but frequently identified abnormalities include:

- Ventricular enlargement (appears to be associated with negative symptoms)
- Reduced brain volumes in particular regions (frontal and temporal lobes, hippocampus, amygdala, parahippocampal gyrus)
- Reduced connectivity between brain regions (particularly frontal and temporal lobes)

Furthermore, people with schizophrenia demonstrate a wide range of cognitive abnormalities, particularly on tasks testing social cognition and memory. They also experience abnormalities of sensory integration leading to 'soft' neurological signs (e.g., abnormalities of stereognosis or proprioception).

Neurotransmitter abnormalities

Abnormalities in a range of neurotransmitter systems have been found in schizophrenia, predominantly glutamate and dopamine. It is not yet known how such abnormalities interact to lead to disorder, and if some abnormalities are a consequence rather than a cause of the disorder. The glutamate hypothesis of schizophrenia suggests that N-methyl-D-aspartic acid (NMDA) receptor hypofunction contributes to the pathogenesis of schizophrenia. The main evidence for this hypothesis is

that genetic variants in NMDA receptor and related genes are associated with schizophrenia, and that giving NMDA receptor blockers (such as ketamine, memantine) to healthy control subjects causes psychotic symptoms.

The dopamine hypothesis suggests that schizophrenia is secondary to overactivity of the mesolimbic dopamine pathway in the brain. The key evidence for this pathway is that the dopamine D_2 receptor has been genetically linked to schizophrenia, antipsychotics block dopamine D_2 receptors, and drugs that potentiate this pathway (e.g., amphetamines, antiparkinsonian drugs) are known to cause psychotic symptoms.

Adverse life events

Exposure to childhood trauma (e.g., sexual abuse, death of a parent, neglect) increases the risk for schizophrenia in adulthood around threefold. Stressful life events in adulthood occur more frequently in the months before a first psychotic episode or relapse and may, therefore, precipitate the illness. However, it may be that the early stages of the illness itself cause the stressful events.

COMMUNICATION

Between the 1940s and 1970s, the concept of the 'schizophrenogenic mother' was common and suggested that schizophrenia was caused by early life difficulties in the relationship between the patient and their family. Although it is true that childhood adversity including emotional abuse and neglect is associated with schizophrenia in adulthood, it is no longer thought that relationship difficulties alone can cause schizophrenia, and families must be reassured on this point.

Cannabis

Chronic cannabis use is associated with an increased risk for schizophrenia (use on more than 10 occasions associated with a twofold increase in risk). Although there may be a degree of 'self-medication' in that people who are becoming unwell try recreational substances in an attempt to normalize their mental state, there is also evidence that cannabis use contributes to the causation of schizophrenia: psychotic symptoms can occur during acute intoxication, an association even when use is several years prior to first presentation, and a dose–response effect. Although cannabis use increases the risk for psychotic disorders, the fact remains that the majority of people who use it do not become mentally unwell. This suggests that it may be particularly detrimental to those who are already predisposed to schizophrenia in some way, for example, through genetic risk.

Assessment, clinical features, investigations and differential diagnosis

Discussed in Chapter 9.

Management

As with many chronic medical conditions, schizophrenia cannot be cured. However, appropriate management can greatly reduce symptoms and relapse. Long-term medication is the mainstay of treatment, although psychosocial treatment is also very important.

Treatment setting

The initial treatment setting depends on the presentation and severity of illness. Home treatment is preferable, but hospitalization is often necessary, especially in cases of first-episode psychosis and when there is a significant risk that psychotic symptoms may lead to harm to self or others, or self-neglect. Detention under mental health legislation may be necessary in patients with reduced insight and impaired judgement.

Long-term community management is usually provided by community mental health teams or assertive outreach teams. Depending on symptoms, patients may have a care coordinator or a CPN, with regular follow-up in a psychiatric outpatient clinic. Patients with schizophrenia who have symptoms that are stable and well controlled can be managed in primary care.

Pharmacological treatment

Antipsychotics are of benefit in reducing positive symptoms (e.g., delusions and hallucinations). However, they have less impact on negative symptoms (e.g., apathy and social withdrawal).

First- or second-line antipsychotics

Differences in efficacy between antipsychotics are small, with the exception of clozapine, which is the most effective antipsychotic known, but is not used first line because of its side effects. Therefore the main factor influencing the choice of antipsychotic is tolerability. Antipsychotics commonly cause side effects, and as they are generally long-term medications, it is important to find one whose side effects the patient feels they can tolerate for the foreseeable future. The National Institute for Health and Care Excellence (NICE; 2014) does not recommend a particular antipsychotic as first line, but rather suggests that patients should be involved as much as possible in the decision. See Table 23.2 for a comparison of some common antipsychotic side effects and see Chapter 2 for more information on antipsychotic side effects and classification.

Treatment-resistant schizophrenia

Around two-thirds of people respond to the first antipsychotic trialled. Treatment-resistant schizophrenia is defined as a lack of satisfactory clinical improvement despite the sequential use of at least two antipsychotics for 6 to 8 weeks, one of which should be a second-generation antipsychotic. If a patient appears treatment resistant, reassess the diagnosis, check concordance, check whether psychological therapies have been offered, and assess for comorbid substance use. If treatment resistance is confirmed, offer clozapine at the earliest opportunity, assuming there are no contraindications and the patient is in agreement with taking oral medication and attending for regular blood tests. Clozapine is not used as a first-line medication due to its significant side effects including life-threatening agranulocytosis in just under 1% of patients. Thus regular haematological monitoring is obligatory (initially weekly, then monthly) and patients are required to be registered with a monitoring service. Clozapine will benefit over 60% of treatment-resistant patients. See Chapter 2 for more details on clozapine prescribing.

Concordance with medication is poor in schizophrenia, with around 75% of patients stopping antipsychotics within 2 years. This frequently leads to relapse. Concordance can be increased using depot intramuscular medication (administered 1–12 weekly), increased social support and patient education.

The length of treatment requires careful consideration as single episodes cannot be predicted and most patients with schizophrenia relapse. After a first episode, prophylactic treatment is recommended for 1 to 2 years but relapse rates are high upon discontinuation (80%–98%). Relapse is less likely if withdrawal of treatment is gradual, over a few weeks. For most patients, antipsychotics are a long-term, lifelong, treatment.

Table 23.2 Side effects of commonly used antipsychotics

Antipsychotic	Sedation	Extrapyramidal side effects	Weight gain/ metabolic syndrome	Hyperprolactinemia	Drug-specific important side effects
First generation					
Chlorpromazine	**Very common**	Common	Common	Common	Photosensitivity
Haloperidol[a]	Common	**Very common**	Common	Common	QTc prolongation on average >20 ms (baseline ECG recommended)
Flupentixol (Depixol)[a]	Common	Common	Common	Common	
Zuclopenthixol (Clopixol)[a]	Common	Common	Common	Common	
Second generation					
Olanzapine[a]	**Very common**	Common	**Very common**	Rare	
Quetiapine	**Very common**	Common	**Very common**	Rare	
Risperidone[a]	Common	**Very common**	Common	**Very common**	
Aripiprazole[a]	Common	Common	Rare	Rare	
Clozapine	**Very common**	Common (tardive dyskinesia very rare)	**Very common**	Rare	Agranulocytosis Hypersalivation

[a]Can be given in long-acting intramuscular injection (depot) form.
ECG, Electrocardiogram.

Other physical treatments

Benzodiazepines can be of enormous benefit in short-term relief of behavioural disturbance, insomnia, aggression and agitation, but they do not have any specific antipsychotic effect.

Antidepressants and lithium are sometimes used to augment antipsychotics in treatment-resistant cases, especially when there are significant affective symptoms, as is the case in schizoaffective disorders or in postschizophrenia depression.

Electroconvulsive therapy is now rarely used in schizophrenia. The usual indication is the rare case with severe catatonic symptoms.

> **HINTS AND TIPS**
>
> Early institution of medication may improve prognosis. Early detection is therefore critical. If uncertain as to whether a patient has psychotic symptoms, be sure to take a collateral history rather than waiting to see what symptoms emerge over time.

Physical health monitoring

Patients with schizophrenia are at increased risk for cardiovascular disease. This risk is increased further by using antipsychotics.

Therefore NICE (2014) recommends that a health screen should be carried out prior to commencing treatment, then at least annually, focusing on cardiovascular risk factors and including enquiry as to diet and activity levels. An electrocardiogram (ECG) is needed prior to commencing an antipsychotic if the patient is in hospital, has a history of cardiovascular disease, has a family history of sudden cardiac death or has evidence of cardiovascular disease on examination (e.g., hypertension). Pretreatment ECGs are also recommended for some antipsychotics at high risk for prolonging the QTc interval (e.g., haloperidol). During treatment initiation, NICE (2014) recommends weekly weights for the first 6 weeks and then again at 12 weeks alongside assessment of serum lipids, glucose, pulse and blood pressure.

Psychological treatments

Historically, psychotic disorders were thought to be unresponsive to psychological interventions, but increasing evidence points towards their value in augmenting drug treatments:

- Schizophrenia can be a devastating condition and is associated with significant social morbidity. Therefore the importance of support, advice, reassurance and education to both patients and carers cannot be overemphasized.
- Cognitive behavioural therapy (CBT) has been shown to be effective in reducing some symptoms in schizophrenia. It is also useful for helping patients with poor insight come to

terms with their illness, thereby increasing concordance with medication. It can also help the patient become aware of early warning signs of relapse. It is recommended by NICE (2014) for all patients with schizophrenia.

- Family psychological interventions focus on alliance building, reduction of expressions of hostility and criticism (expressed emotion), setting of appropriate expectations and limits and effecting change in relatives' behaviour and belief systems. Family intervention has been shown to reduce relapse and admission rates. It is recommended by NICE (2014) for all patients with schizophrenia who live with or are in close contact with their family.

Social support

Issues beyond pharmacological and psychological treatment should be addressed to optimize community functioning; these include financial benefits, occupation, accommodation, daytime activities, support workers and support for carers. A variety of agencies can provide these services, notably health services, social services, local authorities, local support groups and national support groups (e.g., SANE, MIND).

Patients with schizophrenia may benefit from the care program approach, especially if there are concerns about coordination in the delivery of services. Community psychiatric nurses, consultant psychiatrists, occupational therapists, psychologists or social workers may be involved with care. Their primary role is to coordinate the multifaceted aspects of patients' care and to monitor mental state and concordance with medication.

Course and prognosis

The course of schizophrenia is highly variable and difficult to predict for individual patients. In general, the disorder is chronic, showing a relapsing and remitting pattern. About 15% have a single lifetime episode with no further relapses. However, the majority of patients have a poor outcome characterized by repeated psychotic episodes with hospitalizations, depression and suicide attempts.

About 10% of patients with schizophrenia will die by suicide. Those most at risk are young men who have attained a high level of education and who have some insight into their illness. The periods soon after the onset of illness and in the months following discharge from hospital are particularly high risk, although all patients with schizophrenia are at lifelong increased risk for suicide.

The lifespan for patients with schizophrenia is on average 15 years shorter than for the general population. Causal factors include suicide, smoking, socioeconomic deprivation, cardiovascular disease, respiratory disease and accidents.

The overall prognosis for schizophrenia appears to be better in low-income as opposed to middle- and high-income countries; the reasons are unclear but may reflect better extended-family

social support or greater social acceptance once recovered. The factors associated with a good prognosis are:

- Female sex (in younger patients, not in older patients)
- Married
- Older age of onset
- Abrupt onset of illness (as opposed to insidious onset)
- Onset precipitated by life stress
- Short duration of illness prior to treatment
- Good response to medication
- Absence of negative symptoms
- Illness characterized by prominent mood symptoms or family history of mood disorders
- Good premorbid functioning

SCHIZOAFFECTIVE DISORDER

History

In 1933 Jacob Kasanin noted that some of his patients seemed to experience both affective (mood) and psychotic symptoms, which he referred to as 'schizoaffective psychosis'. While it is now considered a diagnosis in its own right, in the original DSM, schizoaffective disorder was a subtype of schizophrenia.

Epidemiology

The prevalence of schizoaffective disorder is estimated to be about a third of that of schizophrenia. It is more common in women than men.

Assessment, clinical features, investigations and differential diagnosis

Discussed in Chapter 9.

Management

Treatment of schizoaffective disorder is often very similar to schizophrenia. As well as management with antipsychotics, patients may be offered a mood-stabilizing agent (such as lithium) or an antidepressant to manage depressive symptoms.

DELUSIONAL DISORDER

Epidemiology

Delusional disorder is considerably rarer than schizophrenia, with an estimated lifetime risk of 0.05% to 0.1%. Delusions of jealousy are more common in men, and erotomania is more common in women.

Assessment, clinical features, investigations and differential diagnosis

Discussed in Chapter 9.

Management

Delusional disorders are difficult to treat, and evidence for efficacy of treatments is limited. A trial of antipsychotics is usually offered, and CBT may be of benefit. Poor insight often limits concordance and engagement with treatment. In cases of delusions of jealousy, consideration needs to be given to the safety of the potential victim, and separation of the partners may be required.

ACUTE AND TRANSIENT PSYCHOSES

Epidemiology

There is limited availability of information on the epidemiology of acute and transient psychotic disorders; however, estimates suggest a prevalence of 3.9 to 9.6 per 100,000 people. It is more common in women (approximately 2:1) and tends to first present later than schizophrenia, in people in their 30s and 40s, although it can occur at any age.

Assessment, clinical features, investigations and differential diagnosis

Discussed in Chapter 9.

Management

There are no specific NICE guidelines for the management of acute and transient psychoses; however, treatment is with antipsychotics. Psychological input such as family therapy or CBT may also be offered.

Course and prognosis

Acute onset, short period of illness and being female are associated with more positive outcomes in acute and transient psychoses. Patients with this condition (particularly male patients or those with a family history of schizophrenia) are significantly more likely to develop schizophrenia than the general population.

● Chapter Summary

- Schizophrenia occurs in around 1% of people worldwide.
- It arises from a combination of genetic and environmental factors influencing neurodevelopment and neurotransmission.
- Schizophrenia is treated with a combination of pharmacological (antipsychotics) and psychological therapy.
- Clozapine is an antipsychotic used for treatment-resistant schizophrenia.
- Schizophrenia is associated with significantly reduced life expectancy: screening for and treating physical health problems are important.
- The majority of people with schizophrenia experience a relapsing and remitting course.
- Patients with schizoaffective disorder may also require treatment with mood stabilizers or antidepressants.

UKMLA Condition
Schizophrenia

UKMLA Presentations
Auditory hallucinations
Fixed abnormal beliefs
Weight gain

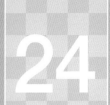

This chapter discusses the disorders associated with the presenting complaints in Chapters 6, 10 and 11, which you might find helpful to read first:

- Suicide and self-harm (Chapter 6)
- Depressive disorders (Chapter 10)
- Bipolar disorder (Chapter 11)
- Cyclothymia and dysthymia (Chapters 10 and 11)

DEPRESSIVE DISORDERS

Epidemiology

Table 24.1 summarizes the epidemiology of the mood disorders.

Aetiology

Depression is a multifactorial disorder, with interacting risk factors from many aspects of a patient's make-up. Genetics, early upbringing and personality can increase vulnerability to depression, with episodes arising depending on the level of acute and chronic stress experienced (see Fig. 24.1).

Genetics

Twin studies show the heritability of depression as 40% to 50%. Over 100 genetic variants have so far been identified as contributing to risk for depression by genome-wide association studies. Interestingly, genome-wide association studies have also found that genetic variants that increase the risk for depression also increase the risk for other major mental disorders. The particular genes involved are only beginning to be identified, but so far include genes involved in calcium signalling, mitochondrial enzymes and regulation of growth of new neurons. To complicate matters further, some genetic influence may only manifest in particular circumstances (gene–environment interactions).

Early life experience

Parental separation (e.g., divorce) during childhood increases the risk for depression in adult life. This may partly relate to the loss of a parent and partly to the disruption of care to the child. Other types of childhood adversity (e.g., neglect, physical and sexual abuse) increase the risk for depression and other psychiatric disorders. Postnatal depression in mothers can be associated with an indifferent early upbringing, leading to poor self-esteem and increased risk for depression in the child.

Personality

Genetics and early upbringing combine to shape personality, so it is unsurprising that some personality features are associated with increased risk for mood disorder. The personality trait 'neuroticism' (anxious, moody, shy, easily stressed) has consistently been found to increase the risk for unipolar depression. Personality disorders with prominent traits of negative affectivity and those with a borderline pattern also increase the risk for depression.

Acute stress

Adverse life events are common around the start of a depressive episode, particularly loss or humiliation events such as bereavement, relationship breakup or redundancy. The life event may not necessarily be causal, as being depressed – or at risk for depression – may also increase the risk for experiencing adverse life events. In recurrent depression, later episodes are less likely to be triggered by life events.

Chronic stress

The psychological and physiological effects of chronic stress may make someone vulnerable to depression and also reduce their ability to cope with more acute stressful life events. Chronic stressors such as poor social support (e.g., lack of someone to confide in), not having employment outside the home and raising young children are associated with depression. Chronic pain and any other chronic illness, particularly heart disease and stroke, are also associated with depression.

Neurobiology

The final common pathway of the multiple aetiological routes to mood disorder is abnormal brain structure and function. It is likely that mood disorders are due to malfunctioning communication between multiple brain regions involved in emotion regulation, rather than just one key abnormal area. Recurrent early onset depression is associated with reduced volume of the hippocampus, amygdala and some regions of frontal cortex. Depression with onset in later life is associated with white matter hyperintensities on neuroimaging, thought to represent small silent infarctions.

Neurochemically, multiple interacting neurotransmitter pathways are likely to be important. The two main abnormalities identified in depression are overactivity of the hypothalamic–pituitary–adrenal axis and deficiency of monoamines (noradrenaline (norepinephrine), serotonin, dopamine).

Table 24.1 Epidemiology of the mood disorders

	Lifetime risk	Average age of onset	Sex ratio (female:male)
Recurrent depressive disorder	10%–25% (women) 5%–12% (men)	Late 20s	2:1
Bipolar affective disorder	1%	20 years	Equal incidence
Cyclothymia	0.5%–1%	Adolescence, early adulthood	Equal incidence
Dysthymia	3%–6%	Childhood, adolescence, early adulthood	2–3:1

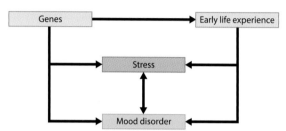

Fig. 24.1 Simplified model of aetiology of mood disorder.

Assessment, clinical features, investigations and differential diagnosis

Discussed in Chapters 6, 10 and 11.

Management

A *biopsychosocial* approach is considered for the management of depression, which means that consideration should be given to treating biological, psychological and social aspects of the illness.

Treatment setting

Most patients with depression can be treated successfully in primary care, or in a psychiatric outpatient clinic with input from the multi-disciplinary team (MDT), including medical staff, mental health nurses, occupational therapists and support workers. Intensive support at home from crisis teams or inpatient admission may be advisable for assessment of patients with:

- Highly distressing hallucinations, delusions or other psychotic phenomena.
- Active suicidal ideation or planning, especially if suicide has previously been attempted or many risk factors for suicide are present (see Chapter 6).
- Lack of motivation leading to extreme self-neglect (e.g., dehydration or starvation).

Detention under mental health legislation may be necessary for patients who need admission but are unwilling to accept inpatient treatment and lack capacity to make decisions regarding their treatment (see Chapter 4).

Lifestyle advice

All patients with low mood should be advised to avoid alcohol and substance use, eat a healthy diet, exercise regularly and practice good sleep hygiene (e.g., avoid caffeine and smoking in the evenings, do not sleep during the day, set regular sleep and wake times, do not use the bedroom for studying/watching TV). Patients can be referred to exercise groups; discounts may be available for those suffering from depression.

Psychological treatment

The National Institute for Health and Care Excellence (NICE; 2022) recommends that psychological treatments are used first line for less severe depression, and in combination with drug treatments for more severe depression (see Fig. 24.2). The severity of depression is determined in part by the number of symptoms (see Chapter 11) and by the degree of functional impairment (i.e., whether the patient is still able to fulfil their normal social and occupational roles). Chapter 3 covers psychological treatments in detail. NICE recommends a range of modalities based on efficacy and cost-effectiveness, with those recommended initially depending on whether the patient has a less severe or more severe depression. However, patient preference and previous response are important to take into account. Modalities recommended by NICE (2022) for use in depression are:

- Guided self-help (usually cognitive behavioural therapy (CBT) based)
- Group CBT
- Group behavioural activation
- Individual CBT
- Individual behavioural activation
- Group exercise
- Group mindfulness-based cognitive therapy and meditation
- Interpersonal therapy (IPT)
- Counselling
- Psychodynamic therapy

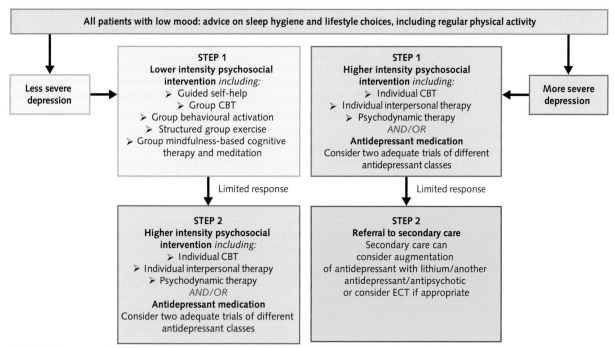

Fig. 24.2 Treatment of depression (summarized from NICE Guidelines (2022)). CBT, *Cognitive behavioural therapy;* ECT, *electroconvulsive therapy.*

Behavioural couples therapy can be considered if the patient's relationship with their partner could be contributing to their depression or involving their partner might help with the treatment of their depression.

COMMUNICATION

Patients reluctant to take medication may prefer the idea of 'talking therapies'. It is worth noting that cognitive behavioural therapy can be as effective as antidepressants in treating moderate depressive episodes and that when used after medication it can reduce the rate of relapse up to 4 years later. You may want to discuss both options with the patient, encouraging the use of both but allowing the patient to make the final decision – this often aids concordance.

Pharmacological treatment

NICE (2022) recommends antidepressants only for patients with more severe depression, patients with persistent sub-threshold depressive symptoms, or patients with less severe depression who have not benefited from a low-intensity psychosocial intervention. Selective serotonin reuptake inhibitor (SSRIs) (e.g., sertraline, paroxetine, citalopram, fluoxetine) are recommended by NICE (2022) as first-line antidepressants because they have the fewest side effects. All antidepressants are similarly effective if prescribed at the correct dose and taken for an adequate length of time. Clinicians therefore tend to choose an antidepressant based not on efficacy, but on its side effect profile (taking into account patient preference and comorbidity), and on which symptoms of depression are most troublesome. Table 24.2 summarizes some of the factors guiding the choice of an antidepressant. See Chapter 2 for more information on antidepressant mechanisms and side effects.

Antidepressants are most effective in moderate–severe depression, where around 50% of patients will respond (compared with 30% on placebo), when prescribed at an adequate dose for a sufficiently long period (usually 4–6 weeks, longer in older adults), with appropriate patient education and encouragement. When an antidepressant has brought remission of symptoms, it should be continued at full dose (i.e., at the dose that induced the remission) for at least 6 months to reduce the relapse rate. Patients with a history of recurrent depressive disorder may benefit from taking antidepressants for a longer period, perhaps even lifelong in severe cases. The prophylactic effect of antidepressants in reducing relapse has been demonstrated for at least 5 years (with imipramine).

Table 24.2 Factors influencing choice of antidepressant

Factor	Considerations
Side effects	SSRIs, in general, are the best-tolerated antidepressants. Side effects should be matched to a patient's symptoms, lifestyle and preferences (e.g., the weight gain caused by mirtazapine may be preferable to the sexual dysfunction caused by the SSRIs); some patients benefit from the sedation caused by some antidepressants (e.g., amitriptyline, trazodone, mirtazapine see Chapter 2).
Previous good response or nonresponse	Prescribe or avoid previous drug, respectively.
Risk for overdose	SSRIs are safer in overdose than venlafaxine, which is safer than TCAs.
Severity of depression	For severe depression requiring hospitalization, antidepressants that affect both noradrenaline (norepinephrine) and serotonin may be preferable, that is, TCAs and high-dose venlafaxine (SSRIs may be slightly less effective in treating depression of severity sufficient to cause hospitalization).
Atypical depression	Atypical depression (i.e., hypersomnia, overeating and anxiety) may respond preferably to MAOIs.
Comorbid physical health problems	SSRIs can cause or worsen hyponatraemia. SSRIs should not normally be prescribed to people taking a nonsteroidal antiinflammatory drug, warfarin or heparin (as SSRIs increase risk for bleeding). SSRIs should be avoided in those taking 'triptan' drugs for migraine. TCAs are contraindicated in patients with a recent myocardial infarction or arrhythmias. Sertraline is the preferred first choice of antidepressant for patients who have had a recent cardiac event. *See NICE (2009) Depression in Adults with a Chronic Physical Health Problem for further details.*
Comorbid mental health problems	Patients with obsessions or compulsions may respond preferably to high-dose SSRIs or clomipramine. A depressive episode with psychotic features usually requires the adjunctive use of antipsychotic medication.

MAOI, *Monoamine oxidase inhibitor;* NICE, *National Institute for Health and Care Excellence;* SSRI, *selective serotonin reuptake inhibitor;* TCA, *tricyclic antidepressant.*

Treatment often fails due to inadequate dose of drug, duration of treatment or poor concordance; therefore these factors should always be ruled out. Box 24.1 describes the strategies that can be used when a patient has not responded to an antidepressant at the correct dose for the correct length of time.

COMMON PITFALLS

- Patients may tell you that they have already taken antidepressants and that they do not work. People often respond to antidepressants from some classes but not others, so it can still be worth trialling a different antidepressant – you may want to explain this before prescribing.
- Remember that patients are often prescribed inadequate doses for inadequate lengths of time before the medication is changed – this does not represent treatment failure, for which a treatment dose needs to have been prescribed for 6 to 8 weeks without a response. You may find it useful to document dose and treatment period in your drug history.

Electroconvulsive therapy

See Chapter 2 for information on the administration and side effects of electroconvulsive therapy (ECT). Indications for ECT in depression include:

- Poor response to adequate trials of antidepressants
- Intolerance of antidepressants due to side effects
- Depression with severe suicidal ideation
- Depression with psychotic features, severe psychomotor retardation or stupor
- Depression with severe self-neglect (poor fluid and food intake)
- Previous good response to ECT

Other management options for treatment-resistant depression

There are other options available for the management of treatment-resistant depression. Ketamine is a fast-acting and effective antidepressant. The first study supporting the use of ketamine in treatment-resistant depression was published in 2000. Since replicated, the study showed that within hours of an IV infusion of ketamine, an antidepressant effect was noted that increased progressively in 3 days following administration. Esketamine nasal spray has also been developed and is licenced for use in the United Kingdom by specialists. There is also a growing interest in the use of psilocybin combined with psychological support for individuals with treatment-resistant depression. Further clinical trials are underway following some promising early data, but psilocybin is not yet licenced in the United Kingdom for treatment of depression.

In addition to pharmacological options, there are other nonpharmacological interventions available. Their use is usually coordinated through highly specialized regional centres in the United Kingdom. Options include repetitive transcranial magnetic stimulation (rTMS) and vagus nerve stimulation. For severe cases of treatment-resistant depression, where all other treatments have been tried and have failed, highly specialized centres can offer an anterior cingulotomy, a surgical procedure.

It is a very rare procedure, with about 3 to 4 cases per year in the United Kingdom.

Management of depression in special circumstances

Depression at the end of life

Depression is common and often underdiagnosed in the palliative care setting due to the overlap between symptoms of depression and symptoms associated with the end of life. Depression is consistently associated with a poor quality of life and reduced physical functioning and can have a significant impact on the patient's relationships with their family at the end of their life. Therefore prompt identification and treatment is important to improve quality of life. See Box 24.2 for a summary of suggested approach to managing depression in a palliative care setting.

Depression in personality disorder

Depression is a common comorbidity for individuals with a personality disorder. Treatment for the depressive episode should not be withheld because of the individual's personality disorder. NICE (2022) recommends a combination of antidepressant medication with behavioural activation, CBT, IPT or short-term psychoanalytical psychotherapy. They also recommend that the treatment may need to be extended for a longer course than would be required for an individual with depression without comorbid personality disorder, with treatment sometimes needing to be extended for up to 1 year.

Psychotic depression

For patients presenting with psychotic features as part of their depressive illness, a combination of an antidepressant and antipsychotic is recommended by NICE (2022). The most evidence is for the addition of quetiapine or olanzapine to antidepressant treatment. If the patient does not respond to pharmacological therapy, ECT can be considered. When the acute symptoms of psychotic depression improve, the patient can be offered psychological therapies.

Course and prognosis

Depression is self-limiting, and without treatment a first depressive episode will generally remit within 6 months to 1 year. However, the course of depression is often chronic and relapsing and around 80% of patients have a further depressive episode, with the risk for future episodes increasing with each relapse.

Depression is one of the most important risk factors for suicide; rates of suicide are over 20 times greater in patients with depression compared with those in the general population.

BIPOLAR DISORDER

Epidemiology

Table 24.1 summarizes the epidemiology of the mood disorders.

Aetiology

Similar to depression, bipolar disorder is thought to arise from an interaction between genes and environmental stress, with genes being particularly important. Twin studies estimate heritability at 65% to 80%. First-degree relatives of a patient with bipolar disorder have a roughly sevenfold increased risk for bipolar disorder (10%), a twofold to threefold increased risk for unipolar depression (20%–30%) and a higher risk for schizophrenia/schizoaffective disorder. Thus genetic susceptibility for severe mental disorder is not disorder-specific: patients with a family history of any of bipolar, schizophrenia or schizoaffective disorder are at increased risk for bipolar disorder. Risk for most patients is likely contributed to by multiple alleles of small individual effect, although some rare high-penetrance alleles probably also exist. Many of the mutations identified so far that slightly increase the risk for bipolar disorder also increase the risk for schizophrenia, including genes related to neuronal development, neurotransmitter metabolism (dopamine and serotonin) and ion channels.

The most important environmental risk factor is childbirth. There is an approximately 37% risk of postpartum relapse in women with bipolar disorder (about two-thirds if untreated, one-quarter if treated) (see Chapter 29). The risk of a severe relapse (e.g., mania, postpartum psychosis) is about 20%. Childbirth can also precipitate the onset of bipolar disorder.

Neurobiologically, structural and functional abnormalities in brain regions linked to emotion and reward (particularly hippocampus, amygdala, anterior cingulate and corpus callosum) have been identified. Multiple neurotransmitter pathways have been implicated, with strongest evidence for dopaminergic pathway hyperactivity in mania and some evidence for dopaminergic hypoactivity in depression.

Assessment, clinical features, investigations and differential diagnosis

Discussed in Chapters 10 and 11.

Management

The main management scenarios are:

- Treatment of acute mania or hypomania
- Treatment of acute depression
- Maintenance treatment (prevention of relapse)

Treatment setting

The initial treatment setting depends on the presentation and severity of illness. An episode of mania needs to be managed by mental health services. In some cases, it may need to be managed by a crisis team or necessitate a period of hospitalization in cases of:

- Impaired judgement endangering the patient or others around them (e.g., sexual indiscretion, overspending, aggression).

- Significant psychotic symptoms.
- Excessive psychomotor agitation with risk for self-injury, dehydration and exhaustion.
- Thoughts of harming self or others.

Detention under mental health legislation is often necessary in those unable to make decisions regarding treatment. Patients with bipolar disorder may also require hospital admission for depressive episodes for reasons outlined in the section on depression.

Pharmacological treatment

The mainstays of acute and maintenance treatment of bipolar illness are mood stabilizers (lithium and some antiepileptics (sodium valproate/valproic acid, lamotrigine and carbamazepine)) and antipsychotics (which stabilize mood as well as reduce psychotic symptoms).

Treatment of acute mania or hypomania or mixed affective state

The environment where a person is managed is important – they should have access to a calm environment and attempts should be made to reduce stimulation. Antidepressants should be discontinued (this may need to be gradual if half-life is short, to avoid discontinuation symptoms). Short-term benzodiazepines are often helpful in reducing severe behavioural disturbance. An antimanic agent should be started. NICE (2014) recommends an antipsychotic (haloperidol, olanzapine, quetiapine or risperidone), in part because of their benefits in reducing behavioural disturbance. If a different mood stabilizer is already being taken, it can be continued, with consideration given to increasing the dose. If there is no improvement, augmentation is recommended with an antipsychotic. Because lithium can be harmful if taken for less than 2 years (discontinuation of lithium can precipitate mania), it is not advisable to start lithium in a manic patient who is unlikely to be concordant with long-term treatment. The addition of valproate can be considered for patients who have not responded to antipsychotics, but it should not be prescribed for people under the age of 55 who are of childbearing potential. Lamotrigine is not used to treat mania.

Treatment of acute depression in context of bipolar disorder

Antidepressants need to be coprescribed with an antimanic agent, to avoid precipitating a hypomanic or manic episode. They should not be prescribed for mild depressive symptoms, only moderate–severe. Doses should start low and increase only gradually. Often, choice will be influenced by what medication someone is already taking. The first-line options are either quetiapine or a combination of fluoxetine and olanzapine (quetiapine and olanzapine have antidepressant properties in addition to antipsychotic effects). If these medications are not of benefit, lamotrigine alone can be given. If someone is already taking lithium or valproate, ensure the dose is providing a level at the upper end of the therapeutic window/is at maximum, and consider augmenting in turn with the three options as earlier. Long-term antidepressants should be avoided, with gradual discontinuation once depression has been in remission for 3 to 6 months.

Maintenance treatment

Not everyone who has suffered from a manic or hypomanic episode needs long-term prophylactic treatment. Maintenance treatment is recommended in those who have had a manic episode associated with serious adverse risk or consequences, a manic episode and another disordered mood episode or repeated hypomanic or depressive episodes with significant functional impairment or risk. Treatment for at least 2 years is recommended but in practice is often required lifelong.

If maintenance treatment is indicated, NICE (2014) recommends lithium as first line. Lithium requires regular blood tests (usually three monthly) to monitor plasma level (see Chapter 3). Discontinuation of lithium can precipitate relapse, meaning net benefit is likely to be gained only after at least 2 years of treatment. Second line is to augment lithium with valproate. If someone is not able to take lithium (e.g., cannot tolerate, cannot attend for routine blood monitoring), alternatives are valproate (not in people of childbearing potential as it is associated with a high risk for neural tube defects), olanzapine or quetiapine. Third-line options are lamotrigine (protects poorly against the manic pole) or carbamazepine (high risk for drug interactions due to induction of liver enzymes).

HINTS AND TIPS

Do not forget to take a comprehensive family history – including the treatment of psychiatric diagnoses. There is evidence to suggest that the level of response to lithium runs in families.

RED FLAG

Different preparations of lithium and valproate (which can mean sodium valproate, valproic acid or semisodium valproate) have different bioavailabilities, so it is important to specify the preparation when prescribing.

RED FLAG

Guidance has recently tightened around the prescription of sodium valproate, and new recommendations will be that no patients (regardless of gender) under the age of 55 should be prescribed sodium valproate, unless two specialists consider and document there is no effective or tolerated alternative to it. For people of childbearing potential prescribed valproate, they must be fully adherent to the Pregnancy Prevention Programme.

Physical health monitoring

People with bipolar disorder are at increased risk for cardiovascular disease, regardless of whether they are taking medication with metabolic side effects or not. NICE (2014) recommends an annual physical health check including weight, pulse, fasting blood glucose, glycosylated haemoglobin, lipids and liver function. Any abnormalities should be proactively treated. Extra monitoring is required for those taking lithium (renal function, thyroid function and calcium).

Psychological treatment

A structured psychological intervention is recommended for all people with bipolar disorder to improve insight and awareness of early warning signs and identify strategies the patients can use themselves to stabilize their mood. If they are in close contact with family members, a family intervention is also recommended. In bipolar depression, a high-intensity psychological intervention is advised (CBT, IPT or behavioural couples therapy). Psychological therapy is not recommended in hypomania or mania, when patients are generally unable to engage. Psychological therapies can harm as well as help, and therapists need to have training specifically to work with people with bipolar disorder.

Electroconvulsive therapy

Although ECT may precipitate a manic episode in patients with bipolar disorder it can be an effective antimanic agent, especially in severe mania and mixed states. It can also be used in a severe depressive episode within bipolar disorder.

Course and prognosis

More than 90% of patients who have a single manic episode go on to have future episodes. The frequency of episodes varies considerably, but on average equates to four mood episodes in 10 years. Between 5% and 15% of patients have four or more mood episodes (depressive, manic or mixed) within 1 year, which is termed *rapid cycling* and is associated with a poor prognosis. Completed suicide occurs around six times more often in people with bipolar disorder than in the general population.

DYSTHYMIA AND CYCLOTHYMIA

Aetiology

The extent to which the aetiologies of dysthymic disorder and cyclothymic disorder resemble those of depression and bipolar disorder is unclear. There are biological similarities between dysthymic disorder and depression; for example, rapid eye movement latency is decreased in both conditions. Genetic studies link cyclothymic disorder and bipolar disorder, as up to one-third of patients with the former have a positive family history of the latter.

Epidemiology and course

Fig. 24.1 summarizes the epidemiology of the mood disorders. Both dysthymia and cyclothymia have an insidious onset and a chronic course, often beginning in childhood or adolescence. A significant number of patients with cyclothymic disorder will go on to suffer more severe affective disorders, most notably bipolar disorder. Dysthymic disorder may coexist with depressive episodes ('double depression'), anxiety disorders and personality disorders.

Assessment, clinical features, investigations and differential diagnosis

Discussed in Chapters 10 and 11.

Management

Dysthymic disorder should be treated according to the NICE guidelines on 'treatment of a new episode of less severe depression', namely, a low-intensity psychological therapy initially, with consideration given to high-intensity psychological intervention or medication if this is ineffective. There are no specific guidelines for treating cyclothymic disorder, but again the emphasis is on psychological intervention, supporting the individual to develop self-management strategies. If medication is felt worthwhile in cyclothymia, the options are a long-term mood stabilizer (most likely lithium) or the short-term use of low doses of mood-stabilizing antipsychotics (e.g., olanzapine, quetiapine) during times of high stress when mood is felt to be least stable. Antidepressants should be used with caution in cyclothymic disorder, owing to their occasional tendency to turn mild depressive symptoms into hypomania.

Chapter Summary

- Mood disorders are common and disabling disorders with onset in early adulthood.
- Risk factors for mood disorders are genetic vulnerability, exposure to childhood adversity and stress.
- Most episodes of depression can be managed in the community, but life-threatening symptoms require hospital admission.
- Most episodes of mania require hospital admission. Hypomania may be manageable in the community.
- Treatment for depression depends on severity. Milder forms benefit from psychological intervention; more severe episodes require both psychological and pharmacological treatments.
- First-line pharmacological treatments for mood disorders are:
  - Depressive episode (unipolar depression): selective serotonin reuptake inhibitor
  - Depressive episode (bipolar depression): olanzapine and fluoxetine, or quetiapine
  - Manic episode: haloperidol or olanzapine or risperidone or quetiapine
  - Maintenance: lithium

UKMLA Conditions
Bipolar affective disorder
Depression

UKMLA Presentations
Behaviour/personality change
Elation/elated mood
End-of-life care/symptoms of terminal illness
Low mood/affective symptoms
Suicidal thoughts

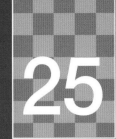
This chapter discusses the most important disorders associated with the presenting complaints in Chapters 12, 13, 14 and 15, which you might find helpful to read first. These disorders are often classed together as 'common mental disorders', along with depression. Historically, obsessive-compulsive disorder (OCD) and post-traumatic stress disorder (PTSD) were classed as anxiety or 'neurotic' disorders but now are considered separately as the aetiology and management overlap, but it is not the same.

ANXIETY DISORDERS

Epidemiology

Anxiety disorders are the most common of all psychiatric disorders with a combined 1-year prevalence rate of 12% to 17%. Epidemiological data collected from different countries have shown varying prevalence rates for individual anxiety disorders, likely reflecting varying thresholds for diagnosis (see Table 25.1 for the epidemiology of anxiety disorders). It is important to remember that anxiety disorders are usually underdiagnosed in primary care settings or only recognized years after onset. A large UK survey found that only a third of people with clinically significant anxiety disorders were receiving treatment of any kind (psychological or pharmacological).

> **COMMUNICATION**
>
> Anxiety disorders are frequent and closely related in aetiology, symptoms and management. For this reason, they are often grouped together along with depression under the heading 'common mental disorders'.

> **HINTS AND TIPS**
>
> In clinical settings, over 95% of patients who present with agoraphobia also have a current diagnosis or a past history of panic disorder. You may want to bear this in mind while screening for symptoms.

> **HINTS AND TIPS**
>
> Anxiety disorders tend to be more common in women than men, except for social anxiety disorder, where the prevalence is about equal.

Aetiology

Genetic and biological factors

Genetic factors contribute moderately to the risk for development of most anxiety disorders, with a heritability of 30% to 50% and common variants identified by genome-wide association studies. There is likely to be considerable genetic overlap with depression. It is possible that different environmental experiences in people with similar genetic vulnerabilities lead to either depression or anxiety, or both.

Panic disorder appears to be the most heritable anxiety disorder, with more than a third of those affected having a first-degree relative with the same diagnosis.

The three main neurotransmitter systems implicated in anxiety disorders are γ-aminobutyric acid (GABA), serotonin and noradrenaline (norepinephrine). Evidence for their role is that these are the neurotransmitters predominantly affected by benzodiazepines, selective serotonin reuptake inhibitors (SSRIs) and tricyclic antidepressants (TCAs).

Amygdala hyperactivation is found in several anxiety disorders, including social anxiety disorder, in response to the relevant anxiety-inducing stimuli. However, anxiety disorders likely reflect abnormalities in networks of brain regions, rather than individual regions alone.

Social and psychological factors

Psychosocial stressors may precede the onset of symptoms in other anxiety disorders.

Cognitive behavioural theories suggest that symptoms are a consequence of inappropriate thought processes and over estimation of dangers, as in the case of panic attacks:

- A cognitive model of the panic attack suggests that an attack may be initiated when a susceptible individual misinterprets a normal body stimulus. For example, a patient may become aware of their heart beating. Instead of dismissing this as

Table 25.1 Epidemiology of the anxiety, stress-related, OCD-related and bodily distress disorders

Anxiety disorder	One-year prevalence	Usual age of onset	Sex ratio (female:male)
Generalised anxiety disorder	3%[a]	Variable: childhood to late adulthood	2–3:1
Panic disorder (with or without agoraphobia)	4%[a]	Late adolescence to mid-30s	2–3:1
Social anxiety disorder	4%[a]	Mid-teens	About equal
Specific phobia	4%[a]	Childhood to adolescence	2:1
Post-traumatic stress disorder	4%[a]	Any age – after trauma	2:1
Complex post-traumatic stress disorder	4%[b]	Any age – after trauma	About 2:1
Obsessive–compulsive disorder	2%[a]	Adolescence to early adulthood	Equal
Hypochondriasis	1%–5% [a]	Early adulthood	Equal
Body dysmorphic disorder	2%[c]	Adolescence to early adulthood (declines with age)	Slight female excess
Bodily distress disorder (somatization disorder in ICD-10)	0.2%–2% [a]	Before 25 years of age, often in adolescence	Far more common in women (about 10:1)
Functional/dissociative disorders	Variation between specific disorders		

[a]One-year prevalence rates from Narrow et al. 2002. Revised prevalence estimates of mental disorders in the United States. Archives of General Psychiatry 59:115–123.
[b]One-year prevalence rates from Cloitre et al. 2019. ICD 11 post-traumatic stress disorder and complex post-traumatic stress disorder in the United States: A population-based study. Journal of Traumatic Stress 32(6):833–842.
[c]Bjornsson et al. 2010. Body dysmorphic disorder. Dialogues in Clinical Neuroscience 12(2):221–232.

normal, they may assume that it is under excessive pressure and that something could be physically wrong. This fear activates the sympathetic nervous system (the 'fight or flight' response), producing a real increase in the rate and strength of the heartbeat. A vicious cycle ensues in which the perception of increasing cardiac effort convinces the sufferer that they are on the point of collapse or a myocardial infarction. The resulting crescendo of symptoms may proceed to a full-blown panic attack involving several of the panic symptoms listed in Box 12.1.

Cognitive behavioural models for phobias suggest a two-step process:

- A neutral stimulus is paired with an aversive stimulus (classical conditioning, e.g., driving and an accident) or anxiety is felt about an intrinsically aversive stimulus (e.g., a snake).
- The neutral stimulus is then associated with anxiety, and avoiding it reduces anxiety (e.g., not driving after an accident, not going into the reptile house in the zoo). The association thus becomes self-reinforcing (operant conditioning) and it becomes increasingly difficult to be exposed to the neutral stimulus (e.g., not getting into a car at all, not going to the zoo at all).

These theories explain why techniques such as graded exposure therapy (see Chapter 3) are effective.

Assessment, clinical features, investigations and differential diagnosis

Discussed in Chapter 12.

Management

Psychological therapies are recommended as first-line treatment for anxiety disorders, particularly milder forms. Pharmacological treatments are also of benefit, but longer-term treatment is generally required, so the risk for side effects and complications is high. Pharmacological treatment can be offered first line for moderate-to-severe anxiety disorders if a patient wishes this, or if psychological treatment has been insufficient. In severe cases, combining the two is required. Fig. 25.1 summarizes the most important concepts in treating anxiety disorders, based on the National Institute for Health and Care Excellence (NICE) guidelines for common mental health disorders (2011), generalised anxiety disorder and panic disorder (2011). It is important that you

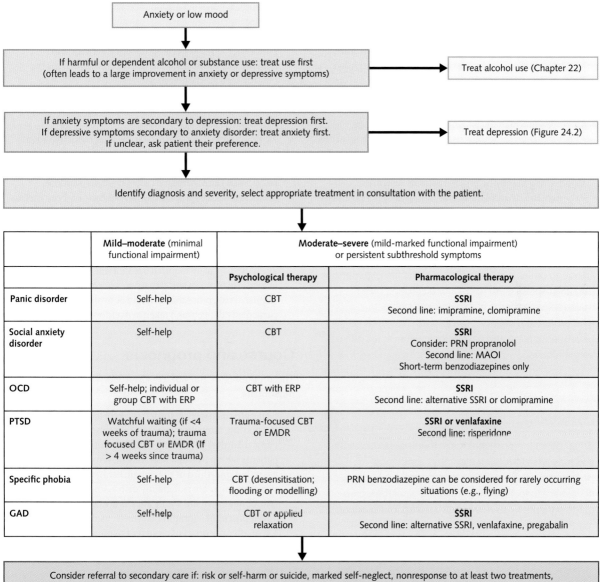

Fig. 25.1 Management of anxiety, stress-related and OCD-related disorders. *CBT,* Cognitive–behavioural therapy; *EMDR,* eye movement desensitization and reprocessing therapy; *ERP,* exposure response prevention; *MAOI,* monoamine oxidase inhibitor; *SSRI,* selective serotonin reuptake inhibitor.

familiarize yourself with this diagram, as anxiety disorders are common in primary care settings and 90% are managed there.

Psychological treatment
- There is strong evidence for the use of cognitive behavioural therapy (CBT) in most anxiety disorders.

- CBT is the first-line treatment for specific phobias, mainly in the form of behaviour therapy, which may involve systematic desensitization, flooding or modelling (see Chapter 3).
- In panic disorder, CBT may help the sufferer to understand that panic attacks can start from a misinterpretation of a normal stimulus, leading to a

'vicious cycle' of spiralling fear and sympathetic activation. When the patient understands this model, the therapist may encourage the patient to break the cycle by challenging the assumption that the original stimulus (e.g., palpitations) is indicative of an impending physical dysfunction (e.g., heart attack).

- Applied relaxation is used in generalised anxiety disorder. This focuses on being able to relax muscularly during situations in which the patient is or may be anxious.
- Other therapies commonly used in anxiety disorders include supportive, psychodynamic and family therapies, although there is less evidence for their efficacy (see Chapter 3).
- Counselling may be helpful for patients who are experiencing stressful life events, illnesses or bereavements (see Chapter 3).

HINTS AND TIPS

Although patients may have genes and life experiences that predispose them to anxiety disorders, often maladaptive patterns of thinking and behaviour exacerbate and maintain symptoms. This means that psychoeducation and psychological therapies can be very effective.

COMMUNICATION

When describing psychological therapies to patients, you may wish to remind them that avoidance perpetuates anxiety. To overcome anxiety, it is necessary to feel anxious. Psychological therapies guide patients to do this in a structured and gradual manner.

Pharmacological treatment

- In general, drugs need to be titrated up to higher doses and take longer to work in anxiety disorders than in depression.
- SSRIs are first-line treatments for most anxiety disorders due to their proven efficacy and tolerable side effect profile. Venlafaxine has a similar side effect profile and also has proven efficacy in generalised anxiety disorder.
- Restlessness, jitteriness and an initial increase in anxiety symptoms may occur in the first few days of treatment with either the SSRIs or the TCAs, which may reduce concordance in already anxious patients. This can be managed by titrating the dose up slowly or by using benzodiazepines in combination with antidepressants during the first few days of treatment.
- Benzodiazepines are highly effective in reducing anxiety. However, the rapid development of tolerance and dependence means they are not recommended for the majority of anxiety disorders.
- Pregabalin is licensed for the treatment of generalised anxiety disorder (often used after an SSRI trial), epilepsy and neuropathic pain.
- TCAs are generally considered only after other treatments have been tried owing to their increased frequency of adverse effects (e.g., dry mouth, sedation, postural hypotension, tachycardia) and increased risk of death in overdose.
- β-Blockers such as propranolol have historically been used to treat anxiety. There is no consistent evidence to suggest that these are effective at treating the anxiety itself; however, many people find they reduce autonomic arousal to anxiety-inducing stimuli, which some people can find very helpful, particularly when used on an as-required basis for intermittent situational or 'performance' anxiety. If there are concerns about suicide or self-harm risk, propranolol should be avoided as it can be particularly dangerous if taken in overdose (see Chapter 7).

Course and prognosis

The prognoses of the anxiety disorders vary greatly between individuals:

- Generalised anxiety disorder: is likely to be chronic, but fluctuating, often worsening during times of stress.
- Panic disorder: depending on treatment, up to one-half of patients with panic disorder may be symptom free after 3 years, but one-third of the remainder have chronic symptoms that are sufficiently distressing to significantly reduce quality of life. Panic attacks are central to the development of agoraphobia, which usually develops within 1 year after the onset of recurrent panic attacks.
- Social anxiety disorder: usually has a chronic course, although adults may have long periods of remission. Life stressors (e.g., a new job) may exacerbate symptoms.
- Specific phobias: have an uncertain long-term prognosis, but it is thought that simple phobias that persist from childhood are less likely to remit than those that begin in response to distress in adulthood.

STRESS-RELATED DISORDERS

Epidemiology

The prevalence of post-traumatic stress disorder (PTSD) and complex post-traumatic stress disorder (complex PTSD) varies between different countries, with the United States having comparatively higher rates of PTSD compared to European countries and upper-middle and lower-middle income countries.

Complex PTSD is a new diagnosis in ICD-11; therefore, there is limited evidence about its epidemiology. Rates of complex PTSD have been found to be high in refugees, asylum seekers, former political prisoners, former child soldiers/gang-members, victims of child abuse and in populations with high levels of violence. Prevalence of complex PTSD among people receiving treatment in mental health facilities has been found to be as high as 50%.

Table 25.1 summarizes the epidemiology of stress-related disorders.

Aetiology

PTSD is quite unique compared to other psychiatric disorders – by nature of the diagnostic criteria, its development can be directly attributed to an external, causative, traumatic event. As discussed in Chapter 14, there are multiple different types of traumatic stressors that can result in an individual developing PTSD. Complex PTSD is also directly linked to a traumatic event or series of traumatic events, but it is more likely to develop after an individual has been exposed to a sustained horrific event or exposed to repeated traumatic events, e.g., following prolonged torture or childhood sexual abuse.

Genetic and biological factors

The neurobiology of PTSD is complex and involves a range of neuroendocrine, neurochemical and anatomical factors. Areas of the brain which are associated with fear and memory have formed the basis for a lot of neurobiological research in PTSD. MRI studies have shown that the amygdala, hippocampus and anterior cingulate cortex have decreased volumes in individuals with PTSD when compared to the general population. One suggestion is that PTSD develops as a result of a failure of the medial prefrontal-anterior cingulate networks to regulate amygdala activity. This results in hyperactivity of the amygdala in response to threat.

The hypothalamic–pituitary–adrenal (HPA) axis coordinates the body's response to stress and has therefore also been a focus for research. Situations that induce fear increase cortisol production through a feedback loop involving the amygdala, hypothalamus and the anterior pituitary gland. However, studies of the HPA axis in PTSD have led to conflicting results, with studies reporting lower, increased or no difference in cortisol levels of individuals with PTSD when compared to healthy controls.

Other neurochemicals have also been implicated in PTSD, including GABA, serotonin and glutamate. The neurobiological basis for PTSD is likely complex, with multiple networks and regions of the brain involved in the development and maintenance of symptoms.

Social and psychological factors

There are various psychological theories that have been suggested to explain the typical patterns of symptoms seen in PTSD. These include:

- Cognitive model: current situations the individual encounters are misinterpreted as threatening, because the individual has developed a view that the world is dangerous, traumatic events will occur more frequently and they are not as able to cope with their emotions after an initial traumatic event.
- Dual representation: this is based on the idea that there are two types of memory – situationally accessible memories (SAMs), which remain unconscious unless triggered, and verbally accessible memories (VAMs), which are easy for the individual to recall. When a person encounters a trigger for a SAM, they re-experience the event in the present, including the emotions which were felt during the traumatic event.
- Emotional processing: following a traumatic event, an individual develops 'fear structure', which when activated by future situations and events results in the individual displaying cognitive, behavioural and physiological symptoms, which are pathological in PTSD. The individual has an altered view of the world and benign stimuli are interpreted as dangerous.

Box 25.1 summarizes the risk factors linked to an increased risk of an individual developing PTSD.

Assessment, clinical features, investigations and differential diagnosis

Discussed in Chapter 14.

Management

Psychological treatment

- Effective treatments in PTSD and complex PTSD include trauma-focused CBT (CBT addressing thoughts and behaviours related to memories of the trauma) or eye movement desensitization and reprocessing therapy (EMDR) (where the patient is asked to think about the trauma while also attending to another sensory stimulus, such as lights or beeps; see Table 3.4).
- Psychological debriefing immediately after trauma is not advised.
- If a patient is struggling significantly with emotional dysregulation and self-harming behaviours, it is usually advisable that some time is spent working with them prior to therapy, to ensure that they have the necessary skills and

FACTORS RELATED TO THE INDIVIDUAL:

- History of previous trauma
- Lower socioeconomic status
- Female sex
- Younger age
- Low social support
- History of a mental disorder prior to the traumatic event
- Multiple major life stressors around the time of the event
- Certain occupations: military personnel, prison officers, emergency service workers, healthcare workers, journalists
- Being a refugee or an asylum seeker

FACTORS RELATED TO THE TRAUMATIC EVENT:

- Higher severity of event
- Intentional rather than accidental event, e.g., rape/assault
- Physical injury as part of the traumatic event
- Longer duration of traumatic event

protections in place to allow them to engage fully. This could include psychoeducation work, helping them with establishing therapeutic relationships, addressing any housing or financial-related issues as far as possible, titrating medication and helping the patient with developing skills that can help them manage periods of distress, e.g., grounding techniques and distress tolerance work.

Pharmacological treatment

- No medication is recommended to try and help 'prevent' the development of PTSD following exposure to a traumatic event.
- NICE (2018) recommends considering SSRI medication or venlafaxine for adults who express a preference for pharmacological treatment of their PTSD symptoms. Commonly used SSRIs include sertraline and paroxetine.
- As with anxiety disorders, when SSRIs/venlafaxine are initiated, restlessness, jitteriness and an initial increase in anxiety symptoms may occur in the first few days of treatment. It might therefore be necessary to prescribe a short course of benzodiazepines to manage these symptoms during the initiation of treatment or to start at a low dose and very gradually increase as tolerated by the patient.

- Antipsychotics, such as risperidone, can be offered alongside psychological therapies for adults with a diagnosis of PTSD if they have severe hyperarousal or psychotic symptoms AND their symptoms have not responded to other treatments.

Other considerations

- Patients with PTSD often have other comorbidities. If they have symptoms of depression, treatment for PTSD should be offered first, as often depressive symptoms resolve with treatment of PTSD. The exception to this would be if the depression is severe enough to be limiting engagement with psychological therapies or if the individual is at risk of harming themselves or others, which is felt to be as a result of their depressive illness.
- Comorbid substance misuse is common in patients with PTSD. This should not prevent them from accessing treatment for PTSD; however, such treatment will need to be tailored to the unique circumstances and may require specialist input for the substance use aspects of the presentation.

Fig. 25.1 summarizes the management of stress-related disorders.

Course and prognosis

PTSD: approximately half of patients will recover fully within 3 months. However, a third of patients are left with moderate-to-severe symptoms in the long term. The severity, duration of symptoms and proximity of a patient's exposure to the original trauma are the most important prognostic indicators.

Complex PTSD: given the additional symptoms associated with complex PTSD (such as unstable sense of self and difficulties in interpersonal relationships), it is associated with a greater functional impairment compared to PTSD. There is limited evidence related to the prognosis for complex PTSD due to its relatively new inclusion in diagnostic guidelines.

OBSESSIVE–COMPULSIVE AND RELATED DISORDERS

Epidemiology

Obsessive–compulsive disorder (OCD) is common. Typical age of onset is in late adolescence, although males tend to show symptoms at an earlier age than females. It is a frequently misdiagnosed and underdiagnosed condition, commonly leading to a significant delay between symptom onset and provision of adequate treatment. The ICD-11 has reconceptualized several other disorders as being related to OCD due to their shared aetiology, clinical features and treatment responsiveness, including body dysmorphic disorder (BDD), hypochondriasis and hoarding disorder. BDD has similar typical age of onset as OCD, although there is a second peak noted in older people as their physical appearance changes with age. The prevalence of BDD is high in people seeking aesthetic or dermatological treatments. The body part, which is the focus of distress, can remain stable, or change over time. Hoarding disorder is more common with increasing age and is commonly comorbid with other mental disorders.

Table 25.1 summarizes the epidemiology of OCD and related disorders.

Aetiology

Genetic and biological factors

OCD is highly heritable, with more than a third of those affected having a first-degree relative with the same diagnosis. OCD shares genetic risk with Tourette syndrome (see Chapter 32). Genes associated with serotonin, dopamine and glutamate neurotransmitter systems have been implicated in OCD, and the efficacy of SSRI medications suggests that abnormalities in serotonin neurotransmission are implicated in the development of OCD and related disorders (including hypochondriasis and BDD). Functional imaging studies have shown increases in metabolic activity and blood flow in the orbitofrontal cortex, limbic structures, caudate and thalamus in individuals with OCD. In some studies, after the individual has received treatment with an SSRI medication, activity in these areas has normalized. In addition, obsessive–compulsive symptoms are often reported following damage to the caudate nucleus in the basal ganglia (e.g., Sydenham chorea).

The perinatal period is a high-risk time for developing OCD (at least a doubling of risk) with an increased incidence during pregnancy and a further increase in incidence postpartum (with risk peaking about 8 weeks). There has been some suggestion that women with OCD experience a worsening of their symptoms during the premenstrual phase of their cycle.

In hoarding disorder, neuroimaging studies have suggested the involvement of fronto-limbic circuits in the brain. Functional neuroimaging has suggested hypometabolism in the cingulate cortex, but results are far from conclusive, and the development of hoarding behaviours is multifactorial.

Social and psychological factors

- Learning theory suggests that compulsive behaviours in OCD temporarily reduce anxiety, therefore are self-reinforcing.
- Cognitive theory suggests that obsessive thoughts represent catastrophic misinterpretations of an individual's thoughts and impulses.
- As with anxiety disorders, individuals with OCD can experience a worsening of their OCD symptoms during times of stress. A stressful life event can also precede the development of OCD symptoms. Hoarding disorder has also been associated with traumatic life events, e.g., grief and loss.
- Individuals with BDD are thought to have maladaptive cognitive processes that over emphasize the importance of perceived attractiveness, which leads them to view themselves negatively, experiencing associated anxiety, shame and low self-esteem. They then use maladaptive coping strategies to deal with these thoughts, including checking physical appearance or avoidance.
- There are different psychological theories that have attempted to explain hoarding behaviours, which include excessive sentimental attachment to possessions, problems with the initiation and completion of tasks and indecisiveness.
- There are high rates of psychiatric comorbidity among individuals with OCD, BDD, hypochondriasis and hoarding disorder.

Assessment, clinical features, investigations and differential diagnosis

Discussed in Chapter 13.

Management

Psychological treatment

OCD and BDD:

- The mainstay of psychological treatment for OCD and related disorders is CBT, including exposure and response prevention (CBT including ERP).
- NICE (2018) recommends that CBT including ERP is initially offered to individuals with OCD or BDD with mild functional impairment in the form of self-help materials, brief individual telephone CBT (including ERP) or group CBT including ERP.
- With increasing functional impairment, the intensity of the psychological therapy offered should be increased.
- For individuals with moderate functional impairment or those with mild functional impairment who have not responded to lower-intensity psychological interventions, either a course of an SSRI medication or more intensive CBT including ERP (i.e., individual CBT) should be offered.
- For individuals with severe functional impairment, a combination of CBT including ERP and SSRI medication should be offered.

Other OCD-related disorders:

- CBT is the recommended treatment modality for individuals with hoarding disorder and hypochondriasis. This can either be alone or in combination with SSRI medication.

Box 25.2 outlines the role of the general practitioner in managing patients with hypochondriasis, which overlaps with the approach for managing patients with bodily distress disorder.

Pharmacological treatment

OCD and BDD:

- SSRI medications are the first-line option in managing OCD. NICE (2005) suggests fluoxetine, paroxetine, sertraline or citalopram for adults with OCD (they also suggest fluvoxamine can be used but this is rarely done in practice). For adults with BDD, NICE (2005) recommends fluoxetine due to the greater evidence base to support its use.

BOX 25.2 ROLE OF THE GENERAL PRACTITIONER IN MANAGING PATIENTS WITH BODILY DISTRESS DISORDER AND HYPOCHONDRIASIS

- Arrange to see patients at regular fixed intervals, rather than reacting to the patient's frequent requests to be seen.
- Increase support during times of stress for the patient.
- Take symptoms seriously, but also encourage patients to talk about emotional problems, rather than just focusing on physical complaints.
- Limit the use of unnecessary medication, especially those that may be abused (e.g., benzodiazepines, opioids).
- Treat coexisting mental disorders (e.g., anxiety, depression).
- Limit investigations to those absolutely necessary, based on objective signs.
- Have a high threshold for referral to specialists.
- Communicate the diagnosis clearly and empathically.
- If possible, arrange that patients are only seen by one or two doctors in the practice to help with containment and to limit iatrogenic harm.
- Help patients to think in terms of coping with their problem, rather than curing it.
- Involve other family members and carers in the management plan.
- Consider referral to a psychiatrist or psychologist.

- In general, drugs need to be titrated up to higher doses and take longer to work in obsessive–compulsive and related disorders than in depression, e.g., up to 12 weeks at the British National Formulary maximum dose for a trial of an SSRI in OCD.
- If a patient responds to SSRI treatment, it should be continued for at least 12 months.
- Clomipramine, the most serotonergic of the TCAs, has proven efficacy in OCD and is recommended if a trial of an SSRI in combination with psychological therapy has failed, or if a patient prefers it, or has had a good response to it previously.
- If a patient does not respond to a full trial of an SSRI at maximum dose, a combination of CBT including ERP plus an SSRI at maximum dose or clomipramine at maximum dose, consideration can be given to the addition of commencing an antipsychotic alongside the SSRI or clomipramine. Most evidence supports the use of risperidone or aripiprazole as augmentation agents.
- If a patient remains treatment resistant, secondary care mental health teams might consider a referral to specialist/tertiary centres at this point for consideration of specialist intervention.

HINTS AND TIPS

Inhibition of serotonin uptake seems to be the essential component of effective drug therapy for obsessive–compulsive disorder as evidenced by the efficacy of the selective serotonin reuptake inhibitors and clomipramine. Clomipramine, which predominantly inhibits serotonin reuptake, is more effective than the other tricyclic antidepressants, which predominantly inhibit noradrenaline (norepinephrine) reuptake inhibition (e.g., desipramine, nortriptyline).

Course and prognosis

- OCD: the majority have a chronic fluctuating course, with worsening symptoms during times of stress. About 70% of patients who receive treatment experience an improvement in their symptoms. About 15% of patients show a progressive deterioration in functioning. Around 5% of patients have a complete remission of symptoms of symptoms between episodes of illness.

- BDD: appropriate treatment with psychological and pharmacological intervention is thought to result in a good prognosis, with one small study reporting 76% of individuals making a full recovery with low rates of recurrence. Other studies have suggested a chronic course, with lasting functional impairment. The presence of beliefs being held with delusional intensity or other comorbid mental disorders is associated with a worse prognosis.
- Hoarding disorder: chronic and progressive course, with symptoms increasing in severity with age.
- Hypochondriasis: usually episodic, with episodes lasting anywhere from months to years. Around one-third of patients are thought to eventually improve significantly. Factors associated with a better prognosis include higher socioeconomic status, anxiety or depressive symptoms that are responsive to treatment and the absence of comorbid personality disorder and physical illness.

DISSOCIATIVE DISORDERS AND BODILY DISTRESS DISORDER

The dissociative disorders are described in Chapter 14. Bodily distress disorder, factitious disorder and malingering are discussed in Chapter 15.

Epidemiology

Table 25.1 includes the epidemiological data for bodily distress disorder. Functional or dissociative disorders are even more common – being seen in around a third of patients seen in hospital medical outpatient clinics. Functional seizures are found in around one in seven people attending a first fit clinic; functional paresis is as common as multiple sclerosis (affecting around 4 in 100,000 people per year), and up to half of presentations with 'status epilepticus' are in fact prolonged functional seizures.

Aetiology

The aetiologies of dissociative disorders and disorders of bodily distress are poorly understood. Childhood sexual abuse increases the risk for both, although the majority of patients with the disorders have not been abused. Growing up in environments where physical distress is more readily acknowledged than psychological distress may have a role. Symptoms often (but not always) have onset or worsen after a stressor, and this may be because emotional states influence the way pain and other bodily sensations are perceived. Symptoms also often follow an actual, minor, physical insult, for example, functional leg weakness following a sprained ankle or irritable bowel syndrome following a viral infection. Similarly, functional seizures occur most often in people who also experience epileptic seizures. There is no convergent pathophysiological explanation, but current theories include:

1. Abnormally intense self-directed attention interferes with normal 'automatic' cognitive processing, causing errors (much like thinking too long about how to spell a word).
2. Abnormal sense of agency or disrupted sensory prediction prevents patients from differentiating self-generated versus involuntary movements, or normal from abnormal sensory input.

Assessment, clinical features, investigations and differential diagnosis

Discussed in Chapters 14 and 15.

Management

Little research is available regarding the treatment of bodily distress disorder. Pharmacotherapy will only alleviate symptoms when the patient has a comorbid drug-responsive condition such as an anxiety disorder or depression. Both individual and group psychotherapy (mainly CBT) may be useful in reducing symptoms by helping patients to cope with their symptoms and develop alternative strategies for managing their emotions. Box 25.2 summarizes the role of the general practitioner in managing patients with bodily distress disorder. A supportive relationship with an empathic doctor able to work with the patient to guide understanding of their condition is likely to be the most important intervention.

In functional/dissociative disorders, a clear and empathically delivered explanation that emphasizes reversibility can often be helpful (see Table 25.2). Treat comorbid psychiatric disorders, consider CBT, and consider physiotherapy for those who are deconditioned.

Course and prognosis

Bodily distress disorder tends to have a chronic episodic course, with waxing and waning symptoms often exacerbated by stress. Functional/dissociative disorders vary widely in outcome. Some patients experience one acute episode, then make a full recovery; others become very disabled.

Table 25.2 Explanation and advice in dissociative/functional disorders

State what is wrong	'You have functional seizures'. 'You have irritable bowel syndrome'.
State what is not wrong	'You do not have epilepsy, coeliac disease, bowel cancer, etc.'.
Describe the mechanism	'Your body is not damaged but it is not working properly'.
Try metaphor	'It's a software not a hardware problem'.
Explain how the diagnosis was made	Demonstrate tremor entrainment, Hoover sign, etc. Share normal investigation results. Point out other symptoms such as derealization/depersonalization.
State you believe them	'I do not think you are making these symptoms up'.
Emphasize the problem is common	'Many people have similar symptoms'.
Emphasize the problem gets better	'There is no damage, so there is potential to make a full recovery'.
Emphasize self-help	'It's not your fault, but there are things you can do to make it better'.

COMMUNICATION

A diagnosis of functional symptoms can be hard to explain. Phrases such as 'you are experiencing a functional, not a structural problem' or 'a software not a hardware problem' may help to reassure patients that you believe they are experiencing symptoms, but these are not driven by a disorder which requires specific treatment.

● Chapter Summary

- Anxiety disorders are common, often chronic conditions, arising more frequently in women than men.
- Self-help is the first-line therapy for the majority of mild anxiety disorders.
- Psychological therapies are first line for moderate-to-severe anxiety disorders.
- Medication, usually selective serotonin reuptake inhibitors, can also be offered for moderate-to-severe anxiety disorders.
- Treatment of OCD and related disorders is CBT with ERP with or without SSRI medication.
- Clomipramine is also a useful pharmacological option in OCD or BDD.
- Principles of treatment in bodily distress disorder and dissociative disorders are to take a holistic approach, give a clear explanation of diagnosis and minimize iatrogenic harm.

UKMLA Conditions
Anxiety
Anxiety disorder (generalised)
Anxiety disorder (post-traumatic stress disorder)
OCD
Phobias
Somatization

UKMLA Presentations
Anxiety
OCD
Phobias
Somatization/medically
Unexplained physical
symptoms

This chapter discusses the disorders associated with the presenting complaints in Chapter 16, which you might find helpful to read first.

ANOREXIA AND BULIMIA NERVOSA

Epidemiology

See Table 26.1

Aetiology

As with the majority of mental disorders, both biological and psychosocial factors have been implicated.

Genetics

Estimates from twin studies suggest that around two-thirds of the variance in the liability to eating disorders is due to genetic factors. Genome-wide association studies in anorexia so far have not identified any common risk variants, but have been underpowered.

Early life experience

Premature birth and some perinatal complications increase the risk for a later eating disorder, potentially implicating epigenetic changes. Childhood adversity (physical, sexual or neglect) also increases the risk for an eating disorder. Relationship difficulties are often (but not always) found within families of patients with anorexia nervosa, including overprotectiveness, enmeshment (overinvolvement, with lack of differentiation between parent and child), conflict avoidance, lack of conflict resolution and rigidity (resistance to change).

Personality

It is possible that the inherited liability might be mediated by certain personality traits, including perfectionism (high attention to detail) and rigidity/obsessionality. High scores in these domains are seen in unaffected relatives of those with anorexia and in those who have recovered and have a normal body mass index (suggesting that these findings do not simply reflect the substantial cognitive changes associated with starvation).

Cultural influences

In Western culture, the widely portrayed notion of the 'ideal body' influences perception of body image, meaning that unusual thinness is often valued more than natural curves. The increase in eating disorders seen in low- and middle-income countries supports the concept that idealized thinness may influence risk for eating disorder, but it is very hard to prove.

Neurobiology

The key neurobiological pathways underlying eating disorder remain to be clarified, but increased volume of the orbitofrontal cortex (involved in reward processing) has been found in anorexia and bulimia, both during and after an episode of illness (suggesting that the findings are not merely a consequence of starvation).

Assessment, clinical features, investigations, complications and differential diagnosis

Discussed in Chapter 16.

BINGE-EATING DISORDER

Epidemiology

See Table 26.1

Table 26.1 Epidemiology of eating disorders

Disorder	Prevalence	Sex ratio	Age of onset
Anorexia nervosa	0.9% of women 0.3% of men	3:1 (10:1 in some studies)	Typically mid-adolescence
Bulimia nervosa	1.5% of women 0.5% of men	3:1	Typically late adolescence or early adulthood
Binge-eating disorder	3.5% of women 2% of men	2:1	Typically in adolescence or early adulthood

Aetiology

As with most mental disorders, there appears to be a combination of biological and psychosocial factors implicated in an individual developing the disorder.

Genetics

Binge-eating disorder appears to have a significant genetic component, with twin studies suggesting that heritability ranges between 41% and 57%.

Early life experience

A history of severe childhood obesity, experiencing bullying as a child or young adult (specifically when the bullying is related to the individual's appearance) and growing up around a family who overeats have all been associated with an increased risk of binge-eating disorder. Childhood adversity (physical, sexual or neglect) is also linked to binge-eating disorder.

Personality

Personality traits in binge-eating disorder are less well defined than those observed in individuals with anorexia nervosa or bulimia nervosa; however, binge eating is often a way for the individual to cope with distress, therefore finding it difficult to handle distress may increase the likelihood of developing binge-eating disorder. Low self-esteem, body dissatisfaction and a tendency towards anxiety and low mood are also associated with binge-eating disorder.

Neurobiology

Neuroimaging studies have suggested differences in corticostriatal circuitry, and other studies have implicated changes in neurotransmitters, in both dopaminergic and opioid systems, in binge-eating behaviours.

Assessment, clinical features, investigations, complications and differential diagnosis

Discussed in Chapter 16.

AVOIDANT RESTRICTIVE FOOD INTAKE DISORDER

At the time of writing, there is limited information available on the prevalence, course and outcomes for avoidant restrictive food intake disorder (ARFID). Small studies have suggested a prevalence of around 1.5% to 3% in school-aged children. ARFID appears to most commonly develop in early childhood, but can develop at any age and persist into adulthood.

Psychiatric comorbidities are common, including neurodevelopmental disorders and anxiety disorders. There is a significant overlap in the sensory sensitivities around food and selective eating patterns seen in individuals with autism spectrum disorder and in those with ARFID.

> **HINTS AND TIPS**
>
> Although depression and obsessive–compulsive disorder may coexist with anorexia nervosa, these symptoms can also result from the effects of starvation. It is helpful to ask, 'what happened first?', and aim to restore weight before treating any remaining mood or anxiety symptoms.

> **RED FLAG**
>
> Binge-eating disorder is associated with physical complications, including obesity, dyslipidaemia, Type-2 diabetes mellitus and hypertension.

Management

Anorexia nervosa

Ambivalence towards treatment coupled with the psychological consequences of starvation (poor concentration, depression, lethargy) means that anorexia nervosa is often difficult to treat. Treatment should be collaborative, with an early aim of establishing a therapeutic alliance. Fig. 26.1 gives an overview of management recommendations (National Institute for Health and Care Excellence (NICE) 2017). Suspected cases should be referred to a specialist eating disorder service for assessment.

Psychotherapy, preferably with familial involvement, is the treatment modality of choice for patients with anorexia nervosa. Table 26.2 lists the psychological interventions recommended by NICE (2017). The interventions for anorexia nervosa differ in detail but have common principles: they are long term (20–40 sessions), they encourage regaining a healthy weight, they involve carers wherever possible and they seek to develop a positive therapeutic relationship. See Chapter 3 for more information about psychological therapies.

The only medication recommended by NICE (2017) in anorexia is a multivitamin. Previously, fluoxetine was often trialled, but this is now felt to be ineffective. A selective serotonin reuptake inhibitor may be of benefit in comorbid anxiety or depressive illnesses, but a return to a normal weight should be attempted first, as this is likely to improve

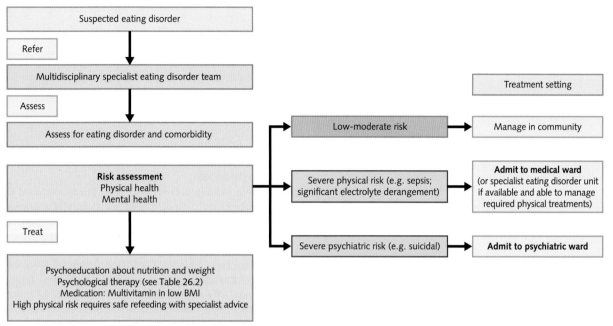

Fig. 26.1 Overview of management of eating disorders. *BMI,* Body mass index.

Table 26.2 Psychological interventions recommended in eating disorders (NICE 2017)

	Anorexia nervosa		Bulimia nervosa		Binge-eating disorder	
	First line	Second line	First line	Second line	First line	Second line
Adult	One of: • CBT-ED • MANTRA • SSCM	• Different first-line therapy • Focal psychodynamic therapy	Guided self-help (CBT informed)	CBT-ED	Guided self-help (CBT informed)	CBT-ED (group or individual)
Young person	Family therapy (anorexia focused)	One of: • CBT-ED • Psychotherapy (adolescent anorexia focused)	Family therapy (bulimia focused)	CBT-ED	Guided self-help (CBT informed)	CBT-ED (group or individual)

CBT-ED, *Individual eating-disorder-focused cognitive-behavioural therapy;* MANTRA, *Maudsley Anorexia Nervosa Treatment for Adults;* NICE, *National Institute for Health and Care Excellence;* SSCM, *specialist supportive clinical management.*

mood and anxiety. When prescribing for anyone who is significantly malnourished, be aware of the additional risks of medications in this group, particularly QTc prolongation. Dose reductions and cautious titration are likely to be required.

Weight should be monitored, and physical complications (see Chapter 16) are actively monitored for.

Hospitalization is necessary in certain medical circumstances (e.g., body mass index less than 13.5 kg/m^2, rapid weight loss, severe electrolyte abnormalities, syncope) and psychiatric circumstances (risk for suicide, social crisis).

In severe cases, patients can lose insight into the severity of their illness, by virtue of both the psychopathology of the illness and the neuropsychological effects of starvation. Where a patient lacks capacity to make decisions regarding his/her care and treatment, it may be necessary to use mental health legislation (see Chapter 4) to effect compulsory admission to hospital and to initiate life-saving treatment.

While mental health legislation in all UK countries only makes provision for the compulsory treatment of mental illness (not physical illness), food is considered to be treatment for mental illness because it leads to improvement in the psychological symptoms (impaired decision-making) caused by starvation. Therefore, as a final resort, in certain cases patients may be force-fed under mental health legislation. In extreme cases, nasogastric or intravenous feeding may be necessary.

> **RED FLAG**
>
> A person with anorexia who is dangerously underweight and refusing to eat should be assessed for compulsory treatment (feeding) under mental health legislation.

> **RED FLAG**
>
> Anorexia nervosa has the highest mortality rate among mental disorders, due to the medical complications associated with the disorder and the increased risk of completed suicide.

Refeeding syndrome

When a patient starts eating after a prolonged (more than 5 days) period of starvation, care must be taken to avoid refeeding syndrome. This arises because of a rapid switch from gluconeogenesis (catabolic state) to insulin release stimulating glycogen, fat and protein synthesis (anabolic state), resulting in rapid intracellular uptake of the cofactors needed for this, such as potassium, phosphate and magnesium (Table 26.3). The associated electrolyte disturbances can be potentially fatal. Management hinges on replacement of fluid and electrolytes, which may need to be intravenous. To avoid it, refeeding is generally commenced cautiously, with frequent electrolyte monitoring for the highest risk period (first week of feeding) and with thiamine replacement.

> **RED FLAG**
>
> Refeeding syndrome can arise in anyone who is malnourished, for example, alcohol dependence, postoperatively, malabsorption syndromes.

Table 26.3 Clinical features of refeeding syndrome

Electrolyte abnormalities	Clinical manifestations
Hypophosphataemia	Muscle weakness
Hypokalaemia	Seizures
Hypomagnesaemia	Peripheral oedema
Hyponatraemia	Cardiac arrhythmias
Metabolic acidosis	Hypotension
Thiamine deficiency	Delirium

HINTS AND TIPS

Hypophosphataemia is the hallmark of refeeding syndrome. If you only remember one thing about it, remember to check for that. If the level is significantly low phosphate should be replaced either orally or intravenously depending on local guidelines.

Bulimia nervosa

Patients with bulimia nervosa tend to be more motivated to address their eating difficulties and are usually of a normal weight. Treatment is predominantly psychological, ranging from psychoeducation, self-help manuals and self-help groups in mild cases to individual cognitive behavioural therapy in more serious cases (Table 26.2). NICE (2017) guidelines recommend up to 20 sessions of cognitive behavioural therapy spread over 20 weeks, with a higher frequency of sessions in the earlier phases of treatment. Management by specialist eating disorder services may be necessary in severe cases. Inpatient treatment is not usually required; however, it may be necessary for the treatment of electrolyte disturbances resulting from purging (which can be fatal) or for management of the risk for suicide or self-harm. Antidepressants are no longer recommended to treat uncomplicated bulimia. However, comorbid substance abuse and depression are common and should be managed as standard. Unlike with anorexia, mood and anxiety symptoms in bulimia are unlikely to be due to malnutrition.

Binge-eating disorder

As with bulimia nervosa, the mainstay of treatment is psychological. Table 26.2 lists the psychological interventions recommended by NICE (2017). Individuals can initially be offered self-help or guided self-help, where they are asked to work through a book, with short, supportive sessions offered periodically with a practitioner. If this has not been successful, individual or group-based cognitive behavioural therapy can be offered. NICE (2017) guidelines suggest between 16 and 20 sessions. No pharmacological treatment is recommended for binge-eating disorder, but any comorbid mental disorders, such as substance use or mood/anxiety disorders, should be identified and treated as per usual clinical practice.

Avoidant-restrictive food intake disorder

There is not one particular form of psychological therapy recommended for individuals with ARFID. The approach to treatment needs to be person-centred and often takes the form of behavioural interventions and systematic desensitization. For individuals with ARFID and significantly low body weight, nutritional deficiencies or associated physical compromise, admission to hospital and parenteral feeding may need to be considered.

Prognosis

Anorexia

Although weight and menstrual functioning usually improve, eating habits and attitudes to body shape and weight often remain abnormal. Recovery is slow; time to complete remission in anorexia nervosa is typically 5 years. Around a fifth of patients make a full recovery, a quarter develop bulimia nervosa and a fifth remain severely unwell. The remainder tend to follow a relapsing–remitting course. Risk for death in those with anorexia is increased sixfold relative to an age-matched population. Premature death is predominantly due to the complications of starvation (e.g., arrhythmia, sepsis), and around a fifth of deaths are due to suicide. Factors associated with a poorer prognosis are described in Box 26.1 and indicate that poorer outcomes are seen in more severe illness.

Bulimia

The course of bulimia is also variable, although generally better than anorexia, with 50% to 70% of patients achieving either full or partial recovery after 5 years. Risk for death in those with

> **BOX 26.1 POOR PROGNOSTIC FACTORS IN ANOREXIA NERVOSA**
>
> - Long duration of illness
> - Age of onset prepuberty or greater than 17 years old
> - Male sex
> - Very low weight
> - Binge–purge symptoms
> - Personality difficulties
> - Difficult family relationships

bulimia nervosa is doubled compared with age-matched controls. Poor prognostic factors include severe bingeing and purging behaviour, low weight and comorbid depression.

Binge-eating disorder

Prognosis for individuals with binge-eating disorder is as yet little studied, but some studies have suggested that around half of those who undergo cognitive behavioural therapy have managed to sustain remission when followed up several years later. Negative predictors of remission include overvaluing weight and body shape and self-blame.

● Chapter Summary

- Eating disorders arise due to a mixture of genetic and environmental risk factors.
- The mainstay of treatment for anorexia nervosa, bulimia nervosa and binge-eating disorder is structured psychological intervention.
- Anorexia nervosa is associated with a high mortality, mainly due to physical complications of starvation.
- Admission to hospital may be required to safely manage high-risk patients with eating disorders, potentially using mental health legislation.
- Recovery is typically slow, and many patients have a relapsing–remitting course.

UKMLA Conditions
Eating disorders

UKMLA Presentations
Abnormal eating or exercise behaviour
Chronic abdominal pain
Decreased appetite
Fatigue
Fixed abnormal beliefs
Palpitations
Weight gain
Weight loss

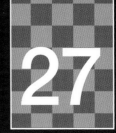

Sleeping is intimately related to mental health. Not only can psychiatric illnesses such as depression and schizophrenia disturb the quantity and quality of sleep, but certain psychiatric drugs can also have the same effect. Furthermore, persistent primary sleep disturbances, which are common, can result in significant psychological consequences in an otherwise mentally healthy individual. Although sleep–wake disorders are not categorized as mental disorders in ICD-11, an awareness of them is helpful in psychiatry, where many patients have sleep complaints.

DEFINITIONS AND CLASSIFICATION

Sleep is divided into five distinct stages as measured by polysomnography (see discussion later): four stages of non–rapid eye movement (non-REM; stages 1, 2, 3 and 4) and an REM stage. Fig. 27.1 summarises the key characteristics of the stages of sleep.

Sleep can be disrupted due to:

1. Primary sleep disorders
2. Sleep disorders secondary to a mental illness
3. Sleep disorders secondary to another medical condition
4. Sleep disorders secondary to the use of a substance

This chapter will focus principally on primary sleep disorders, which are not caused by another medical condition (e.g., arthritis) or mental illness (e.g., depression), and do not occur secondary to the use of a substance (e.g., alcohol). These disorders are presumed to arise from some defect of an individual's endogenous sleeping mechanism (the reticular activating system) coupled with unhelpful learned behaviours (e.g., worrying about not sleeping). The primary sleep disorders, in turn, are divided into the dyssomnias and the parasomnias.

The dyssomnias are characterized by abnormalities in the amount, quality or timing of sleep. They include:

a. Insomnia disorders – chronic or short term
b. Hypersomnolence disorders (narcolepsy, idiopathic hypersomnolence and Kleine–Levin syndrome)
c. Sleep-related breathing disorders (central or obstructive sleep apnoea)
d. Circadian rhythm sleep–wake disorders
e. Sleep-related movement disorders (restless leg syndrome, REM sleep behaviour disorder)

The parasomnias are characterized by abnormal episodes that occur during sleep or sleep–wake transitions. They include non-REM sleep arousal disorders (night terrors and sleepwalking), nightmares and REM sleep behaviour disorder.

Insomnia

Insomnia describes sleep of insufficient quantity or poor quality due to:

- Difficulty falling asleep
- Frequent awakening during the course of sleep
- Early morning awakening with subsequent difficulty getting back to sleep
- Sleep that is not refreshing despite being adequate in length.

In addition to daytime tiredness, persistent insomnia can have significant effects on mood, behaviour and performance. It has been shown that insomnia can also lead to an impairment of health-related quality of life similar to heart failure or depression.

Primary insomnia is diagnosed when present for at least 3 months and not attributable to medical or psychiatric illness, substance misuse or other dyssomnia or parasomnia. The numerous causes of insomnia as summarised in Box 27.1 include primary sleep disorders, medical and psychiatric illness and substance use.

Assessment of insomnia

Assessment involves excluding a medical, psychiatric or substance-related cause of insomnia. Many cases of primary insomnia are related to poor sleep hygiene (see Box 27.2 for advice to offer patients). Therefore, it is essential to enquire about sleeping times and patterns, and caffeine consumption. It is also useful to obtain collateral information from the patient's sleeping partner regarding sleeping patterns, snoring and movements during the night.

The following questions might be helpful in eliciting the key symptoms of insomnia:

- Do you fall asleep quickly or do you find yourself tossing and turning for some time before dropping off?
- Do you wake up repeatedly in the night or can you sleep through once you have managed to get to sleep?
- Do you sometimes awaken too early in the morning and then find that you are unable to get back to sleep?
- Is your sleep refreshing or do you still feel tired in the morning?

Stage of sleep	Duration spent in this phase during night	Characteristics and electroencephalogram (EEG) findings
Stage 1	5%	• Transition from wakefulness to sleep **EEG: theta waves** 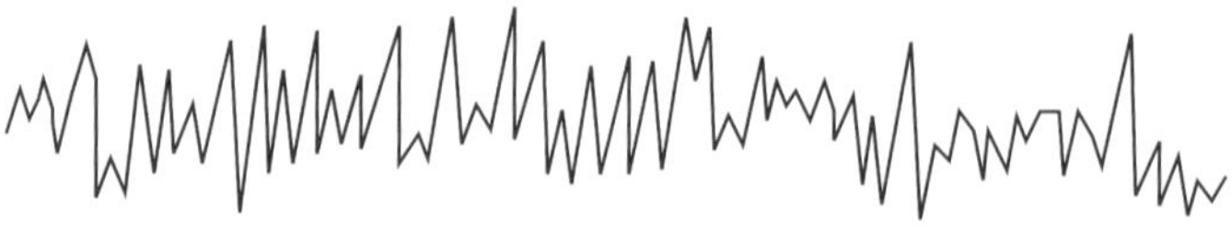 Theta waves: low amplitude, spike-like waves, 4–7 Hz
Stage 2	45%	**EEG: sleep spindles and K-complexes** 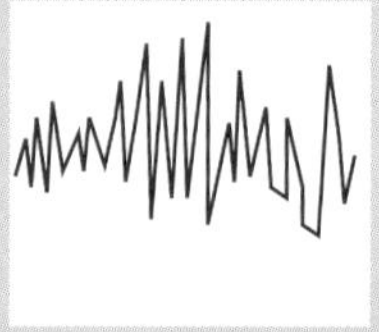 Sleep spindles: short rhythmic waveform clusters of 12–14 Hz 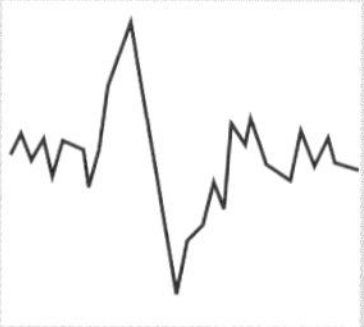 K-complex: sharp negative wave followed by a slower positive component
Stages 3 and 4 (slow wave sleep)	25%	• Deep sleep • Unusual arousal characteristics: disorientation, sleep terrors, sleepwalking • Occur in first third to half of night **EEG: delta waves** *Stage 3 – delta waves <50%* *Stage 4 – delta waves >50%* 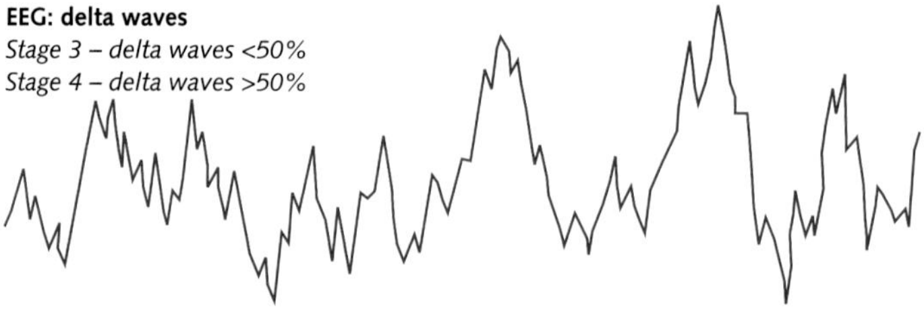 Delta waves: high amplitude, low frequency (<4 Hz)
REM	25%	• Occurs cyclically through the night, every 90 minutes alternating with non-REM sleep • Each episode increases in duration – most episodes occur in last third of night • Features penile erection, skeletal muscle paralysis and surreal dreaming (including nightmares) **EEG: low amplitude, high frequency, with sawtooth waves** 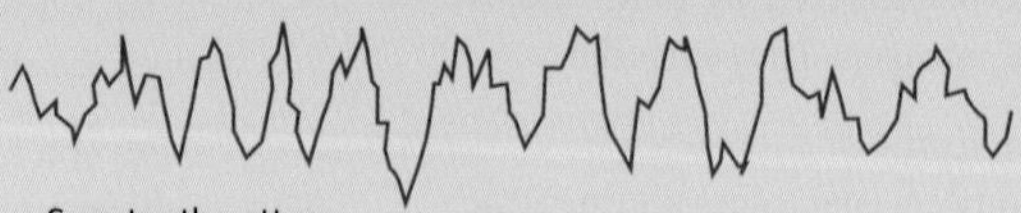 Saw-tooth pattern

Fig. 27.1 Stages of sleep. *REM*, Rapid eye movement.

246

BOX 27.1 COMMON CAUSES OF INSOMNIA

PRIMARY SLEEP DISORDERS

- Dyssomnias
  a. Insomnia disorders
  b. Circadian rhythm sleep–wake disorders (jet lag, shift work)
  c. Sleep-related breathing disorders (sleep apnoea syndromes)
  d. Sleep-related movement disorders (restless legs syndrome)
- Parasomnias (all)

PSYCHIATRIC DISORDERS

- Anxiety
- Depression
- Mania
- Schizophrenia

PHYSICAL DISORDERS

- Painful conditions (malignancies, arthritis, reflux disease)
- Cardiorespiratory discomfort (dyspnoea, coughing, palpitations)
- Nocturia (prostatic hypertrophy, urinary tract infections)
- Metabolic or endocrine conditions (thyroid disease, renal or liver failure)
- Central nervous system lesion (especially brainstem and hypothalamus)

SUBSTANCES

- Caffeine and other stimulants
- Alcohol
- Prescribed drugs (e.g., selective serotonin reuptake inhibitors, some antipsychotics)
- Substance withdrawal syndrome

BOX 27.2 GOOD SLEEP HYGIENE

- Avoid sleeping during the day.
- Exercise during the day (but not within 4 hours of bedtime) and maintain a healthy diet.
- Eliminate the use of stimulants (e.g., caffeine, nicotine, alcohol) within 6 hours of bedtime.
- Condition the brain by only using the bed for sleeping and sex – not for reading, watching TV, etc.
- Go to bed and awaken at the same time each day.
- Avoid stimulating activities before bedtime (e.g., television, games, mobile phone). NICE (2022) recommends 2 hours of screen-free time before bed. Instead, engage in relaxation techniques or reading.
- Try having a hot bath or drinking a cup of warm milk near bedtime.
- Avoid large meals within 2 hours of bedtime.
- Ensure that the bed is comfortable and that the bedroom is quiet.
- Ensure bedroom is not too hot or too cold.
- Do not lie in bed awake for longer than 15 minutes (but do not watch the clock!). Get up and do another relaxing activity and try sleeping later.

oxygen saturation, chest and abdominal excursion, mouth and nose air entry rates and the loudness of snoring.

Chronic insomnia can be diagnosed when the patient experiences difficulty getting off to sleep or maintaining sleep at least several times over the course of a week, and the difficulty has been present for at least three months. If the difficulties have been present for less than three months, short-term insomnia would be diagnosed.

COMMUNICATION

When considering insomnia, ask what the normal amount of sleep is for the patient in order for them to feel refreshed in the morning and what time they normally wake up. There is significant individual variation.

If, after a full history, the cause of insomnia remains unclear, the National Institute for Health and Care Excellence (NICE; 2022) recommends asking the patient to complete a sleep diary. Refer the patient to a sleep specialist for further investigation if there is diagnostic uncertainty or a suspicion of sleep apnoea, circadian rhythm disorders, parasomnias or narcolepsy. Further investigation is likely to include polysomnography: the simultaneous process of monitoring various physical parameters during sleep, including electroencephalogram, electrocardiogram, electromyogram, electrooculogram (eye movement), blood

Management of insomnia

The most important aspect of management is providing education about correct sleep hygiene (see Box 27.3). There is a limited role for medication in the treatment of insomnia. Hypnotics may help in the short term, but the development of tolerance to

PRIMARY SLEEP DISORDERS
- Dyssomnias
  a. Idiopathic hypersomnia
  b. Narcolepsy
  c. Kleine–Levin syndrome
  d. Sleep-related breathing disorders (sleep apnoea syndromes)
  e. Sleep-related movement disorders (restless legs syndrome)
  f. Circadian rhythm sleep disorders (jet lag, shift work)
- Parasomnias (all)

PSYCHIATRIC DISORDERS
- Depression

PHYSICAL DISORDERS
- Encephalitis and meningitis
- Stroke, head injury, brain tumour
- Degenerative neurological conditions
- Toxic, metabolic or endocrine abnormalities

SUBSTANCES
- Alcohol
- Prescribed drugs (e.g., antipsychotics, benzodiazepines, tricyclic antidepressants)
- Substance withdrawal syndrome

SECONDARY TO INSOMNIA OR SLEEP DEPRIVATION

their effects (usually within 2 weeks), possible dependence and their propensity to cause rebound insomnia limit their use. They should therefore only be prescribed on a time-limited basis, ideally for use on alternate or occasional nights rather than every night. Drugs with a long half-life should be avoided, to prevent leaving patients feeling drowsy the next day (the 'chemical hangover') and to avoid accumulation with repeated doses. Commonly used agents include the 'Z-drugs' (zopiclone, zolpidem, zaleplon) and benzodiazepines with a short half-life (such as temazepam). NICE (2022) advises that if there is no response to one hypnotic, an alternative should not be prescribed.

Hypersomnia

Hypersomnia describes excessive sleepiness that manifests as either a prolonged period of sleep or sleep episodes that occur during normal waking hours.

Hypersomnolence is diagnosed when patients present with hypersomnia for at least a month not attributable to a medical or psychiatric condition, substance use or other dyssomnia (especially narcolepsy and sleep apnoea) or parasomnia. The numerous causes of hypersomnia as summarized in Box 27.3 include primary sleep disorders, medical and psychiatric illness, substance use and sleep deprivation.

Hypersomnolence disorders

Narcolepsy

Narcolepsy typically presents in young people aged 10 to 20 years who report an abrupt onset of pervasive daytime sleepiness. It affects around 1 in 2000 people. Symptoms of narcolepsy are the tetrad of:

1. Irresistible attacks of refreshing sleep that may occur at inappropriate times (e.g., driving)
2. Cataplexy (sudden, bilateral loss of muscle tone usually precipitated by intense emotion leading to collapse and lasting for seconds to minutes)
3. Hypnagogic or hypnopompic hallucinations (see Chapter 9)
4. Sleep paralysis at the beginning or end of sleep episodes

The symptoms arise from elements of REM sleep intruding into wakefulness. Diagnosis is confirmed by observing rapid onset of REM on polysomnography during sleep latency studies.

In type 1 narcolepsy, cataplexy always occurs. It is due to a deficiency of hypocretin, a neuropeptide that regulates the initiation of REM sleep. Levels are low in cerebrospinal fluid obtained via lumbar puncture. It is thought to arise following autoimmune-mediated damage to hypocretin-producing cells in the hypothalamus, triggered following an infection. Over 98% of people with type 1 narcolepsy have a particular human leukocyte antigen haplotype. In type 2 narcolepsy (which is even rarer), cataplexy either does not occur or is atypical. Its aetiology overlaps with type 1 narcolepsy but, in general, is less well understood.

The treatment of narcolepsy includes taking naps at regular times and ensuring sufficient duration of night-time sleep. Typically, stimulants are needed to reduce daytime sleepiness (modafinil is first line). Cataplexy, sleep paralysis and hallucinations at the sleep–wake boundary can be improved by low-dose antidepressants (usually venlafaxine or clomipramine). Noradrenaline and serotonin suppress REM sleep, and so do antidepressants.

Kleine–Levin Syndrome

This extremely rare disorder (around 1 in a million people) is characterized by recurrent episodes of severe sleepiness (up to 20 hours per day), which typically last for around 10 days. The sleepiness is associated with hyperphagia (excessive food intake), hypersexuality, childish behaviour, depression and anxiety and sometimes hallucinations and delusions. Patients return to their usual baseline in between periods of sleepiness. It mainly affects teenage boys.

Circadian rhythm sleep–wake disorders

Circadian rhythm sleep–wake disorders are characterized by a lack of synchrony between an individual's endogenous circadian rhythm for sleep and that demanded by their environment, resulting in the individual being tired when they should be awake (hypersomnia) and being awake when they should be sleeping (insomnia). This disorder results from either a malfunction of the internal 'biological clock' that regulates sleep or from an unnatural environmental change (e.g., jet lag, night-shift work). Actigraphy can be used to measure sleep for a period to help inform management. Treatment comprises of sleep hygiene, enhancing environmental cues regarding time of day (e.g., having a dark bedroom) and bright light therapy. Melatonin is also licensed for short-term management of jet lag.

Sleep-related breathing disorders

Abnormalities of ventilation during sleep can cause repeated disruptions to sleep. This results in unrefreshing sleep and excessive sleepiness during the day. Obstructive sleep apnoea syndrome, the most common breathing-related sleep disorder, is characterised by obstruction of the upper airways during sleep, despite an adequate respiratory effort. Typically, an individual will have noisy breathing during sleep with loud snoring interspersed with apnoeic episodes lasting from 20 to 90, sometimes associated with cyanosis. It is an increasingly common condition, affecting around 10% of men, 5% of women and 1% of children. The prevalence is much higher in obese, elderly or hypertensive individuals and is also prominent in some patients with intellectual disabilities. The repeated stress of sudden arousals has significant cardiovascular and neuropsychiatric morbidity and should be actively excluded when an at-risk patient presents with hypersomnia, impairment of concentration and memory or other psychiatric symptoms. Collateral history from a bed partner, who is often aware of the sleeping difficulties, is extremely useful. The Epworth Sleepiness Scale is a set of eight questions related to the individual's likelihood of falling asleep during different activities that can be used to screen for obstructive sleep apnoea.

The diagnosis is confirmed by polysomnography with concurrent monitoring of electroencephalogram and respiration. Treatment comprises lifestyle advice (weight loss, avoidance of alcohol, sleep on one's side, not back) and provision of nasal continuous positive airway pressure.

RED FLAG

Obstructive sleep apnoea increases the risk for road traffic accidents around sevenfold and also increases the risk for systemic hypertension. It is a useful diagnosis to make as the majority of patients respond well to treatment with continuous positive airway pressure. However, most cases go undiagnosed.

HINTS AND TIPS

Medication and substances increase the risk for obstructive sleep apnoea, particularly opiates, benzodiazepines and alcohol. Always take a substance history in someone presenting with symptoms of sleep apnoea.

Sleep-related movement disorders

Restless legs syndrome is the commonest sleep-related movement disorder. Patients report uncomfortable sensations in their legs when at rest (typically crawling, burning, tingling or itching), which are relieved by movement. Because inactivity is required for sleep, restless leg syndrome can delay sleep onset and precipitate awakenings. The disorder arises most frequently in young adults and generally worsens slowly over time, affecting around 1 in 50 people. It runs in families, is twice as common in women and often occurs transiently during pregnancy. Medication can cause it, particularly lithium, antidepressants, antihistamines and dopamine antagonists (e.g., metoclopramide, antipsychotics). Key differentials are peripheral neuropathy (not worse at night), vascular disease (worsened by movement, not relieved) and akathisia (movement driven by an inner restlessness, not a specific need to move legs). Ferritin levels should be checked, as restless legs are a rare presentation of iron deficiency, which impacts on dopamine metabolism. Nonpharmacological management includes sleep hygiene, exercise and avoidance of agents which may worsen symptoms (e.g., alcohol, caffeine, medication). Pharmacological management is reserved for severe cases for short periods (e.g., 6 months) and includes dopamine agonists (e.g., pramipexole, ropinirole) or antiepileptics which bind voltage-gated calcium channels (gabapentin, pregabalin).

Parasomnias

Non-REM sleep arousal disorders

Non-REM sleep arousal disorders are recurrent incomplete awakenings from sleep during sleep stages outwith REM, generally slow wave sleep and generally during the first third of the night. The duration of the incomplete awakening is generally 1 to 10 minutes but can be up to an hour. The two main subtypes are night terrors and sleepwalking. They are thought to share a common pathophysiology. Management is to exclude other diagnoses, offer reassurance and advise good sleep hygiene. It is not necessary to attempt to terminate episodes, but it may be useful to remove potentially harmful objects or routes from around someone who sleepwalks frequently.

Sleep terrors (night terrors)

Sleep terrors are episodes that feature an individual (usually a child) abruptly waking from sleep, usually with a scream, appearing to be in a state of extreme fear. These episodes are associated with:

- Autonomic arousal, for example, tachycardia, dilated pupils, sweating and rapid breathing.
- A relative unresponsiveness to the efforts of others to comfort the person, who appears confused and disorientated.

Upon full awakening, there is amnesia for the episode and no recall of any dream or nightmare. Sleep terrors are seen in up to 6% of children aged 4 to 12 years and usually resolve by adolescence. Sleep terrors should be distinguished from nightmares, panic attacks and epileptic seizures. Panic attacks tend not to be associated with confusion, and amnesia is uncommon.

Sleepwalking disorder (somnambulism)

Sleepwalking is characterised by an unusual state of consciousness in which complex motor behaviour occurs during sleep. While sleepwalking, the individual has a blank staring face, is relatively unresponsive to communication from others and is difficult to waken. When sleepwalkers do wake up, either during an episode or the following morning, they have no recollection of the event ever having occurred. Sleepwalking is not associated with impairment of cognition or behaviour, although there may be an initial brief period of disorientation subsequent to waking up from a sleepwalking episode. The peak prevalence of sleepwalking occurs at the age of 12 years, with an onset between the age of 4 and 8 years. About 2% to 3% of children and about 0.5% of adults have regular episodes. Sleepwalking runs in families, with 80% of sleepwalkers having a positive family history for sleepwalking or sleep terrors.

Nightmares

Between 10% and 50% of children, aged 3 to 5 years, experience repeated nightmares, and they also occur occasionally in up to 50% of adults. Nightmares are characterised by an individual waking from sleep due to an intensely frightening dream involving threats to survival, security or self-esteem. Nightmares are distinguished from sleep terrors by the observation that not only is the individual alert and orientated immediately after awakening but is able to recall the bad dream in vivid detail. Furthermore,

nightmares tend to occur during the second half of the night because they arise almost exclusively during REM sleep, which tends to be longer and have more intense, surreal dreaming during the latter part of the night. Nightmares can be precipitated by withdrawal from REM-suppressing agents (such as antidepressants or alcohol) or by commencing β-blockers or dopamine agonists. Management is to reassure, avoid medications that may precipitate nightmares and advise avoidance of stress.

HINTS AND TIPS

Upon awakening from a rapid eye movement (REM) parasomnia, the patient is alert and recalls a dream. Patients who are woken from a non-REM parasomnia are disorientated and confused, with no recollection of a dream or their behaviour.

REM sleep behaviour disorder

Unlike the other parasomnias, REM sleep behaviour disorder is more common in older adults, typically presenting in men in their 50s. There is a failure of muscle atonia during REM, allowing dreams to be acted out. The dream content is often of a negative and violent nature, so sufferers may jerk, punch, shout, get out of bed or attack their partner. This occurs regardless of whether the sufferer has a history of violence and aggression. When awakened, patients often report very vivid, intense, threatening dreams. Often, patients present because of injuries to themselves or their partner. The behaviours are more frequent in the last third of the sleep period and can occur cyclically (as REM sleep occurs approximately every 90 minutes).

There is a strong association between REM sleep behaviour disorder and neurodegenerative conditions involving abnormal deposition of synuclein protein (Parkinson disease, Lewy body dementia, multisystem atrophy). Over half of patients will go on to be diagnosed with Parkinson disease, potentially up to 10 years later. The sleep disorder can improve as the neurodegeneration progresses.

Management includes environmental modification to reduce injury (e.g., cushions around the bed and removal of potentially dangerous objects from the bedroom). Clonazepam is highly effective in reducing the behaviours (up to 90% of cases). Interestingly, tolerance does not seem to arise, so it can be continued long term.

RED FLAG

Rapid eye movement sleep behaviour disorders often arise in the early stages of neurodegenerative conditions such as Parkinson disease and Lewy body dementia. Careful assessment and monitoring of neurological status are needed.

Chapter Summary

- Sleep can be disrupted due to a primary sleep disorder, a psychiatric condition, a medical condition or substance use (prescribed medications or recreational).
- Dyssomnias are characterised by abnormalities in the amount, quality or timing of sleep.
- Parasomnias are characterised by abnormal episodes that occur during sleep or sleep–wake transitions.
- Good sleep hygiene, ensuring sufficient duration of sleep and avoiding recreational substances are recommended for all patients with sleep problems.
- Hypnotics can be helpful for short-term use in insomnia but lose effectiveness if continued long term.

UKMLA Presentation
Sleep problems

FURTHER READING

Sleep diary sample.
https://www.nhs.uk/livewell/insomnia/documents/sleepdiary.pdf.
Epworth Sleepiness Scale.
http://epworthsleepinessscale.com/about-the-ess/.

Sexual problems and disorders · 28

Physical or psychological problems (or a combination of the two) can cause a wide variety of sexual problems. Mental health workers may be consulted about sexual problems that are largely due to psychological difficulties (not predominantly due to a biological problem) – that is, psychosexual problems.

This chapter will discuss three aspects of sexuality that you may come across in psychiatry:

- Sexual dysfunction
- Disorders of sexual preference (paraphilias)
- Gender incongruence

SEXUAL DYSFUNCTION

Clinical features

Sexual stimulation is summarized in a four-phase sexual response cycle. Sexual dysfunction describes pain associated with intercourse or abnormalities of the sexual response cycle that lead to difficulties in participating in sexual activities. Although this chapter is focused on psychological dysfunction, the sexual response cycle consists of both psychological and

biological processes and it is rarely possible to identify cases of sexual dysfunction with a purely physiological or purely psychological aetiology. Table 28.1 summarizes the sexual dysfunction disorders.

> **HINTS AND TIPS**
>
> Women have a large interindividual variability in the type and duration of stimulation that results in orgasm. The diagnosis of female orgasmic disorder (anorgasmia in the ICD-11) should only be made if the dysfunction results in clinically significant distress.

Epidemiology

Sexual dysfunction is very common. A large UK survey found that 42% of men and 51% of women reported one or more problems with sexual response lasting at least 3 months, but only around 10% of people were distressed about their sexual function. The self-report cross-sectional prevalence (not clinical diagnoses) of

Table 28.1 Sexual dysfunction disorders

Phase of cycle	Dysfunction[a]	Description
Desire	Hypoactive sexual desire dysfunction (male hypoactive sexual desire disorder; female sexual interest/arousal disorder)	Loss of desire to have or to fantasize about sex – not due to other sexual dysfunction (e.g., erectile dysfunction, dyspareunia). Avoidance of sex due to negative feelings (fear, anxiety, repulsion) or lack of enjoyment. Inability to sustain desire once sex is initiated.
Excitement	Sexual arousal dysfunction (male erectile disorder; female sexual arousal disorder)	Absent or reduced response to adequate sexual stimulation when sex is desired. In men, an erection that is insufficient to allow intercourse. In women, a reduction in genital response (e.g., vulvovaginal lubrication), nongenital response (e.g., nipple hardening) and feelings of arousal.
Orgasm	Orgasmic dysfunction (female orgasmic disorder; delayed ejaculation) Ejaculatory dysfunction (premature ejaculation)	Recurrent absence, or delay, of orgasm or ejaculation despite adequate sexual stimulation and desire for sex. Recurrent ejaculation with minimal sexual stimulation before the man wishes.
Sexual pain	Sexual pain–penetration disorder (genito-pelvic pain/penetration disorder)	Genital pain during sex in men or women – not due to other sexual dysfunction (e.g., poor lubrication–swelling response) or medical condition (e.g., atrophic vaginitis). May occur due to involuntary tightening of pelvic floor muscles during attempted penetration (vaginismus).

[a]DSM-5 terms are in square brackets; ICD-11 terms are not.

Table 28.2 Reported frequency of sexual dysfunction in Britons aged 16–74 years

		(%)[a]
Men	Premature ejaculation	15
	Lack of sexual interest	15
	Erectile difficulties	13
	Unable to achieve orgasm	9
Women	Lack of sexual interest	34
	Unable to achieve orgasm	16
	Trouble lubricating	13
	Pain during sex	8

[a]Problem present for 3 or more months in those who have had sex within previous year.
(Data from Sexual function in Britain: findings from the third National Survey of Sexual Attitudes and Lifestyles (Natsal-3). Mitchell KR et al., Lancet. 2013 Nov 30;382(9907):1817–29. doi:10.1016/S0140-6736(13)62366-1.)

> **BOX 28.1 PRESCRIBED AND RECREATIONAL DRUGS ASSOCIATED WITH SEXUAL DYSFUNCTION**
>
> Psychiatric drugs
> - Antidepressants (tricyclics, selective serotonin reuptake inhibitors (SSRIs) and monoamine oxidase inhibitors (MAOIs))[a]
> - Antipsychotics (especially first-generation antipsychotics)
> - Benzodiazepines
> - Lithium
>
> Recreational drugs
> - Alcohol
> - Amphetamines
> - Cannabis
> - Cocaine
> - Opiates
>
> Medical drugs
> - Antiandrogens
> - Anticonvulsants
> - Antihistamines
> - Antihypertensives (including β-blockers)
> - Digoxin
> - Diuretics
>
> [a] The antidepressant least likely to be associated with sexual dysfunction is mirtazapine.

specific sexual dysfunctions is shown in Table 28.2. The evidence suggests that:

- The prevalence of sexual problems in women tends to decrease with increasing age, except for those who report trouble lubricating.
- Men, by contrast, have an increased prevalence of erectile problems with increasing age.
- Sexual dysfunction is more likely among people with poor physical and emotional health (particularly depression).
- Sexual dysfunction is highly associated with negative experiences in sexual relationships.
- Sexual dysfunction is associated with relationship difficulties: being unhappy in a relationship, not being in a steady relationship and difficulties communicating with a partner about sex.

Aetiology

There are many, often interrelated, psychosocial factors that may result in psychogenic sexual dysfunction:

- Ambivalent attitude about sex or intimacy (e.g., anxiety, fear, guilt, shame).
- History of rape or childhood sexual abuse.
- Fears of consequences of sex (e.g., pregnancy, sexually transmitted diseases).
- A poor or deteriorating relationship (e.g., feeling undesirable, finding the partner undesirable, lack of trust, feelings of resentment or hostility, lack of respect, fear of rejection).

- Anxiety about sexual performance or physical attractiveness.
- Fatigue, stress or difficult psychosocial circumstances.

Frequently, there is more than one psychosocial problem that can affect more than one of the phases of the sexual response cycle. For example, the belief that sex is inherently sinful in the context of an abusive relationship may lead to a lack of desire, a poor lubrication–swelling response and difficulty in reaching orgasm.

Differential diagnosis

Other causes of sexual dysfunction should be excluded when assessing a patient with sexual dysfunction. These include:

- Medical conditions (e.g., diabetes mellitus, vascular disease, vaginitis, endometriosis, spinal cord injuries, pelvic fractures, prostatectomy, multiple sclerosis, thyroid disease, hyperprolactinemia).
- Prescribed or recreational drugs (see Box 28.1).
- Psychiatric illness: mental disorders such as depression, anxiety and alcohol dependence are frequently associated

with sexual dysfunction. In addition, psychiatric medication often results in sexual dysfunction as a side effect. However, sexual functioning frequently improves as the patient's mental illness (e.g., depression) improves, even though the medication (e.g., antidepressants) may have adverse sexual effects.

RED FLAG

Erectile dysfunction is a strong predictor of coronary artery disease and is a common presenting symptom of diabetes mellitus. Assess cardiovascular risk and glucose in all men presenting with erectile dysfunction.

HINTS AND TIPS

The clear presence of a biological cause of sexual dysfunction does not rule out a psychological contribution to sexual dysfunction, as the two are often interrelated. For example, a 55-year-old man with diabetes and advanced atherosclerosis notices a weakened erection; he subsequently becomes anxious during sex, fearing that he is losing his virility. This leads to a complete loss of his ability to experience an erection.

RED FLAG

If it is necessary to perform an examination of or around patient's genitalia, consider how to minimize the reliving of any previous sexual trauma (see text for suggestions). Take these steps with everybody, whether or not they have disclosed sexual trauma. Remember that 23% of women and 4% of men in the United Kingdom have been sexually assaulted at least once since age 16.

Assessment considerations

- The wide differential diagnosis requires a comprehensive history including medical, psychiatric, sexual and relationship histories as well as current medication and recreational substance use. Questions regarding sexual activities outside the problematic context (e.g., morning erections, masturbation, sexual fantasy) can be very helpful.
- A thorough physical examination, including genitalia, should be conducted. In addition, gynaecological examination may be needed for cases of sexual pain in women.
- Trauma-informed examination: it is important to consider how any previous sexual trauma might influence the examination, and how the examination may trigger memories of difficult sexual experiences or even symptoms of post-traumatic stress disorder. Trauma-informed practice suggests sensitively asking the patient whether they have a history of sexual trauma prior to commencing the examination, while they are clothed and seated. If the patient's notes already document sexual trauma consider sensitively acknowledging this. A chaperone should always be offered, and if possible the patient should be asked which gender they would prefer, or whether they would prefer to be joined by a friend or family member. If informed consent is given to proceed with the examination, ensure that you affirm that the patient is in control and offer explanations of what you are doing during each step of the examination. Ask the patient to remove or position their clothing rather than doing it for them and avoid placing your hands underneath their clothing. If the patient asks you to stop at any point during the examination, respect this and only continue if the patient tells you they feel able to. Other suggestions include only exposing the parts of the patient's body that are absolutely necessary for the examination and allowing the patient time to get used to the presence of any examination equipment, e.g., a speculum, before proceeding with the next stage of the examination.
- Blood tests should be performed to assess for medical causes of sexual dysfunction, particularly hyperprolactinemia, hypotestosteronaemia and in erectile dysfunction, glucose and lipids. Rarely, further investigations may be necessary to exclude medical causes of erectile dysfunction (e.g., monitoring of nocturnal penile tumescence (excludes physiological causes of impotence if able to have erection during rapid eye movement sleep) and monitoring penile blood flow with Doppler ultrasonography).

COMMUNICATION

Taking a sexual history can be embarrassing for both patients and doctors, and basic communication skills are very important. Privacy should be ensured, and nonverbal aspects of communication should be utilized (e.g., body language, use of silence). Straightforward terminology should be used (e.g., 'vagina', rather than 'down below'; 'condom', rather than 'protection'). Reassurance and acknowledgement of discomfort (e.g., 'I can see how difficult this is for you to talk about') can be very helpful.

Management considerations

- Many patients need no more than reassurance, advice and sexual education. Patients who have significant relationship difficulties may benefit from relationship counselling before attempting specific treatment for sexual dysfunction.
- Some couples with minor problems benefit from self-help materials, particularly those with no major relationship difficulties.
- Urology clinics deal mainly with physiological sexual dysfunction, particularly erectile problems.
- Sexual dysfunction clinics have multidisciplinary teams that focus on both psychological and physical aspects of sexual dysfunction and are best equipped to deal with cases that do not respond to nonspecific measures.
- Some couples benefit from sex therapy, in which partners are treated together and are taught to communicate openly about sex, in addition to receiving education about sexual anatomy and the physiology of the sexual response cycle. They also take part in graded assignments, beginning with caressing of their partner's body, without genital contact, for their own and then their partner's pleasure. These behavioural tasks progress through a number of stages with increasing sexual intimacy, with the focus remaining on pleasurable physical contact as opposed to the monitoring of sexual arousal or the preoccupation with achieving orgasm. Couples suitable for sex therapy include those with a significant psychological component to their problem, those with reasonable motivation and those with a reasonably harmonious relationship.
- Table 28.3 summarizes some of the specific exercises often used in the context of sex therapy that may be helpful with particular problems.

Table 28.3 Specific exercises useful in sexual dysfunction

Sexual dysfunction	Exercise
Female orgasmic disorder	Exercises in sexual fantasy and masturbation, sometimes with a vibrator or dildo.
Premature ejaculation	Squeeze technique: partner or individual squeezes the glans of penis for a few seconds when he feels that he is about to ejaculate. Start–stop method: stimulation is halted and arousal is allowed to subside when the man feels that ejaculation is imminent. The process is then repeated. Quiet vagina: man keeps penis motionless in vagina for increasing periods before ejaculating.
Vaginismus	Desensitization, first by finger insertion followed by dilators of increasing size.

- Biological treatments may be very effective, especially for erectile problems (e.g., oral sildenafil (Viagra), intracavernosal injections, vacuum devices, prosthetic implants and surgery for venous leakage). See Box 28.2. Testosterone may increase sexual drive in patients with low levels of the hormone. For difficulties with premature ejaculation, selective serotonin reuptake inhibitors may delay ejaculation, but this is rarely a long-term solution.

Prognosis

Vaginismus has an excellent prognosis. Premature ejaculation and psychologically driven erectile dysfunction also respond fairly well to treatment. Problems associated with low sexual desire, especially in men, seem more resistant to treatment.

DISORDERS OF SEXUAL PREFERENCE (PARAPHILIAS)

A paraphilic disorder is when a person experiences recurrent, sexually arousing fantasies, urges or behaviours which cause distress or harm, or where the subject is unable to consent (such as a child or an animal). To meet criteria for a paraphilic disorder a patient must have either acted on these feelings or be distressed by them. The paraphilic disorders include the following:

- Exhibitionistic disorder: patients become sexually aroused by exposing their genitals to nonconsenting people.
- Voyeuristic disorder: patients become sexually aroused by watching an unaware person engaging in sexual acts.

BOX 28.2 MANAGEMENT OF MEN WITH ERECTILE DYSFUNCTION

- Check testosterone level.
- Calculate 10-year cardiovascular risk and manage appropriately.
- Lifestyle advice:
  - Weight loss, stop smoking, reduce alcohol, increase exercise.
  - If a man cycles more than 3 hours a week: advise a trial without cycling.
- Medication:
  - Consider substituting potentially contributory medication (see Box 28.1).
  - Consider a phosphodiesterase inhibitor (sildenafil, tadalafil or vardenafil), regardless of the cause.

- Paedophilic disorder: patients experience sexual thoughts, urges or behaviours related to children.
- Coercive sexual sadism disorder: patients become aroused by inflicting (or the thought of inflicting) suffering on a nonconsenting person.
- Frotteuristic disorder: patients become aroused by rubbing their genitals on a nonconsenting person.

HINTS AND TIPS

Paraphilias have been significantly revised in the ICD-11. In the ICD-10, sexual preferences which may be enjoyed by consenting adults such as fetishism or sadomasochism were classified as paraphilias. In the ICD-11 a preference must cause distress or harm to be classified as a paraphilia.

RED FLAG

Paraphilias can emerge due to medical or psychiatric conditions: mania, frontal lobe injury, neurodegenerative conditions or as a rare side effect of high-dose dopaminomimetic medication. Always ask about the duration of an unusual sexual preference.

Management options include behaviour therapy (covert sensitization, where patients attempt to pair paraphilic thoughts with humiliating consequences) and aversion therapy (pairing paraphilic thoughts with a noxious stimulus such as an unpleasant odour or taste). Individual psychodynamic and group therapies are also used. Cognitive behavioural therapy programmes and antiandrogens (e.g., cyproterone acetate) have shown some efficacy in the treatment of some paedophiles and exhibitionists; however, there is little evidence that any treatment is consistently effective in either of these conditions. It should be noted that, dependent on risk for offending, management within a forensic setting may be required (see Chapter 34).

Paraphilias associated with a young age of onset, a high frequency of acts, no remorse about acts and a lack of motivation for change have a particularly poor prognosis.

GENDER INCONGRUENCE

Gender incongruence is a new diagnosis in the ICD-11 and refers to a marked and persistent incongruence between an individual's experienced gender (the gender they identify as being) and their assigned sex (based on their genital appearance or karyotype at or before birth). ICD-11 has redefined gender identity-related health, replacing now outdated diagnostic categories like ICD-10's 'transsexualism' and 'gender identity disorder of children' with 'gender incongruence of adolescence and adulthood' and 'gender incongruence of childhood'. See Box 28.3 for definitions of terms in current use in relation to gender.

Trans-health care is provided by a wide range of specialists and it is common for psychiatrists to have input into specialised gender identity clinics. Individuals to whom the description of gender incongruence applies are more visible now than in the past and as such may be perceived as more common than before by doctors in their day-to-day practice. This section has been included to provide some basic information around trans-health care and transpeople which may enhance the quality of care provided through influencing approach and understanding.

The exact prevalence of gender incongruity is unknown and studies have reported quite different figures across different cultures and countries. In the 2021 UK census, 0.5% of people answered the question, 'Is your gender the same as your registered sex at birth?' with 'No'. In 2023, there were 10 Gender Identity Clinics in England, 4 in Scotland, 2 in Wales and 1 in Northern Ireland.

Assessment and treatment

The assessment of gender incongruence is usually carried out within a gender identity clinic. The diagnosis relies on a comprehensive biopsychosocial history, with particular focus on the

---

BOX 28.3 DEFINITIONS RELATED TO GENDER

Gender identity is the personal sense of one's own gender. It is an individual's sense of being female, male, neither, both or anywhere along the gender spectrum.

Gender incongruence is a marked and persistent incongruence between an individual's gender identity and their assigned sex.

Gender dysphoria is the feeling of discomfort or distress that may occur in some people who do not identify with their assigned gender. The degree of dysphoria experienced varies greatly between people and may be felt more intensely during certain stages of life.

Gender nonconformity is not the same as gender dysphoria: it refers to the extent to which a person's gender identity, role or expression differs from cultural norms prescribed for people of a particular sex. Only some gender nonconforming people experience gender dysphoria.

---

developmental aspects of the individual's gender experience. Dysphoria may be social in nature (i.e., the negative feeling attached to being gendered by others incorrectly) or physical (i.e., negative feelings towards the appearance or function of their body).

There are a range of treatments available on the NHS across the United Kingdom which may include hormone-affirming therapy, speech therapy, hair removal, genital-affirming surgery or gender-affirming chest surgery. Other surgeries which may be sought include facial feminization surgery, breast augmentation, cricothyroid prominence reduction or vocal cord surgery.

In the United Kingdom, an individual seeking genital-affirming surgery will require two supportive opinions from a nonsurgical gender specialist prior to surgery. In some areas, only one is required if the individual has been granted a gender recognition certificate (Box 28.4).

BOX 28.4 THE GENDER RECOGNITION ACT 2004

The Gender Recognition Act 2004 (and its many amendments and orders) is an act of Parliament which enables people to apply to receive a Gender Recognition Certificate (GRC). People with a GRC are able to obtain a birth certificate showing their recognized legal sex.

In order to obtain a GRC, the person must be at least 18 years of age, have lived in their acquired gender for at least two years, have a diagnosis of gender dysphoria and provide two medical reports (one must be from a specialist in the field of gender dysphoria). The person is not required to have had surgery.

● Chapter Summary

- Sexual dysfunction is common, particularly in those with poor physical or emotional health.
- It often arises due to a combination of physical and psychological factors.
- It is important to exclude potentially serious causes, particularly cardiovascular disease and diabetes in erectile dysfunction.
- Management of any psychological component hinges on reassurance, psychoeducation and graded intimate contact.
- Paraphilias are unusual sexual interests that are viewed as disorders when associated with significant harm, or risk for harm, to the individual or others.
- Gender incongruence is a mismatch between a person's assigned sex and experienced gender. Rarely, this arises due to mental disorder.

UKMLA Presentations
Erectile dysfunction
Loss of libido

PREMENSTRUAL SYNDROME

Clinical features

The premenstrual syndrome (PMS) has been defined as the recurrence of symptoms during the premenstruum, with their absence in the postmenstruum. Symptoms include mood symptoms (depressed mood, irritability), somatic symptoms (lethargy, joint pain, overeating) and cognitive symptoms (concentration difficulties, forgetfulness). Typically, symptoms begin several days before menstruation and will start to improve a few days afterwards. They are absent again from around 1 week after the onset of menstruation. Symptoms must have been present during a majority of menstrual cycles within the preceding year, prior to a diagnosis being made.

The DSM-5 and the ICD-11 describe *premenstrual dysphoric disorder* (PMDD), which in essence are the mental health symptoms of PMS combined with significant distress or functional impairment. Prospective evaluation of symptoms over at least two cycles is recommended prior to making the diagnosis, as retrospective recall is unreliable.

The National Institute for Health and Care Excellence (NICE; 2019) classifies PMS as mild, moderate or severe depending on its impact on personal, social or professional life. Mild PMS does not interfere with normal functioning in these domains, moderate PMS causes interference and severe PMS causes withdrawal from these domains.

Epidemiology/aetiology

Up to 40% of women report experiencing some symptoms of PMS; however, only around a fifth seek medical help and around 3% to 8% of women experience symptoms of a severity sufficient to interfere with their work or lifestyle. The prevalence is higher in women who experience significant degrees of psychosocial stress, have a history of trauma, smoke, are obese, have a family history of PMS or who have a history of depression or anxiety. In those who have a history of mental health problems, it is important to confirm that the luteal phase symptoms are not merely an exacerbation of difficulties that are present continuously. If this is the case, management should focus on the primary mental health problem.

The exact cause of PMS is unknown. PMS occurs in women who are ovulating, and symptoms do not occur during puberty, pregnancy or postmenopause. This suggests a link between changing levels of oestrogen and progesterone and the symptoms of PMS. However, previous theories about oestrogen excess and progesterone deficiency are now thought to be incorrect. Some studies have suggested that women with PMS might have an exaggerated response to normal hormonal fluctuations, but other studies have also suggested that the symptoms of PMS might be linked to low levels of serotonin, as PMS symptoms can respond to SSRIs. Twin studies have also suggested there is a genetic component.

Management

Management is informed by aetiology, with the principles being stress reduction, ovulation suppression (which prevents the cyclical changes in gonadal hormone levels) and central nervous system serotonin enhancement.

For all women with PMS, NICE (2019) recommends advice on healthy eating, stress reduction, regular sleep and regular exercise. They also recommend smoking cessation and reducing alcohol intake where applicable. Simple analgesia is recommended for pain, including headaches. For cyclical breast pain, simple analgesia or topical NSAIDs can be offered. In moderate PMS, NICE (2019) recommends a new-generation combined oral contraceptive (first-line treatments are those containing the progestogen drospirenone). If the patient is interested in psychological intervention, refer for cognitive behavioural therapy (CBT). In severe PMS (which would include anyone with a diagnosis of PMDD), the strategies for moderate PMS should be trialled first, and a selective serotonin reuptake inhibitor (SSRI) tried if these are ineffective. This can be given either continuously or during the luteal phase only (days 15–28, stopping on first day of menses). Standard doses of common SSRIs are recommended (e.g., fluoxetine 20 mg). If these treatment options do not work, further treatments can be initiated under specialist supervision including gonadotropin-releasing hormone analogues with add-back hormone replacement therapy (HRT) or even surgical treatment with add-back HRT.

MENOPAUSE

The menopause and perimenopausal period have been linked to an increased risk of mental illness, including schizophrenia and depression. This is particularly the case for women who have had previous hormone-related mood disorders such as postnatal depression or PMDD. As well as undergoing profound physiological changes, women of perimenopausal age are often experiencing psychosocial stressors (e.g., caring responsibilities for parents/children, relationship problems, first significant physical health problems in themselves/partners/friends). NICE (2019) advises that HRT can be considered to treat low mood arising around the time of menopause, but if a woman meets criteria for depression, standard management of a depressive episode in adults should also be followed (i.e., a combination of talking therapy and antidepressants, see Chapter 24).

PSYCHIATRIC CONSIDERATIONS IN PREGNANCY

- The development of most psychiatric illnesses during pregnancy is no more common than in the general population (the exception is OCD, where risk is increased about twofold). However, both psychosocial stressors and changing or stopping maintenance medications in women with a history of major mental illnesses carries a degree of risk, and the puerperium is a very high-risk period for relapse in major mental illness, particularly bipolar disorder.
- Domestic violence is more common during pregnancy, and this can impair mental health and resilience.
- Women with a major mental illness (bipolar disorder, schizophrenia, severe depression) or a history of puerperal psychosis who are pregnant or planning pregnancy should be referred to perinatal psychiatry services, even if they have been stable for some years. Box 29.1 summarizes the indications for referral to a specialist perinatal mental health team.
- For patients prescribed psychotropic medication during pregnancy, a judgement needs to be made – in conjunction with the patient – weighing up the risk of relapse against the risk of medication-induced teratogenic or adverse effects for the mother or child. Risks associated with various psychotropic medications are summarised in Table 29.1. Decisions should be made prior to conception (if possible). Up-to-date information on the use of medications during pregnancy should always be sought.
- There is an increased incidence of adverse life events in the weeks prior to a spontaneous abortion (miscarriage).
- Following miscarriage and termination of pregnancy, there is an increased risk for adjustment and bereavement reactions (see Chapter 14). In addition, the risk for puerperal psychosis remains.

HINTS AND TIPS

It is easy to be put off by the potential consequences of medication on a developing foetus but remember that a psychiatrically unwell mother is harmful for a baby's gestation and infancy also: risks of stopping medication often outweigh risks of continuing. This decision needs to be made in conjunction with the patient, and any partners or family the patient wishes to involve.

HINTS AND TIPS

General principles of prescribing in pregnancy are:
- Use the drug with the lowest known risk to mother and foetus.
- Use the lowest effective dose.
- Use a single drug rather than multiple drugs, if possible and be aware that doses may need to be adjusted due to physiological consequences of pregnancy.

HINTS AND TIPS

Pseudocyesis is a rare condition when a nonpregnant woman has the signs and symptoms of pregnancy (e.g., abdominal distension, breast enlargement, cessation of menses, enlargement of the uterus). Couvade syndrome describes the condition in which men develop typical pregnancy-related symptoms during their partner's pregnancy (e.g., morning sickness, vague abdominal pains, labour pains). Both of these conditions are psychosomatic and should be distinguished from delusion of pregnancy. Pseudocyesis and delusion of pregnancy may occur together.

Table 29.1 Psychiatric medication during pregnancy and breastfeeding[a]

Drug group	Pregnancy	Breastfeeding
Selective serotonin reuptake inhibitors	Can be associated with withdrawal symptoms in neonates, which are generally mild and self-limiting. Rarely associated with persistent pulmonary hypertension when given after first trimester.	Paroxetine and sertraline: very small amounts excreted in breast milk; short half-life fluoxetine and citalopram are excreted in relatively larger (but still small) amounts. Fluoxetine has a long half-life and thus may accumulate.
Tricyclic antidepressants	Have been used during pregnancy for many years. Commonly result in mild and self-limiting withdrawal reactions in neonates.	Tricyclics are excreted in small amounts only but avoid doxepin (accumulation of metabolite).
Mood stabilizers	All are associated with teratogenicity. Valproate and carbamazepine increase the risk for neural tube defects and should be avoided in pregnancy. Valproate also increases the risk for developmental disorders (30%–40% of babies). Lithium increases the risk for cardiac defects but may be taken during pregnancy.	Risk for neonatal lithium toxicity as breast milk contains 40% of maternal lithium concentration. Avoid if possible. Consider the use of carbamazepine if necessary, but bear in mind risk for infant hepatotoxicity.
Antipsychotics	Most antipsychotics have no established teratogenic effects but may cause self-limiting extrapyramidal side effects in neonates. Olanzapine increases risk for gestational diabetes.	Only small amounts excreted but possible effects on developing nervous system. Avoid high doses due to risk for lethargy in infant. Clozapine should be avoided due to the risk of agranulocytosis in the infant.
Benzodiazepines and other hypnotics	Associated with floppy infant syndrome (hypotonia, breathing and feeding difficulties) and neonatal withdrawal syndrome.	May cause lethargy in infant. Choose drugs with short half-lives (e.g., lorazepam) if necessary.

[a]*Information on the risks of medication during pregnancy and breastfeeding is constantly evolving. Seek up-to-date advice.*

HINTS AND TIPS

Useful sources of up-to-date information regarding medication during pregnancy and breastfeeding are
- UK teratology information service (UKTIS; http://www.uktis.org/)
- Best use of medicines in pregnancy (BUMPS; http://www.medicinesinpregnancy.org/)
- Drugs and Lactation Database (LACTMED; https://www.ncbi.nlm.nih.gov/books/NBK501922/)

PUERPERAL DISORDERS

Any mental disorder can arise during or be exacerbated by pregnancy, delivery or new motherhood. These experiences are anxiety provoking, stressful and potentially life-threatening. They can be difficult for anyone to deal with, even without previous mental health problems, and can worsen symptoms or maladaptive behaviours in those with existing mental health problems. This chapter covers the most common and important perinatal psychiatric disorders, but all the other mental disorders can and do occur in the perinatal period.

In general, the symptoms of a mental disorder are the same within and without the perinatal period, but management can be different as treatment decisions involving medication during pregnancy or breastfeeding require a careful risk–benefit analysis.

The incidence of psychiatric illness in the puerperium is exceptionally high. In primiparous women, there is up to a 35-fold increased risk for developing a psychotic illness and needing hospital admission in the first month following childbirth. Women with bipolar disorder have a 50% chance of relapse during the postpartum period, with about 25% experiencing a severe relapse (the risk is greater in bipolar I than II). There is also an increased risk of depression and anxiety disorders. Suicide is one of the leading causes of maternal death in the United Kingdom.

RED FLAG

Women who are within the first few months postpartum, particularly primiparous women, are at higher risk of developing a psychiatric disorder than probably any other time in their life.

The services available to women and families during the perinatal period have greatly expanded over recent years (see Box 29.2).

Postnatal 'blues'

Also known as 'maternity blues' and 'baby blues', this occurs in at least 50% of postpartum women. It presents within the first 10 days postdelivery, symptoms peak between days 3 and 5 and it resolves within 2 weeks. It is characterized by episodes of tearfulness, mild depression or emotional lability, anxiety and irritability. There appear to be no links with life events, demographic factors or obstetric events, which is suggestive of an underlying biological cause (e.g., a sudden fall in progesterone postdelivery). Postnatal blues is self-limiting, resolves spontaneously and usually only requires reassurance. However, an apparent bad case of postnatal blues may mark the onset of postnatal depression. Symptoms lasting longer than 2 weeks should raise suspicion of a depressive episode.

Perinatal depression

Clinical features

Postnatal depression usually develops within 3 months of delivery, with peak time of onset at 3 to 4 weeks. Around a third of cases begin during pregnancy (antenatal depression). A depressive episode arising more than 12 months after delivery is not generally viewed as postnatal depression. The symptoms are similar to a nonpuerperal depressive episode: low mood, loss of interest or pleasure, fatigability and suicidal ideation (although suicide is rare). Note that sleeping difficulties, weight loss and decreased libido can be normal for the first few months following delivery. Additional features of postnatal depression may include:

- Anxious preoccupation with the baby's health, often associated with feelings of guilt and inadequacy.
- Reduced affection for the baby with possible impaired bonding.
- Obsessional phenomena, typically involving recurrent and intrusive thoughts of harming the baby (it is crucial to ascertain whether these are regarded as distressing (ego-dystonic), as obsessions usually are, or whether they pose a potential risk).
- Infanticidal thoughts (thoughts of killing the baby) require urgent psychiatric assessment. True infanticidal thoughts are different from obsessions in that they are not experienced as distressing (ego-syntonic as opposed to ego-dystonic) and (worryingly) may involve active planning.

Epidemiology and aetiology

In high-income countries, postnatal depression is the most common complication of childbirth, with rates of around 10% to 15%. Risk factors for developing postnatal depression include a past history of mental illness during pregnancy, a lack of social support, poor partner relationship, stressful recent life events and having baby blues. A previous history of depression is an important risk factor. In women with a history of depression, obstetric complications during delivery are associated with an increased rate of postnatal depression.

Management

The diagnosis and management of antenatal and postnatal depression are often undertaken within primary care. Psychological and social measures, such as mother-and-baby groups, relationship counselling and problem solving, are often helpful. Midwives and health visitors can be very helpful. In mild cases, NICE (2014) recommends facilitated self-help. For more severe illness, NICE (2014) recommends a high-intensity psychological intervention (e.g., CBT) or antidepressant medication (an SSRI, SNRI or tricyclic). In pregnant women, consideration of the risks to the foetus from exposure to medication needs to be weighed against the risks to the foetus and mother of untreated mental illness (Table 29.1). Postnatally, antidepressants may be transmitted in small quantities to the baby via breast milk, and a judgement needs to be made, in conjunction with the patient, of the risks versus benefits of medication. It should be noted that (with the exception of doxepin) there has never been evidence to suggest that antidepressants transmitted via breast milk have caused long-term harm to a baby, but there are significant risks for the baby's cognitive and emotional development if the mother has untreated depression. Table 29.1 provides information on the use of psychotropic medication in breastfeeding mothers. Mothers with severe postnatal depression with suicidal/infanticidal ideation may require hospital admission, with admission alongside the baby to a mother-and-baby unit usually being preferable. Electroconvulsive therapy may be indicated and usually results in a rapid improvement, which is important to allow the mother to resume contact with her baby as soon as possible. Remember that the assessment of the infant's well-being is an additional part of the comprehensive psychosocial and risk assessment.

> **RED FLAG**
>
> If a woman taking an antidepressant becomes pregnant and seeks advice about continuing the medication or not, do NOT automatically advise to stop it (with the exception of sodium valproate). The risks of a perinatal relapse of depression are significant and need to be weighed against the generally low risks of teratogenicity and neonatal adaptation syndromes.

> **HINTS AND TIPS**
>
> If a woman has been on an antidepressant during pregnancy, do not change after delivery to a different antidepressant that is 'better for breastfeeding'. Doing this means the child is exposed to two medications, instead of one. The foetus is exposed to far greater levels of antidepressant in utero than levels transmitted in breast milk, so if they are healthy at delivery they are unlikely to be harmed by further, lower, exposure.

Prognosis

Most women respond to standard treatment and episodes resolve within 3 to 6 months; however, around 20% of women are still depressed at 1 year post delivery and may require long-term treatment and follow-up. Women who develop postnatal depression have around a 40% increased risk for developing a similar illness following childbirth in the future. Postnatal depression is associated with disturbances in the mother–infant relationship, and this can lead to short- and long-term problems with the child's social, behavioural, cognitive and emotional development.

> **RED FLAG**
>
> Suicide is a leading cause of maternal death, even though it is fortunately rare (1 in 100,000 pregnancies). About 60% of cases were experiencing a severe affective or psychotic illness at the time of death. Always ask about thoughts of suicide in a new mother who is mentally unwell.

> **RED FLAG**
>
> Eliciting red flags for maternal suicide:
> - Do you have new feelings or thoughts that you have never had before, which make you disturbed or anxious?
> - Are you experiencing thoughts of suicide or harming yourself in violent ways?
> - Are you having severe struggles to sleep?
> - Are you feeling incompetent, as though you cannot cope, or estranged from your baby? Are these feelings persistent?
> - Do you feel you are getting worse?
>
> MBRRACE-UK 2022 (Mothers and Babies: Reducing Risk through Audits and Confidential Enquiries across the UK)

Perinatal anxiety disorders

Clinical features

Anxiety disorders in the perinatal period present very similarly to anxiety disorders outside the perinatal period and can include generalized anxiety disorder, obsessive–compulsive disorder, phobias and post-traumatic stress disorder, which may have onset following a highly distressing delivery. Tokophobia is a specific phobia of childbirth and can be primary (nulliparous) or secondary (often following a difficult first delivery). Anxiety disorders can occur on their own or comorbidly with depression.

Epidemiology and aetiology

Anxiety disorders occur in around 13% of women who are pregnant or postpartum. Many of these disorders arise prior to pregnancy rather than being triggered by it; however, there is some evidence that the risk for new-onset obsessive–compulsive disorder is increased antenatally and postpartum (approximately doubled). Risk factors for perinatal anxiety disorders are unclear but are probably similar to those for anxiety disorders outside the perinatal period (see Chapter 23), combined with the natural increase in anxiety that responsibility for a vulnerable new infant brings. Around 50% of women feel that their labour was traumatic, but only about 5% of women go on to develop post-traumatic stress disorder.

Management

The diagnosis and management of perinatal anxiety disorders is often done within primary care. As with postnatal depression, midwives and health visitors can be very helpful in identifying psychosocial supports such as community groups and classes. The first-line intervention in all cases is a psychological therapy (NICE 2014). The nature of the therapy depends on the type of anxiety disorder and its severity, following the general NICE guidance for adults (see Chapter 23). Medication may also be required, particularly if a woman is already taking this or has required it in the past. In post-traumatic stress disorder, attending a birth reflections clinic may be helpful, along with trauma-focussed psychotherapy.

Prognosis

With the exception of post-traumatic stress disorder, anxiety disorders tend to be chronic, relapsing/remitting conditions. Anxiety disorders during pregnancy are a risk factor for postnatal depression. Prenatal maternal anxiety is associated with altered stress-induced cortisol responses in 7-month-old infants and subsequently in adolescence, potentially influencing the child's own risk for anxiety and depression.

Failure to bond

Some women struggle to form a loving bond with their baby. Mothers at particular risk include those whose own mother–infant attachment was insecure (see Table 30.1), women who experienced childhood neglect or sexual abuse and women with perinatal psychiatric difficulties (e.g., postnatal depression). The woman may seek help, or difficulties may be identified by a health visitor. Management is to involve an early year's or parent–infant mental health service who can provide guidance to the mother regarding positive infant interactions.

Postpartum (puerperal) psychosis

Clinical features

The postpartum period is an extremely high-risk period for the development of a psychotic episode. Postpartum (puerperal) psychotic episodes characteristically have an abrupt onset with rapid deterioration. About 50% of cases experience onset of symptoms within postnatal days 1 to 3 and the vast majority within 2 weeks of delivery. Episodes typically begin with insomnia, restlessness and perplexity, later progressing to suspiciousness and marked psychotic symptoms (often with content related to the baby). The symptoms can be polymorphic and frequently fluctuate dramatically in their nature and intensity over a short space of time. Mood symptoms are prominent and can comprise elation, depression or both (mixed affective state). Patients often retain a degree of insight and may not disclose certain bizarre delusions or suicidal/homicidal thoughts.

> **RED FLAG**
>
> Postpartum psychosis is a psychiatric emergency. The rapidly fluctuating nature of symptoms, alongside the significant risk to both the mother and the baby, means that a very cautious approach to management needs to be taken – a person who seems reasonably well at interview could deteriorate rapidly. Admission is required in nearly all cases.

> **BOX 29.3 RISK FACTORS FOR POSTPARTUM PSYCHOSIS**
>
> - Previous postpartum psychosis
> - History of psychotic illness or bipolar disorder
> - Family history of postpartum psychosis or bipolar disorder
> - Primiparous mother
> - Delivery associated with perinatal death

Epidemiology and aetiology

Postpartum psychosis develops in 1 to 2 per 1000 childbirths. It occurs more frequently in primiparous women and those who have a personal or family history of bipolar disorder or postpartum psychosis. If a close family member has bipolar disorder, the risk can be as high as 15 in 500 childbirths. If the woman has a personal history of bipolar disorder the risk is about 20%, and if they have a personal history of postpartum psychosis the risk is about 30%. Psychosocial factors seem less important, unlike in postnatal depression. Occasionally, a postpartum psychosis may be precipitated by a systemic illness (e.g., eclampsia, puerperal infection) or medication. Delirium secondary to such complications is an important differential. Box 29.3 summarizes the risk factors for postpartum psychosis.

Management

Postpartum psychosis is a psychiatric emergency. Assessing for the risk of infanticide and suicide is crucial. Concerning symptoms include:

- Thoughts of self-harm or harming the baby
- Severe depressive delusions (e.g., belief that the baby is, or should be, dead)
- Command hallucinations instructing the mother to harm herself or her baby

Hospitalization is invariably necessary, with joint admissions to a mother-and-baby unit being preferable where the mother is able to look after her infant under supervision. Detention under mental health legislation may be necessary. Depending on presentation, antipsychotics, antidepressants and mood-stabilising medications are indicated. Benzodiazepines may be needed in cases of severe behavioural disturbance. All psychotropic drugs should be used with caution in breastfeeding mothers (see Table 29.1), but many women are too unwell to breastfeed in any case. Electroconvulsive therapy can be particularly effective in severe or treatment-resistant cases. Psychosocial interventions are similar to those for other psychotic episodes, but also include providing support for the father where appropriate.

The prevalence of postnatal blues, postnatal depression and puerperal psychosis is inversely related to their severity:

- Postnatal blues develops after 1 in 2 childbirths.
- Postnatal depression develops after around 1 in 10 childbirths.
- Puerperal psychosis develops after around 1 to 2 in 1000 childbirths.

Prognosis

It can take anywhere between 6 and 12 months to recover from puerperal psychosis, but the most severe symptoms tend to last for 2 to 12 weeks. Around 70% of women will go on to further nonpuerperal mood episodes and develop bipolar disorder. There is about a 30% chance of experiencing a recurrence of postpartum psychosis after future childbirths, which can be reduced by prophylactic therapy. Women who have had both puerperal and nonpuerperal depressive or manic episodes (i.e., have an established mood disorder) have a >50% chance of future puerperal psychotic episodes.

PERINATAL SUBSTANCE MISUSE

Despite increasing awareness about the risks of using substances during pregnancy, some women continue to use recreational drugs, alcohol and tobacco in the perinatal period and there can be significant implications to the health of the woman and her foetus from their continued use. It is therefore crucial that women are asked, in a nonjudgemental way, about substances, particularly as pregnancy may be a motivator for the woman to stop or reduce her substance use. It is also important to recognize that women may be fearful of repercussions from social services if they disclose substance misuse, and having early conversations with the woman around this, and aiming to include them in decisions about referrals to social services can help.

Epidemiology and aetiology

It is estimated at the time of their booking appointment that around 10% of women are using tobacco, around 5% are using alcohol (although this may be an underestimate) and around 1% of women are misusing other substances. Tobacco smoking and drug misuse are more common in younger women, whereas alcohol use in pregnancy is more common in women over 35 years.

Management

All women with significant alcohol use and/or substance misuse during pregnancy should be referred to specialist substance misuse services for support and management.

Alcohol

The use of alcohol during pregnancy is associated with an increased risk of premature delivery and low birth weight. It is also associated with foetal alcohol syndrome (see Chapter 8). There is no safe level of alcohol consumption during pregnancy, so all women should be supported to reduce and stop their alcohol consumption. For women who are alcohol dependent, it is important that they are advised not to stop drinking suddenly, as this can precipitate alcohol withdrawal and seizures. They can be offered inpatient alcohol detoxification using benzodiazepines, preferably as early in their pregnancy as possible.

Opioids

The use of opioids in pregnancy is associated with overdose, malnutrition, domestic violence and poor engagement with services for the pregnant woman. For the foetus, there is an increased risk of low birth weight, premature delivery and perinatal mortality. There is also the potential for withdrawal after delivery and neonatal abstinence syndrome, which occurs in approximately 70% to 95% of babies exposed to opioids in utero.

Given the often complex medical and social issues surrounding a pregnant woman dependent on opioids, it is important that their care is delivered by a multidisciplinary team including obstetricians and midwives, substance misuse services, GPs and social services. The focus of care should be on stabilization, and the risk of initiating substitute prescribing at any point in the pregnancy is lower than continued illicit substance misuse. Women should therefore be encouraged to abstain from illicit opioid misuse during pregnancy and commence opioid substitute therapy. NICE Guidelines (2022) recommend methadone, rather than buprenorphine for substitute prescribing for women who are not already established on a substitute prescription. The dose of methadone should be titrated to a level that prevents illicit opioid misuse as far as possible. Once established on a substitute prescription, the woman should be encouraged to remain on a maintenance prescription, rather than undergoing detoxification. This is because detoxification during pregnancy is associated with an increased risk of relapse into illicit opioid misuse compared to maintenance treatment, and there are also increased risks to the foetus associated with detoxification. These include a risk of spontaneous abortion if undertaken in the first trimester, and foetal distress and stillbirth if undertaken in the third trimester.

Despite the risks, many women request detoxification upon finding out they are pregnant. If, after being counselled about the risks associated with detoxification, the patient still wishes to try, it should be attempted in the second trimester in the form of small, frequent reductions in their substitute prescription.

After delivery, women who are stable on opioid substitute therapy should be encouraged to breastfeed their baby, unless contraindicated.

HINTS AND TIPS

Breastfeeding when on opioid substitute therapy may actually reduce the intensity and length of neonatal abstinence syndrome and has been associated with improved outcomes.

● Chapter Summary

- Premenstrual dysphoric disorder describes mood and cognitive symptoms during the luteal phase only, which are severe enough to cause functional impairment.
- Treatment of premenstrual dysphoric disorder includes lifestyle advice, preventing ovulation via oral contraception, cognitive behavioural therapy and selective serotonin reuptake inhibitors.
- Postnatal blues is a common and self-limiting episode of mood and anxiety symptoms, which resolve within 2 weeks of delivery.
- Perinatal depression is a common and potentially serious episode of depression arising during pregnancy or within 1 year of delivery.
- Management of perinatal depression is very similar to standard management of depression, but in severe cases admission to a mother-and-baby unit may be required and electroconvulsive therapy is recommended at an early stage.
- Postpartum psychosis is a rare but very serious illness generally arising within 2 weeks of delivery.
- In all cases of postpartum psychosis, admission to a mother-and-baby unit is required for risk management.
- Women who are pregnant and dependent on opioids should be encouraged to avoid illicit opioid misuse and commence opioid substitute therapy, and to maintain this during the course of their pregnancy and beyond.
- Detoxification during pregnancy is associated with increased risk of relapse into illicit opioid use and risks to the foetus.

UKMLA Conditions
Anxiety/phobias/OCD
Bipolar affective disorder
Depression
Substance use disorder

UKMLA Presentations
Addiction
Anxiety/phobias/OCD
Behaviour/personality change
Elation/elated mood
Low mood/affective problems
Mental health problems in pregnancy or postpartum
Substance misuse
Suicidal thoughts

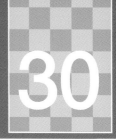

This chapter discusses the disorders associated with the presenting complaints in Chapter 18, which you might find helpful to read first.

THE PERSONALITY DISORDERS

Epidemiology

There is a lack of consensus about the definition of personality disorders and the diagnostic concepts have undergone significant revision in recent years, with the DSM-5 and the ICD-11 now diverging significantly. It is unclear whether there is any correlation between diagnostic criteria and the subjective experiences of people identified as having disordered personality. While a number of structured interview schedules and diagnostic instruments have been validated, the level of correlation between these is generally poor. Mental health professionals also remain divided as to how personality disorders should be conceptualised, with some clinicians questioning whether the diagnosis is of any clinical benefit.

Patients with personality disorders have a significantly increased mortality, as well as physical and psychiatric morbidity. Relationships with relatives and friends are often adversely affected, and there is a strong association between some types of personality disorder and involvement with healthcare and criminal justice services.

Community studies have shown the prevalence of any personality disorder to be 4% to 13%, with an increased prevalence in younger age groups (particularly 25–44 years), and an equal distribution between the sexes. This varies according to the population group sampled. It is higher in patients frequently consulting general practitioners (GPs; 10%–30%), even higher in psychiatric outpatient clinics (30%–40%) and higher still in psychiatric in-patients (40%–50%), patients who self-harm (40%–80%) and prisoners (50%–80%).

Aetiology

Genetic, biological and environmental factors have been shown to have an effect on the development of personality disorders.

Genetic and biological factors

- Monozygotic twins show a higher concordance for personality disorders than dizygotic twins, suggesting a heritability of 30% to 60%.

- One study has shown that there is a strong association between childhood trauma and genetic polymorphisms associated with the hypothalamus–pituitary–adrenal axis in individuals with a diagnosis of personality disorder with a borderline pattern.
- Other genetic studies have found abnormalities of the serotonin (5-HT) transporter and the 5-HT$_{2A}$ receptor gene in individuals with personality disorders with a borderline pattern.
- Exposure to maternal stress when an individual is in utero or an infant leads to increased sensitivity of their pituitary–adrenal responses when they are exposed to stressors at a later age. Depressive disorders are more common in the relatives of patients with personality disorders with a borderline pattern.
- Emotional dysregulation and impulsivity can be features of personality disorders. The prefrontal cortex and the amygdala play a role in emotional regulation and behavioural responses. One theory is therefore that decreased prefrontal regulation or increased amygdala activation might be linked to the emotional dysregulation seen in personality disorders.

Early life experience

- Early adverse social circumstances (such as parental substance use, physical or emotional neglect, violence, sexual abuse) are associated with the development of personality disorders.
- There is a strong association between personality disorders with a borderline pattern and childhood sexual abuse, although this is not universal.
- Various psychoanalytical theories suggest that disordered attachment between infants and their caregivers leads to difficulties in relationships throughout the rest of life, which may manifest as personality disorders.

Table 30.1 summarizes the epidemiology of personality disorders. It refers to the DSM-5 diagnoses that can be approximately mapped onto the new the ICD-11 diagnostic system, for which no epidemiology is as yet available.

Assessment, clinical features, classification and differential diagnosis

Discussed in Chapter 18.

Table 30.1 Epidemiology of personality disorders using the DSM-5 diagnostic criteria.

Personality disorder	Prevalence in general population (%)	Comments
Paranoid	0.7–4.4	More common in males and lower socioeconomic classes More common in relatives of patients with schizophrenia
Schizoid	0.7–4.9	More common in males and offender populations May be more common in relatives of patients with schizophrenia
Schizotypal	1.6–3.9	More common in relatives of patients with schizophrenia May be slightly more common in males
Emotionally unstable (borderline)	1.2–5.9	More prevalent in younger age groups and females Aetiological link with childhood sexual abuse Most contact with services in mid-20s 40-fold increase in suicide rate Associated with poor work history and single marital status Often comorbid with depression, substance abuse, bulimia and anxiety
Antisocial (dissocial)	0.6–4.5	Much more common in men Highest prevalence in 25- to 44-year-olds Associated with school dropout, conduct disorder and urban settings Very high prevalence in prisons and forensic settings Highly comorbidity with substance abuse
Histrionic	0.4–2.9	Recent research shows equal gender ratio (previously thought to be more common in women)
Narcissistic	0.1–6.2	More common in males and forensic settings
Dependent	0.3–0.6	Often comorbid with borderline personality disorder
Avoidant (anxious)	1–5.2	Equal gender ratio Comorbid with social phobia
Obsessive compulsive (anankastic)	1.2–7.9	More common in white, male, highly educated, married and employed individuals

Management

There continues to be considerable debate concerning how (and by whom) patients with personality disorders should be managed. Previously, personality disorders were generally considered to be untreatable. However, advances in diagnosis, psychotherapy and psychopharmacology have equipped clinicians with a variety of treatment options that can be useful in maximising engagement with services, reducing distress, managing comorbid mental illness and substance misuse, improving relationships and optimising quality of life.

Patients with a diagnosis of a personality disorder with a borderline pattern are frequently encountered in clinical practice, and the most is known about what treatments do, and do not, help people with this diagnosis. This will therefore be the focus of this section.

Principles of managing patients with personality disorders with a borderline pattern

Patients with a personality disorder with a borderline pattern should not be excluded from health or social care services because of their diagnosis or because they have self-harmed. A consistent and tolerant approach should be taken. Autonomy and choice should be encouraged, with the patient being actively involved in deciding treatment options and in finding solutions to their problems. An optimistic, trusting and nonjudgemental relationship should be developed. Endings and transitions may evoke strong emotions and reactions in patients with personality disorder, and as such should be carefully planned and structured to minimise distress. A multidisciplinary approach to care should be considered, as psychological, social and biological treatment modalities all have an important role. A comprehensive assessment should be made of sources of distress to self and others (thoughts, emotions, behaviour and relationships), other comorbid mental illnesses and specific impairments of functioning at work or home.

PRINCIPLES OF CARE IN MANAGING PATIENTS WITH A DIAGNOSIS OF A PERSONALITY DISORDER WITH A BORDERLINE PATTERN

- Be positive, kind and nonjudgemental (many are survivors of abuse).
- Be accessible, consistent and reliable (do what you say you will do).
- Encourage autonomy; facilitate the patient to find their own solutions to problems.
  - What is the problem right now?
  - What has worked in the past?
  - What would you like to do?
  - What is an achievable change?
- Manage transitions and changes carefully, in a planned way.
- Monitor for comorbid mental illness (e.g., depression or substance use)

Crisis management

It can be useful to develop a crisis management plan in conjunction with the patient, detailing self-management strategies, sources of support (family, friends, telephone-based services) and details on how to access emergency care. This should be shared with the patient and other relevant professionals (GPs, assessment and crisis teams).

EXAMPLE CRISIS PLAN IN PERSONALITY DISORDER WITH A BORDERLINE PATTERN

Triggers that might lead to a crisis
e.g., Losing job, drinking too much alcohol, argument with partner

Things I can do to help myself
e.g., Talk to my friend, watch favourite TV shows, exercise, get enough sleep, avoid drugs and alcohol

When I should seek help
e.g., If I injure myself badly, if I am having very strong thoughts of suicide, if I feel so sad that I can't go to work, if my friend advises me to

Who I should contact and how
e.g., Samaritans, general practitioner, community psychiatric nurse, crisis team, NHS24, best friend, mother

---

Short-term drug treatments can be useful to alleviate distress during a crisis. If possible, this should be agreed in advance with the care team and the patient. Drugs with acceptable side effects, low risk of dependence, and low toxicity in overdose profiles are preferable, and should be dispensed in small quantities (e.g., weekly dispensing). Drugs should not be used in place of other more appropriate interventions.

Before admission to acute in-patient psychiatric care, crisis resolution or home treatment teams should be considered. Admission may be necessary if the management of the crisis involves significant risk to self or others that cannot be managed within other services. If possible, actively involve the patient in the decision, and ensure that it is based on an explicit, joint understanding of the potential benefits (and likely harm) that may result from admission. Agree the length and purpose of the admission in advance. If the patient is detained under mental health legislation, ensure that this is regularly reviewed and that management on a voluntary basis is resumed at the earliest opportunity.

After a crisis has resolved, ensure that the care plan is updated. If drug treatment was started, review this and discontinue if possible. If this is not possible, ensure that it is regularly reviewed to monitor effectiveness, side effects, misuse and dependency.

Short-term management

While treatment of personality disorders should be considered to be a long-term process, various biological, psychological and social management strategies can be employed in the shorter term, with the aim of facilitating trust, building a positive relationship with health and social care services and identifying and alleviating sources of distress.

Psychopharmacology

There are no medications that are currently either recommended or licenced specifically for the treatment of personality disorders with a borderline pattern (National Institute for Health and Care Excellence (NICE) 2009 – referred to as borderline personality disorder in these guidelines). However, drugs can be useful to treat comorbid mental illness, or to manage cases of behavioural disturbance and suicidal behaviour during the more severe phases. In addition, there is some evidence that some drugs may be efficacious in targeting specific symptoms. For instance, antipsychotics may be of some use in treating the pseudo-psychotic symptoms that are sometimes experienced, in reducing agitation and in stabilizing mood. Antidepressants may be useful in treating depressive symptoms. Selective serotonin reuptake inhibitors may help with obsessive-compulsive symptoms as well as impulsivity and self-harming behaviour. Mood stabilizers such as lithium, sodium valproate and lamotrigine may be useful in treating aggression, impulsivity and mood instability. Benzodiazepines should be used with caution due to the potential for abuse, dependence and diversion.

Psychosocial

Supportive psychotherapy provides patients with an authority figure during times of crisis. Regular contact with a healthcare professional can also provide the patient with a sense of containment. Members of the multidisciplinary team can provide psychoeducation, as well as facilitating development of coping strategies, relaxation and distraction techniques, improving disturbed relationships and development of skills and hobbies. In cooperation with social services, issues such as housing, finances and employment can be addressed.

COMMUNICATION

People with personality disorders by definition have difficulties forming and maintaining relationships, and that includes doctor–patient relationships. Misunderstandings and frustration are common on both sides. Remember to be calm, clear and consistent and try to take the long view; do not let one difficult encounter dominate your relationship with the patient.

Longer-term management

The long-term management of patients with personality disorders with a borderline pattern involves addressing and modifying maladaptive traits of personality. This generally involves psychological therapy. Because traits and behaviours tend to be deeply engrained, this process can take many years. Around 40% of people with personality disorder with a borderline pattern disengage with psychotherapy, and so it is important to build a trusting relationship and to be prepared for therapeutic change taking a long time.

There is evidence suggesting the efficacy of various modalities of psychotherapy in the treatment of personality disorder with a borderline pattern. It may be that the consistency of therapy, the maintenance of boundaries, and the empathic and nonjudgemental stance of the therapist allow for the successful development of a therapeutic relationship, which may in itself be more important than the specific type of therapy. For more information on psychotherapy, see Chapter 3. The following psychological treatments can be helpful in personality disorder with a borderline pattern:

- Dialectical behaviour therapy (DBT) uses a combination of cognitive and behavioural therapies, with relaxation techniques and mindfulness. It involves both individual and group therapy, and can be helpful in reducing self-harming and improving functioning. It is recommended by NICE (2009).

- Mentalization-based therapy (MBT) focuses on allowing patients to better understand what is going on in both their minds and in the minds of others. It can utilize both individual and group components.
- Cognitive behavioural therapy (CBT) has been adapted for use as 'schema-focused therapy'.
- Cognitive analytical therapy (CAT).
- Psychodynamic psychotherapy, as both individual and group therapy, which focuses on the relationship with the therapist.
- Therapeutic communities are a residential form of therapy, where the patient may stay for weeks or months. The community tends to run as a 'democracy', with patients often having as much say as the staff. Most of the therapeutic work is done in groups, and patients learn from getting on (or not getting on) with others. It differs from 'real life' in that any disagreements or upsets happen in a controlled and safe environment. These placements tend to be reserved for those with severe functional impairment or very high service usage, because of their high cost.

HINTS AND TIPS

Remember that personality disorders involve long-standing personality traits. While they are 'treatable', pharmacotherapy is not the mainstay, but is used to alleviate specific symptoms (e.g., comorbid depression, anxiety or impulsivity). Medications are unlikely to affect maladaptive personality traits. With appropriate psychosocial interventions, these may significantly improve with time. You may want to consider this when discussing management with patients.

Course and prognosis

The course and prognosis of personality disorders, is now considered more optimistic than previously. Some 78% to 99% of patients with personality disorders with a borderline pattern will show signs of sustained symptomatic remission at 16-year follow-up. Patients with a personality disorder with prominent features of dissociality may also improve with time, especially if they have formed a relationship with a therapist.

Patients with personality disorder have a greater incidence of other mental illnesses such as depression, bipolar disorder, anxiety and schizophrenia. Furthermore, these tend to be more severe and have a worse prognosis than if the personality disorder was not present. Patients with personality disorder also have far higher rates of suicide and accidental death than the general population.

Chapter Summary

- Personality disorders are common, particularly in users of health services.
- Comorbid mental illnesses are more frequent and difficult to treat in those with personality disorder.
- When managing personality disorder with a borderline pattern:
  - Take a consistent, nonjudgemental approach.
  - Help the patient to make a crisis plan and share it with everyone involved in the patient's care.
  - Symptoms can be improved by long-term psychological treatments such as dialectical behavioural therapy.
  - Medication is only recommended in crises and for comorbid mental illnesses.
- Personality disorders generally gradually improve over decades.

UKMLA Conditions
Personality disorder
Self-harm

UKMLA Presentations
Behaviour/personality change
Overdose
Self-harm
Suicidal thoughts

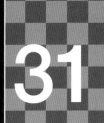
EPIDEMIOLOGY AND AETIOLOGY

Intellectual disabilities affect approximately 1% of the population, with a sex ratio of approximately 1:1.5 for females: males. Some common causes of intellectual disability are shown in Table 31.1. No clear aetiology can be determined in at least a third of patients with mild intellectual disability, suggesting they may represent the lower end of the normal distribution curve for intellectual functioning. Specific causes are more likely to be found in people with severe or profound intellectual disabilities, as well as a greater number of comorbidities and increasing likelihood of an underlying genetic diagnosis.

Assessment, clinical features, investigations and differential diagnosis

See Chapter 8.

Management and prognosis

Prevention and detection

Primary prevention includes genetic screening and counselling for higher-risk groups, prenatal testing (e.g., amniocentesis, rhesus incompatibility), improved perinatal and neonatal care and early detection of metabolic abnormalities that may contribute to intellectual impairment (e.g., phenylketonuria, neonatal hypothyroidism). Milder intellectual disabilities may be less obvious, and early detection requires the ability of teachers and family doctors to be able to identify difficulties as soon as possible.

Secondary prevention aims to maximise the young person's potential, by providing compensatory education and early attempts to reduce behavioural problems. Some children take longer than others to meet developmental milestones (referred to as Global Developmental Delay if aged under five); however, not all of these children subsequently meet criteria for intellectual disability. If you suspect a child has an intellectual disability, this should be discussed with either a community paediatrician or a child and adolescent mental health specialist, who will be able to provide guidance on local services. If you suspect an adult has an undiagnosed mild intellectual disability, this should be discussed with the local intellectual disabilities team, who may suggest an initial referral for neuropsychological assessment.

> ### HINTS AND TIPS
>
> To make a diagnosis of intellectual disability in an adult there must be evidence that the issues began in childhood.

Table 31.1 Causes of intellectual disability	
Genetic	Trisomies or large structural variants (e.g., Down syndrome, fragile X syndrome, Prader–Willi syndrome) Inherited point mutations (e.g., phenylketonuria, neurofibromatosis, tuberous sclerosis, Lesch–Nyhan syndrome, Tay–Sachs disease, other enzyme-deficiency diseases) De novo (sporadic) point mutations have been identified in over 700 genes, potentially all with the capacity to contribute to intellectual disability
Prenatal	Congenital infections (e.g., TORCH infections (toxoplasmosis, rubella, cytomegalovirus, herpes simplex and zoster (chicken pox)), also syphilis and human immunodeficiency virus (HIV)) Substance use during pregnancy (e.g., foetal alcohol syndrome, prescribed drugs with teratogenic effects) Complications of pregnancy (e.g., preeclampsia, intrauterine growth restriction, antepartum haemorrhage)
Perinatal	Birth trauma (e.g., intracranial haemorrhage, hypoxia) Prematurity (e.g., intraventricular haemorrhage, hyperbilirubinaemia (kernicterus), infections)
Environmental	Neglect, malnutrition (e.g., iodine deficiency in developing countries), poor linguistic and social stimulation
Medical conditions in childhood	Infections (e.g., meningitis, encephalitis) Head injury Toxins (e.g., lead, other heavy metals)

There are also methods specifically developed for people with intellectual disability to communicate, including signing (e.g., Makaton and Signalong) and use of images (e.g., Talking Mats and the Picture Exchange Communication System).

Help for families

As well as coming to terms with diagnosis and behaviour, parents of young people with intellectual disabilities often have to cope with other challenges, including social stigma, lack of sleep, and insecure attachment patterns, increasing risk of complex relationship and adjustment problems. In addition, parents of young people with disabilities have increased rates of psychiatric disturbance. From the time the diagnosis is made, families should be provided with support and information, which may take the form of individual counselling, family therapy, practical support, respite care and assistance in supporting their child to achieve their full potential. This may need to be increased at the more challenging times, such as puberty, starting or leaving school, times of stress (e.g., bereavement or illness) and the transition to adult services.

Communication

Many patients with intellectual disabilities may struggle with reading and writing, or with verbal communication with others. Making sure patients have accessible information (often in simple 'Easy Read' format), free from jargon can empower them to make their own decisions as far as possible. Speech and language therapists can help develop individual strategies for patients depending on their preferences and needs, for example, a patient may struggle to speak verbally but can write or draw.

Education, training and occupation

If the needs of a child with intellectual disability can be met by mainstream education, this should be encouraged due to the benefits of societal inclusion and mutual understanding. Mainstream schools often have additional support, such as access to an education support worker. However, around 1% of school places in the United Kingdom are in specialist schools that support those with more complex needs. Later, vocational guidance should be offered. Around 5% of adults with intellectual disability are in paid work. People may be able to work for 'mainstream' employers with additional support (e.g., specialist equipment, altered hours); however, there are also organisations (often social enterprises) that focus on providing contracts to people with intellectual disabilities.

Housing and social support

Many people with mild intellectual disabilities are able to live independently, with varying degrees of social and familial support. If people need to live outside of their family and social group, assessment of tasks of daily living will be necessary to ensure that people are appropriately placed. For people with more severe difficulties, residential care may be considered. People with intellectual disabilities should be considered valuable contributors to their community, and provided with resources allowing them to be so.

COMMUNICATION

Patients with intellectual disabilities are all different, and what one patient understands another patient may struggle with. Use simple language when speaking, keep sentences short with only one concept per sentence and remember to check understanding and rephrase if necessary.

Medical care

People with intellectual disabilities should have the same access to medical services as everyone else, although communication difficulties and false attribution of symptoms to the intellectual disability (diagnostic overshadowing) mean care is often suboptimal. Extra medical care is often required due to comorbidities such as physical disability or epilepsy. Many general hospitals have specialist nurses who are experienced in the management of individuals with intellectual disabilities attending outpatient departments, or being admitted for medical treatment or surgery.

Those with intellectual disabilities die on average around 20 years younger than those without. Sometimes this is due to unavoidable factors, such as people with Down syndrome often developing Alzheimer dementia at a young age, however, many deaths are due to 'avoidable' issues (e.g., aspiration, seizure, respiratory infection). A study comparing causes of deaths in children with and without intellectual disabilities found that those with intellectual disabilities were five times more like to have died from an 'avoidable' cause.

RED FLAG

'Diagnostic Overshadowing' refers to the assumption that a person's presentation is due to their intellectual disability, rather than a comorbid condition, e.g., assuming someone rubbing their abdomen is behavioural rather than considering alternatives such as pain or constipation. People with intellectual disability have an increased risk for many physical health conditions, so be sure to get a collateral, and assess and investigate thoroughly.

Sexual Health

Many people with intellectual disabilities are able and want to engage in sexual relationships, and should be provided with the same resources as the wider community to be able to do so

safely. Obtaining a sexual history should never be assumed to be irrelevant. People with intellectual disabilities may also have children, and wherever possible should be supported to be able to care for their children like any parent.

RED FLAG

Patients with intellectual disabilities are at higher risk than the general population of sexual abuse. If you elicit that they are sexually active (e.g., through disclosure of pregnancy, sexually transmitted infection), consider sensitive enquiry about the nature of the relationship (especially if this is not known) and involve the multidisciplinary team (e.g., social work/adult protection) if there are concerns which necessitate further exploration.

HINTS AND TIPS

Epilepsy is a common comorbidity in individuals with intellectual disabilities and can often complicate assessment and management. Remember that a number of different psychotropic medications can lower seizure threshold, and that 'mood stabilizers' (with the exception of lithium) are antiepileptic medications.

Psychiatric care

Given the higher prevalence of comorbid mental illness in this group, people with intellectual disabilities should have access to specialist care (usually on an outpatient, community or day-patient basis) as and when required. It can be difficult to assess and manage psychiatric illness and behavioural disturbances in individuals with intellectual disability. This is why most areas have multidisciplinary specialist teams. These teams can address not only major mental illnesses (e.g., schizophrenia, bipolar disorder, depression) but can also help manage autism and challenging behaviours, such as self-harm, hurting others, destroying objects or difficult sexual behaviours.

Psychotropic medication may be indicated; however, given the common difficulties with unusual presentations, polypharmacy, comorbidities and sensitivity to medication, there should be a low threshold for seeking advice from, or referral to, a specialist doctor. The NHS initiative STOMP (Stopping the

Overmedication of People with a Learning Disability, Autism or Both) acknowledges that these medications are more likely to be used in people with intellectual disability, and promotes alternative strategies to medications.

Psychological treatments including behavioural therapy may be useful in the management of maladaptive or otherwise difficult behaviours, and positive behavioural support aims to understand and prevent difficult behaviours rather than using punishment or restrictions after they have happened.

People with intellectual disabilities may require admission to psychiatric hospital if acutely mentally unwell. Many areas have specialist wards for intellectual disabilities, with nurses specially trained in managing these patients. Additionally some areas may have specialist home treatment teams as an alternative to hospital admission.

Where medication is required, often lower doses are required than in the general adult population. Risperidone is often favoured if antipsychotic medication is indicated. Sleep difficulties are common in this patient cohort, and melatonin is often used 'off-license' for this indication.

HINTS AND TIPS

Learning disability nursing is a separate training pathway to mental health nursing in which nurses are trained specifically to care for and support those with intellectual disabilities. Learning disability nurses may work in both inpatient and outpatient settings helping to deliver medical/psychiatric care, and providing support to patients to lead as full lives as possible.

COMMUNICATION

Collateral histories are invaluable when assessing someone with an intellectual disability. When a change in behaviour occurs, it is useful to ask about what else has changed in the patient's life or their daily routine. The prevalence of other psychiatric disorders is three to four times higher, so these must also be carefully assessed for.

● Chapter Summary

- Around 1% of the population meet criteria for intellectual disability, and it is slightly more common in males than females.
- Families should be supported to care for children with intellectual disabilities as much as possible.
- People with intellectual disabilities may need alternative strategies to help them with communication.
- Children may be educated in mainstream education or require a place at a special school.
- People with intellectual disabilities die on average 20 years earlier than those without.
- Psychiatry input is offered through specialist intellectual disability services.

UKMLA Conditions
Learning disability
Self-harm
Speech and language problems

UKMLA Presentations
Developmental delay
Down syndrome
Learning disability
Self-harm
Struggling to cope at home

The neurodevelopmental disorders

32

Neurodevelopmental disorders are a large and diverse group. This chapter covers those that most commonly present to psychiatry: autism spectrum disorder (ASD), attention deficit hyperactivity disorder (ADHD) and Tourette syndrome. Intellectual disability is discussed in Chapter 31.

AUTISM SPECTRUM DISORDER

Epidemiology and aetiology

Key epidemiology is shown in Table 32.1. Autism is a highly heritable condition (heritability of around 80%). A substantial proportion of this genetic risk is not inherited but arises from sporadic mutations – de novo (sporadic) variants occur four times as often in people with autism as their unaffected siblings. Rare variants in over 800 genes have been linked to autism in this manner and are thought to be the cause in around one in five cases. Common genetic variants of small effect also exist. Analyses of biological processes influenced by the numerous implicated genes have highlighted a range of core cellular functions underlying synaptic formation and signalling: cell adhesion, chromatin remodelling and regulation of transcription and translation. It seems likely that what is currently referred to as 'autism spectrum disorder' is made up of many different sorts of disorder influencing distinct but related basic neuronal functions.

Although genetics may seem far removed from clinical practice at present, it can provide clinically relevant information. For example, if parents have one child with autism, the overall risk for having a second child with autism is 10% to 15%. However, if genetic testing identifies a causative genetic variant as de novo or inherited, this risk can be much more accurately estimated at 1% or 50%, respectively (if the variant is 100% penetrant).

Autism is diagnosed more often in men (with most studies suggesting a ratio of 2:1 or 3:1); however, the proportion of women being diagnosed increases with age. The reasons for this are unclear. It may be that women are more motivated to appear social and develop relationships, which may make the diagnosis less apparent initially.

In recent years the number of adults being assessed for autism is increasing, likely due to increased awareness of autism and more standardised assessment pathways.

HINTS AND TIPS

Many of the genes linked to autism have also been associated with intellectual disability, epilepsy, schizophrenia and attention deficit hyperactivity disorder: the same genetic variants can influence risk for many neurodevelopmental disorders.

COMMUNICATION

There is no evidence to support the claim that the measles, mumps, rubella (MMR) vaccine results in autism. The small study that did suggest there was a link has since been conclusively discredited.

Assessment, clinical features, investigations and differential diagnosis

See Chapter 8.

Management and prognosis

No pharmacological treatments are recommended for the core symptoms of autism (National Institute for Health and Care Excellence (NICE) 2012, 2013). Instead, the emphasis is on

Table 32.1 Epidemiology of neurodevelopmental disorders

Disorder	Population prevalence[a]	Sex ratio (female:male)
Autism spectrum disorders	1%	1:3
Attention deficit hyperactivity disorder	5% in children 2.5% in adults	1:2
Tourette syndrome	0.3%	1:3

[a]These estimates are approximate but taken from meta-analysis where possible. Different diagnostic systems give different prevalence estimates.

BOX 32.1 PSYCHOSOCIAL INTERVENTIONS IN ADULTS WITH AUTISM (NICE 2012)

Everyone

- Self-help or support groups – for individuals, and for their families, partners or carers.
- Social learning program (group or individual). Should include modelling of useful social behaviour, explicit statement of social rules and strategies for difficult social situations.

If appropriate to individual

- Supported employment programme
- Structured leisure activity, with a facilitator
- Anger management
- Antivictimization intervention
- Crisis plan

BOX 32.2 ENVIRONMENTAL MODIFICATIONS TO OPTIMIZE FUNCTIONING IN ADHD (CHILDREN OR ADULTS)

- Changes to seating arrangements
- Reducing distractions, e.g., use of headphones
- More frequent movement breaks
- Reinforcing verbal instructions in writing
- Support from teaching assistants (for those at school)

---

psychosocial interventions (see Box 32.1, adults). In children, a social–communication intervention that is play based and designed to maximise joint attention and reciprocal communication between the child and their parents, carers or teachers is recommended (NICE 2013). Comorbid mental health problems (e.g., anxiety or depression) should be treated as normal, except that psychological interventions should focus more on changing behaviour rather than cognitions and avoid the use of metaphor and hypothetical situations.

The functional impact of ASD symptoms fluctuates in response to stressors such as change (school, relationships, employment) and physical illness. The prognosis is extremely variable, reflecting the great variability between those with a diagnosis. An intelligence quotient (IQ) above 70, communicative language by age 5 years and absence of epilepsy are predictors of better long-term outcome. Some people can learn to develop strategies to work around their difficulties and make use of their strengths; however, many continue to have difficulty in finding employment or friendship and require family support into adulthood. Those with a comorbid intellectual disability are unlikely to be able to live independently in adulthood.

ATTENTION DEFICIT HYPERACTIVITY DISORDERS

Epidemiology and aetiology

Key epidemiology is shown in Table 32.1. Twin studies have shown that ADHD has one of the highest heritabilities of all psychiatric illnesses, at around 80%. A first-degree relative of someone with ADHD has a 20% chance of also having ADHD. Replicated candidate gene studies and genome-wide association studies of copy number variants implicate variants in genes encoding dopaminergic, serotonergic and glutamatergic pathways as influencing risk.

Prenatal, perinatal and postnatal environmental factors also modestly increase risk: maternal smoking, alcohol consumption and heroin use during pregnancy; very low birth weight; foetal hypoxia; perinatal brain injury and prolonged emotional deprivation during infancy.

Assessment, clinical features, investigations and differential diagnosis

See Chapter 8.

Management and prognosis

Children

First-line interventions in all cases are environmental modifications and parenting skills psychoeducation (NICE 2019). Environmental modifications are changes to the physical environment which aim to minimise the impact of ADHD (Box 32.2).

If despite the above a school-age child is still experiencing significant impairment due to ADHD, medication can be offered (NICE 2019).

The central nervous system stimulant methylphenidate (Ritalin) is normally tried in the first instance. It comes in short-acting form (Ritalin) and modified release preparations which have a range of release profiles to suit different needs (Concerta XL, Equasym XL, Medikinet XL, Xaggitin XL). Lisdexamfetamine can be considered if a 6-week trial of methylphenidate at adequate doses has not resulted in sufficient improvement or side effects are intolerable. Atomoxetine (Strattera) and guanfacine are third-line options.

If a young person has benefited from medication but still has ongoing significant impairment, consider offering a course of CBT focussing on social skills, problem-solving, self-control, active listening and dealing with feelings.

Oppositional defiant disorder and conduct-dissocial disorder are commonly comorbid with ADHD in young people, in which case a specific parent-training programme should be offered (NICE 2019; see also Chapter 33).

HINTS AND TIPS

Lisdexamfetamine is a prodrug that is metabolised to dexamfetamine by an enzyme in red blood cells. This limits the rate at which dexamfetamine is generated, reducing its potential for abuse. However, some patients benefit from the faster on-and-off times that dexamfetamine provides. NICE (2019) recommends trying lisdexamfetamine first, and changing to dexamfetamine if the longer effect profile cannot be tolerated (in both children and adults).

Improvement usually occurs during adolescence, particularly in hyperactivity. Unstable family dynamics and coexisting conduct-dissocial disorder are associated with a worse prognosis. Around two-thirds of patients have symptoms persisting into later life, and around half of these patients may need to continue medication long term. Children with ADHD are at increased risk for substance use and imprisonment in adult life, although this risk is moderated by treatment. With improvements in awareness and diagnosis in recent years many successful individuals such as professional athletes, doctors, journalists and actors have publicly stated they have ADHD.

COMMUNICATION

Parents' concerns need to be addressed as well as the patient's. Treatment of attention deficit hyperactivity disorder has received much media interest, especially potential side effects – be aware of this.
Methylphenidate is associated with growth suppression with prolonged use. It is only prescribed in specialist settings with regular weight and height monitoring. Drug holidays can be used to allow children to make-up growth gains. Rarely, atomoxetine is associated with liver dysfunction and suicidality.

RED FLAG

Before starting attention deficit hyperactivity disorder drug treatment, assess height, weight, blood pressure and heart rate and personal or family history of cardiovascular disease. Then monitor these parameters during treatment. Stimulants are sympathomimetic and can suppress appetite.

COMMUNICATION

One way to sum up management of severe childhood attention deficit hyperactivity disorder (ADHD), or adult ADHD, is to tell patients they need both 'pills and skills'. 'Pills' can provide a window of opportunity to allow people to develop organisational 'skills' they struggled to achieve before.

Adults

First-line treatment in adults is also environmental modifications (Box 32.2) (NICE 2019). Pharmacological management can be offered if symptoms are still causing significant impairment. Psychological interventions can be offered instead of medication if patients prefer it, and are recommended if impairment persists despite medication. The psychological intervention should be structured, ADHD focussed and may contain elements of CBT. Methylphenidate or lisdexamfetamine are recommended first line. If one is ineffective, try the other. Atomoxetine is third line.

Diversion of stimulant medication is a risk in young people and adults. If someone is actively using recreational substances, advise them that they should stop doing so before a trial of ADHD medication. If fears remain regarding diversion, try atomoxetine or lisdexamfetamine (Elvanse).

RED FLAG

Stimulant medications have a street value, and therefore are at risk of being diverted. If a child needs stimulant medication prescribed and there is a past or current history of parental substance misuse, the school can be asked to dispense medication, or an alternative used. If a young person or adult is actively using recreational substances, they need to stop before any stimulants can be prescribed. If this is not possible, or if diversion is suspected at any point, a nonstimulant alternative can be tried.

Nearly half of individuals with ADHD in childhood continue to experience symptoms in adolescence and approximately one-third into adulthood. Hyperactivity-impulsivity behaviours often decrease with age and inattentive behaviours become more apparent. It seems reasonable that symptoms might become more tolerable as people learn additional coping strategies (e.g., diaries, reminders), or modify their environment to minimise functional impairment (e.g., get a job that requires brief bursts of sustained attention only). 'Drug holidays' every couple of years to assess whether medication is still of benefit are probably worth trying.

ADHD is often comorbid with other psychiatric disorders (bipolar disorder, depression, anxiety disorders, substance use), so ensure these are assessed and treated also.

TOURETTE SYNDROME

Tourette syndrome is classified under 'Diseases of the Nervous System' in the ICD-11 rather than under 'Mental, Behavioural or Neurodevelopmental Disorders'. It is however a common comorbidity for neurodevelopmental conditions (particularly ADHD), and has been left in this book for reference.

Epidemiology and aetiology

Key epidemiology is shown in Table 32.1. Aetiology is unclear but abnormalities in dopaminergic neurotransmission have been found.

Assessment, clinical features, investigations and differential diagnosis

See Chapter 8.

Management and prognosis

Often tics do not require treatment, particularly if they are not interfering with daily life. Tourette syndrome is very commonly comorbid with other conditions (anxiety, obsessive-compulsive disorder, ADHD), and these should be treated first, according to standard guidelines. If tics remain problematic after other disorders are treated, psychological treatments should be tried first (psychoeducation, habit reversal and exposure and response prevention). If tics persist, clonidine (an alpha 2 adrenergic agonist) is recommended first. Antipsychotics can also help (haloperidol, pimozide, risperidone or aripiprazole). Risk for side effects should always be balanced against benefits on an individual basis.

Around two-thirds of children and young people with Tourette syndrome go on to have no or very mild tics in adulthood.

● **Chapter Summary**

- Neurodevelopmental disorders are common, particularly attention deficit hyperactivity disorder (ADHD).
- Neurodevelopmental disorders are often comorbid with Tourette syndrome, other mental disorders and epilepsy. It is important to treat comorbid conditions.
- Autism spectrum disorder is managed primarily with psychosocial interventions.
- ADHD is managed with a combination of psychosocial and pharmacological interventions.

UKMLA Conditions
Attention deficit hyperactivity disorder
Autism spectrum disorder

UKMLA Presentations
Behavioural difficulties in childhood
Substance misuse

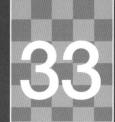

Child and adolescent psychiatry 33

This chapter covers the assessment and management of problems with mood, anxiety or conduct in children and young people. Neurodevelopmental disorders, including intellectual disability, can cause similar symptoms or be comorbid with these disorders, but are covered separately in Chapters 8, 31 and 32. Mental illnesses that commonly affect adults such as eating disorders, bipolar disorder and schizophrenia can also present in adolescence; these are predominantly covered in their own chapters but also briefly here. Finally, this chapter briefly covers child abuse. Mental disorders in children can both be caused by child abuse and increase the risk of experiencing abuse, and it is important to always be alert to this possibility.

CHILD AND ADOLESCENT MENTAL HEALTH SERVICES

Child and Adolescent Mental Health Services (CAMHS) provide emotional and mental health support, diagnosis and treatment to individuals up to the age of 18 years. In some areas CAMHS services also continue to provide input up to the age of 25 for certain groups of patients, e.g., care-leavers and those under the care of the early onset psychosis teams, although this is not widespread and dependent on funding.

Children often find it difficult to explicitly verbalise psychological distress. Instead, the presenting problem can commonly be a nonspecific concern about a child's abnormal behaviour or performance (e.g., 'being disruptive in the classroom'), often raised by someone other than the young person (e.g., parent, schoolteacher, paediatrician). This means the ability to take a good history and synthesize information from multiple sources is particularly important in CAMHS. While multiple sources of information can be helpful to give different perspectives on the child or young person's difficulties, it is important to ensure that the voice of the young person is heard and taken into consideration throughout their care and treatment, and not lost among the sometimes-conflicting voices of the adults involved in their care.

Family and wider community are important in assessing and maintaining a young person's well-being and this is reflected in the broad composition of multidisciplinary teams in CAMHS, which are likely to include psychiatrists, psychologists, occupational therapists, community mental health workers, social workers, community psychiatric nurses, family therapists and creative therapists. Fig. 33.1 shows an overview of the tiered approach to CAMHS services common in the United Kingdom.

ATTACHMENT

Attachment refers to the bond between an infant and their primary caregiver. How the primary caregiver responds to a young child's needs during their early years sets the tone for that child's expectations for the rest of their life: how others are likely to behave towards them and how they should behave in return. Put simply, if a child is shown kindness and understanding, they are more likely to become a kind and empathic adult. If a child is ignored and neglected, they are less likely to be social or caring towards others. If a child is treated inconsistently, sometimes with love, sometimes with disdain, they will expect the world to be unpredictable and chaotic, people in authority to be untrustworthy and themselves as unable to be in control. Disrupted attachment during early childhood can often lead to behavioural difficulties in children and potentially personality disorders in adulthood (see Table 33.1).

Importantly, not everyone who has a difficult upbringing will have a difficult adulthood; behaviour and thinking patterns can change (sometimes with the help of psychological therapy). It is also important to note that primary caregivers do not always provide an optimal early environment for a range of reasons, some within and some outwith their control (e.g., postnatal depression, substance use, poverty, bereavement, war). Nonetheless, encouraging parents and care providers to provide a loving and responsive environment for infants and young children has become a key governmental priority.

HINTS AND TIPS

As you meet children, young people and adults who seem to be behaving in harmful ways, it can often be helpful to try to understand how their early experiences have shaped them. Often thoughts or behaviours that are helpful during times of adversity (e.g., not trusting others when experiencing abuse) can become unhelpful in other times and contexts (e.g., difficulty forming close relationships).

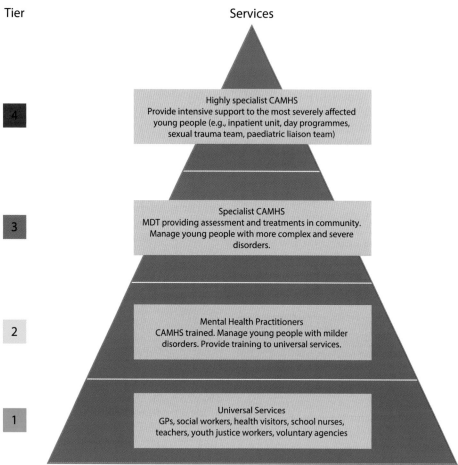

Fig. 33.1 Tiered structure of CAMHS. *CAMHS,* Child and Adolescent Mental Health Services; *GP,* general practitioner; *MDT,* multidisciplinary team.

Table 33.1 Attachment styles

Child attachment style	Caregiver behaviour	Child behaviour	Adult attachment style	Adult behaviour
Secure (two-thirds)	Responsive, understanding, consistent	Happy, curious	'Autonomous'	Able to self-soothe, but also able to maintain relationships.
Insecure (a third)				
'Avoidant' (21%)	Aloof, unresponsive, ridiculing	Emotionally distant, withdrawn	'Dismissive'	Desire to be independent. Avoidance of intimacy.
'Ambivalent/resistant' (16%)	At times sensitive, at times ignores	Anxious, uncertain, angry	'Preoccupied'	Hypersensitive to rejection, care-seeking.
'Disorganised' (rare)	Abusive, scary, scared	Sad, angry, fearful	'Disorganised'	Fearful, abusive, dissociative.

EPIDEMIOLOGY

Mental health problems affect around 1 in 6 children and young people between the ages of 6 and 19. See Table 33.2 for individual disorders. Research conducted by NHS England suggests that there has been a significant increase in rates of probable mental disorders in children and young people between 2017 and 2021. Rates in 6- to 16-year-olds have increased from 1 in 9 young people to 1 in 6. For 17- to 19-year-olds, rates of probable mental disorders have also increased from 1 in 10 young people to 1 in 6 over the same period. CAMHS services in the United Kingdom have therefore seen a significant increase in referrals, with the Royal College of Psychiatrists quoting a 96% increase in 2021 referral rates, when compared to the same period in 2019. The effects of the COVID-19 pandemic have been suggested as one contributing factor.

MENTAL ILLNESS IN CHILDREN AND ADOLESCENTS

Formulation

Concrete diagnoses are used less frequently in CAMHS compared to adult services. Instead, a descriptive and formulation-based approach is much more common. A formulation is a way of understanding the 'how' of a child or young person developing a mental illness or disorder. One common approach is the 'biopsychosocial' approach, which looks at how biological, psychological, and social factors contribute to the young person developing symptoms of mental illness. Each of the '5 Ps' can then be considered for each of these factors: the problem, then predisposing, precipitating, perpetuating and protective factors. See Fig. 33.2 for further information about the '5 Ps'.

A formulation is usually developed collaboratively between the clinician and the young person and can be used to inform and guide interventions and approaches to treatment. While developing a formulation can be helpful for all children and young people presenting with symptoms of mental illness, it remains appropriate to assign a diagnosis of a mental illness or mental disorder for some young people, particularly when this can help them access appropriate services and treatments.

Anxiety disorders

The anxiety disorders in childhood are often thought to be exaggerations of normal developmental trends rather than discrete illnesses in themselves. They tend to have a good prognosis, and do not commonly persist into adulthood, however there is an increased risk of the child or young person

Table 33.2 Epidemiology of mental disorders in childhood and adolescence

Disorder	Typical age of presentation	Prevalence in under 18-year-olds (posttypical age of onset)
Intellectual disability	Infancy or preschool	3%
Autism spectrum disorder	Preschool or primary	1%
Attention deficit hyperactivity disorder	Preschool or primary	5%
Anxiety disorders	Primary or older	5% (up to 20% have a phobia)
Conduct-dissocial disorder	Primary or older	8% males, 4% females
Oppositional defiant disorder	Primary or older	4%
Eating disorders	Adolescence	2%–3%
Depression	Adolescence	4%
Bipolar disorder	Late adolescence	1%
Schizophrenia	Late adolescence	Rare
Personality disorder	Late adolescence	Around 3% (for personality disorder with a borderline pattern)

developing anxiety or depressive disorders in adulthood. The treatment of these disorders is focused on behavioural and family therapy. In late adolescence common anxiety disorders of adulthood (generalized anxiety disorder, panic disorder and obsessive-compulsive disorder (OCD)) emerge; diagnosis and management are very similar to adulthood (see Chapters 12, 13 and 25) but with an even stronger emphasis on psychological therapy.

Separation anxiety disorder

Normal separation anxiety usually occurs in children from 6 months to 3 years of age. It usually peaks between the ages of 10 and 18 months. However, some children experience inappropriate and excessive anxiety about separation from attachment figures. They may display clinging behaviour or temper tantrums when their attachment figures attempt to separate from them. This disorder is only diagnosed when the anxiety is of such a severity that it is markedly different from other children of a similar age or when it persists beyond the usual age period (e.g., a 6-year-old girl becoming incredibly distressed when her mother drops her off at school).

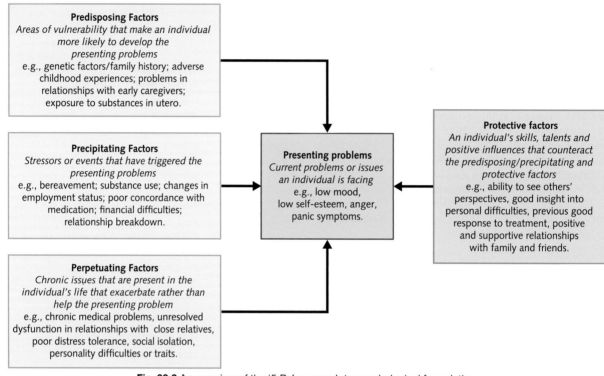

Fig. 33.2 An overview of the '5 Ps' approach to psychological formulation.

Phobic anxiety disorder

Minor phobic symptoms are common in childhood, and the object of the phobia varies with developmental stage (e.g., fear of animals or monsters in preschool children). Phobic anxiety disorder is diagnosed when the phobic object is age inappropriate (e.g., a 9-year-old boy who is afraid of monsters under the bed), or where levels of anxiety are clinically abnormal. Nondevelopmental phobias (e.g., agoraphobia) do not fall under this category, but under the adult phobia category (see Chapters 12 and 25).

Obsessive-compulsive disorder

Median age of onset is 10 years but can be from age 5 years. About two-thirds of young children have various rituals/habits (e.g., lining up toys, specific stories before bed) that parents may be concerned is OCD. What is important to bear in mind is the developmental stage of the child. Rituals/habits help children to make sense of the world around them as they grow and develop. OCD is suggested if the ritual/habit is very intense or frequent, impairs the child's ability to function or causes them distress. Another key difference between diagnosis in adults and children is that children are not required to recognise their thoughts as abnormal. Treatment is largely psychological, primarily cognitive-behavioural

therapy (CBT) with exposure response prevention (ERP). There is a low threshold for considering commencing selective serotonin reuptake inhibitor (SSRI) medication alongside continuing CBT with ERP, if psychological therapy alone has been ineffective. Sertraline has been shown to be effective in treating children and young people with OCD and is usually first line if medication is being considered.

Social anxiety disorder

Normal stranger anxiety occurs in well-adjusted children from 8 months to 1 year of age. Social anxiety disorder is a persistent and recurrent fear and/or avoidance of strangers. This disorder is only diagnosed when the anxiety is of such a severity that it is markedly different from other children of a similar age or when it persists beyond the usual age period. A large majority of cases emerge between the ages of 8 and 15 years.

School refusal

School refusal is the refusal to go to school because of anxiety. It is not a diagnosis in itself, but is a common symptom of many different conditions and disorders. It can be caused by separation anxiety in younger children, another mental illness or disorder (e.g., depression, social anxiety disorder, autism spectrum disorder, attention deficit hyperactivity disorder (ADHD)), occur as a result of difficulties in the classroom (e.g., due to undiagnosed dyslexia or developmental coordination disorder) and/or as a result of negative psychosocial factors (e.g., bullying, teasing, abuse). In contrast, *truancy* would be defined as absence from school by choice. While truancy has associations with poor academic performance, a family history of antisocial behaviour and large family sizes, it is important that professionals do not just attribute behaviour to the child or young person being 'bad'. A young person's behaviour is part of their communication and truancy can be a response to trauma they have experienced at home or be related to their experience at school. Professionals should try to understand what is driving the behaviour, diagnose and treat any mental illness or disorder and optimise the young person's school and home environment as far as possible to give them the best possible chance of attending school.

Selective mutism (elective mutism)

Selective mutism is a selectivity in vocal communication depending on the social circumstances. The young person speaks normally in some situations (e.g., at home), but is mute in others (e.g., at school). These children have adequately developed language comprehension and ability (although a minority may have slight speech delay or articulation problems). It is not uncommon for children to be reluctant to speak in the first few weeks of starting school, so the diagnosis should only be made if the behaviour persists for several months. It usually presents before the age of 5 years, is slightly more common in girls and is associated with psychological stress, social anxiety and oppositional behaviour.

COMMUNICATION

It can often be helpful to include other members of the multidisciplinary team (MDT) in an assessment of a child with elective mutism, such as speech and language therapy. They can support the child or young person to communicate in nonverbal ways, e.g., using Talking Mats.

HINTS AND TIPS

Social anxiety is common in children with neurodevelopmental disorders. Remember to screen for autism and attention deficit hyperactivity disorder (see Chapter 8) in a child presenting with anxiety.

HINTS AND TIPS

All behaviour is communication – if a child is not attending school, for whatever reason, consideration needs to be given to the reasons why, the child's experience of school, attachment, anxiety, trauma history (child and family) and undiagnosed neurodevelopmental disorder. These are not just 'bad kids'.

Disruptive behaviour disorders

Disruptive behaviour is a common reason children and young people are referred to CAMHS. If, after initial assessment appointments, it is felt that their disruptive behaviour is not a result of a mental illness or disorder, the child or young person is redirected to other supports, e.g., social work. In some cases, the patterns of behaviour seen can warrant a diagnosis of a disruptive behaviour disorder. Disruptive behaviour disorders include conduct-dissocial disorder and oppositional defiant disorder.

There is debate around these disorders, as some professionals feel that the diagnostic criteria for the disorders do not necessarily take into account the child or young person's internal experience and the underlying cognitive and emotional processes that are driving their disruptive behaviour, and are instead based on behavioural symptoms. There is also significant overlap between the aetiological risk factors for disruptive behaviour disorders and complex trauma, with a history of trauma or attachment problems being very common among children and young people with disruptive behaviour disorders. The impact of previous traumatic experiences can be overshadowed by a diagnosis of a disruptive behaviour disorder.

It is also important to remember that a disruptive behaviour disorder diagnosis can be very stigmatising for the child or young person and their family, and some clinicians have moved away from diagnosing these disorders. Conversely, if the child or young person meets criteria for the disorder, having a diagnosis can make it easier to access appropriate services and support from external services and agencies.

Conduct-dissocial disorder

Conduct-dissocial disorder is characterised by a pattern of repetitive, severe, and persistent behaviour where age-appropriate societal expectations and the rights of others are disregarded. This can take the form of aggression towards people and animals, destruction of property (including fire setting), deceitfulness or theft and rule violations, e.g., truancy, running away from home and staying out at night. Typically, symptoms of conduct-dissocial disorder may be mild, e.g., lying but can then progress to more severe symptoms, e.g., assault. Conduct-dissocial disorder can commonly co-occur with ADHD and they share similar risk factors. A diagnosis of both can be made, but if the observed behaviours are because of direct and severe noncompliance with rules and societal expectations, rather than due to inattentiveness and hyperactivity, the additional diagnosis of conduct-dissocial disorder can be appropriate.

The prevalence of conduct-dissocial disorder is estimated to be around 3% in school-aged children and young people. Rates among populations in young offender institutions have been estimated to be as high as 87%. The male-to-female ratio is approximately 2:1. Aetiological factors include genetics, parental psychopathology (mental illness, substance abuse, dissocial personality traits), child abuse and neglect, poor socioeconomic status and poor educational attainment. Many adolescents improve by adulthood; however, a substantial proportion go on to develop personality disorders with dissocial traits and substance-related issues, particularly when the disorder has had an earlier rate of onset. NICE (2013) recommends parental skills training programmes for parents/carers, cognitive-behavioural problem-solving programmes for young people and multimodal interventions (e.g., multisystemic therapy) aiming to influence how the young person interacts with their family, school, community and criminal justice system. Input from social work is often required as the young person can be outside of parental control.

Oppositional defiant disorder

Oppositional defiant disorder is defined as a persistent pattern of negative, defiant, hostile and disruptive behaviour *in the absence of* behaviour that violates the law or the basic rights of others as occurs in conduct-dissocial disorder (e.g., theft, cruelty, bullying, assault). Young people with this disorder deliberately defy requests or rules, are angry, extremely irritable and resentful and annoy others on purpose. The behaviour must have been present for at least 6 months prior to the diagnosis being made. The behaviour also needs to be present in multiple settings and across different relationships. For example, it would be inappropriate to diagnose oppositional defiant disorder if the defiant behaviours are only noted when a certain authority figure, e.g., a parent interacts with them. Management is very similar to conduct-dissocial disorder.

HINTS AND TIPS

It helps to remember that family histories should relate to both genetic lineage and factors that influence psychological development: the risk of developing conduct-dissocial disorder is increased if a first-degree relative suffers from it, but also if there is a history of personality disorder with prominent features of dissociality in a close family member, regardless of whether they are a biological relative.

Attachment disorders

Reactive attachment disorder

Reactive attachment disorder (RAD) occurs in children under 5 years of age who have been severely neglected and unable to form a secure attachment to a primary caregiver. The affected child does not seek out their primary caregiver for comfort or support during periods of distress, and they do not respond when they are offered comfort. Children with RAD do not display security-seeking behaviours towards any adult, and they can display unexplained irritability, sadness and fearfulness during interactions with other caregivers. They can also present as listless and withdrawn.

With adequate care, children with RAD can experience a complete remission of their symptoms. However, if the child remains in the environment in which the disorder develops and/or their care remains inadequate, the disorder can persist for several years, and difficulties forming relationships can persist into adulthood. They are also at a higher risk of developing a depressive illness compared to their peers, and they are also at risk for developing comorbid post-traumatic stress disorder or complex post-traumatic stress disorder related to chronic and repetitive maltreatment.

HINTS AND TIPS

'Quiet' signs of reactive attachment disorder, e.g., withdrawal, can easily be missed in care environments where resources are directed towards children and young people with the 'noisier' signs, e.g., aggression.

Disinhibited social engagement disorder

Disinhibited social engagement disorder also occurs in the context of grossly insufficient care of a child under the age of 5. It manifests with abnormal social behaviours, where a child will display reduced or absent reservations about approaching and interacting with unfamiliar adults. They can present as overly familiar, e.g., asking age-inappropriate questions or seeking comfort from unknown adults. They show no preference for their primary caregiver, with diminished or absent 'checking back' behaviour when they have ventured into unfamiliar settings. They can also display willingness to venture off with unfamiliar adults with little hesitation.

Disinhibited social engagement disorder is rare, and unlike RAD, the symptoms tend to be more persistent after the child starts to receive appropriate care. As the child gets older, they often develop superficial peer relationships and have difficulties with social interactions. As with RAD, children with disinhibited social engagement disorder are at increased risk of developing comorbid Post-traumatic stress disorder or complex Post-traumatic stress disorder. There is also a high rate of co-occurrence with ADHD.

Disorders of elimination

Disorders of elimination are most commonly managed by community paediatrics and school nurses. CAMHS services often only become involved if there is thought to be underlying psychopathology.

Nonorganic enuresis

This condition is characterised by the involuntary voiding of urine in children who, according to their developmental stage, should have established consistent bladder control (therefore ordinarily not diagnosed before the age of 5 years). It may occur during the day or night and is not directly caused by any medical condition (e.g., seizures, diabetes, urinary tract infection, constipation, structural abnormalities of the urinary tract) or use of a substance (e.g., diuretic). Two types of enuresis have been described: primary enuresis means that urinary continence has never been established; and secondary enuresis means that continence has been achieved in the past. Secondary enuresis most commonly develops between the ages of 5 and 8 years. Nonorganic enuresis occurs in around 7% of 5-year-olds; 4% of 10-year-olds and around 1% of adolescents over 15 years. Gender distribution is equal in younger patients; however, cases that persist into adolescence tend to be males. Aetiological factors include genetics, developmental delays, psychosocial stressors (moving house, birth of a sibling, start or change of school, divorce, bereavement and inadequate toilet training). About 75% of children with nonorganic enuresis have a first-degree biological relative who has had the same problem. Management (NICE 2010) involves exclusion of physical cause, parental education about toilet training (especially in primary enuresis), behavioural therapy (pad and buzzer apparatus, star chart, bladder training) and – as a last resort – pharmacotherapy (imipramine, nasal desmopressin). Most cases of nonorganic enuresis resolve by adolescence.

Nonorganic encopresis

This condition is characterized by the deposition of normal faeces (i.e., not diarrhoea) in inappropriate places, in children who – according to their developmental stage – should have established consistent bowel control (therefore ordinarily not diagnosed before the age of 4 years). It may be due to unsuccessful toilet training where bowel control has never been achieved (primary encopresis) or may occur after a period of normal bowel control (secondary encopresis). Encopresis may result from a developmental delay; coercive or punitive potty training; emotional, physical or sexual abuse; a disturbed parent–child relationship; parental marital conflict or can feature as a symptom of a neurodevelopmental disorder (e.g., autism or intellectual disability). About 1% of 5-year-olds have the condition and it is more common in males. Management includes ruling out an organic cause (constipation with overflow incontinence, anal fissure, gastrointestinal infection), assessing and treating disturbed family dynamics (ruling out child abuse), parental guidance regarding toilet training and behaviour therapy (e.g., star chart). Stool softeners may be used for constipation. The prognosis is good with 90% of cases improving within a year.

Disorders arising in adolescence and adulthood

Eating disorders

Eating disorders (see Chapters 16 and 26) often commence in adolescence. Symptomatology and diagnosis are the same as in adulthood. The management is very similar to that recommended for adults – the first-line treatment is always psychological therapy (family-based therapy is the gold standard in young people), rather than medication. For cases of treatment-resistant anorexia, low-dose olanzapine is sometimes used, and fluoxetine can be considered alongside psychological therapy (usually CBT) for bulimia nervosa. When assessing physical risk from eating disorder in adolescents it is important to refer to age-specific guidelines (e.g., Medical emergencies in eating disorders (MEED), which contains age-adjusted parameters to assess the young person's physical health).

HINTS AND TIPS

Supporting a young person with an eating disorder can be enormously stressful. There are lots of third-sector organisations that can provide advice and support for parents and carers. One of the largest is BEAT, an eating disorder charity.

Depression

Depression also arises frequently in adolescence. The treatment is similar to adults, but psychological therapies are first line, and a far smaller range of antidepressants are recommended.

Mild depression: NICE (2019) suggests watchful waiting for mild depression. If symptoms persist, NICE then recommends group-based psychological treatment CBT, nondirective supportive therapy (NDST) or interpersonal therapy (IPT)). This would usually be offered in a Tier 2 setting (Fig. 33.1). If this is ineffective, the next step would be a referral to a Tier

3 CAMHS service for individual CBT or attachment-based family therapy. Medication is not recommended for mild depression.

Moderate-to-severe depression: Young people with moderate-to-severe depression should be reviewed by a CAMHS team. For 5- to 11-year-olds, the first-line psychological therapies recommended include family-based IPT, family therapy, individual CBT or psychodynamic psychotherapy, adapted where possible to suit their developmental stage. For 12- to 18-year-olds, individual CBT is recommended for at least a 3-month period. If this is not effective, IPT for adolescents, family therapy or psychodynamic psychotherapy are recommended. Psychological therapy can be combined with fluoxetine after four to six sessions, following a multidisciplinary team review and if the team feel that the young person's limited response to psychological therapy is not the result of external factors, e.g., comorbid conditions. Second-line antidepressants are sertraline and citalopram, but this is an off-label use of the medications and there is not a large amount of evidence for their use.

> **RED FLAG**
>
> Selective serotonin reuptake inhibitors should be started at lower doses in adolescents than adults. Young people should be monitored closely for thoughts of self-harm or suicide weekly for the first month of commencing treatment or after a dose increase.

Bipolar disorder and schizophrenia

Severe and enduring mental illnesses such as bipolar disorder and schizophrenia often begin to manifest in adolescence (60% of bipolar disorder has onset before age 20) but are uncommonly fully symptomatic or diagnosed until late adolescence. Suspected cases are generally managed in early intervention for psychosis teams. Classification is the same as in adulthood. Treatment follows the same principles as in adults but focusses on psychological treatments and family interventions rather than pharmacological treatments, with a smaller range of medications used in young people. Management of acute mania remains pharmacological and follows similar principles to the management of the disorder in adults. Common medications used include olanzapine, risperidone, aripiprazole and lurasidone–the choice of medication is often guided by most tolerable side effect profile to help with concordance Physical monitoring preinitiation and during treatment is also required. This includes weight, BP/pulse, ECG and blood monitoring (lipids, glucose, renal function, liver function and prolactin).

> **HINTS AND TIPS**
>
> Comorbidities are common in young people with bipolar disorder, with 40% to 90% of young people also meeting diagnostic criteria for ADHD. Other common comorbidities include disruptive behaviour disorders, substance use problems and anxiety disorders.

Personality disorder

From as early as three years old, children begin to exhibit personality traits that gradually become more stable over the course of their lives. Early life experiences, particularly traumatic events, influence the trajectory of how an individual's personality develops. While it can be harmful to label a young person with a personality disorder diagnosis which turns out to be incorrect, it can also be harmful to misattribute problems due to personality traits to a different mental disorder, or to minimise them. There is increasing evidence that there are benefits to making an early diagnosis of personality disorder. Due to the malleability of the brain during adolescence, it is a key period for intervention. A sensitively communicated diagnosis can help a young person and their family and friends make sense of their experiences and symptoms. Treatment of personality disorder in CAMHS is very similar to that in adulthood (see Chapter 30), with the mainstay of treatment being psychological rather than pharmacological. Due to the historical reluctance to diagnose personality disorders in childhood and adolescence, there is limited evidence as to the most appropriate treatment modality.

CHILD ABUSE

Child abuse includes the overlapping concepts of physical, sexual and emotional mistreatment, as well as neglect or deprivation of the child. Child abuse is very common: around 1 in 4 adults report severe abuse of some kind as a child, with 1 in 20 children in the United Kingdom experiencing sexual abuse. Table 33.3 lists the risk factors associated with child abuse. In addition to the physical manifestations, victims of abuse may present with failure to thrive and symptoms of depression, anxiety, aggression, age-inappropriate sexual behaviour and self-harm. They are also at an increased risk for the development of a substantial range of psychiatric problems in later life.

Table 33.3 Risk factors for child abuse

Parent/environmental factors	Child factors
• Parents who were abused • Parental substance abuse • Parental mental illness (intellectual disability, depression, schizophrenia, personality disorders) • Caregiver in the home who is not a biological parent • Young, immature parents • Parental criminality • Poor socioeconomic status and overcrowding • Familial isolation from wider social supports	• Low birth weight or prematurity • Early maternal separation • Unwanted child • Excessive crying • Challenging behaviour • Intellectual or physical disability • Hyperactivity

All National Health Service Trusts in the United Kingdom have specific child protection guidelines which should be easily accessible and consulted before they are needed. Box 30.7 provides some general principles. All healthcare staff (not just child psychiatrists and paediatricians) have a duty to protect children from harm, and the safety of a child should always take priority. If a child discloses ongoing abuse (of any sort), or if you suspect that they are being abused or neglected, confidentiality cannot be maintained, and this should (if appropriate) be explained to the child. Comprehensive notes should be kept, and care should be taken to allow the child to make the disclosure in their own words without suggestion from others (either family or healthcare staff). Concerns should be reported as soon as practically possible. While local procedures vary slightly, the police, social workers and the duty paediatrician should be able to offer guidance. In some cases, the child may be in imminent danger (e.g., being taken home by the alleged perpetrator). It may be necessary to involve the police to prevent further harm and to remove the child to a place of safety, e.g., admitting them to hospital overnight.

RED FLAG

Children have the same right to confidentiality as adults. However, if you believe or suspect a child is being abused, you have a duty to break confidentiality and report this promptly to authorities as per local guidelines (generally a social worker or a paediatrician). If there is imminent risk, you should contact the police.

RED FLAG

What to do if a child discloses abuse to you

Listen carefully – do not interrupt or express surprise or your own views

Say
• 'You've done the right thing to tell me' ·
• 'It's not your fault'
• 'I believe you'
• Ask open and nonleading questions

Share
• Tell a senior doctor
• Share the information with authorities
• Consider if the child is safe to go home
• Tell the child what you plan to do, if age appropriate
• Document carefully using child's own words
• Do not challenge the alleged abuser

ASSESSMENT CONSIDERATIONS IN YOUNG PEOPLE

• Problems need to be considered in the context of a child's developmental stage; for example, 'temper tantrums' are normal for a 2-year-old child but should have subsided by age 5 years.
• Parents or carers usually accompany children and young adolescents. It is often useful to interview them – with or without the child present – to obtain a full description of the current concerns, as well as a complete history (psychiatric, neurodevelopmental, educational and medical). An indirect evaluation of the parents' personalities, relationship and style of parenting often creates another perspective from which to understand the context of the presenting complaint.
• The ability of youngsters to provide a candid account of their difficulties varies dramatically. The assessment style should be tailored to the individual abilities of the young person rather than to their age. In children who are unable to articulate their inner experiences (usually younger children), it is often necessary to observe them in play situations.
• The child's own understanding of their difficulties should (if possible) be taken into consideration, as this can affect their management (in terms of motivation to engage with psychosocial interventions, and concordance with medication).
• It may be useful to change the order of the assessment to build rapport. For example, start with open and general questions about school and home rather than the presenting complaint.

- The importance of obtaining collateral information cannot be overstated. This is extremely important in fully understanding the development of the presenting problem, and the young person's premorbid functioning. It includes obtaining academic, educational or psychological reports as well as discussions with teachers and any other agencies involved. Remember to obtain consent from the parent/carer (and the child, if they are able).

- Further information can be obtained from structured and semistructured interviews (e.g., Kiddie Schedule for Affective Disorders and Schizophrenia (K-SADS-P), Revised Children's Anxiety and Depression Scale (RCADS), Diagnostic Interview Schedule for Children (NIMH-DISC-IV)), objective assessment instruments (Autism Diagnostic Observation Schedule (ADOS)) and parent/teacher/self-rating scales (strengths and difficulties questionnaire (SDQ), ADHD rating Scale IV).

Chapter Summary

- Mental health problems are common in children and adolescents.
- Collateral histories and multidisciplinary working are particularly important in Child and Adolescent Mental Health Services.
- Anxiety disorders in childhood often resolve by adulthood.
- First-line treatment of mental health problems in young people is generally psychological, not pharmacological.
- Childhood and adolescence is a key window for therapeutic intervention.
- Child abuse is common. Communicating concerns is key.

UKMLA Conditions
Anxiety
Bipolar affective disorder
Depression
Eating disorders
OCD
Personality disorder
Phobias
Schizophrenia

UKMLA Presentations
Behaviour/personality change
Behavioural difficulties in childhood
Child abuse
Low mood/affective problems

FURTHER READING

Medical emergencies in eating disorders (MEED) guidelines. https://www.rcpsych.ac.uk/docs/default-source/improving-care/better-mh-policy/college-reports/college-report-cr233-medical-emergencies-in-eating-disorders-(meed)-guidance.pdf?sfvrsn=2d327483_55.

Websites with useful resources for carers of young people with mental health problems. https://www.minded.org.uk/ and https://www.youngminds.org.uk/.

Forensic psychiatry is concerned with assessment and treatment of mentally disordered offenders, as well as the assessment of the risks posed by some individuals who may not yet have committed an offence. In practice, forensic psychiatric services tend to assess and manage those who pose a high risk to the safety of others (typically, those who have committed murder, attempted murder, severe sexual assault or arson). Some patients may be managed in the community; however, others may require treatment and rehabilitation in a secure environment. Levels of security can vary from a locked ward in a psychiatric hospital to a high-security 'special hospital' (Broadmoor, Rampton/Ashworth Hospitals or The State Hospital in Scotland).

MENTAL DISORDER AND CRIME

The vast majority of patients suffering from a mental illness have never committed an offence, and most offences are not committed as a result of a mental illness. Indeed, patients with mental disorders are four times more likely to fall victim to violence than members of the general population. However, there is a significantly higher prevalence of mental disorders among prisoners than in the general population for all mental disorders investigated (Table 34.1). Longitudinal studies suggest that most mental disorders manifest prior to imprisonment, not as a consequence of it. Substance use is extremely common in prisoners, with around a quarter of patients misusing alcohol and a third to a half misusing substances. Around one in six prisoners has a major depressive or psychotic illness. Female inmates are more likely to have a mental disorder than male inmates.

Identifying mental disorder in prisoners is important not least because the suicide rate in custody is around nine times that of the general population and could potentially be reduced by care plans to support inmates at high risk. Patients who are very unwell can be transferred from prison to a secure psychiatric hospital. This is essential when compulsory treatment under mental health legislation is required, as this cannot be given in prison.

Although those who commit crimes are more likely to have a mental disorder than the general population, it is important to note that the mental disorder alone is rarely sufficient to result in offending behaviour.

More commonly, risk factors that predispose to mental disorder also predispose to offending, for example, childhood abuse and chronic stress. Prison inreach mental health services therefore offer a good opportunity to alleviate suffering in those with mental health problems but will not necessarily reduce the risk of reoffending.

How best to manage offenders with personality disorders is particularly controversial. Personality disorder is more common in offenders, but it is unclear whether treating personality disorder reduces offending. This is at least in part because personality disorder is hard to treat, requiring long-term psychological therapy and motivation on the part of the patient (see Chapter 30). Government initiatives focused on those with 'dangerous and severe personality disorders' (now termed 'offending personality disorders') aimed to reduce offending rates by focusing resources on offenders with personality disorders (predominantly antisocial and emotionally unstable), and providing specialist units in which such individuals can be detained while they receive the treatment. The problem with this approach is that it may have led to those with personality disorder being detained for longer than those without personality disorders who had committed similar offences, potentially indefinitely, in the hope that treatment would reduce risk of offending, but without evidence that this was a likely outcome. Attempting to improve assessment and access to treatment for those with personality disorder in prisons seems sensible, but indefinite detainment while waiting for treatments to work does not.

HINTS AND TIPS

Mental disorders associated with violent crime (alcohol and substance dependence, attention deficit hyperactivity disorder, personality disorders and paranoid psychotic disorders) have a multiplicative effect for the risk of future violence when they occur in combination.

HINTS AND TIPS

Delusional jealousy (Othello syndrome) is often associated with alcohol abuse and linked to violent crime such as assault and homicide.

Table 34.1 Mental disorders associated with crime

Mental disorder	% of Prison population	Associations with crime
Personality disorder	10–65	Associated with violent crime, especially those with prominent dissocial traits. Personality disorders with dissocial traits, disinhibition or a borderline pattern are frequently diagnosed in forensic settings, often in association with comorbid substance abuse.
Alcohol and substance use	10–60 Substance misuse 10–30 Alcohol misuse	Substance misuse is a key factor that significantly increases the risk of violence in those with or without an existing mental disorder. Alcohol intoxication may also lead to driving offences and breaches of the peace, and offences may be committed to fund drug habits.
Neurodevelopmental disorders	ADHD 11–25 Intellectual disability 0.5–1.5	Impulsivity and mood instability in ADHD is associated with both violent and nonviolent crimes. There is an association between intellectual disabilities and sexual offences (especially indecent exposure), as well as arson. The prevalence of autism spectrum disorders in offenders is uncertain.
Psychotic disorders	5	Schizophrenia increases the risk of violent acts by a factor of 4. Many offences committed by people with schizophrenia are minor and are manifestations of impaired social skills. More people with schizophrenia are victims of crime than perpetrators
Mood disorders	Depression 10 Bipolar affective disorder 2–7	Depression is rarely associated with homicide. These cases are usually due to mood-congruent delusions (e.g., everyone would be better off dead) and are often followed by suicide. Postnatal depression is sometimes a cause of maternal filicide. Offences by manic patients usually reflect financial irresponsibility or acts of aggression.

ADHD, *Attention deficit hyperactivity disorder.*

HINTS AND TIPS

The term 'psychopath' is frequently misused. It is not a diagnosis in the Diagnostic and Statistical Manual of Mental Disorders, 5th edition, or the International Statistical Classification of Diseases and Related Health Problems, 11th edition (ICD-11). It is defined using the Hare Psychopathy Checklist – Revised, and in essence is a diminished ability to feel empathy coupled with antisocial behaviour. Only around 1 in 10 people with personality disorders with dissocial traits meet criteria for psychopathy.

ASSESSING AND MANAGING RISK OF VIOLENCE

The key principle in assessing the risk of violence that a patient with a mental disorder poses to others presents an ethical conflict between protecting the community from a potentially violent offender and respecting the human rights of the individual in question (see Chapter 4). This is often a very difficult balance to achieve. Forensic multidisciplinary teams in the United Kingdom have moved from simply trying to predict the risk of future violence (generally unsuccessful) to looking at the evidence-based risk factors present in an individual patient. This enables a formulation of scenarios in which future violence would be more likely to occur, facilitating the creation of management plans which will decrease the risk in a proactive fashion. Approaches to assessment include:

- Unaided clinical risk assessment: this involves drawing on the experience of the clinician involved. This has been demonstrated to be associated with a less effective and less accurate risk assessment than evidence-based methods.
- Actuarial methods: assessment using predetermined static actuarial or statistical variables (e.g., demographic factors). These methods do not take into account the specific factors of the case, and – used in isolation – can be misleading.
- Structured clinical judgement: assessment utilizing both empirical actuarial knowledge and clinical expertise. The Historical/Clinical/Risk Management 20-item (HCR-20) scale is by far the predominant mode of risk assessment used in the United Kingdom, and is particularly useful in assisting with risk management. Some newer tools have been developed that take protective factors significantly into account.

Box 34.1 summarises some of the factors that have been associated with the risk of violence.

A clinician confronted with an individual who poses a serious risk of violent behaviour will need to discuss the case with colleagues, including social workers and forensic mental health specialists. Compulsory hospitalisation may be required in some cases.

ETHICS

Clinicians have a duty to breach confidentiality to warn potential victims of serious threats that have been made (in consultation with the police), as per the Tarasoff ruling. The Tarasoff case was a case heard by the Supreme Court of California in 1974 and 1976, where a student (Tarasoff) was murdered by her ex-partner, who had disclosed his intent to kill her during sessions with his treating psychologist.

COMMUNICATION

A history of violent behaviour is the best predictor of future violent behaviour. It is important to both ask the patient about this and seek verification from other sources (police, social workers, family members and medical records).

BOX 34.1 SOME FACTORS ASSOCIATED WITH RISK OF VIOLENCE[a]

Historical (History of problems with…)
  H1. Violence
  H2. Other antisocial behaviour
  H3. Relationships
  H4. Employment
  H5. Substance use
  H6. Major mental disorder
  H7. Personality disorder
  H8. Traumatic experience
  H9. Violent attitudes
  H10. Treatment or supervision response
Clinical (Recent problems with…)
  C1. Insight
  C2. Violent ideation or intent
  C3. Symptoms of major mental disorder
  C4. Instability
  C5. Treatment or supervision response
Risk management (Future problems with…)
  R1. Professional services and plans
  R2. Living situation
  R3. Personal support
  R4. Treatment or supervision response
  R5. Stress or coping

[a] HCR-20 v3 items, from HCR-20 2013 by the Mental Health, Law, and Policy Institute, Simon Fraser University. Reprinted with permission from the copyright owner.

CONSIDERATIONS IN COURT PROCEEDINGS

Where there are grounds to believe that the accused may have been suffering (or is currently suffering) from a mental disorder, a psychiatric defence may be used. This means that the presence of mental disorder may have been a mitigating factor in the offence or may interfere with court proceedings. Throughout the UK, this is mainly based on case law rather than legislation. The role of the forensic psychiatrist is to act as an expert witness to the court. While the psychiatrist can make recommendations, the ultimate decision comes from the court.

Fitness to plead

Individuals with mental disorder are not exempt from taking responsibility for their actions. However, defendants should be competent to stand trial and mount a defence against their charges. The term 'fitness to plead' is used in English law to describe this capacity (with similar criteria in Scots and Northern Irish Law). Using psychiatric and/or psychological evidence, the court determines this by assessing whether the accused can:

- understand the nature of the charge;
- understand the difference between a plea of guilty and not guilty;
- instruct counsel (legal representation);
- follow the evidence brought before the court;
- challenge a juror.

Criminal responsibility

Before a defendant can be convicted, criminal responsibility needs to be determined. It should be determined whether, at the time of the offence, the person was able to control their own behaviour and choose whether to commit an unlawful act or not. Integral to this process is the concept of *mens rea* ('guilty intent' or 'guilty mind'), which means that the individual realised the nature of, and intended to commit, the unlawful act. Varying levels of *mens rea* are recognised, known as 'modes of culpability'. *Actus reus* ('guilty act' or 'crime') means the person is guilty of committing the act, whatever their intent. A defendant may be deemed to have decreased criminal culpability due to:

- Age: in England and Wales, children are only deemed legally responsible for their actions after the age of 14 years. Children under the age of 10 years are deemed incapable of criminal intent (*doli incapax*). Children aged 10 to 14 years are not considered criminally responsible unless the prosecution can prove *mens rea*.
- Reason of insanity: in English law, legal insanity (not a psychiatric term) is defined in terms of the M'Naghten Rules, which state that 'at the time of committing the act, the party accused was labouring under such a defect of reason, from disease of the mind, as to not know the nature and quality of the act he was doing, or, if he did know it, that he did not know what he was doing was wrong.' It is a defence that is rarely successful due to the high threshold of the legal definition of insanity.
- Diminished responsibility: in English law, a defence of diminished responsibility is only available in relation to charges for murder. If successful, this will lead to the accused being found guilty of manslaughter rather than murder, which allows for flexible sentencing (murder carries a mandatory life sentence). It depends upon the presence of 'an abnormality of mind (whether arising from a condition of arrested or retarded development of mind or any inherent causes or induced by disease or injury)'. An 'abnormality of mind' is not a psychiatric term and is open to wide

interpretation, leading to successful defences such as 'emotional immaturity' and 'premenstrual tension'.

- Automatism: an act committed without presence of mind (e.g., during sleepwalking or epileptic seizure) may warrant this rare defence.

HINTS AND TIPS

Self-induced (voluntary) intoxication with alcohol or other drugs cannot be used as a defence on the grounds of insanity or diminished responsibility.

HINTS AND TIPS

It is the responsibility of the Court (taking into consideration advice from expert witnesses) to decide upon sentencing or 'disposal' (i.e., what happens to the individual after trial). In cases where psychiatric defences are successfully used, the Court may utilise mental health legislation to transfer the individual to a secure hospital. In other cases, the Court may decide to impose a custodial sentence, or to place conditions upon the individual (e.g., to adhere to a drug treatment programme).

Chapter Summary

- Forensic psychiatrists assess and treat mental disorders in people who have committed serious offences.
- Mental disorders are more common in offenders, but usually do not directly cause offending.
- Misuse of drugs and alcohol is a major risk factor for offending.
- Assessment of risk of future violence is imprecise, but is aided by a structured approach.
- Forensic psychiatrists act as expert witnesses regarding the impact of mental disorder on criminal responsibility.

UKMLA Presentations
Mental capacity concerns
Threats to harm others

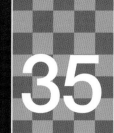
OVERVIEW OF SAMPLE QUESTIONS

1. History of cognitive decline from a relative
2. History of low mood
3. Risk assessment following self-harm
4. Alcohol history and brief alcohol intervention
5. Explanation and advice on schizophrenia
6. History of anxiety

HISTORY OF COGNITIVE DECLINE FROM A RELATIVE

Candidate instructions

You are a medical student attached to a GP practice. Mrs Jones attends alone to discuss concerns she has about her mother (Margaret) who has been found wandering and more confused lately. You are asked to take a history from them, then report your findings and discuss management with a more senior doctor.

There are two parts to this station:

1. Take a collateral history focussing on Margaret's cognitive decline and possible contributing factors.
   Do not take a full psychiatric history.
2. With 2 minutes remaining, the examiner will ask you to:
   • Suggest your differential diagnosis
   • Explain your reasoning based on your findings from the history
   • Suggest an initial management plan, including investigations

   You have 8 minutes for this station.

CHECKLIST

Communication

- Introduce yourself
- Confirm to whom you are speaking and their relationship with patient
- Use open questions to elicit their concerns

History

- Clarify key features of cognitive decline
  - Nature of problems (memory and/or other domains)?
  - Acute, chronic, acute on chronic?
  - Associated with functional impairment?
  - Associated with risk? (e.g., wandering, cooking)
- Screen for precipitants of decline
  - Medication changes
  - Physical health changes
  - Depression

Differential diagnosis is of delirium, dementia or depression.

Initial management should include:

- Same-day review (GP home visit or A&E attendance).
- Initial investigations to include a full physical exam, urine dipstick and blood tests.

A good student would specify most of the required blood tests (FBC, U&E, LFT, TFT, glucose, Ca, PO_4, Mg, B_{12}/folate), an excellent student would specify them all. An excellent student would also suggest other investigations that may be indicated by the patient's physical symptoms/signs (e.g., MSU, ECG, CXR, CT head).

A good student would also suggest a structured cognitive assessment. A very good student would specify an appropriate test (4AT, AMT, ACE-III, MOCA).

Discriminating viva questions

1. What are the causes of delirium?
   (see Table 19.1)
2. Where should delirium be managed?
   (see Chapter 20, Delirium: management)
3. What medication can be of benefit in delirium?
   (see Chapter 20, Delirium: management and Fig. 20.2)
4. What environmental modifications can be of benefit in delirium?
   (see Chapter 20, Delirium: management and Fig. 20.2)
5. What is the prognosis of delirium?
   (see Chapter 20, Delirium: course and prognosis)

HISTORY OF LOW MOOD

Candidate instructions

You are a medical student attached to a General Practice. Your next patient is Mr Smith, a 57-year-old man with COPD. His sister has booked him an appointment because she is concerned about his mood.

There are two parts to this station:

1. Take a history of the presenting complaint and relevant background from Mr Smith in order to establish the most likely diagnosis.
   Do not take a full psychiatric history.
2. Conduct a mental state examination alongside taking a history.
3. With 2 minutes remaining, the examiner will ask you to:
   • Suggest your differential diagnosis
   • Explain your reasoning based on your findings from the history
   • Suggest an initial management plan

You have 8 minutes for this station.

CHECKLIST

Communication

- Introduce yourself
- Clarify to whom you are speaking
- Communicate sensitively with someone who is depressed

History

- The three clusters of depression symptoms:
  - Affective: Depressed mood, anhedonia
  - Cognitive-behavioural: Impaired concentration, low self-esteem/guilt, hopelessness, thoughts of death or suicide
  - Neurovegetative: Sleep disturbance, appetite changes, psychomotor agitation/ retardation, fatigue
- Screen for psychotic symptoms
- Possible triggers (e.g., stress, chronic pain, social circumstances)
- Substance use
- Past psychiatric history
- Family psychiatric history
- Past medical history

Initial management.

This will depend on severity of depressive episode and patient preference.

- Lifestyle advice (sleep hygiene, physical activity, avoid substances)
- Psychological therapies
- Pharmacological treatments

Discriminating viva questions

1. How common is depression?
   (see Table 24.1)

2. What is the heritability of depression?
   (see Chapter 24, Depressive disorders: aetiology, genetics)
3. What would a first-line antidepressant be?
   (see Chapter 24, Depressive disorders: management, pharmacological treatment)
4. What would a first-line high-intensity psychological intervention be?
   (see Fig. 24.2)
5. How would you distinguish mild from moderate-severe depression?
   (see Chapter 11, Depressive episode specifiers)

ASSESSING RISK TO SELF

Candidate instructions

You are a medical student in A&E. A 37-year-old patient is in the department after taking an overdose. The A&E team have assessed them and they do not require any medical treatment. You are asked to assess whether they are safe to go home, then report your findings to a senior doctor.

There are three parts to this station:

1. Take a history focusing on their recent overdose, and relevant background information.
   Do not take a full psychiatric history.
2. Conduct a mental state examination alongside taking a history.
3. With 2 minutes remaining, the examiner will ask you to:
   • Estimate the patient's risk to themselves
   • Explain your reasoning based on findings from your history and mental state examination
   • Present a brief initial management plan

You have 8 minutes in total for this station.

CHECKLIST

Communication

- Introduce yourself
- Clarify to whom you are speaking
- Communicate sensitively with someone who is distressed

History

- Assess the presence of ongoing suicidal intent or not (pass/fail)
  - Circumstances of the overdose
    - Planning
    - Final acts
    - Intent
    - Method used
    - Perceived lethality
    - Circumstances of discovery
    - Whether regretful
    - Role of substances
- Assess for contributory factors (stress, relationships, employment, physical illness)
- Assess for protective factors
- Assess for current social support
- Past psychiatric history (including previous self-harm)
- Evidence for current mental disorder

Initial management

Initial management will depend greatly on the severity of risk the patient presents, and on the contributing and positive factors. Consider a short- and long-term plan which may include:

- Crisis contact details (e.g., helplines, mental health services)
- Reducing access to means of self-harm (e.g., removal of unnecessary medication)
- Involvement of existing social supports
- Low-intensity support (e.g., GP review, referral to psychiatric outpatients)
- High-intensity support (e.g., crisis team, hospital admission)

Discriminating viva questions

1. What are the risk factors for suicide?
   (see Box 6.1)
2. Which methods of suicide place the patient at highest risk of death?
   (see Chapter 6, Assessment of patients who have inflicted harm upon themselves: suicidal intent)
3. What mental disorders are associated with an increased risk of suicide?
   (see Table 6.1)
4. How many times more likely is someone with a borderline pattern personality disorder to end their life via suicide?
   (see Table 6.1)
5. Are people who self-harm at increased risk of suicide?
   (see Chapter 6, Assessment of patients who have inflicted harm upon themselves: introductory paragraph)

BRIEF ALCOHOL INTERVENTION

Candidate instructions

You are a medical student attached to a general practice. Your next patient is Mr Brown, a 47-year-old man who had abnormal liver function tests (mildly elevated gamma GT and transaminases) noted as part of a routine medical exam for insurance purposes. You have been asked to meet with him to take an alcohol history and offer a brief alcohol intervention if indicated.

There are two parts to this station:

1. Take an alcohol history, establishing how many units Mr Brown drinks per week and any harm caused by alcohol.
   Do not take a full psychiatric history.
   Do not take a full history regarding causes of abnormal liver function tests.
2. Provide a brief alcohol intervention, covering Mr Brown's motivation to change and options for how to do so.
   You have 8 minutes for this station. You are advised to spend around 4 minutes on each part.

CHECKLIST

Communication

- Check patient's understanding, e.g., are they aware of the abnormal LFTs? What do they think caused them?
- Use non-judgemental tone and language
- Demonstrate empathy
- Encourage self-efficacy of patient: express confidence in their ability to change. An excellent student would elicit confident statements from patient
- Use a mixture of open and closed questions

History

- Use of alcohol
  - Typical weekly alcohol consumption in sufficient detail to allow calculation of units (e.g., size of bottles, typical strength of beer or wine)
  - Pattern of drinking: every day? Binges?
  - Duration of drinking
  - Used alongside any other substances?
- Harm caused by drinking
  - Livelihood – problems with employment?
  - Liver – health: physical or mental harm?
  - Love – problems with relationships?
  - Law – criminal charges?
- Features of dependence.
- *Impaired control* over substance use, including how often, how much, and when to stop.

Continued

- *Increasing priority* given to substances, over, e.g., relationships, work, school, or activities of daily living.
- *Physiological features* of dependence such as increasing tolerance or withdrawal symptoms.

Initial management (provision of a brief alcohol intervention using aspects of FRAMES)

(Appropriate feedback, advice and menu will depend on history. The below is appropriate if Mr Jones is a harmful drinker but not dependent)

- Feedback – the harm caused by alcohol (abnormal LFT, potentially other harms from history).
- Responsibility – emphasize to the patient the decision is theirs. Ask the patient what they would like to do.
- Advice – advise to cut back on use to within low-risk drinking guidelines (see Fig. 17.2).
- Menu – offer a range of patient-centred practical steps. An excellent candidate would come up with options collaboratively with the patient, including options to circumvent things the patient sees as barriers to change. Potential next steps are:
  - Alcohol diary
  - Alcohol-free days
  - Putting money that would have been spent on alcohol aside for a treat
  - Alternative activity to alcohol, e.g., going to sports class on Friday night instead of pub
  - Attending third-sector alcohol counselling or mutual aid

Empathy and self-efficacy are covered under communication.

Discriminating viva questions

1. What are maximum weekly units for men and for women advised by the low-risk drinking guidelines? (see Fig. 17.2)
2. What type of cancers is Mr Brown at increased risk of? (see Box 17.2)
3. What stage is Mr Brown at in the Prochaska and DiClemente model of change? (see Fig. 22.3)
4. If Mr Brown decides he wishes to become abstinent, will he need a detoxification with benzodiazepines? (see Chapter 22, Management: treatment of alcohol withdrawal)
5. If Mr Brown decides he wishes to become abstinent, what medication could help him? (see Chapter 22, Management: maintenance after detoxification, pharmacological therapy)

SCHIZOPHRENIA EXPLANATION AND ADVICE

Candidate instructions

Background

You are a 5th-year medical student on your Psychiatry attachment where you meet Alex White, a 23-year-old man who has recently been diagnosed with schizophrenia. For a year he has experienced auditory hallucinations of three CIA agents talking about him amongst themselves. He holds the delusional belief that the CIA have placed a brain chip in him that broadcasts his thoughts to them. He has made a cut in his scalp to try to remove the chip. He does not believe he is unwell and last week was admitted to hospital using the mental health act. He has not yet received any treatment. He has never used recreational substances.

You have been asked to speak to Alex's mother about his diagnosis and what treatment may be available.

Your task is to explore her understanding of schizophrenia and answer her questions. Alex has given permission for you to share information with his mother.

You have 8 minutes in total for this station.

CHECKLIST

Communication

- Check mother's initial understanding – of Alex's symptoms, diagnosis and treatment options
- Demonstrate empathy
- An excellent student will summarize information
- An excellent student will check mother's understanding at end

Explanation and advice

Likely questions to cover would be:

- What is schizophrenia?
- What are the symptoms of schizophrenia?
- What is a hallucination?
- What causes schizophrenia?
- Why has the mental health act been used to keep Alex in hospital?

(Note risk and poor insight highlighted in history)

- How can schizophrenia be treated?
- What are the common side effects of medication?
- What happens if Alex refuses medication?
- What is the long-term outcome likely to be for Alex?
- If Alex has a child, what is their chance of having schizophrenia?

Discriminating viva questions

1. What is the mechanism of action of antipsychotics?
   (see Chapter 2, Antipsychotics: mechanism of action)
2. What is the management of treatment-resistant schizophrenia?
   (see Chapter 21, Management, pharmacological treatments, treatment-resistant schizophrenia)
3. Does Alex have any first-rank symptoms of schizophrenia?
   (see Box 9.3)
4. What psychological therapies are used in schizophrenia?
   (see Chapter 23, Management, psychological treatments)
5. What physical health monitoring should Alex receive if he remains on antipsychotics?
   (see Chapter 23, Management, physical health monitoring)

HISTORY OF ANXIETY

Candidate instructions

You are a medical student attached to a General Practice. Your next patient is Lisa Johnson, a 27-year-old woman with anxiety.

There are two parts to this station:

1. Take a history of the presenting complaint and relevant background from Lisa in order to establish the most likely diagnosis.
   Do not take a full psychiatric history.
2. Conduct a mental state examination alongside taking a history.
3. With 2 minutes remaining, the examiner will ask you to:
   - Suggest your differential diagnosis
   - Explain your reasoning based on your findings from the history
   - Suggest an initial management plan

You have 8 minutes for this station.

CHECKLIST

Communication

- Introduce yourself
- Clarify to whom you are speaking
- Communicate sensitively with someone who is anxious

History

Check for core symptoms of range of anxiety disorders.

- Onset after life event?
(Adjustment disorder, acute stress reaction, PTSD – if considering PTSD, screen for hypervigilance, re-experiencing and avoidance)

- Onset unrelated to life event?
  - Anxious only following clear trigger?
  - Particular situations? (specific phobia, social anxiety, agoraphobia)
  - Intrusive thought or image? (OCD or related disorder – check for compulsions)
  - Anxious unpredictably, in range of situations?
  - Panic attacks (panic disorder)
  - Free-floating, multiple topics (GAD – check for motor tension and autonomic overactivity)
- Assess for low mood
- Check for thoughts of self-harm or suicide
- Screen for psychotic symptoms
- Possible triggers (e.g., stress, chronic pain, social circumstances)
- Substance use
- Past psychiatric history
- Family psychiatric history
- Past medical history

Initial management:

This will depend on severity of anxiety and patient preference.

- Lifestyle advice (sleep hygiene, avoid substances).
- Psychological therapies – these are first line for all anxiety disorders. Primarily self-help for milder cases and CBT for moderate-severe cases.
- Pharmacological treatments – second line. SSRIs are recommended first.

Discriminating viva questions

1. What investigations would you perform in someone presenting with anxiety for the first time? (see Chapter 12, Investigations)
2. Which anxiety disorders have the highest heritability? (see Chapter 25, Anxiety disorders, aetiology)
3. What would a first-line medication be for GAD? (see Chapter 25, Anxiety disorders, management)
4. What would a first-line high-intensity psychological intervention be for OCD? (see Chapter 25, Obsessive-compulsive disorders, management)
5. What is the role of benzodiazepines in managing anxiety disorders? (see Chapter 25, Anxiety disorders, management)

CLINICAL CASES

CASE 1 – First episode psychosis in a young person

A 22-year-old man presents with auditory hallucinations.

Q1. What differential diagnoses would you consider for this patient?

- Psychosis secondary to a general medical condition
- Substance intoxication
- Substance withdrawal
- Substance-induced psychotic disorder
- Schizophrenia
- Acute and transient psychotic disorder
- Other primary psychotic disorder
- Schizoaffective disorder
- Mania with psychotic symptoms
- Depressive episode with psychotic symptoms

Psychosis secondary to a general medical condition – suggested by presence of a physical health problem associated with psychosis (e.g., temporal lobe epilepsy, Huntington's, HIV) or presence of severe systemic disease leading to delirium. Treatment of the physical health problem (where possible) should improve the psychosis.

Substance intoxication/withdrawal/substance-induced psychotic disorder – use of a psychoactive substance prior to onset of symptoms, particularly one known to be associated with psychotic symptoms (cocaine, amphetamines, cannabis, extensive alcohol use) or withdrawal from a psychoactive substance (e.g., alcohol withdrawal).

Schizophrenia – suggested by *gradual onset associated with social and occupational decline.* Symptoms lasting longer than 1 month. Must have at least two of the key diagnostic features, which include persistent delusions, persistent hallucinations, disorganized thinking, experiences of influence, passivity or control or negative symptoms. First-rank symptoms are highly suggestive of schizophrenia but not essential to diagnosis.

Acute and transient psychotic disorder – *acute onset without a prodrome, with symptoms typically lasting less than 1 month.* Symptoms change rapidly and negative symptoms are not present. Often follow acute stress. If symptoms are not polymorphic or negative symptoms are present consider other primary psychotic disorder.

Schizoaffective disorder – prominent mood symptoms (sufficient to diagnose mania or depression) and symptoms typical of schizophrenia (bizarre delusions or hallucinations) arise around the same time and within the same episode of illness.

Mania with psychotic symptoms – presence of manic symptoms (e.g., elated or irritable mood, reduced sleep, reduced appetite, increased energy, poor concentration). Mood congruent psychotic symptoms (e.g., grandiose delusions, encouraging auditory hallucinations).

Depression with psychotic symptoms – presence of core depressive symptoms (low mood, fatigue, anhedonia). Mood congruent psychotic symptoms (e.g., nihilistic delusions, derogatory second-person auditory hallucinations)

Q2. What information would you seek in the clinical examination?

a. Mental state examination

Appearance and behaviour:

- Poor self-care suggests an insidious onset with social decline, suggesting schizophrenia.
- Abnormal movements may suggest catatonia.
- Agitation can suggest intoxication, withdrawal, mania or psychosis.

Speech: pressured speech or wordplay suggests mania, delayed speech or poverty of speech in single-episode depressive disorder with psychotic symptoms.

Mood: lowered or elated mood suggests depression or mania.

Thought form: flight of ideas suggests mania, loosening of associations suggests psychosis.

Thought content: bizarre delusions (e.g., thought insertion/withdrawal/broadcast or passivity phenomena) suggest schizophrenia. Grandiose delusions suggest mania with psychotic symptoms. Nihilistic delusions suggest single-episode depressive disorder with psychotic symptoms.

Perception: visual hallucinations are more common in psychosis secondary to a medical condition/delirium.

Cognition: distractibility suggests mania or delirium.

b. General examination

Inspection:

- Injection sites suggestive of substance use
- Intoxication with a substance, e.g., constricted pupils, slurred speech, ataxia

Endocrine: goitre may suggest hypo or hyperthyroidism

Neurological:

- Symptoms of catatonia suggestive of schizophrenia
- Abnormal movements suggestive of Huntington's
- Peripheral neuropathy suggestive of vitamin B_{12}/folate deficiency or prolonged alcohol excess

Q3. What investigations would you request?

a. For everyone

- Full blood count (FBC), urea and electrolytes (U&E), liver function test (LFT), Ca, thyroid function test (TFT), prolactin, glucose, C-reactive protein/erythrocyte sedimentation rate (CRP/ESR) – to screen for potential general medical causes of psychosis and to establish pretreatment baselines.
- Toxicology – typically an oral or urine drug screen, to screen for common psychoactive substances.
- ECG to provide pretreatment baseline, particularly if any cardiac history.

b. Consider

- Consider Computed tomography (CT) or magnetic resonance imaging (MRI) head if case is atypical, not responding to treatment or any neurological abnormalities.
- Syphilis or HIV serology if indicated by history.

CASE 2 – Weight loss in an adolescent

A 16-year-old female presents with weight loss.

Q1. What differential diagnoses would you consider for this patient?

- Weight loss secondary to a general medical condition
- Substance use (including alcohol)
- Psychotic disorder
- Depression
- Obsessive-compulsive disorder
- Anorexia nervosa
- Bulimia nervosa
- Avoidant restrictive food intake disorder

Weight loss secondary to a general medical condition – check for past history and assess for current symptoms of systemic illness, gastrointestinal illness, endocrine disorders (e.g., hyperthyroidism, diabetes) or malignancy.

Substance use – alcohol can lead to weight loss if patients spend money on alcohol rather than food, and through malabsorption. Amphetamines and other stimulants suppress appetite.

Psychotic disorder – this is unlikely in a 16-year old but important not to miss. Psychotic symptoms can lead to weight loss directly (e.g., delusional belief that food is poisoned or that person already dead) or indirectly (distress due to psychotic experiences reducing appetite).

Depression – a severe depression can reduce appetite. In anorexia, appetite is usually maintained until late in illness. Check for core symptoms of depression (*low mood, fatigue,*

anhedonia). These symptoms are also caused by severe weight loss, so a longitudinal history is important (low mood then weight loss is more suggestive of depression).

Obsessive-compulsive disorder – obsessions can lead to weight loss directly (e.g., fears of contamination) or indirectly (e.g., time spent on time-consuming rituals around meal times leaving little time to eat).

Anorexia nervosa – *significantly low body weight with persistent pattern of behaviours aimed to prevent restoration of normal body weight.* Commonly used threshold is body mass index (BMI) < 18.5 kg/m^2 for adults and BMI for age under 5th centile for young people under 18. Often accompanied with physical complications of starvation, including amenorrhoea, bradycardia, postural hypotension, hypothermia and biochemical abnormalities.

Bulimia nervosa – *over-valued idea of being fat* coupled with episodes of binge eating and compensatory behaviours, e.g., self-induced vomiting. Behaviours usually result in a normal or increased weight. This diagnosis is unlikely given the presentation with weight loss.

Avoidant restrictive food intake disorder – *avoidance or restriction of food* resulting in significant weight loss *without preoccupation with low body weight.*

Q2. What information would you seek in the clinical examination?

a. Mental state examination

- Mood: lowered mood suggests depression or response to starvation.
- Thought content: overvalued idea about body shape being too fat suggests anorexia nervosa or bulimia nervosa. Obsessions suggest OCD and delusions suggest a psychotic illness.
- Cognition: concentration and memory are likely to be impaired in someone who is significantly underweight.

b. General examination

Inspection:

- Observations, including weight and height (BMI < 18.5 or loss of >20% of body weight in 6 month period suggests anorexia in adults, hypothermia suggests anorexia)
- Lanugo hair (anorexia)
- Callused knuckles (self-induced vomiting (Russel sign))
- Poor dentition (frequent vomiting)
- Signs of puberty (delayed if anorexia of early onset)
- Signs of dehydration (anorexia)

Cardiovascular: pulse, erect and supine blood pressure (dehydration in anorexia).

Gastrointestinal: faecal loading common in anorexia (dehydration).

Musculoskeletal: sit-up, stand-squat (SUSS) test – proximal muscle wasting suggests anorexia.

> **RED FLAG**
>
> See Red Flag box in Chapter 16 for high-risk physical findings in anorexia. When assessing physical risk of eating disorders in people under 18 years old, refer to age-specific guidelines.

Q3. What investigations would you request?

a. For everyone

- FBC, U&E, LFT, amylase, TFT, glucose, lipids, CRP/ESR – to screen for potential general medical causes of weight loss and to assess for complications of weight loss.
- ECG (to assess for conduction changes secondary to starvation).

b. Consider

- DXA scan to assess bone density.
- Toxicology – typically an oral or urine drug screen to screen for common psychoactive substances.

CASE 3 – Inattention in a child

A 7-year-old boy presents with trouble paying attention at school.

Q1. What differential diagnoses would you consider for this patient?

- Normal for age
- Secondary to sensory impairment
- Secondary to mental or physical health problem
- Secondary to psychosocial adversity
- Intellectual disability
- Attention deficit hyperactivity disorder
- Disruptive behaviour disorders
- Specific learning difficulty, e.g., dyslexia

Normal for age – children are less able to sustain attention than adults. Check with the caregivers and teacher as to whether the child's behaviour is different to his peers.

Secondary to sensory impairment – difficulty hearing or seeing can make a child appear inattentive. They may also be bored and stop paying attention if they cannot fully participate in an activity, e.g., cannot hear a story.

Secondary to mental or physical health problem – if a child is preoccupied or distracted by pain, anxiety or any other sort of discomfort, they will be less able to pay attention.

Secondary to psychosocial adversity – if a child is hungry, or worried about a caregiver's behaviour towards them (e.g., abuse) or experiencing illness or bereavement in the family, this may result in them not focussing on schoolwork.

Intellectual disability – if schoolwork is too hard, or too easy, a child will not be able to engage with it.

Attention deficit hyperactivity disorder – the core symptoms are *impaired attention, impulsivity and hyperactivity*. These should be present and persistent in multiple settings.

Disruptive behaviour disorders (oppositional defiant disorder or conduct-dissocial disorder) – a child has the ability to pay attention but something in their life or upbringing is making it hard for them to do so. A history of trauma or attachment problems are very common among children and young people with disruptive behaviour disorders. Associated features are limited expression of emotions, limited remorse or guilt about their behaviour and limited capacity for empathy towards others.

Specific learning difficulty – a child with a specific learning difficulty is able to sustain attention in most areas and at home but may struggle with lessons related to a topic they find particularly difficult, e.g., dyscalculia may lead to inattention during maths, dyslexia to inattention during reading.

Q2. What information would you seek in the clinical examination?

a. Mental state examination

Appearance and behaviour:

- Dysmorphic features suggest an intellectual disability.
- Excess activity (e.g., noisy play, running around) during the consultation suggests ADHD.
- Abnormal caregiver–child interaction (e.g., child appears scared of parent) raises possibility of child abuse.
- Challenging behaviour during consultation suggests disruptive behaviour disorder (e.g., refusing to enter room, running away, assaultative behaviour).

Speech: over-talkativeness and interrupting suggest ADHD. Cognition:

- Not paying attention to information and asking repetitive questions suggest ADHD.
- Distractibility by external stimuli suggests ADHD.
- Difficulty comprehending questions suggests intellectual disability.

b. General examination

Inspection:

- Dysmorphic signs suggest intellectual disability.
- Signs of general medical disorder may suggest pain or discomfort.
- Signs of malnutrition (e.g., low weight, rickets) suggest child neglect.

Test hearing and vision.

Q3. What investigations would you request?

a. For everyone

- No investigations are mandatory in assessment for neurodevelopmental disorder.

b. Consider

- Genetic testing for known causes of intellectual disability
- Blood tests as indicated if general medical cause suspected
- Structured rating scales for symptoms of ADHD completed by parents and teachers can be useful

CASE 4 – Memory problems in an older adult

A 77-year-old woman presents with trouble remembering names.

Q1. What differential diagnoses would you consider for this patient?

- Delirium
- Dementia
- Mild neurocognitive disorder
- Subjective cognitive impairment
- Stable cognitive impairment post insult
- Depression
- Psychotic disorders
- Amnestic disorder

Delirium – this is important not to miss. Check for its core features: acute or fluctuating cognitive impairment, altered conscious level and inattention.

Dementia – trouble remembering names by itself is not a big problem. If it is associated with objective cognitive impairment which is *generalized, progressive* (over several months) and associated with *functional impairment*, consider the diagnosis of dementia. Fluctuations in impairment or consciousness level make delirium more likely.

Mild cognitive impairment – *objective cognitive impairment which is not associated with functional impairment*. This is a risk state for later onset of dementia.

Subjective cognitive impairment – if a patient scores normally on standardized cognitive testing but still feels they have a problem with their cognition.

Stable cognitive impairment post insult – objective impairment on standardized test following a one-off insult to the brain, e.g., stroke, viral encephalitis. Impairment should not be progressive. If affecting memory, it may be termed an amnestic disorder.

Depression – depression impairs concentration and memory. Assess for the core features (low mood, fatigue, anhedonia). These features can occur with advanced dementia but are unlikely to be prominent in early dementia.

Psychotic disorders – negative symptoms in schizophrenia can include marked cognitive deficits but these will have gradually worsened from the time of the onset of the psychotic illness.

Amnestic disorder – suggested if objective cognitive impairment only involves anterograde memory and there is strong evidence of a brain disease known to cause the amnesic disorder (e.g., Korsakoff's, head injury, stroke).

Q2. What information would you seek in the clinical examination?

a. Mental state examination

Appearance and behaviour:

- Poor self-care or poor punctuality suggests functional impairment.
- Disinhibition or abnormal social manner suggests frontotemporal dementia.

Speech: increased latency or word-finding difficulties suggest dementia (particularly frontotemporal dementia).
Mood: low mood suggests depression. Anxiety may precipitate subjective cognitive impairment.
Thought content: negative cognitions suggest depression.
Perceptions: hallucinations suggest Lewy body dementia or delirium.
Cognition:

- Altered conscious level suggests delirium.
- Inattention or distractibility suggests delirium.
- Impairment on standardized cognitive test excludes subjective cognitive impairment.
- Confabulation (plausible recounting of untrue autobiographical information) suggests amnestic syndrome.

b. General examination

Check hearing and vision.
Inspection:

- Signs of malnutrition (e.g., low weight) or injury suggest functional impairment.
- Abnormal gait suggests vascular dementia, Parkinsonism (Lewy body dementia), Huntington's.

Cardiovascular:

- Hypertension and atrial fibrillation are risk factors for dementia.

Neurological:

- Focal neurological signs suggest vascular dementia.
- Parkinsonism (bradykinesia, rigidity, tremor) suggests Lewy body dementia.
- Abnormal movements (e.g., dystonia, chorea) suggest Huntington's.

Q3. What investigations would you request?

a. For everyone

If diagnosis is subjective cognitive impairment, psychosis or depression, these investigations are not needed, but if there is any doubt it is safer to perform them.

- U&E, Ca, TFT, glucose, vitamin B_{12}/folate to exclude reversible causes of dementia.

b. Consider

- Structural brain imaging (CT or MRI) to exclude reversible causes of dementia.
- In delirium, further tests as indicated e.g., ECG, CXR, urinalysis.
- Syphilis or HIV screening if indicated by history (can cause dementia).
- Genetic testing in young onset dementia, e.g., Huntington's, Alzheimer's.
- Functional brain imaging to support diagnosis of subtypes of dementia, e.g., hypoactivation of frontal lobes in frontotemporal dementia.

Q4. What potential reversible cause of dementia should be further investigated given these blood results (see table 35.1 below for example blood results)?

Table 35.1 Example blood results		
Blood test	**Result**	**Normal value**
Sodium	129 mmol/L	133–146 mmol/L
Potassium	5.9 mmol/L	3.5–5.3 mmol/L
Calcium (adjusted)	2.4 mmol/L	2.2–2.6 mmol/L
Magnesium	0.89 mmol/L	0.7–1.0 mmol/L
Chloride	99 mmol/ L	98–106 mmol/L
Phosphate	1.2 mmol/ L	0.74–1.4 mmol/L
Urea	6.9 mmol/L	2.5–7.8 mmol/L

Answer: Addison's disease.

CASE 5 – Medically unexplained symptoms in an adult

A 37-year-old woman repeatedly presents with extreme concern about tingling in her arm, which has been appropriately investigated with no problems identified.

Q1. What differential diagnoses would you consider for this patient?

- Undiagnosed unknown medical condition
- Undiagnosed known medical condition
- Dissociative neurological symptoms disorder (functional disorder)
- Hypochondriasis
- Bodily distress disorder
- Body dysmorphic disorder
- Factitious disorder/malingering
- Anxiety disorder
- Mood disorder
- Psychotic disorder

Undiagnosed unknown medical condition – this is *impossible to exclude.* Positive features of other conditions (see later) can make this unlikely.

Undiagnosed known medical condition (e.g., systemic lupus erythematosus, multiple sclerosis) – *known conditions should always be excluded* with minimally invasive tests proportionate to the symptom and its associated features.

Dissociative neurological symptom disorder (functional disorder) – this is the most likely diagnosis given the brief details given. It would be supported by a nondermatomal pattern of paraesthesia and positive signs of other functional symptoms (such as Hoover sign and tremor entrainment (see Table 14.1)). The diagnosis would also be supported by past trauma or a recent stressful event, although this is not essential to the diagnosis. 'Functional disorder' is an umbrella term for *presumed dysfunction in high-level cortical processing* of motor and sensory information leading to symptoms which are genuinely experienced and involuntary, even though no structural or physiological abnormality is identified.

Bodily distress disorder – this is suggested by bodily symptoms that are *distressing to the individual, with excessive attention being directed toward the symptoms.* The patient could have had multiple other symptoms from multiple other systems which have also been investigated without finding physiological abnormality (e.g., diarrhoea, urinary frequency, muscle pain).

Hypochondriasis – persistent *preoccupation about the possibility of having a serious illness* suggests hypochondriasis. Associated with repetitive and excessive health-related behaviours, e.g., repeatedly checking body or researching the illness.

Body dysmorphic disorder – concern about one or more *subjectively perceived defects with appearance* with associated *repetitive and excessive behaviours* associated with the body part, e.g., checking in mirror would suggest body dysmorphic disorder. What does the patient think about the appearance of their arm?

Factitious disorder/malingering – these are suggested by evidence that the *symptom is fabricated*. Given the intrinsically subjective nature of paraesthesia, this could only be proven if the patient reported they had been lying about their experiences. If the gain is to receive health care, this is factitious disorder. If the gain is secondary (e.g., access to disability benefits as a result of symptoms) the diagnosis is malingering.

Anxiety disorder – *paraethesia is a common symptom of anxiety*. Screen for other physical symptoms of anxiety (e.g., muscle tension, palpitations) and ask about anxious cognitions. Check if the paraesthesia is continuous or episodic, if episodic, what is the trigger?

Mood disorder – sometimes patients attend GPs regarding minor symptoms when the true problem is a mood problem, or a psychosocial stressor. Check for common symptoms of depression (*low mood, fatigue, anhedonia*) and ask what else is going on in the patient's life.

Psychotic disorder – this is unlikely but important not to miss. Carefully assess the patient's beliefs about the origin of the sensation. It could potentially be a passivity symptom (a delusion that others are controlling what the patient thinks or feels).

Q2. What information would you seek in the clinical examination?

a. Mental state examination

Appearance and behaviour:

- Evidence of functional symptoms, e.g., atypical ataxia?
- Evidence of abnormal illness behaviour, e.g., holding the arm in a sling? (which would not be expected to alleviate paraesthesia).

Mood: low mood suggests depression. Check also for anxiety. Thought content: assess the patient's concerns carefully. Are they worried about the tingling itself (bodily distress disorder), the possibility of a serious underlying illness (hypochondriacal disorder) or about an effect on their appearance (body dysmorphic disorder)? Are they delusional?

b. General examination

A thorough physical examination on the relevant system is required when a patient first presents with a symptom. However, if the symptom is unchanged there is no benefit in repeating the examination.

Consider assessing for positive signs of other functional neurological conditions (see Table 14.2).

Q3. What investigations would you request?

a. For everyone

- No investigations can be used to diagnose a functional or bodily distress disorder.

b. Consider

- Relevant investigation of the symptom in a proportionate and minimally invasive way.

High yield association table

Presentations

Topic	If this...	Then that...
Neurodevelopmental disorders	A female with normal development until 5 months, with gradual loss of skills/functioning after 6 months	Rett syndrome
	A child with an intellectual disability, a long face, prominent ears and jaw, and machroorchidism (if male)	Fragile X
	A child with an intellectual disability, congenital cardiac defects, a high-pitched voice, a cleft palette	22q11.2 deletion syndrome (DiGeorge/velocardiofacial syndrome)
	A child with a narrow face, almond-shaped eyes, excessive weight gain and hunger, hypogonadism	Prader-Willi syndrome
	Lifelong difficulties in social interactions and rigid/inflexible patterns of behaviour	Autism spectrum disorder
	Lifelong difficulties with inattentiveness and hyperactivity	Attention deficit hyperactivity disorder
	A patient with an intellectual disability, microcephaly, growth restriction, executive functioning problems	Foetal alcohol syndrome
Mood disorders	Irritability, disinhibition, pressured speech, grandiosity, increased energy	Mania
	Low mood, early morning wakening, impaired concentration and anhedonia	Depression
Psychotic disorders	Persistent delusions, auditory hallucinations, thought disorder, experiences of external control, disorganized behaviour WITHOUT mood symptoms	Schizophrenia
	Persistent delusions, auditory hallucinations, thought disorder, experiences of external control, disorganized behaviour WITH mood symptoms	Schizoaffective disorder
Anxiety disorders	Anxiety symptoms when in a situation from which escape might be difficult, e.g., crowded shop	Agoraphobia
	Anxiety symptoms in social situations or when expected to perform in front of others (e.g., giving a speech)	Social anxiety disorder
	Anxiety symptoms when exposed to one specific stimulus (e.g., spiders, heights)	Specific phobia
	Panic symptoms unrelated to a particular situation	Panic disorder
	Free-floating anxiety	Generalised anxiety disorder
Obsessions/compulsions	Ego-dystonic intrusive thoughts, compulsive rituals/behaviours	Obsessive-compulsive disorder
	Preoccupation with a perceived defect in personal appearance	Body dysmorphic disorder
Reaction to stress	Reexperiencing a previous traumatic event in the present, avoidant behaviour and persistent perceptions of heightened threat	Post traumatic stress disorder
	Reexperiencing a previous traumatic event in the present, avoidant behaviour and persistent perceptions of heightened threat AND with affect regulation difficulties, low self-worth and difficulties in interpersonal relationships	Complex post traumatic stress disorder
	Pervasive grief, intense emotional pain, longing for deceased individual, symptoms lasting longer than cultural norms	Prolonged grief disorder

Continued

Topic	If this...	Then that...
Abnormal response to physical symptoms	Significant distress related to physical symptoms that have no identified physical cause	Bodily distress disorder
	Concern about having a serious illness with associated excessive health-related behaviours	Hypochondriasis
Eating or weight problems	Low body weight, amenorrhea, lanugo hair	Anorexia nervosa
	Normal or increased body weight, binge-purging	Bulimia
	Normal or increased body weight, binging without purging	Binge eating disorder
Alcohol/substance use	Tremors, nausea, vomiting, tachycardia, increased anxiety, seizures/hallucinations	Alcohol withdrawal
	Altered conscious level, confusion and hallucinations approximately 48 hours after admission	Delirium tremens
	Ataxia, ophthalmoplegia and acute cognitive impairment	Wernicke encephalopathy
Impairment in cognition/consciousness	Acute and fluctuating confusion with impaired cognition and sleep/wake cycle	Delirium
	Gradual onset, executive functioning and progressive memory problems, word finding difficulties and functional impairment	Alzheimer dementia
	Stepwise deterioration in memory and functioning	Vascular dementia
	Parkinsonism, visual hallucinations, fluctuating cognition	Lewy body dementia
	Significant personality and behaviour change, language problems, apathy, emotional blunting	Frontotemporal dementia

Management		
Topic	If this...	Then that...
Neurodevelopmental disorders	Attention deficit hyperactivity disorder (ADHD) in <18s	Parent training programme (1st line) Methylphenidate (2nd line)
	Attention deficit hyperactivity disorder (ADHD) in >18s	Methylphenidate or lisdexamfetamine
Mood disorders	Acute mania in >18s	Haloperidol, olanzapine, risperidone or quetiapine
	Bipolar affective disorder – long-term management	Lithium (1st line) Valproate (2nd line if patient >55/not of childbearing potential)
	Choosing an antidepressant in <18s	Fluoxetine
	Treatment of less severe depression in >18s	Psychological therapy
	Treatment of more severe depression in >18s	Psychological therapy + SSRI
Psychotic disorders	Schizophrenia	Atypical antipsychotic
	Schizoaffective disorder	Atypical antipsychotic
Obsessions/compulsions	Obsessive-compulsive disorder with mild functional impairment	CBT with ERP
	Obsessive-compulsive disorder with moderate/severe functional impairment	CBT with ERP + SSRI
Reaction to stress	Post traumatic stress disorder	Trauma-focused CBT

Topic	If this...	Then that...
Eating or weight problems	Anorexia nervosa in <18s	Family-based treatment (FBT; 1st line), individual eating-disorder-focused cognitive behavioural therapy (CBT-ED; 2nd line)
	Anorexia nervosa in >18s	Individual eating-disorder-focused cognitive behavioural therapy (CBT-ED), Maudsley anorexia nervosa treatment for adults (MANTRA) or specialist supportive clinical management (SSCM)
	Bulimia nervosa in <18s	FBT
	Bulimia nervosa in >18s	CBT-ED
Alcohol/substance use	Alcohol withdrawal	Supportive management, benzodiazepines, Pabrinex
	Wernicke encephalopathy	Pabrinex
	Opioid dependence	Harm reduction, methadone or buprenorphine
	Opioid overdose	Naloxone
	Alcohol dependence	Psychological intervention, acamprosate, naltrexone – 1st line, disulfiram – 2nd line
Impairment in cognition/consciousness	Delirium	Identify and treat underlying cause
	Distress in delirium	Identify and treat underlying cause, verbal and nonverbal de-escalation if distressed – 1st line, short-term low dose haloperidol – 2nd line
	Alzheimer dementia	Acetylcholinesterase inhibitors, e.g., donepezil/rivastigmine/galantamine – 1st line, memantine – 2nd line
	Vascular dementia	No specific pharmacological treatment
	Dementia with Lewy bodies	Rivastigmine or donepezil
	Frontotemporal dementia	No specific pharmacological treatment
	Symptoms of stress and distress in dementia	Exclude physical or environmental cause, verbal, and nonverbal de-escalation – 1st line, risperidone – 2nd line (except in Lewy body dementia or Parkinson dementia)

Single best answer (SBA) questions

Chapter 2 Pharmacological therapy and electroconvulsive therapy

1. A 37-year-old woman with treatment-resistant schizophrenia is considering commencing clozapine. What should she be advised regarding haematological monitoring that is initially required?
   A. Weekly renal function checks.
   B. Weekly liver function tests.
   C. Weekly full blood counts.
   D. Weekly lipid profiles.
   E. Weekly fasting glucose assays.

2. A 45-year-old woman has recently started phenelzine. She is out for lunch with her friend who is a doctor. She asks her friend which of these options can she safely eat from the menu?
   A. Broccoli and stilton soup.
   B. Pickled herring on a bed of salad.
   C. Marmite and sesame toast.
   D. Smoked mackerel pâté.
   E. Egg mayonnaise toastie.

3. Which of the following is an indication for ECT?
   A. A patient with body dysmorphic disorder not responding to SSRI medication.
   B. A patient presenting with first-episode psychosis and associated acute behavioural disturbance.
   C. A patient with a severe depressive episode with significant weight loss and no oral intake for the past 3 days.

D. A patient with established bipolar affective disorder on lithium presenting with depressive symptoms and a subtherapeutic lithium level.
E. A patient with no past psychiatric history who has been admitted after jumping from a local bridge with suicidal intent.

4. Which of these mood stabilizers should NOT be used in people under the age of 55?
   A. Lithium
   B. Carbamazepine
   C. Quetiapine
   D. Sodium valproate
   E. Topiramate

5. A 22-year-old woman recently commenced on an antipsychotic is pacing her bedroom and says she feels very restless. What would be the most appropriate pharmacological agent to trial to manage her symptoms?
   A. Procyclidine
   B. Olanzapine
   C. Propranolol
   D. Quinine
   E. Haloperidol

6. A 26-year-old man commenced antipsychotics a month ago. You review him in your outpatient clinic. His face shows little expression, and he does not swing his arms when he walks. He does not have a tremor, and his gait is not shuffling. What would be the most appropriate medication to manage his side effects?
   A. Intramuscular procyclidine
   B. Oral procyclidine
   C. Oral diazepam
   D. Oral propranolol
   E. Oral quinine

7. A 34-year-old man has been on an intramuscular zuclopenthixol decanoate depot and regular procyclidine for over a decade. His mother contacts you as she has become concerned about unusual facial movements, she has noticed the patient making. When you review him in clinic, you notice that he makes frequent darting movements with his tongue but seems unaware of this. Which of the following would be the most appropriate management option?
   A. Increase the dose of his zuclopenthixol decanoate depot – he is responding to unseen stimuli.
   B. Watch and wait.
   C. Stop procyclidine.
   D. Commence low dose aripiprazole in addition to his zuclopenthixol decanoate depot.
   E. Refer to neurology.

8. Which of the following describes the mechanism of action of venlafaxine?
   A. 5-HT 2C receptor antagonist and melatonin receptor agonist.
   B. Inhibits serotonin and noradrenaline reuptake pumps; does not affect acetylcholine receptors.
   C. Inhibits serotonin and noradrenaline reuptake pumps; also blocks acetylcholine receptors.
   D. Reversible inhibition of monoamine oxidase A.
   E. Inhibits dopamine and noradrenaline reuptake pumps.

Chapter 3 Psychological therapy

1. A 49-year-old man has been struggling to move on with his life after his son died in a car accident 8 months ago. Which of the following would be the most appropriate psychological therapy in the first instance?
   A. Psychodynamic therapy
   B. Cognitive-behavioural therapy
   C. Person-centred counselling
   D. Exposure and response prevention
   E. Mindfulness-based cognitive therapy

2. A 35-year-old man is undergoing psychodynamic psychotherapy, and a letter from his therapist describes his 'transference'. Which of the following is the most accurate description of transference?
   A. The level of trust in the patient-therapist relationship.
   B. Good eye contact throughout sessions.
   C. Patient response towards the therapist based on previous relationships.
   D. The level of empathy in the patient–therapist relationship.
   E. Therapist attitude towards the patient based on previous relationships.

3. A 25-year-old male student has a history of depression and has been referred for cognitive-behavioural therapy. He reports that 'my life is over because I failed my final exams.' Which of the following most accurately describes this cognitive distortion?
   A. Emotional reasoning
   B. Fortune telling
   C. Personalization
   D. Labelling
   E. Magnification

4. A 57-year-old teacher attends her general practitioner requesting a referral for interpersonal therapy after reading about it in a magazine. In which of the following conditions has interpersonal therapy proven to be of benefit?
   A. Alzheimer disease
   B. Moderate depression

C. Generalized anxiety disorder
D. Paranoid schizophrenia
E. Panic disorder

5. A 57-year-old lady has a depressive disorder of moderate severity. She attributes her symptoms to the fact that her father has been taken into a nursing home, her daughter has left home to attend university and she was recently made redundant from her job in a bank. Which of the following would be the most appropriate modality of psychological therapy to suggest?
   A. Dialectical behavioural therapy (DBT)
   B. Counselling
   C. Psychoanalysis
   D. Interpersonal therapy (IPT)
   E. Eye movement desensitization and reprocessing (EMDR)

6. A 42-year-old gentleman has a diagnosis of obsessive-compulsive disorder and is mainly troubled by having to check switches and locks in his home. He feels that a therapy that is 'more practical than talking' would be helpful. Which of the following would be the most appropriate modality of psychological therapy to suggest?
   A. Cognitive behavioural therapy with exposure and response prevention
   B. Cognitive behavioural therapy
   C. Mindfulness-based cognitive therapy
   D. Interpersonal therapy
   E. Art therapy

Chapter 4 Mental health and the law

1. A 72-year-old woman has recently been diagnosed with dementia. She continues to drive and gets shopping for her and her partner every week. He says there are no problems with her driving. What should she be advised?
   A. She should stop driving immediately.
   B. She should stop driving once she feels her driving is not as good as it used to be.
   C. She should stop driving once her partner feels her driving is not as good as it used to be.
   D. She should continue driving but notify the Driver and Vehicle Licencing Agency (DVLA).
   E. She should continue driving but her general practitioner will notify the DVLA.

2. A 23-year-old man has suffered a head injury in a road traffic accident and has a Glasgow Coma Scale (GCS) score of 8. A decision needs to be made as to whether he should be ventilated or not. What is the best description of his capacity to make this decision?
   A. Capacity should be assumed to be present.
   B. Capacity is absent because of impaired communication.
   C. Capacity is absent because of impaired understanding.
   D. Capacity is absent because of impaired retention of information.
   E. Capacity is absent because of impaired ability to balance and weigh up information.

3. A 59-year-old man has suffered from Wernicke encephalopathy and now cannot remember any new information. A decision needs to be made regarding which accommodation option he should choose. What is the best description of his capacity to make this decision?
   A. Capacity should be assumed to be present.
   B. Capacity is absent because of impaired communication.
   C. Capacity is absent because of impaired understanding.
   D. Capacity is absent because of impaired retention of information.
   E. Capacity is absent because of impaired ability to balance and weigh up information.

4. A 34-year-old woman is experiencing a manic episode with psychotic features. She broke her leg jumping off a bus shelter but denies the need for surgery as she thinks she can heal her leg herself. The decision is whether she needs surgery or not. What is the best description of her capacity to make this decision?
   A. Capacity should be assumed to be present.
   B. Capacity is absent because of impaired communication.
   C. Capacity is absent because of impaired understanding.
   D. Capacity is absent because of impaired retention of information.
   E. Capacity is absent because of impaired ability to balance and weigh up information.

5. A 55-year-old man has schizophrenia with chronic auditory hallucinations and negative symptoms. The decision is whether he should take a statin or not. What is the best description of his capacity to make this decision?
   A. Capacity should be assumed to be present.
   B. Capacity is absent because of impaired communication.

C. Capacity is absent because of impaired understanding.
D. Capacity is absent because of impaired retention of information.
E. Capacity is absent because of impaired ability to balance and weigh up information.

Chapter 5 Mental health service provision

1. Which patient is MOST likely to need secondary mental health services?
   A. A 34-year-old woman with a first episode of depression, responding well to cognitive behavioural therapy
   B. A 34-year-old woman with a first episode of depression, who has not responded to cognitive behavioural therapy or two antidepressants
   C. A 34-year-old woman with generalized anxiety symptoms, on the waiting list for cognitive behavioural therapy.
   D. A 34-year-old woman who is frequently tearful following the death of her mother 2 months ago
   E. A 34-year-old woman who says she has been depressed for years but objectively seems euthymic

2. A 21-year-old man with no past psychiatric history is experiencing odd beliefs that he has some special power and that things around him are of special significance. He struggles to explain these beliefs further and says they cannot be true. He has stopped going out with his friends and his personal hygiene has deteriorated. He has no thoughts of harm to himself or others. Which team should he be referred to?
   A. Community mental health team
   B. Early intervention in psychosis team
   C. Assertive outreach team
   D. Home treatment team
   E. Inpatient unit

Chapter 6 The patient with thoughts of suicide or self-harm

1. A 45-year-old policeman with a history of self-harm, depression and alcohol dependence discloses that he has been thinking about ways of killing himself since his wife left him a month ago. Which ONE of the following preparatory measures would suggest strong suicidal intent?
   A. Internet research
   B. Contacting the Samaritans
   C. Telling his ex-wife of his plans
   D. Making a will and paying bills
   E. Telling his general practitioner of his plans

2. A 29-year-old builder with a diagnosis of depression states that he is considering various methods of suicide. Which ONE of the following plans places him at highest risk of suicide?
   A. Jumping from a height
   B. Paracetamol overdose
   C. Suspension hanging
   D. Making cuts to wrists
   E. Carbon monoxide poisoning

3. Which of the following mental disorders is associated with the highest relative risk compared to the general population of completed suicide?
   A. Personality disorders
   B. Generalised anxiety disorder
   C. Anorexia nervosa
   D. Schizophrenia
   E. Obsessive-compulsive disorder

4. A 19-year-old woman states that she is going to kill herself because 'the voices in my head are telling me to'. These started troubling her this morning after an argument with her mother. Yesterday, she felt fine with no voices. She has no symptoms of depression. She insists that 'it will be all your fault when I commit suicide' and demands admission to a psychiatric ward. She has a history of self-harm by cutting and is well known to mental health services from previous emergency presentations. What is the most likely diagnosis?
   A. Schizophrenia
   B. Personality disorder with prominent features of disinhibition and a borderline pattern
   C. Bipolar affective disorder, current episode manic with psychotic symptoms
   D. Single episode depressive disorder
   E. Personality disorder with prominent features of detachment

5. A 50-year-old female bank manager who tried to gas herself in her car is found in a remote forest clearing at 4:30 a.m. by a dog walker. Typed letters to her wife and children (currently on holiday) were found on the passenger seat. She has no psychiatric history. She appeared intoxicated; however, she states she is not a big drinker. She described recent weight loss and wakening early in the morning. She is also convinced that a recent financial crisis is all her fault. What is the most likely diagnosis?
   A. Alcohol dependency
   B. Schizophrenia
   C. Single episode depressive disorder, severe with psychotic symptoms

D. Single episode depressive disorder, moderate without psychotic symptoms

E. Severe personality disorder with prominent traits of negative affectivity

Chapter 7 Psychiatric Emergencies

1. A 23-year-old woman presents at the accident and emergency department stating that she is feeling suicidal and has taken an overdose of paracetamol several hours ago. What is the most appropriate initial management step?

   A. History of circumstances leading to overdose
   B. Mental state examination
   C. Physical health assessment including serum paracetamol levels
   D. Determination of suicidal intent
   E. Evaluation of current social supports

2. Nursing staff ask for you to urgently review a 24-year-old man who is a psychiatric inpatient and is hypertensive, tachycardic and pyrexial. He is very drowsy and has rigid limbs. What action will most help distinguish between neuroleptic malignant syndrome and serotonin syndrome?

   A. Checking serum creatinine kinase levels.
   B. Looking at his prescription.
   C. Checking his past medical history.
   D. Formally assessing his cognition.
   E. Monitoring his condition over time.

3. Nursing staff ask for you to urgently review a 24-year-old man who is a psychiatric inpatient and is hypertensive, tachycardic and pyrexial. He is very drowsy and has rigid limbs. He was admitted a week ago with a first episode of psychosis and has received large doses of haloperidol since. What is the most appropriate first management step?

   A. Discontinue all antipsychotics.
   B. Work up for electroconvulsive therapy.
   C. Give dantrolene.
   D. Give bromocriptine.
   E. Assess ABCDE.

4. A 37-year-old woman who takes lithium for bipolar affective disorder has recently completed a course of ibuprofen for a knee injury. She now feels very tired and weak. She is unsteady on her feet and has a coarse tremor. A random lithium level is assessed. What is the lowest result that would suggest her symptoms are due to lithium toxicity?

   A. 0.2 mmol/L
   B. 0.4 mmol/L

   C. 0.8 mmol/L
   D. 1.0 mmol/L
   E. 1.8 mmol/L

5. A 23-year-old woman has been admitted to the general adult psychiatry ward due to experiencing persecutory delusional ideas about the NHS and a belief that health professionals are trying to steal her DNA in order to perform experiments on her. She has been detained under the mental health act at the time of admission. She has become acutely distressed, has barricaded herself in the nurse's office and is threatening to hit anyone who tries to enter with a fire extinguisher. Which of these options would be the most appropriate first step to manage the situation

   A. I.M. lorazepam
   B. Ask security to restrain the patient and return her to her room
   C. Contact the police and ask that the patient be taken to custody
   D. Verbal de-escalation techniques
   E. Oral haloperidol

6. A 35-year-old woman experiencing a manic episode with psychotic features had been attempting to make the voices go away by repeatedly banging her head against her sink. De-escalation techniques had not worked, and she had refused oral medication, so in view of the significant risk to herself she received intramuscular rapid tranquillization. She has no past medical history. It is now 30 minutes post administration and she is sitting dozing peacefully in the quiet room. What monitoring does she now require?

   A. No monitoring is required
   B. General observations
   C. Temperature, pulse, blood pressure, respiratory rate, hydration status and consciousness level every hour
   D. Temperature, pulse, blood pressure, respiratory rate, hydration status and consciousness level every 15 minutes
   E. Continuous monitoring of pulse, blood pressure and respiratory rate with regular temperatures

7. A 35-year-old woman has received intramuscular rapid tranquillization. Which of the following complications is least important to monitor for?

   A. Respiratory depression
   B. Inability to protect her own airway
   C. Hyperglycaemia
   D. Acute arrhythmia
   E. Life-threatening hypotension

8. A 22-year-old woman was recently commenced on an antipsychotic. You are called to review her as the nurses are concerned as she has been staring at the ceiling and clenching her jaw tightly. After completing an ABCDE assessment, what would be the most appropriate pharmacological management?

   A. Intramuscular procyclidine
   B. Oral procyclidine
   C. Propranolol
   D. Quinine
   E. Intramuscular haloperidol

Chapter 8 The patient with neurodevelopmental differences

1. A 7-year-old boy keeps getting up at school and walking to the front of the classroom. His mother is worried he has attention deficit hyperactivity disorder (ADHD). He is not restless at home and sits calmly during the interview. What is the most appropriate initial step in management?

   A. Check thyroid function
   B. Collateral history from teacher
   C. Ensure he has an up-to-date eye test
   D. Genetic testing to exclude ADHD
   E. Refer for ADHD assessment

2. A 1-year-old girl has stopped crawling. She used to cry a lot but is now calm and placid. She had developed a social smile but has not done this for a few weeks. She also makes less eye contact than she used to. What is the most likely diagnosis?

   A. Autism spectrum disorder
   B. Heller syndrome
   C. Intellectual disability
   D. Muscular dystrophy
   E. Rett syndrome

3. A 23-year-old man reports he is very anxious in social situations. He recently lost his job because he talked too much in the office. Now he is worried about talking to others at all. He says he 'doesn't get the rules' and he thought his workmates were enjoying what he was telling them about the history of photocopiers. What is the most likely diagnosis?

   A. Personality disorder with prominent traits of anankastia
   B. Autism spectrum disorder
   C. Depressive episode
   D. Generalized anxiety disorder
   E. Social anxiety disorder

4. A 24-year-old woman lives alone with input from a support worker twice a week and works in a bakery. She required extra induction sessions at the bakery before she could independently serve customers as she found it very difficult to use the cash register or give the correct change. She needed extra help at school with reading and writing and did not achieve any qualifications. What would her most likely diagnosis be?

   A. No diagnosis
   B. Mild intellectual disability
   C. Moderate intellectual disability
   D. Severe intellectual disability
   E. Profound intellectual disability

5. A 22-year-old man lives with his family, who are his main carers. He requires some assistance getting dressed and tending to his personal hygiene; however, he can do this by himself on good days. He can feed himself and spends his days watching children's television programmes and playing with Lego. What would his most likely diagnosis be?

   A. No diagnosis
   B. Mild intellectual disability
   C. Moderate intellectual disability
   D. Severe intellectual disability
   E. Profound intellectual disability

6. A 39-year-old man struggles to concentrate on tasks such as paying his bills. He has started gambling. At interview his speech is hard to interrupt and his thought form is tangential. He has had to give up his job as an accountant following involvement in a road traffic accident. What is the most likely driver of his difficulties?

   A. ADHD
   B. Intellectual disability
   C. Traumatic brain injury
   D. Generalized anxiety disorder
   E. Substance misuse

Chapter 9 The patient with psychotic symptoms

1. A 78-year-old widow with macular degeneration is brought to her general practitioner by her daughter who is concerned that her mother has been asking her to move nonexistent dogs and cats off her couch. Her mother is otherwise alert, orientated and in good health. What is the most likely diagnosis?

   A. Brain tumour
   B. Charles Bonnet syndrome
   C. Delirium
   D. Dementia
   E. Schizophrenia

2. A 62-year-old man with schizophrenia attends his general practitioner. He is dishevelled and smells strongly of tobacco. He reports feeling that someone is pressing on his chest, particularly when he approaches the church at the top of the hill. He wonders if it is the devil. What is the most probable cause of the sensation in his chest?

   A. Delusion of control
   B. Ischaemic heart disease
   C. Persecutory delusion
   D. Tactile hallucination
   E. Thought disorder

3. A 43-year-old man tells his general practitioner, 'I think my wife is having an affair'. When asked about why he thinks this, he tells his GP that 2 weeks ago his wife had her hair cut, and since then he has realized that she is being unfaithful to him. He is very upset by this and determined to get conclusive evidence to confront her with. He has quit his job to follow her and taken out a personal loan to purchase cameras to place in her car, workplace and handbag. He becomes annoyed when his GP suggests an alternative explanation for his belief. What is the psychopathology described here?

   A. Delusions of infidelity
   B. Erotomania
   C. Visual hallucination
   D. Obsession
   E. Over-valued idea

4. A 19-year-old man is brought to accident and emergency by his flatmates because for the last fortnight, he has been complaining the neighbours are talking about him and tonight stated 'enough was enough' and picked up his cricket bat to go and confront them. His friends cannot hear the neighbours. The man has smoked cannabis every day for the last 6 months and has recently been experimenting with some 'stimulant medication' he bought online. What is the most likely diagnosis?

   A. Delusional disorder
   B. Depressive episode, severe, with psychotic features
   C. Substance-induced psychotic disorder
   D. Schizophrenia
   E. Acute and transient psychotic disorder

5. A 43-year-old woman is referred to the community mental health team because she has been seeing shadowy figures in her room at night as she is going to sleep. She denies experiencing auditory hallucinations, and she reports that the figures are only present in this specific setting. What is the most likely explanation for her symptoms?

   A. Schizophrenia
   B. Hypnogogic hallucination
   C. Severe depressive episode with psychotic symptoms
   D. Hypnopompic hallucination
   E. Pseudohallucination

6. A 45-year-old man has recurrent episodes of low mood associated with third-person auditory hallucinations in the form of an abusive running commentary. These symptoms do not occur separately. What is the most likely diagnosis?

   A. Personality disorder
   B. Single episode depressive disorder with psychotic symptoms
   C. Schizophrenia
   D. Schizoaffective disorder
   E. Delusional disorder

7. A 47-year-old teacher presents to his GP for the 25th time in 6 months convinced he has bowel cancer, despite having had a normal colonoscopy and abdomen/pelvis computed tomography. His conviction arose after he smelt some dog faeces on the pavement and felt this was a sign. He tells his GP he knows logically he cannot have bowel cancer but at the same time he is certain he does. His mood is normal and he is still working. What is the most likely diagnosis?

   A. Hypochondriasis
   B. Single episode depressive disorder with psychotic symptoms
   C. Schizophrenia
   D. Schizoaffective disorder
   E. Delusional disorder

8. A 37-year-old man is brought to accident and emergency by the police for assessment after he called them to say his neighbour is persecuting him by refusing to move her wheelie-bin. The police note multiple previous calls over the last decade about previous neighbours. The man agrees it is possible the neighbour has some other reason for not wanting to move the wheelie-bin, but thinks it is most likely because she wants to spite him. He is angry with the police for bringing him to see a doctor, stating he plans to contact his lawyer about their behaviour. What is the most likely diagnosis?

   A. Personality disorder
   B. Single episode depressive disorder with psychotic symptoms
   C. Schizophrenia
   D. Schizoaffective disorder
   E. Delusional disorder

9. A woman requests a GP home visit for her 78-year-old father who has no previous psychiatric history. She is concerned that he has told her he can hear his mother and sister, who are both dead, talking. She is also concerned that he seems very forgetful and does not seem to be looking after himself properly. He is quite cheerful and enjoys speaking with his relatives. What is the most likely diagnosis?

   A. Huntington disease
   B. Vitamin B12 deficiency
   C. Cocaine use
   D. Hyperthyroidism
   E. Neurosyphilis

Chapter 10 The patient with elevated or irritable mood

1. Reception staff ask the general practitioner to see a 29-year-old man with a history of bipolar disorder who has arrived 2 hours late for his appointment. He is speaking very quickly and the words don't make sense. He also appears to be talking to someone who the reception staff cannot see. What is the most likely cause for his presentation?

   A. Manic episode with psychotic symptoms
   B. Hypomanic episode
   C. Single episode depressive disorder
   D. Cyclothymia
   E. Schizophrenia

2. A 55-year-old man has had several admissions to hospital with elated episodes when he believes he is Jesus Christ but has never been depressed. What is the diagnosis?

   A. Recurrent hypomania
   B. Bipolar disorder
   C. Schizoaffective disorder
   D. Cyclothymia
   E. Recurrent mania

3. A 25-year-old farmer is brought to accident and emergency by the police after he tried to steal a tractor. He is agitated, but shows no remorse, stating loudly that it rightfully belongs to him as he is the King of Tractors. He has no past psychiatric history, past medical history or previous criminal offences. Which investigation will be most important diagnostically?

   A. Computed tomography (CT) scan
   B. Electroencephalogram (EEG)
   C. Full blood count
   D. Urine drug screen
   E. Thyroid function

4. A 24-year-old unemployed woman presents to her general practitioner asking to be treated for bipolar disorder. She has looked it up on the internet and thinks it may explain why she is always losing her temper with people. Her mood swings frequently, sometimes several times in a day. She often does things she later regrets and has never managed to maintain a long-term relationship or job. She has had these mood swings from when she was a child. What is the most likely diagnosis?

   A. Bipolar disorder
   B. Dysthymia
   C. Cyclothymia
   D. Personality disorder
   E. Substance use

5. A 40-year-old lawyer attends his general practitioner (GP) asking for a medication to reduce his sex drive because his wife is complaining. He is smartly dressed in a new suit and says he feels 'on top of the world'. He has been finding it hard to stay focused at work but so far no one has commented. Fortunately, he is able to stay up late catching up on work without feeling tired the next day. He denies any drug or alcohol use. What is the most likely diagnosis?

   A. Manic episode with psychotic features
   B. Manic episode without psychotic features
   C. Hypomanic episode
   D. Acute and transient psychotic disorder
   E. No mental illness

6. A 28-year-old doctor is brought to A&E by his flatmates. He has recently started a stressful new job and his flatmates are worried because he doesn't seem to be eating or sleeping well, despite seeming quite cheerful. He paces the flat at night talking about new operative techniques he is designing, at times they wondered if he was on the phone as this sounded like a conversation, but they soon realized he was alone in his room. His consultant sent him home from work because he refused to scrub for theatre, stating 'I'm pristine already'. What is the most likely diagnosis?

   A. Manic episode with psychotic features
   B. Manic episode without psychotic features
   C. Hypomanic episode
   D. Acute and transient psychotic disorder
   E. No mental illness

Chapter 11 The patient with low mood

1. A 40-year-old woman who was started on a new medication a month ago presents with a 4-week history of depression. Which of the following might account for her presentation?

A. Paracetamol
B. Omeprazole
C. Salbutamol
D. Verapamil
E. Prednisolone

2. A 35-year-old woman presents with mild depression. On examination you notice a midline neck swelling. What is the most appropriate initial step in patient care?
   A. Refer to psychiatry
   B. Check thyroid function
   C. Start an antidepressant
   D. Request a neck ultrasound
   E. Advise her to return if the symptoms persist

3. A 55-year-old man with no previous psychiatric history presents with low mood, anhedonia and fatigue. He has come for help as he believes his organs are rotting away. What is the most likely diagnosis?
   A. Bipolar disorder
   B. Schizoaffective disorder
   C. Schizophrenia
   D. Single episode depressive disorder with psychotic features
   E. Dementia

4. A 25-year-old student turns up late for her appointment. She gives a 1-month history of low mood, anhedonia and fatigue. What is the most important area to cover in what remains of the appointment time?
   A. Presence of neurovegetative symptoms of depression
   B. Drug history
   C. Family history of mood disorder
   D. Suicidal ideation
   E. Past medical history

5. A 19-year-old shop assistant presents in tears because her boyfriend broke up with her the day before. She did not sleep well last night and did not feel like having breakfast. She feels hopeless about the future and thinks she will never meet anyone else. She says she feels really depressed. She denies suicidal ideation. What is the most appropriate initial step in patient care?
   A. Start an antidepressant
   B. Refer to psychiatry
   C. Ask her to complete a mood diary
   D. Watchful waiting
   E. Check full blood count, urea and electrolytes, liver function test and thyroid function test

6. A 26-year-old veterinary student presents with tingling in her left arm. She becomes tearful during the consultation, admitting she is finding the fourth year of her studies much more difficult than the previous years. You see she attended 3 months ago with a sore eye and blurred vision which resolved spontaneously. What is the most likely diagnosis?
   A. Multiple sclerosis
   B. Thrombocytopenia
   C. Cushing syndrome
   D. Systemic lupus erythematosus
   E. Hypothyroidism

7. A 76-year-old widowed retired headmistress is brought to accident and emergency by her family who are concerned she has not been eating. She paces the cubicle, keeps buttoning and unbuttoning her coat and does not sit down when offered a chair. Which term best describes the observed finding in the mental state examination?
   A. Poor self-care
   B. Psychomotor retardation
   C. Psychomotor agitation
   D. Reduced range of reactivity
   E. Incongruous affect

Chapter 12 The patient with anxiety, fear or avoidance

1. A 21-year-old student calls an ambulance because of chest pain, shortness of breath and a feeling she is about to die. This settles by the time she reaches the accident and emergency department. On all occasions, her examination, electrocardiogram and cardiac enzymes are normal. She has her final exams in a fortnight and admits she is very worried. What is the most likely diagnosis?
   A. Acute coronary syndrome
   B. Thyrotoxicosis
   C. Hypoglycaemia
   D. Panic attack
   E. Asthma

2. A 57-year-old obese man keeps cancelling appointments with the practice nurse to have bloods taken for cholesterol and glucose. Although he is normally very cheerful and relaxed, he becomes pale, sweaty and tremulous when you offer to take his bloods during the consultation. What is the most likely diagnosis?
   A. Myocardial infarction
   B. Hyperglycaemia
   C. Blood-injection-injury phobia
   D. Panic disorder
   E. Hypochondriasis

3. A 63-year-old woman with a history of depression presents to the accident and emergency department and

tells you she has a dry mouth, a choking sensation, butterflies in her stomach, palpitations and shortness of breath. She tells you she had some bad news recently. What is the most appropriate first step in management?

A. Electrocardiogram (ECG)
B. Airway, breathing, circulation, disability, exposure (ABCDE)
C. Psychiatry referral
D. Bloods: full blood count, urea and electrolytes, liver function tests and troponin
E. Arterial blood gas (ABG)

4. A 24-year-old man who was recently diagnosed with type 1 diabetes attends his general practitioner (GP). Over the last month he has experienced recurrent attacks of anxiety associated with sweating and tachycardia. The episodes do not seem to have any triggers, last for about 20 minutes, and resolve when he sits down with his girlfriend and has a cup of tea and a biscuit. What should the GP advise the patient to do next time it happens?

A. Deep breathing exercises
B. Note it in a diary
C. Take diazepam
D. See a counsellor
E. Check blood sugar

5. A 44-year-old businessman presents to his general practitioner (GP) because for the last month he has felt anxious, sweaty and shaky in the mornings. He feels better when he has lunch and generally his mood is good. He admits to drinking a bottle of red wine every night, and usually having champagne during business lunches. What is the most likely diagnosis?

A. Depressive episode
B. Diabetes
C. Panic disorder
D. Alcohol withdrawal
E. Work phobia

6. A 28-year-old secretary presents to her general practitioner with weight loss. Six months ago in a supermarket she suddenly felt like she was going to die. She had pain in her chest, was short of breath and her arms and lips tingled. She rushed outside and the feeling subsided, but now she does not like to go into any large shops and is eating less well. She is still going to work but now walks 5 miles each way as she does not want to be on a bus and have another attack. As long as she is in her house or with her friends she is relaxed. What is the most likely diagnosis?

A. Agoraphobia without panic attacks
B. Agoraphobia with panic attacks

C. Social phobia with panic attacks
D. Generalized anxiety disorder with panic attacks
E. Panic disorder

7. Over the last 3 months, a 35-year-old builder has experienced several episodes of sudden onset shortness of breath, palpitations, sweatiness, nausea, feeling that the world is unreal and feeling he is about to die. These feelings resolve spontaneously over 20 minutes. He cannot identify any triggers. In particular, they are not brought on by exercise and he can continue to do his active job. His electrocardiogram (ECG) is normal. What is the most likely diagnosis?

A. Panic disorder
B. Social phobia
C. Agoraphobia without panic attacks
D. Agoraphobia with panic attacks
E. Generalized anxiety disorder

8. A 23-year-old man has started a new job with a finance company. He has noticed that he gets very irritable and anxious by the end of the day and has had to go home early a couple of times. He drinks a lot of his favourite soft drink, 'Go-Man'. What substance is the most likely driver of his anxiety?

A. Caffeine
B. Cocaine
C. Cannabis
D. Alcohol
E. Amphetamine

Chapter 13 The patient with obsessions and compulsions

1. A 29-year-old woman mentions she is obsessed with a TV talent show. She watches each episode multiple times and has pictures of all the contestants on her bedroom wall. She called in sick the day of the final as her shift clashed with the showing. She enjoys watching and thinking about the show and thinks she might audition next year. What is the most likely diagnosis?

A. No mental illness
B. Social anxiety disorder
C. Personality disorder with prominent traits of anankastia
D. Obsessive-compulsive disorder
E. Delusional disorder

2. A 36-year-old man keeps thinking about his own death. He sees repetitive images of his body in a coffin. He tries to distract himself, but it does not work. The images started about 3 months ago, around the time he started

to feel low in mood associated with fatigue, less pleasure in life, insomnia and anorexia. What is the most likely diagnosis?

A. Obsessive-compulsive disorder
B. Generalised anxiety disorder
C. Depressive disorder
D. Hypochondriasis
E. Nihilistic delusion

3. A 44-year-old man has had intrusive thoughts for several years regarding security. He keeps thinking his house is unlocked and has developed a routine of checking every door and window nine times before leaving the premises. This means he has to get up half an hour early and sometimes come home from work early to recheck. This has caused friction with a new manager at work and over the last month he has noticed his mood is lower. He no longer enjoys playing football, is very tired all the time, and is struggling to concentrate at work. What is the most likely diagnosis?

A. Depressive disorder
B. Obsessive-compulsive disorder (OCD)
C. Generalised anxiety disorder
D. OCD with comorbid depressive episode
E. Personality disorder with prominent features of anankastia

4. A 33-year-old graphic designer is driven to produce perfect images. She has always been very conscientious, even at primary school. The thought of a mistake in one of her designs makes her feel so anxious she often stays late at work checking them through. She is proud of the quality of work, and feels her colleagues are sloppy and should work harder. She had to leave her last two companies because she told the manager this. She has recently separated from her partner as they said she was not 'spontaneous enough'. What is the most likely diagnosis?

A. Obsessive-compulsive disorder
B. Mild personality disorder with prominent features of anankastia
C. No mental illness
D. Autistic spectrum disorder
E. Obsessive-compulsive disorder with comorbid depressive episode

5. A 23-year-old woman reports a voice inside her head telling her to harm herself. She is not sure where it comes from as no one is around when she hears it. What is the psychopathology she displays?

A. Obsession

B. Pseudohallucination
C. Rumination
D. Thought insertion
E. Hallucination

6. A 25-year-old woman insists that she wants plastic surgery on her nose, as she feels it is crooked and deformed. She has stopped leaving the house for fear of other people noticing. She cannot stop thinking about how ugly it is, and this often keeps her awake at night. On examination, her nose is entirely normal, and she does appear slightly reassured when told this. Which of the following is the most likely diagnosis?

A. Somatic delusional disorder
B. Factitious disorder
C. Malingering
D. Body dysmorphic disorder
E. Hypochondriasis

7. For the last few years, a 27-year-old nurse has been influenced by an NHS advertising campaign featuring soiled hands spreading COVID-19. Washing her hands reduces her fear that they are contaminated. Now she washes her hands before and after every patient contact, up to 100 times a day, and is developing contact dermatitis. What is the most likely diagnosis?

A. Phobia
B. Panic disorder
C. Obsessive-compulsive disorder
D. Hypochondriasis
E. No mental illness

8. During an assessment a patient discloses that 'When I saw a picture on TV of germs crawling on someone's skin, I knew that I was fatally ill. The doctor told me I was fine, but I know my days are numbered'. What is the mostly accurate descriptor for this experience?

A. Delusion
B. Obsession
C. Over-valued idea
D. Rumination
E. Hallucination

Chapter 14 The patient with a reaction to a stressful event

1. A 23-year-old man with a history of schizophrenia appears confused and withdrawn the morning after he was severely assaulted by a group of youths in the local park. He has no recollection of the event. Which of the following diagnoses should be initially considered?

A. Acute stress reaction
B. Adjustment disorder
C. Relapse of schizophrenia
D. Intracranial haemorrhage
E. Posttraumatic stress disorder

2. A 57-year-old woman has been referred urgently by her general practitioner for symptoms of low mood, weight loss and insomnia. These have been troublesome for the past 10 weeks, since she watched her husband drown while on a yachting holiday. Which of the following would be suggestive of a diagnosis of depression rather than a normal bereavement reaction?
   A. Thinking that she would be better off dead
   B. Difficulty concentrating on watching the television
   C. Inability to tend to her self-care or get out of bed
   D. Extreme guilt for not making her late husband wear a lifejacket
   E. Hearing the voice of her late husband while lying alone in bed

3. A 28-year-old woman was signed off her job in a call centre 2 weeks ago with 'work-related stress', a month after she was promoted to a supervisory position in a new department. She has no psychiatric history and denies substance misuse. At interview, she tells you she feels 'unable to cope' with the demands of her new role. She is sleeping well, and continues to enjoy jogging on a daily basis. Which of the following would be the most appropriate diagnosis?
   A. Depressive disorder
   B. Adjustment disorder
   C. Dissociative neurological symptom disorder
   D. Acute stress reaction
   E. No mental illness

4. A 19-year-old female asylum seeker is brought to hospital by a social worker regarding concerns with her memory. She recalls her entire life until 3 months ago when she received news that government militia were coming towards her former hometown in Sierra Leone. She has memory of the last 4 weeks of her life in the UK and is able to tell you about her current address, social circle and circumstances. You see from her medical notes that she had a termination of pregnancy 6 weeks ago; however, she has no recollection of either the conception or the procedure. Physical examination and investigations reveal no abnormalities, and she seems indifferent to her difficulties. Which ONE of the following is the most likely diagnosis?
   A. Dissociative amnesia
   B. Anterograde amnesia following head trauma

C. Transient global amnesia
D. Posttraumatic stress disorder
E. Wernicke–Korsakoff syndrome

5. A 19-year-old woman presents to A&E for the seventh time in the past year after taking an overdose with suicidal intent. She has a history of repeated childhood sexual abuse. She re-experiences the abuse in the form of vivid, intrusive images, triggered by the smell of certain aftershaves. She is easily startled by loud noises in the department and tries to avoid being alone with male members of staff. She describes difficulties since the event with controlling her emotions, maintaining friendships and with feelings of worthlessness. What is the most likely diagnosis?
   A. Depressive disorder
   B. Post traumatic stress disorder
   C. Acute and transient psychotic disorder
   D. Obsessive-compulsive disorder
   E. Complex post traumatic stress disorder

6. A 46-year-old businessman from a distant city is brought to hospital by the police, after apparently trying to withdraw money from a building society and being unable to remember his name. At interview, he seems unable to recall any personal details about himself and has no idea where he is. He is carrying a bundle of business cards for a company that was recently reported to have gone bankrupt. What is the most likely diagnosis?
   A. Dissociative identity disorder
   B. Depersonalization disorder
   C. Dissociative amnesia with dissociative fugue
   D. Posttraumatic stress disorder
   E. Trance disorder

7. A 29-year-old mother of two, with a history of depression and a family history of epilepsy, has recently started having episodes, during which she falls to the floor, moving all her limbs, with her eyes squeezed tight shut. The episodes last at least 5 minutes. They do not cause tongue-biting, incontinence or postictal confusion. She can remember 'shaking all over'. She denies alcohol or drug use. Her husband tells you that this started when he told his wife of his new job on an oil rig. He now feels he cannot leave home for fear that she will be seriously harmed by the seizures. What is the most likely diagnosis?
   A. Dissociative amnesia
   B. Dissociation secondary to psychoactive substance use
   C. Epilepsy
   D. Functional paralysis
   E. Nonepileptic seizures

8. A 27-year-old woman is referred from the neurosurgical unit 4 months after a fall from a first-floor balcony. She reports episodes of derealization, followed by visual hallucinations, loss of memory and extreme tiredness
   A. Posttraumatic stress disorder
   B. Temporal lobe epilepsy
   C. Adjustment disorder
   D. Musculoskeletal injury
   E. Dissociative neurological disorder

Chapter 15 The patient with medically unexplained physical symptoms

1. A 26-year-old male teacher attends his general practitioner requesting tests to confirm that he is suffering from multiple sclerosis. He thinks that he has this because he had some stabbing pain in his upper arm last week. The pain has now resolved and examination is unremarkable. Which ONE of the following should the GP do?
   A. Watchful waiting
   B. Refer for urgent neurology appointment
   C. Organize magnetic resonance imaging scan and lumbar puncture
   D. Tell the patient that he is worrying too much
   E. Organize another appointment in 3 days

2. A 32-year-old former nurse complains of pelvic pain. Despite the apparent severity of the pain and the presence of multiple abdominal surgical scars, her physical appearance, examination and basic investigations are entirely normal. She tells you in detail about her previous diagnoses and invasive investigations, and requests pethidine and a diagnostic laparoscopy. She is visiting from a distant town. Which of the following should be the next step in her management?
   A. Urgent diagnostic laparoscopy
   B. Prescribe pethidine
   C. Tell her that she is lying
   D. Contact previous centres of care
   E. Refer to psychiatry

3. A 72-year-old man is referred to psychiatry because of dyspnoea and stabbing pain in his chest. He has not seen a general practitioner for years, and examination and routine blood tests are normal. The medical doctor feels that he has panic attacks. Which ONE of the following should be the next step in his management?
   A. Cognitive-behavioural therapy
   B. Further physical investigations
   C. Explanation of functional illness

D. Antidepressant medication
E. Watchful waiting

4. A 41-year-old woman is a frequent visitor to her general practitioner. She has had numerous investigations over several years for a multitude of physical symptoms, including abdominal pain, dysmenorrhoea, dysuria and difficulty swallowing. She refuses to accept her GP's explanation that there is no physical cause for her symptoms. She is now requesting a referral to a neurologist because she has a persistent tingling sensation in her legs. Which of the following is the most likely diagnosis?
   A. Multiple sclerosis
   B. Factitious disorder
   C. Bodily distress disorder
   D. Hypochondriasis
   E. Generalised anxiety disorder

Chapter 16 The patient with eating, feeding or weight problems

1. A 22-year-old female medical student is brought to your clinic by her mother, who discovered she was making herself vomit after meals. Which of the following is suggestive of a diagnosis of anorexia nervosa rather than bulimia nervosa?
   A. Significantly low body weight
   B. A dread of fatness and a distorted image of being too fat
   C. Use of herbal dieting medications
   D. Tendency to exercise excessively
   E. A preoccupation with being thin

2. The weight of a 13-year-old boy is 25% lower than expected, having previously been on the 50th percentile for both height and weight. He has not started puberty. He reports that he eats well and denies any concerns regarding body image. What is the most appropriate next management step?
   A. Refer for psychiatric assessment
   B. Refer for cognitive-behavioural therapy
   C. Investigate for physical causes of growth restriction
   D. Try to establish rapport to facilitate assessment
   E. Ask him to keep a food diary

3. A 32-year-old barmaid is worried that she has lost a great deal of weight recently (body mass index 17). She describes feeling tired all the time and having no appetite. Her mood has been low for the last 3 months, and she is anhedonic. She drinks six vodkas and cokes when she is working, and three on her days off. If she doesn't have a

drink she feels anxious and gets palpitations. She is sometimes sick, not always after meals. Physical examination and investigations reveal no abnormalities. What is the most likely diagnosis?

A. Bulimia nervosa
B. Depressive episode
C. Panic disorder
D. Anorexia nervosa
E. Alcohol dependence

4. A 25-year-old female lawyer has a diagnosis of anorexia nervosa, with a body mass index of 14.5 kg/m². Which of the following investigation results requires urgent treatment?

A. Glucose 3.7 mmol/L
B. Haemoglobin 95 g/L
C. Total cholesterol 7 mmol/L
D. Phosphate 0.7 mmol/L
E. Potassium 2.1 mmol/L

5. A 19-year-old female accountant describes a dread of fatness and feels that she is overweight despite having a body mass index of 13.6 kg/m². She describes a 1-year history of severely restricting her dietary intake. She reports amenorrhoea (secondary) and has lanugo hair. Which of the following is the most likely diagnosis?

A. Depressive episode
B. Bulimia nervosa
C. Schizophrenia
D. Anorexia nervosa
E. Obsessive-compulsive disorder

6. A 19-year-old boy has anorexia nervosa and is receiving weekly weights and physical examination. Which of the findings below places him at high physical risk?

A. Blood pressure 95/65 mm Hg supine, 88/60 mm Hg erect
B. Capillary refill time <2 seconds
C. Heart rate 58 bpm, regular
D. Temperature 36.5°C
E. Unable to rise from squatting without assistance

Chapter 17 The patient with alcohol or substance use problems

1. A 57-year-old woman described auditory hallucinations telling her that she was evil. These started a week ago, after several months of heavy alcohol use. She is socially isolated. Her mood, concentration and memory were normal. Other than slightly abnormal liver function tests, physical examination and investigations were normal, and breath alcohol was undetected. What is the most likely diagnosis?

A. Delirium tremens
B. Late-onset schizophrenia
C. Hepatic encephalopathy
D. Alcoholic hallucinosis
E. Wernicke–Korsakoff syndrome

2. A 62-year-old salesman is admitted to an orthopaedic ward following a fractured neck of femur. Two days later (before surgery to repair his hip), he appears shaky, confused and disorientated, and tells you that he can see a small horse on the table. His wife discloses that he had been drinking a bottle of whisky per day in the 3 months prior to admission. Which of the following aspects of his management should be delayed?

A. Benzodiazepines
B. Parenteral thiamine
C. Full physical exam
D. Neck of femur repair
E. Consistent nursing care

3. A 27-year-old man comes to your outpatient clinic and tells you that he has been injecting heroin on a daily basis for several months and wants you to restart his methadone to help him stop. What is the most appropriate initial step in patient care?

A. Prescribe his previous dose of methadone
B. Give him some dihydrocodeine to use first
C. Obtain a urine sample for drug testing
D. Refer him to the drug counselling service
E. Contact the police because he has been using illegal drugs

4. A 35-year-old woman asks you about 'safe' limits for drinking alcohol. You know the answer is 14 units per week; however, she asks you to explain this in terms of how many drinks she can safely take. What would you tell her?

A. Six pints (568 mL) of continental lager (5.3% alcohol by volume (ABV)) per week
B. A 'half bottle' (350 mL) of premium gin (40% ABV) per week
C. Two bottles (2 × 750 mL) of red wine (12.5% ABV) per week
D. A large (3 L) bottle of strong white cider (8.4% ABV) per week
E. Six bottles (6 × 330 mL) of 'alcopops' (4.9% ABV) per week

5. A 24-year-old accountant confides in you that he has tried cocaine on a work night out. He experienced some strange feelings and wants to know whether these were likely to be due to cocaine, or whether he was sold

something else. Which of the following symptoms is not suggestive of cocaine intoxication?

A. Chest pain
B. Fast heart rate
C. Fever
D. Hallucinations
E. Drowsiness

6. A 34-year-old musician presents to the ED asking to speak to a psychiatrist. He reports feeling like he is not real and that he is floating outside of his body. He does report some substance use earlier in the day but cannot remember what he has taken. What is the most likely drug he has used
A. Cocaine
B. Buprenorphine
C. Ketamine
D. MDMA
E. LSD

Chapter 18 The patient with personality problems

1. A 20-year-old woman frequently attends her GP reporting low mood and difficulties maintaining romantic relationships due to frequent arguments and fear of abandonment from her partner. She reports that she has poor self-esteem. She has a successful job but has few friends. She has a good relationship with her parents. She also describes difficulties in managing confrontation and feels as though she is quick to anger. These difficulties with friendships and relationships have been present throughout her adolescence. What is the most likely diagnosis?
A. No mental disorder
B. Mild personality disorder
C. Moderate personality disorder
D. Severe personality disorder
E. Social anxiety disorder

2. A 35-year-old man is assessed in police custody after he has been arrested following an assault. He reports longstanding difficulties with experiencing intense, and at times unbearable emotions, being extremely quick to anger and being prone to making impulsive and often later regretted decisions. He has been arrested several times before for assault and breach of the peace, with his first arrest at the age of 13. He describes a sense of self-loathing that has been present since his teenage years and he frequently uses alcohol and drugs to help him manage his emotions. He has been in several short-term relationships, but struggles to maintain friendships and is

no longer in touch with his family. He is unemployed. He also has a history of self-harm and previous presentations to A&E following impulsive overdoses with suicidal intent. What is the most likely diagnosis?
A. Social anxiety disorder
B. Polysubstance dependence
C. Mild personality disorder
D. Moderate personality disorder
E. Severe personality disorder

3. A 55-year-old librarian attends a psychiatric outpatient clinic. She reports that she has, since her teenage years, been a 'perfectionist'. She describes finding it difficult to tolerate her new colleague, who she feels does 'half a job' as they do not follow the extensive guidelines she prepared for them. She lives alone after separating from her partner of 2 years, as they argued too frequently about cleaning tasks in the household and the patient's lack of spontaneity. What is the most likely prominent personality trait?
A. Personality disorder with prominent features of detachment
B. Personality disorder with prominent features of negative affectivity
C. Personality disorder with prominent features of dissociality
D. Personality disorder with prominent features of anankastia
E. Personality disorder with prominent features of disinhibition

4. A 25-year-old prisoner is reviewed in clinic after pushing a fellow prisoner down a flight of stairs. When challenged about this, he stated that the person had been walking too slowly and was preventing them from getting dinner. He states that he does not feel guilty, as the fellow prisoner is not as important as him, and his needs are more important than theirs. You look back through their medical records and can see that this is not the first time they have done something like this, with the earliest entry being from when they were 17 and had punched their social worker for suggesting they would not be entitled to increased benefits. What is the most likely diagnosis?
A. Personality disorder with prominent features of detachment
B. Personality disorder with prominent features of negative affectivity
C. Personality disorder with prominent features of dissociality
D. Personality disorder with prominent features of anankastia
E. Personality disorder with prominent features of disinhibition

5. A 21-year-old woman is seen in the emergency department. This is her fourth presentation with a paracetamol overdose in the past 2 months. At assessment, she describes difficulties with maintaining relationships, constantly worrying that people are going to abandon her. She describes feeling 'empty' and feels as though she does not know who she is as a person. She has a history of self-harm dating back to the age of 11, and states she uses self-harm as a way to deal with her emotions going 'all over the place' and manage her distress after arguments. She also describes making impulsive decisions and acting based on immediate emotional responses to situations, rather than thinking through her actions. She 'never' plans anything and becomes distracted by what is going on around her during the assessment. What is the most likely diagnosis?
   A. Personality disorder with prominent features of detatchment and a borderline pattern
   B. Personality disorder with prominent features of negative affectivity and a borderline pattern
   C. Personality disorder with a prominent features of dissociality and a borderline pattern
   D. Personality disorder with prominent features of anankastia and a borderline pattern
   E. Personality disorder with prominent traits of disinhibition and a borderline pattern

Chapter 19 The patient with impairment of consciousness, memory or cognition

1. An 82-year-old woman is brought to A&E by her family. They are concerned that over the last couple of days she has been very suspicious of them, has mentioned seeing wolves in her kitchen and has been pacing her sitting room all night. She scores 4/10 on the Abbreviated Mental Test. She normally functions well, living alone with no carers. What is the most likely diagnosis?
   A. Late onset schizophrenia
   B. Lewy body dementia
   C. Alzheimer dementia
   D. Delirium
   E. Charles Bonnet syndrome

2. A woman brings her 62-year-old father to register at a new GP practice as he has recently moved to the area to be closer to her. He tells the GP about upcoming events and occasions he has planned, but his daughter says none of this is true, and that for some years now he has had a very poor memory for new information. He can spell 'WORLD' backwards and draw a clock face without difficulty. By the end of the consultation, he is not able to recall what you said to him or why he is in the practice. He

used to be a heavy drinker. What is the most likely diagnosis?
   A. Korsakoff syndrome
   B. Dementia
   C. Alcohol excess
   D. Malingering
   E. Fugue state

3. A 75-year-old retired fisherman presents to his general practitioner with a 12-month history of gradual onset, gradually worsening memory impairment confirmed by his wife. He is no longer able to cook or help mend nets like he used to. ACE-III is 76/100. He has a past medical history of hypertension and is an ex-smoker. Physical examination is normal. He has had normal full blood count, U&Es, calcium, HbA1c, vitamin B12, folate CRP, ESR and thyroid function tests in the last month. Which of these investigations would be the most appropriate next step?
   A. Computed tomography (CT) of the head
   B. Chest X-ray
   C. Syphilis and HIV serology
   D. Electroencephalogram (EEG)
   E. Cerebrospinal fluid examination

4. A 77-year-old woman is an inpatient on a general medical ward. She was admitted 2 weeks ago with a severe urinary tract infection (UTI) requiring intravenous antibiotics. In A&E her Abbreviated Mental Test (AMT) was 2/10. Since admission she has been disorientated and hallucinating. Her antibiotics finished a week ago and her inflammatory markers returned to normal. Four days ago she was almost discharged, but became very confused and agitated the night before going. Repeat AMT was 4/10. Prior to admission she functioned well and was cognitively normal. What is the most likely diagnosis?
   A. Delirium
   B. Late-onset schizophrenia
   C. Lewy body dementia
   D. Alzheimer dementia
   E. Charles Bonnet syndrome

5. A 74-year-old man is admitted to hospital because he has acute cognitive impairment and is hypervigilant and agitated. Past medical history is of insomnia and ischaemic heart disease. His medications are amitriptyline 50 mg nocte, aspirin 75 mg mane, lisinopril 5 mg, omeprazole 20 mg mane, simvastatin 20 mg nocte. His daughter thinks he has recently started a new medication. Physical examination, blood tests, electrocardiogram, chest X-ray and head computed tomography are normal. What is the most likely cause of his presentation?

A. Amitriptyline
B. Aspirin
C. Lisinopril
D. Omeprazole
E. Simvastatin

6. A 74-year-old woman presents to her general practitioner (GP) with her husband who is concerned that over the last 8 weeks she has become increasingly forgetful and disorientated. She has burnt a couple of pans after leaving them unattended. Some days she takes afternoon naps, which is new for her. When pressed he recalls she was hit on the head by a football around 3 months ago while watching her grandson's team but seemed fine afterwards. Past medical history includes atrial fibrillation and asthma. ACE-III is 70/100 and neurological exam shows normal conscious level and a subtle right hemiparesis. What is the most likely diagnosis?
A. Hypothyroidism
B. Vitamin B12 deficiency
C. Space occupying lesion
D. Addison disease
E. Chronic subdural haematoma

7. An 81-year-old man has an 18-month history of fluctuating cognitive impairment on a background of a gradual cognitive deterioration. He has been investigated for delirium but no cause found. Sometimes he is very drowsy during the day. He is increasingly stiff and finds it hard to roll over in bed. He also finds it hard to keep his balance and has had a lot of falls recently. Sometimes he experiences visual hallucinations of cats and mice. Head CT shows generalized cerebral atrophy. Which is the most likely diagnosis?
A. Lewy body dementia
B. Alzheimer dementia
C. Alcohol-related brain damage
D. Vascular dementia
E. Frontotemporal dementia

8. A 62-year-old teacher presents to her GP because she feels she is not remembering the names of the children in her class as well as she used to. She is worried she has dementia like her mother. She has no difficulties in activities of daily living and her mood is normal. She scores 82/100 on ACE-III.
A. Alzheimer dementia
B. Mild neurocognitive impairment
C. Vascular dementia
D. Factitious Disorder
E. Delirium

Chapter 20 Dementia and delirium

1. A 91-year-old nursing home resident with severe Alzheimer dementia frequently shouts unintelligible words. Physical examination and investigations are normal, and she does not seem low in mood. Staff can detect no pattern or triggers to her shouting. She appears mildly distressed by it. What option should be tried first to reduce her shouting?
A. Assess for changes to physical health
B. Antipsychotic
C. Antidepressant
D. Cholinesterase inhibitor
E. Referral to speech and language therapy

2. A 75-year-old man has Lewy body dementia. His carers are worried that he is not eating well. He tells his general practitioner that he is certain his carers are trying to poison him. What management strategy should be avoided if possible?
A. Antipsychotics
B. Nutritional supplements
C. Cholinesterase inhibitors
D. Antibiotics
E. Antidepressants

3. A 77-year-old man was admitted 3 days ago with abdominal pain of uncertain aetiology. Initially he was alert and orientated but nurses are concerned that he is now acutely disorientated and agitated. Which medication is most likely to explain his behaviour?
A. Paracetamol
B. Metoclopramide
C. Co-codamol
D. Omeprazole
E. Cyclizine

4. A general practitioner (GP) is asked to visit a 71-year-old woman in her home. She is disorientated in time, does not recognize the GP (whom she has known for years) and is very drowsy. She is plucking at her bedclothes and refuses to let the GP examine her because she thinks he wants to hurt her. Her husband states she was fine until 2 days ago, but now he cannot cope with her. Where should the GP manage this lady with acute onset psychotic symptoms?
A. Her own home
B. Day hospital
C. Emergency respite via social work
D. Acute medical ward
E. Acute psychiatric ward

5. A 78-year-old woman has a recent diagnosis of Alzheimer dementia. She continues to live at home with support workers visiting daily. Her past medical history includes sick sinus syndrome, chronic obstructive pulmonary disease (COPD) and an active peptic ulcer. Which of the following is the most appropriate treatment to try and maintain her current level of cognitive functioning?

   A. Donepezil
   B. Memantine
   C. Fluoxetine
   D. Quetiapine
   E. Rivastigmine

6. A 67-year-old man presents with a change in his personality, trouble communicating and his wife has concerns that he has been making sexually inappropriate comments to their cleaner. He is diagnosed with frontotemporal dementia. Which of the following options would be the most appropriate treatment to try and maintain his current level of cognition?

   A. No medication recommended by current guidelines
   B. Memantine
   C. Donepezil
   D. Trazodone
   E. Olanzapine

Chapter 21 Older adult psychiatry

1. A 74-year-old woman gives a 6-month history of low mood, anhedonia and fatigue associated with difficulty concentrating and remembering. Neighbours have noticed she is forgetting to put her bins out and no longer cooks meals for herself. Her score on the Addenbrooke's Cognitive Examination (ACE-III) is 72/100. What is the best management option?

   A. Antidepressant
   B. Cholinesterase inhibitor
   C. Memantine
   D. Refer for cognitive reminiscence therapy and occupational therapy
   E. Refer for counselling

2. A 72-year-old widow has presented to her general practitioner 20 times in the last month with minor physical concerns. Previously she attended infrequently. During consultations she is restless, wrings her hands and seems to struggle to remember advice given to her. Her friends are struggling to cope as she telephones them throughout the night to check they are alright. Her score on the Montreal Cognitive Assessment (MoCA) is 29/30. What is the most likely diagnosis?

   A. Mild neurocognitive impairment
   B. Generalised anxiety disorder
   C. Single episode depressive disorder
   D. Late-onset schizophrenia
   E. Hypochondriasis

3. A 71-year-old widower has a 3-month history of low mood, fatigue and anhedonia associated with anorexia. He was transferred from a general hospital to a psychiatric hospital 4 weeks ago after an episode of acute kidney injury precipitated by poor oral intake. He has been commenced on an antidepressant but is poorly concordant and his presentation has changed little. His kidney function has not returned to baseline as he continues to drink little fluid. What is the best management option?

   A. Electroconvulsive therapy (ECT)
   B. Continue current oral antidepressant
   C. Commence depot medication with antidepressant properties
   D. Change to an alternative oral antidepressant
   E. Change to lithium

4. An out-of-hours general practitioner calls for advice about a patient who has been 'behaving oddly'. The computer system is down, so their past psychiatric history is unknown. Which of the patients below is most likely to have late-onset schizophrenia?

   A. A diabetic man who reports that the police are stealing his thoughts. He cannot say what day it is or where he is
   B. A deaf woman who lives alone and reports that the police are trying to rob her
   C. A woman who lives alone and is seeing 'shadow figures'
   D. A blind woman who lives alone and reports seeing policemen in her living room every night
   E. A man with ischaemic heart disease who feels like he is going to die

5. A 76-year-old woman who started mirtazapine for a depressive episode 4 weeks ago attends her general practitioner. Her son also has depression and noticed improvement after 2 weeks of an antidepressant. She has not noticed any benefit or side effects from mirtazapine and is wondering if she should change treatment. What would be the best management option?

   A. Change to the antidepressant that worked for her son
   B. Augment mirtazapine with the antidepressant that worked for her son

C. Change to a tricyclic antidepressant
D. Continue mirtazapine for at least 8 weeks
E. Discontinue mirtazapine and observe without antidepressant

6. A 77-year-old lady with a history of bipolar affective disorder no longer requiring medication is brought to the accident and emergency department by her family. In the past 24 hours she has started behaving very oddly – getting dressed in the middle of the night, dropping to the ground and shaking her leg about and shouting irritably at people when she is asked questions about her orientation. Her Abbreviated Mental Test score is 2/10. What is the most likely diagnosis?
    A. Lithium toxicity
    B. Manic episode
    C. Hypomanic episode
    D. Bodily distress disorder
    E. Delirium

7. A general practitioner (GP) pays a home visit to a 74-year-old man with a long history of schizophrenia. The man mentions that he is more bothered by auditory hallucinations than normal. The GP notices little piles of olanzapine tablets on saucers in the kitchen and living room. The man admits that he is struggling to keep track of whether he has taken his medication or not. What would be the best way to improve concordance?
    A. Start a depot antipsychotic
    B. Dispense medication weekly in a labelled compliance aid
    C. Refer for a support worker to prompt medication
    D. Arrange daily dispensing at the local pharmacy
    E. Change the time of olanzapine so he can take it in the morning with his other medication

8. An 82-year-old widow with no past psychiatric history presents to her general practitioner (GP) requesting a repeat prescription of trazodone. Her supply should not have run out yet, and she admits she took six extra tablets last night in the hope of 'going to sleep and not waking up'. In the event she just overslept, and no harm was done. She feels foolish now and would just like to go home and stop wasting the GP's time. What is the best management option?
    A. Ask her to attend accident and emergency (A&E)
    B. Review by GP in a week
    C. Refer to the local lunch club
    D. Refer to psychiatric outpatients
    E. Refer for urgent, same day, psychiatric review

Chapter 22 Alcohol and substance-related disorders

1. A 29-year-old man with alcohol dependence syndrome tells you that he wants to give up drinking, but he is worried that he will lose all his friends from the pub. At which stage of the Prochaska and DiClemente Transtheoretical Model of Change would you consider him to be?
    A. Precontemplation of change
    B. Contemplation of change
    C. Preparation for change
    D. Action for change
    E. Maintenance of change

2. A 21-year-old homeless woman tells you that she uses £20 of heroin per day via intravenous injection. She is keen to be prescribed methadone. Which of the following measures would be essential prior to starting methadone?
    A. History from a friend to corroborate her usage
    B. Viral serology for HIV and hepatitis B and C
    C. Thorough physical examination with focus on injection sites
    D. Admission to psychiatric hospital
    E. Urine drug test to confirm presence of opioids

3. A 45-year-old man is being treated by the alcohol problems team. He has successfully been 'detoxified' using chlordiazepoxide. Which of the following is true regarding his future pharmacological treatment?
    A. Trazodone can be prescribed to treat his alcohol dependence
    B. Long-term, low-dose chlordiazepoxide is the treatment of choice
    C. Naltrexone can be helpful even if he relapses to drinking
    D. Acamprosate causes an unpleasant reaction when taken with alcohol
    E. Disulfiram should control his cravings for alcohol

4. A 26-year-old woman asks you for help with her heroin dependence. She does not want to receive methadone, as she feels this is more addictive than heroin. Which of the following drugs might she prefer to try as substitution therapy?
    A. Lofexidine
    B. Diazepam
    C. Buprenorphine
    D. Clonidine
    E. Naltrexone

5. A 21-year-old former gymnast presents to addiction services for support with her excessive use of dihydrocodeine. She was prescribed this following an injury three years ago, and her use has escalated to the degree she is buying dihydrocodeine from street dealers. She has tried to stop 'cold turkey' but experienced significant withdrawal symptoms. She is willing to attend the chemist regularly if required. What would be the first-line treatment?

A. Methadone prescription
B. Ongoing dihydrocodeine prescription
C. Disulfiram
D. Naltrexone
E. Subcutaneous buprenorphine (Buvidal)

Chapter 23 The psychotic disorders

1. A pregnant woman with schizophrenia asks how likely her child is to develop schizophrenia. Her partner does not have a mental illness.

A. 1%
B. 12.5%
C. 2.5%
D. 37.5%
E. 50%

2. A pregnant woman with schizophrenia asks how likely her child is to develop schizophrenia. Her partner also has schizophrenia.

A. 1%
B. 12.5%
C. 25%
D. 37.5%
E. 50%

3. A 22-year-old man was started on olanzapine 4 months ago for a first episode of schizophrenia. He is now symptom free, but troubled by weight gain. He asks how long in total he needs to stay on an antipsychotic.

A. 6 months
B. 9 months
C. 1–2 years
D. 3–5 years
E. Lifelong

4. A 27-year-old woman has developed schizophrenia. She is interested in talking therapies. What type of psychological therapy does NICE (2014) recommend to her?

A. Psychodynamic psychotherapy
B. Interpersonal therapy
C. Dialectical behaviour therapy

D. Cognitive-behavioural therapy
E. Cognitive analytic therapy

5. A 32-year-old woman with an established diagnosis of schizoaffective disorder is admitted to hospital. She describes grandiose delusional beliefs that she is the wife of a prominent religious figure and has healing powers. She has pressured speech and is not sleeping. She is noted to be very irritable in her interactions with staff and fellow patients on the ward. She is not currently prescribed any medication as she has had a long period of stability in the community. What would be the most appropriate first management step?

A. Commence lithium
B. Commence sodium valproate
C. Commence olanzapine
D. Electroconvulsive therapy (ECT)
E. Watch and wait approach

6. A 28-year-old model has been admitted to an inpatient ward with a first episode of psychosis. She is very keen to avoid weight gain and states she would not be concordant with any treatment that causes her to gain weight. Which would be the most appropriate antipsychotic to trial first?

A. Olanzapine
B. Risperidone
C. Aripiprazole
D. Quetiapine
E. Zuclopenthixol

7. A 43-year-old woman with a diagnosis of schizophrenia presents to her GP complaining of a new 'rash' on her face, hands and upper chest. She was recently prescribed an 'as required' medication by her psychiatrist to help with periods of agitation in the context of a resolving psychotic episode. On examination she has widespread redness to the skin which is painful to touch. Which of the following medications is the most likely to have been prescribed and has cause of her symptoms?

A. Chlorpromazine
B. Olanzapine
C. Quetiapine
D. Risperidone
E. Diazepam

8. A 26-year-old woman with a diagnosis of schizophrenia remains troubled by distressing psychotic experiences associated with functional impairment. Her pharmacological management so far has included a 3-month trial of olanzapine and a 3-month trial of

risperidone at optimum doses. What would be the most appropriate next management step?

A. Switch to aripiprazole
B. Switch to clozapine
C. Work up for consideration of ECT treatment
D. Argument risperidone with lithium
E. Augment risperidone with amisulpride

Chapter 24 The mood (affective) disorders

1. Which of the following patients with depression would be the highest priority for electroconvulsive therapy (ECT)?

A. Someone who is not eating or drinking
B. Someone who believes they are already dead, so there is no point taking medication, but they are drinking fluids
C. Someone who has experienced no benefit from two antidepressants
D. Someone who has benefited from ECT in the past
E. Someone who has experienced no benefit from several antidepressants but does not want ECT

2. A 24-year-old man is brought to accident and emergency by the police. He has a 1-week history of irritable mood, insomnia and grandiose delusions that he has superpowers. The police found him about to jump off some scaffolding to prove he is invincible. He does not believe he is unwell and says there is no way he is coming into hospital. What is the best initial step in management?

A. Appointment with general practitioner later that day
B. Informal admission
C. Admission under mental health legislation
D. Urgent outpatient psychiatric review
E. Police custody after arrest for breach of the peace

3. A 45-year-old man is admitted to hospital with a 6-week history of low mood. He plans to kill himself at the first opportunity because he believes the world is going to end soon and wants to die quickly. He is not currently on any medication. What would be the best management option?

A. Citalopram
B. Amitriptyline
C. Quetiapine
D. Citalopram and quetiapine
E. Amitriptyline and quetiapine

4. A 29-year-old postgraduate student with a diagnosis of bipolar affective disorder is admitted with a manic episode after stopping medication. She is very agitated on the ward, pacing, being verbally aggressive to staff and fellow patients, and punching her wardrobe. What is the best medication to commence?

A. Lithium
B. Olanzapine
C. Citalopram
D. Sodium valproate
E. Lamotrigine

5. A 36-year-old lecturer with moderate to severe depression wants to try a psychological therapy for depression. Which of the following should be offered?

A. Self-help cognitive-behavioural therapy (CBT)
B. Structured group physical activity
C. Individual CBT
D. Dialectical behaviour therapy
E. Graded exposure therapy

6. A 55-year-old man with a mild depressive episode has not benefited from self-help CBT. He is not keen to try further psychological therapies. What would be the next most appropriate management step?

A. Refer to secondary care mental health services
B. Commence venlafaxine
C. Refer for psychodynamic psychotherapy
D. Commence clomipramine
E. Commence fluoxetine

Chapter 25 The anxiety, stress related, OCD related and bodily distress disorders

1. A 35-year-old woman has been recently diagnosed with bodily distress disorder. How should this diagnosis change her management by her general practitioner?

A. She should not be allowed access to urgent appointment slots
B. She should be seen on a planned, regular schedule
C. She should not be investigated for physical complaints
D. She should never be prescribed benzodiazepines
E. She should be reassured that her symptoms do not really exist

2. A 17-year-old school pupil has a phobia of bodily fluids but aspires to be a nurse. What treatment can she be offered?

A. None – she should change her career plans
B. Cognitive-behavioural therapy (CBT) with desensitization
C. CBT focused on trauma
D. Diazepam when necessary (PRN) – to be taken before any possible contact with bodily fluids
E. Selective serotonin reuptake inhibitor (SSRI)

3. A 29-year-old chemist has obsessive-compulsive disorder (OCD) regarding orderliness. She has been tidying up her colleagues' laboratory benches and spoilt some experiments. She has been threatened with dismissal. She does not want to try any talking therapies. What treatment can she be offered?

   A. Clomipramine
   B. Mirtazapine
   C. Selective serotonin reuptake inhibitor (SSRI)
   D. Pregabalin
   E. Self-help

4. A 35-year-old former soldier has been diagnosed with post traumatic stress disorder. He does not have a preference for either pharmacological or psychological therapy. What would be the most appropriate first step in his management?

   A. Inpatient admission
   B. Selective serotonin reuptake inhibitor (SSRI)
   C. CBT with a trauma focus
   D. Quetiapine
   E. Diazepam

5. A 44-year-old zookeeper has generalised anxiety disorder and is unable to work. He has tried CBT in the past and would now like to try a different talking therapy. Which would be the next most appropriate management option?

   A. Interpersonal therapy (IPT)
   B. Dialectical behavioural therapy (DBT)
   C. Mindfulness-based cognitive therapy (MBT)
   D. Psychodynamic psychotherapy
   E. Applied Relaxation

Chapter 26 Feeding and eating disorders

1. A 17-year-old boy has a median percentage body mass index (m% BMI) of 80%, wears baggy clothes, and states that he is worried about being overweight. He is diagnosed with anorexia nervosa, although he does not feel that he has a problem. However, he is agreeable to meeting a therapist, mainly to please his mother. Which of the following modalities of psychotherapy would be recommended in the first instance?

   A. Maudsley model of anorexia treatment for adults
   B. Family therapy
   C. Focal psychodynamic psychotherapy
   D. Cognitive-behavioural therapy
   E. Specialist supportive clinical management

2. A 20-year-old man has a body mass index of 16 kg/m², wears baggy clothes, and states that he is worried about being overweight. He was diagnosed with anorexia

nervosa as a 17-year-old. After a period of treatment and remission his symptoms have returned. Which of the following modalities of psychotherapy would be recommended in the first instance?

   A. Exposure-response prevention therapy
   B. Family therapy
   C. Focal psychodynamic psychotherapy
   D. Interpersonal therapy
   E. Individual eating-disorder-focused cognitive behavioural therapy (CBT-ED)

3. A 29-year-old female actuary is diagnosed with anorexia nervosa. Which of the following factors is associated with a poor prognosis?

   A. Early age of onset
   B. Rapid weight loss
   C. Binge–purge symptoms
   D. Family history of anorexia
   E. Slow to engage with psychotherapy

4. A 17-year-old woman has been diagnosed with anorexia nervosa. Which medication should she be advised to take until she regains a healthy nutritional intake?

   A. Citalopram
   B. Fluoxetine
   C. Multivitamin
   D. Paroxetine
   E. Sertraline

5. A 21-year-old woman with severe anorexia nervosa was found collapsed in the street secondary to heart failure due to malnutrition. She has subsequently been admitted to a specialist eating disorder unit to receive nasogastric feeding under mental health legislation. Which of the following blood test results raises concern that she is experiencing refeeding syndrome?

   A. Calcium 2.4 mmol/L
   B. Magnesium 1.7 mEq/L
   C. Phosphate 0.3 mmol/L
   D. Potassium 3.7 mmol/L
   E. Sodium 141 mmol/L

Chapter 27 The sleep–wake disorders

1. A 33-year-old woman describes creeping, burning sensations in her legs which keep her awake at night. She finds getting up and walking around eases them. Her mother had the same problem. She has tried nonpharmacological management and would like to try medication. Which medication is recommended first line?

A. Fluoxetine
B. Haloperidol
C. Lithium
D. Metoclopramide
E. Pramipexole

2. A 33-year-old woman describes creeping, burning sensations in her legs which keep her awake at night. The pain also affects her throughout the day. She finds getting up and walking around makes little difference. She has poorly controlled type one diabetes. What is the most likely diagnosis?

A. Akathisia
B. Intermittent claudication
C. Iron deficiency
D. Neuropathy
E. Restless legs syndrome

3. A 33-year-old woman describes trouble sleeping at night, with early morning wakening. She has recently been diagnosed with depression and started on fluoxetine (20 mg) 2 weeks ago. Her mood is slightly better, but she is worried that her sleep is not. What is the next best management step?

A. Increase fluoxetine dose
B. Keep a sleep diary
C. Refer for polysomnography
D. Sleep hygiene advice
E. Short course of temazepam

Chapter 26 Sexual problems and disorders

1. A 24-year-old woman presents to her general practitioner concerned that she achieves orgasm infrequently during penetrative sex with her partner. What should she be advised?

A. Caressing without genital contact can improve sex
B. Sexual dysfunction is rare in young people
C. She is likely to have a physical problem preventing orgasm
D. She should stop any medication which could be contributing
E. Talking about sexual problems with her partner is likely to increase anxiety in the bedroom

2. A 57-year-old man tells his general practitioner he is unable to have an erection, even when masturbating. He occasionally found it hard to achieve an erection as a younger man but it has got much worse recently. He was previously obese but has lost weight recently. What is the most important next management step?

A. Advise to lose more weight and return if problem persists
B. Check blood glucose
C. Direct to self-help resources regarding sexual dysfunction
D. Prescribe sildenafil
E. Refer to urology

3. A 63-year-old man with Parkinson disease has recently started making obscene phone calls. He becomes sexually aroused during this. He has been working his way through his wife's address book and several of her friends have been very distressed. Which of the medications below is least likely to have caused this behaviour?

A. Levodopa
B. Olanzapine
C. Pergolide
D. Pramipexole
E. Selegiline

4. A 23-year-old woman with obsessive-compulsive disorder attends her GP reporting that she is having difficulty achieving orgasm during sex with her long-term partner. Which of the following medications is the most likely to have contributed to this problem?

A. Mirtazapine
B. Pregabalin
C. Propranolol
D. Sertraline
E. Bupropion

Chapter 29 Disorders relating to the menstrual cycle, pregnancy and the puerperium

1. A 27 year old schoolteacher reports increased irritability in the week prior to menstruation. This quickly resolves within a day of starting her period. Most of the time the irritability does not cause her any problems apart from when she recently had an argument with her boyfriend. What is the best management option?

A. Encourage exercise
B. Prescribe combined oral contraceptive pill
C. Prescribe ibuprofen
D. Prescribe selective serotonin reuptake inhibitor (SSRI)
E. Refer for cognitive-behavioural therapy (CBT)

2. A 53-year-old company director reports low mood, increased fatigability and early morning wakening for the past 2 months, accompanied by increased suicidal thoughts. She has had to take some time off work. She attributes her symptoms to her menopause. What is the best management option?

A. Hormone replacement therapy
B. Dietary and lifestyle advice
C. Omega-3 fish oils
D. Counselling
E. Psychological therapy

3. A 25-year-old artist has a history of bipolar disorder. She has been taking lithium and has been well for the past 3 years. She presents to her GP and explains that she wants to start a family with her partner and has heard that lithium can cause problems with foetal malformations. What is the most appropriate management?
A. Switch to semisodium valproate
B. Switch to carbamazepine
C. Discontinue lithium and continue without treatment
D. Switch to olanzapine
E. Refer to perinatal mental health team

A. A 33-year-old woman previously experienced a protracted episode of postnatal depression following the birth of her first child, which necessitated admission to a mother-and-baby unit. The episode responded well to antidepressant medication. She has recently become pregnant and is incredibly anxious that she will become unwell again postnatally. What is the most appropriate management?
A. Reassure that becoming unwell again would be unlikely
B. Restart antidepressant treatment immediately
C. Referral to psychologist to identify relapse signature
D. Watchful waiting
E. Referral to perinatal mental health team

5. A 22-year-old lady is found by the police. She was found walking near a river with her 2-week-old baby boy. She reported that the infant was possessed by the devil, and that she had thoughts that she needed to drown him to save humanity. At interview, she appears perplexed and is openly responding to auditory hallucinations. She does not want to be admitted to hospital as she does not think she is unwell. She has a very supportive family who are keen to look after her at home. What is the most appropriate initial management option?
A. Detention in hospital under mental health act
B. Treatment at home under care of crisis team
C. Transfer to police cells
D. Urgent referral for outpatient follow-up by perinatal mental health team
E. Urgent referral to social work

Chapter 30 The personality disorders

1. A 19-year-old hairdresser has a diagnosis of a moderate personality disorder with prominent features of negative affectivity and disinhibition and a borderline pattern. She requests information on drug treatment that may be beneficial. What should she be advised?
A. Sodium valproate is effective for reducing interpersonal problems
B. Omega-3 fatty acids are effective in reducing impulsivity
C. Risperidone is effective for reducing anger
D. Amitriptyline reduces chronic feelings of emptiness
E. Drug treatment is not the main intervention

2. A 34-year-old man has a diagnosis of a personality disorder with prominent features of disinhibition and dissociality, and requests information on different types of psychotherapy that may be beneficial. Which of the following psychological treatments does NICE (2009) recommend?
A. Dialectical behaviour therapy
B. Mentalization-based therapy
C. Psychodynamic
D. Cognitive-analytical therapy
E. Therapeutic communities

3. A 27-year-old female postgraduate student has a diagnosis of a personality disorder with prominent features of negative affectivity and a borderline pattern. She reported low mood and insomnia for the past month and has subsequently been absent from university (which is unusual for her). Normally, she is easily angered, but relatively cheerful. At assessment she reports increased thoughts of suicide, but no immediate plans. What is the most appropriate next step in management?
A. Refer for dialectical behaviour therapy
B. Request a urine drug screen
C. Prescribe diazepam
D. Admit to an acute psychiatric ward
E. Suggest 'weekly dispensing' of medication

4. A 29-year-old man has a diagnosis of a severe personality disorder with prominent features of dissociality. He coldly tells his psychiatrist of his intention to kill his landlord following an argument about rent arrears, before describing a detailed plan on how he would stab him in the throat. What is the most appropriate next management step?
A. Ask him to return for review in 1 week
B. Prescribe diazepam
C. Alert the police and the intended victim
D. Admit to psychiatric hospital under detention
E. Refer for anger management

Chapter 31 The neurodevelopmental disorders

1. A 23-year-old man is diagnosed with an autism spectrum disorder. Which medication can be prescribed to reduce the core symptoms of his disorder?
   A. Fluoxetine
   B. Methylphenidate
   C. None
   D. Risperidone
   E. Sodium valproate

2. A 7-year-old boy has recently been diagnosed with attention deficit hyperactivity disorder (ADHD). It is having a substantial impact on his behaviour at school, and he is at risk of expulsion. His parents have already attended a parent-training programme. What should be the next management option trialled?
   A. Atomoxetine
   B. Cognitive-behavioural therapy
   C. Dexamphetamine
   D. Methylphenidate
   E. Referral to social work for consideration of a place at a special educational needs school

3. A 12-year-old boy has multiple motor tics and repeatedly shouts 'Batman!' when he is stressed or excited. He had to leave the cinema once because of this but is otherwise not troubled by his symptoms. What is the first-line treatment for this disorder?
   A. Clonidine
   B. No treatment
   C. Pimozide
   D. Psychoeducation
   E. Risperidone

Chapter 32 Intellectual Disability

1. A 24-year-old man with a moderate intellectual disability is referred to his local Community Learning Disability team by the manager of his care home. He has become increasingly distressed at mealtimes, and is at times hitting out at staff. What would be the appropriate first step in management?
   A. Commence risperidone 0.5 mg twice daily
   B. A physical examination
   C. Arrange care in a secure facility
   D. Suggest he is placed under 1:1 supervision
   E. Contact the police to report the assaults on staff

2. A 32-year-old woman with a mild learning disability who lives in supported accommodation is admitted to hospital following an overdose of paracetamol. She is reviewed with her support worker, and presents as very withdrawn and appears to startle easily when her support worker moves closer to her. The support worker has requested that they are present to 'help with communication'. You notice some unusual bruising on her arms. What would be the most appropriate first step?
   A. Discharge her home
   B. Refer to the community learning disability team
   C. Continue trying to assess her with her support worker present
   D. Ask the support worker to leave the room so you can speak to the patient alone
   E. Admit to an inpatient psychiatric ward for further assessment

Chapter 33 Child and adolescent psychiatry

1. For the past 6 months, a 12-year-old boy has repeatedly been in trouble with the police. Recently, he has been violent towards his sister and has killed her pet hamster. His mother sought help after he deliberately set the garden shed on fire. What is the most likely diagnosis?
   A. Personality disorder with prominent traits of dissociality
   B. Conduct-dissocial disorder
   C. Oppositional defiant disorder
   D. Reactive attachment disorder
   E. Substance misuse

2. An 8-year-old girl presents with encopresis. During examination by the junior doctor, genital warts and vaginal trauma are noted. What is the next most appropriate step in management?
   A. The child should be sent home and seen in outpatients
   B. The parents should be confronted by the nurses
   C. The child should be directly asked what happened
   D. Police should be contacted to question the girl
   E. The duty social worker and on-call paediatrician should be alerted

3. A 16-year-old girl presents with a 2-month history of low mood and fatigue. She no longer enjoys playing netball and feels her friends do not like her anymore. She is still attending school but is no longer doing well academically. What treatment should she be offered first line?
   A. Citalopram
   B. Cognitive-behavioural therapy
   C. Fluoxetine
   D. Sertraline
   E. Watchful waiting

4. A 16-year-old girl presents with low mood. She has had episodes of low mood for most of her life, often varying from good to bad and back again within a day. She has never had any close friends because she feels her peers have always rejected her. She has self-harmed by cutting since the age of 13 years, and often makes herself sick after meals. She says she feels angry and empty at the same time. After her father took an overdose she started hearing his voice inside her head telling her to do it too. Her body mass index is 22 kg/m². What is the most likely diagnosis?
    A. Bipolar disorder
    B. Bulimia nervosa
    C. Depressive episode
    D. Personality disorder prominent features of negative affectivity and a borderline pattern
    E. Schizophrenia

5. A 4-year-old boy has recently been adopted by his aunt and uncle after his parents died in a road traffic accident. He had normal language development and initially he seemed to settle in well to his new home. However, he gradually stopped speaking at home. Nursery staff report he speaks normally there. During the consultation he initially does not speak but does so when his adoptive parents leave the room. His adoptive parents appear caring but anxious and unsure what to do. They have been arguing recently. What is the most likely diagnosis?
    A. Selective mutism
    B. Posttraumatic stress disorder
    C. Social anxiety disorder
    D. Autism spectrum disorder
    E. Reactive attachment disorder

6. A 4-year-old girl watches other children playing at nursery but does not attempt to join in. When she falls over in the playground she cowers away when an adult offers first-aid. She has a sad demeanour but otherwise shows little emotion. She has been taken into care after experiencing physical abuse from both parents. What is the most likely diagnosis?
    A. Selective mutism
    B. Posttraumatic stress disorder
    C. Social anxiety disorder
    D. Autism spectrum disorder
    E. Reactive attachment disorder

Chapter 34 Forensic psychiatry

1. A 32-year-old man with substance misuse problems reports he is thinking of taking up mugging to fund his habit. Which of the following factors in his history places him at highest risk of future violence?
    A. Having a mental disorder
    B. Using substances
    C. Previous violence
    D. Experiencing command hallucinations
    E. Childhood abuse

2. A 19-year-old gentleman has been charged with a serious assault. He appears incredibly distracted and distressed and is openly responding to auditory hallucinations. The forensic psychiatrist has been asked to assess his fitness to plead. What finding on mental state exam would suggest he was fit to plead?
    A. He is unable to say why he is in custody
    B. He asks for most questions to be repeated as he is distracted by hallucinations
    C. He is thought disordered, with loosening of associations such that his answers are very hard to follow
    D. He believes he has been abducted by aliens and his answers will determine the fate of the universe
    E. He is able to give a coherent account of events leading up to the offence but denies memory of the offence itself

3. A 36-year-old man with schizophrenia has committed a crime. He asks his lawyer if he can be considered to have had diminished responsibility. What is the only charge diminished responsibility applies to?
    A. Arson
    B. Rape
    C. Theft
    D. Grievous bodily harm
    E. Murder

4. A 21-year-old man has been charged with assaulting a police officer. He has a lengthy history of police contacts from adolescence onwards, mainly for impulsive acts of aggression. He dropped out of school at 14 years of age because he struggled to concentrate. He is angry with himself for getting into trouble with the police again and is asking for help in controlling his bursts of anger. What diagnosis should he be further assessed for?
    A. Personality disorder with prominent features of dissociality
    B. Attention deficit hyperactivity disorder (ADHD)
    C. Autism spectrum disorder
    D. Bipolar disorder
    E. Personality disorder prominent features of disinhibition and a borderline pattern

5. A 35-year-old man was arrested after he assaulted a bus driver. He believed that the driver was trying to procure the services of his wife, who he is convinced is working as a prostitute. He has dismissed extensive reassurances from his wife and his own siblings. He reports that he has a sword in the back of his car and intended to 'get the truth out of her'. He has a history of alcohol abuse. What is the most likely diagnosis?
   A. Delusional disorder (delusional jealousy)
   B. Schizophrenia
   C. Schizoaffective disorder
   D. Personality disorder with a borderline pattern and prominent traits of dissociality
   E. Single episode depressive disorder

SBA answers

Chapter 2 Pharmacological therapy and electroconvulsive therapy

1. C. Weekly full blood counts (FBCs). Without monitoring, just under 3% of patients treated with clozapine develop neutropenia (low neutrophil count), and just under 1% develop agranulocytosis (negligible neutrophil count). This is most likely to occur early in treatment. Therefore, weekly FBCs are advised initially. As for all antipsychotics, she will also require regular checks of blood pressure, liver function, lipid profile and glucose. These parameters should be checked every 1 to 3 months initially, then annually.

2. E. Egg mayonnaise toastie is the only safe option, given the dietary restrictions required for irreversible monoamine oxidase inhibitors such as phenelzine. See Box 2.2. She should also avoid drinking Chianti wine with lunch.

3. C. This patient is at significant risk of harm related to their severe depression due to their lack of oral intake. Due to the life-threatening nature of this presentation ECT would be indicated.

4. D. Sodium valproate must not be used in women or men of childbearing potential due to the risks of congenital abnormalities in an unborn foetus (neurodevelopmental disorders including malformation of the spinal cord) and risks of infertility in men.

5. C. Propranolol. This woman is probably experiencing akathisia. This is hard to treat, but propranolol or benzodiazepines can help. Procyclidine does not help akathisia and may make it worse as it is an alerting medication. Ideally, the dose of antipsychotic is reduced. Quinine can be used for restless leg syndrome when in bed. The differential includes agitation secondary to psychosis.

6. B. Oral procyclidine. This man has drug-induced parkinsonism. In the early stages, the features are different to idiopathic parkinsonism. Anticholinergics such as procyclidine can help, but ideally the dose of antipsychotic would be reduced or an alternative antipsychotic trialled.

7. C. Stop anticholinergics, such as procyclidine. This man has tardive dyskinesia. This is hard to treat but stopping anticholinergics and reducing or withdrawing antipsychotics, if possible, can help.

8. B. Venlafaxine is an SNRI. SNRIs work by inhibiting reuptake of serotonin and noradrenaline back into cells and do not affect acetylcholine. Duloxetine is another of the SNRIs.

Chapter 3 Psychological therapy

1. C. This man is likely suffering from prolonged grief disorder. In the first instance, it would be helpful to direct him to bereavement counselling, which most commonly takes the form of person-centred counselling. In the United Kingdom, Cruse is a large voluntary sector service offering bereavement counselling. Psychodynamic therapy, cognitive-behavioural therapy and mindfulness-based cognitive therapy have little evidence to support their use in this instance. Exposure and response prevention is a behavioural therapy used in the treatment of obsessive-compulsive disorder.

2. C. Transference is the theoretical process by which the patient transfers feelings or attitudes experienced in an earlier significant relationship onto the therapist. Counter-transference refers to the feelings that are evoked in the therapist during the course of therapy. The therapist pays attention to these feelings, as they may be representative of what the patient is feeling, and so helps the therapist to empathize with the patient. Often, the therapist has undergone therapy themselves as part of their training: this helps the therapist to separate out what feelings belong to them, and what feelings belong to the patient.

3. E. This cognitive distortion is an example of magnification (also known as 'catastrophization or catastrophizing'), where things get 'blown out of proportion.' An example of emotional reasoning in this context would be 'I feel so miserable, so I must have failed my exam.' An example of fortune telling would be 'I failed my exam, so in the future no one will employ me.' An example of personalization would be 'It is all my fault: I failed my exams.' An example of labelling would be 'I am stupid.' Note that more than one type of cognitive distortion can exist in the same patient in the same circumstances. See Table 3.3.

4. B. There is a strong evidence base to support the use of interpersonal therapy in the treatment of mild to moderate depression. See Table 3.5 for modalities of benefit in the other conditions listed.

5. D. Interpersonal therapy is based on the assumptions that problems with interpersonal relationships and social functioning contribute significantly to mental illness. Main areas of focus include role disputes, role transitions, interpersonal deficits and grief. She may also find cognitive-behavioural therapy of benefit, for example, if interpersonal therapy is not available.

6. A. Exposure and response prevention is a type of cognitive-behavioural therapy in which the patient is encouraged not to respond to the obsessional thought with a compulsive act. Relaxation techniques are used instead to overcome the anxiety associated with not carrying out the compulsion.

Chapter 4 Mental health and the law

1. D. She needs to notify the DVLA of her diagnosis. They will then ask for a doctor's report and potentially a driving assessment and are likely to arrange more frequent reviews of the licence than otherwise (e.g., annually). It is the DVLA's decision as to whether she is fit to drive or not. Many patients with mild dementia are found fit to continue to drive. Patient and partner reports of driving can be unreliable as patients can have poor insight and partners may not want to act in a way they perceive as harming the patient, or themselves. It is the patient's responsibility to notify the DVLA although doctors may need to do so if patients ignore this advice and present a significant risk to others through driving.

2. B. The patient lacks capacity as his low GCS means he will not be able to communicate his decision. He is also unlikely to be able to understand, to retain and to weigh up information, but this cannot be assessed in the absence of communication.

3. D. He is likely to lack capacity for any decisions requiring more consideration than is available in working memory as he will not be able to retain information for long enough to weigh it up. As a guide, someone should be able to retain information for as long as necessary to make a decision. A quick decision, e.g., meal choice, does not require a long time to make. A big decision, e.g., where to live, would normally be something that a person would consider and mull over for a few days at least.

4. C. She lacks capacity for the decision about surgery, as she does not believe the information because of a

delusion. However, she is likely to have the capacity to make decisions about which she does not have delusions.

5. A. He should be assumed to have the capacity to make a decision about a statin, unless his psychotic symptoms relate to cholesterol (which is unusual) or he is very thought disordered.

Chapter 5 Mental health service provision

1. B. Patient B has evidence of treatment resistance, and would be most appropriate for CMHT input.

2. B. Early intervention in psychosis team. This man may be experiencing prodromal psychosis. He does not currently appear to be at high enough risk to require home treatment or admission. As he does not have an established diagnosis of mental illness, an assertive outreach team is not appropriate. A community mental health team could manage him, but early intervention teams are expert at identifying early psychosis and are therefore best placed to monitor him.

Chapter 6 The patient with thoughts of suicide or self-harm

1. D. While researching methods is also worrying, acts of closure (such as making a will, organizing finances, writing suicide notes) are the most worrying signs and suggest strong suicidal intent. Contacting voluntary support agencies (such as the Samaritans) suggests emotional distress but also a degree of ambivalence. Telling his wife of his plans may be a way of communicating his feelings to her but is not necessarily a final act. Disclosing plans to a healthcare professional does not reduce his risk.

2. C. Suspension hanging is the most common method of completed suicide in England, Wales and many other countries. Means are widely available and lethality is high. Paracetamol is the most common drug of overdose in the UK; however, advances in medical treatment and public health measures have reduced mortality associated with this. Jumping from height is a fairly 'public' method of suicide and thus is often reported in the news (although media coverage of all suicides has reduced in recent years due to campaigns to reduce 'advertising' of suitable locations). Carbon monoxide poisoning used to be fairly common; however, catalytic converters on modern motor vehicles has reduced fatality of this method.

3. A. Personality disorders with a borderline pattern carries a 45-fold risk of completed suicide compared to the

general population. Personality disorders without a borderline pattern are also associated with elevated, but lower, risk. Anxiety disorders carry a 3-fold risk, anorexia carries an 8-fold risk, schizophrenia has a 13-fold risk and OCD is not associated with increased risk of completed suicide. There is some variation in these figures depending on the source.

4. B. Personality disorder with a borderline pattern and prominent traits of disinhibition. She is a young woman with a long history of self-harm, difficulties with interpersonal relationships and auditory pseudohallucinations at times of stress. She has no symptoms suggestive of a depressive illness.

5. C. This woman has made a serious suicide attempt. Note that she went to some effort to prevent discovery (remote location, unsocial hour) and made acts of closure (typed letters imply that some thought had gone into these). She has neurovegetative and psychotic symptoms of depression. She may have intoxicated herself to reduce her inhibitions prior to the act and is not necessarily alcohol dependent.

Chapter 7 Psychiatric emergencies

1. C. Physical health assessment including measurement of serum paracetamol levels (plus INR, liver function, other baseline bloods) to determine the requirement for potentially life-saving treatment is the priority in this case. This can be measured from 4 hours postingestion although levels become harder to interpret after 15 hours. The other options are all important aspects of psychiatric evaluation and risk assessment but are not urgent.

2. B. Looking at his prescription. Although the two syndromes have features in common, they can nearly always be easily distinguished by medication history (see Table 2.8). Clonus is another useful distinguishing factor, as it is present in serotonin syndrome but absent in neuroleptic malignant syndrome (where lead-pipe rigidity is common).

3. E. Assess ABCDE. This man is likely to be experiencing neuroleptic malignant syndrome. After ABCDE has been addressed, all antipsychotics should also be discontinued. The other answers are all possible treatment options, but none are first line. Before they are considered, he needs initial resuscitation, and then is likely to need transfer to a general hospital for investigation and monitoring. See Table 2.8.

4. E. 1.8 mmol/L. Her symptoms are consistent with lithium toxicity in the 1.5–2.0 mmol/L range. However,

symptoms of toxicity can manifest at lower levels, particularly in older adults. Toxicity is likely to have been precipitated by the recent course of nonsteroidal antiinflammatory drugs. See Table 2.3.

5. D. If safe to do so verbal de-escalation techniques should always be attempted in the first instance. If these fail more restrictive measures such as oral/IM medication or restraint can be considered. As this patient believes staff are trying to perform experiments on her, touching her against her will (such as during a restraint or IM) may escalate the situation rather than diffuse it.

6. D. Temperature, pulse, blood pressure, respiratory rate, hydration status and consciousness level should be checked every 15 minutes following parenteral administration of rapid tranquillization (until there are no further concerns about the patient's physical health status) where any of the following apply (NICE 2015):

Patient appears to be asleep or sedated

Patient has recently taken recreational drugs or alcohol

BNF maximum doses for medication have been exceeded

Patient has a preexisting physical health problem

Patient experienced any harm as a result of the intervention

If none of the above have occurred, observations should be hourly until the patient is able to walk and interact normally. If the patient refuses or remains too behaviourally disturbed to allow observations, they should be regularly observed for respiratory effort, airway and consciousness level. See Fig. 21.2.

7. C. Transient hyperglycaemia secondary to stress may arise but is unlikely to be clinically important. All the other options are potentially life-threatening: benzodiazepines can cause respiratory depression, oversedation by any means can cause loss of airway, antipsychotics and hyperarousal increase the risk of arrhythmia, and benzodiazepines and antipsychotics can both cause hypotension. Additional life-threatening complications of antipsychotic use include seizures and dystonias. All these complications can occur with oral formulations also, but are more likely when large doses are given via a fast-acting method.

8. A. Intramuscular procyclidine. This woman is experiencing a dystonia with an oculogyric crisis and trismus (sustained contraction of muscles of mastication). Her clenched jaw means administering oral procyclidine is not possible. Baclofen and dantrolene should be used for chronic spasticity.

Chapter 8 Patient with neurodevelopmental differences

1. C. Ensure he has an eye test. This boy may not be able to see the blackboard. Children can be embarrassed to admit this. ADHD and thyroid dysfunction are unlikely given that the symptoms are only present in one setting. Genetic testing is not yet indicated in ADHD and certainly cannot be used to exclude it. A collateral history from the teacher would be helpful if his eye test comes back normal.

2. E. Rett syndrome. The fact that she initially developed normally, then regressed, excludes autism and intellectual disability. Heller syndrome (childhood disintegrative disorder) is possible but unlikely as it is more common in males and usually has onset after the age of 2 years. Muscular dystrophy is also possible, but the child would be more likely to present with generalized muscle weakness, rather than only a reduced use of those muscles important for social interaction. It also mainly affects boys.

3. B. Autism spectrum disorder. This is suggested by his poor understanding of social cues and the hint that he has an unusually intense interest. To make this diagnosis definitive, a much fuller history would be required. Social anxiety is unlikely as the problem is his poor social understanding, not him feeling that others are critical of him. Social anxiety is nonetheless common as a consequence of autism. A personality disorder with prominent traits of anankastia is unlikely as this does not impair the ability to interact socially. A depressive episode might follow his redundancy but it is not the primary problem. Generalized anxiety is unlikely as he has not mentioned worrying about anything except social situations.

4. B. This woman has a mild intellectual disability. It will take her longer to learn tasks than her peers without an intellectual disability, but she is able to work and live independently with appropriate support in place. Individuals in this group represent the majority (85%) of all people with intellectual disabilities.

5. D. This man has a severe intellectual disability. He lives with his family, who are his main carers and is able to perform simple tasks under supervision. His self-care skills are limited, but sometimes he seems able to contribute to these.

6. C. Traumatic brain injury. This would need to be confirmed by checking the details of his injuries in the road traffic accident. ADHD is excluded by the lack of significant difficulties prior to the accident (suggested by his ability to work as an accountant). He may be suffering neuropsychological sequelae post damage to his frontal lobes.

Chapter 9 The patient with psychotic symptoms

1. B. Charles Bonnet syndrome. Based on the information given here, Charles Bonnet syndrome is the most likely diagnosis. However, it is crucial to exclude delirium with a physical examination and cognitive assessment.

2. B. Ischaemic heart disease. This man has risk factors for ischaemic heart disease (age, male, smoker) and gives a description of exercise-induced chest pain with a classic 'weight on chest' description typical of cardiac ischaemia. People with schizophrenia are at increased risk of cardiovascular disease. Although this symptom could also be a tactile hallucination, it is important to exclude a physical origin before making this attribution.

3. A. Delusions of infidelity. This man has developed a delusion that his wife is having an affair based on a seemingly illogical factor (in this case how she is doing her hair), and this is fixed, as shown by his upset when questioned by his GP. The impact of this delusion on this man's life is substantial as he has become preoccupied with it to an unreasonable extent.

4. B. Substance-induced psychotic disorder. Substance intoxication is also a differential, particularly if he has been using the new stimulants every day or nearly every day – more information is needed as to timing and pattern of his substance use. A definite diagnosis of substance-induced psychotic disorder is the most likely diagnosis but requires a longitudinal assessment. The diagnosis would be confirmed if he stops using substances and his symptoms resolve. However, chronic cannabis use is a risk factor for developing schizophrenia and if his symptoms persist despite abstaining from substances this may emerge as the diagnosis. At present he has not had the symptoms long enough to meet criteria for schizophrenia in any case.

5. B. Hypnogogic hallucinations are hallucinations that occur as a person is falling asleep. A hypnopompic hallucination occurs as a person is waking up. These hallucinations do not occur at any times other than when she is falling asleep, so schizophrenia or a severe depression with psychotic symptoms are unlikely. A pseudohallucination is an abnormal perception that the patient is able to recognize as being from their own mind.

6. D. Schizoaffective disorder is the most likely diagnosis. This man has concurrent mood symptoms and first-rank symptoms of schizophrenia. His mood and psychotic symptoms are equally prominent, making a recurrent psychotic depression unlikely.

7. E. Delusional disorder is the most likely diagnosis. This man has a longstanding unshakeable belief arrived at through faulty reasoning: a delusion. He has insight into this. Schizophrenia is unlikely because the delusion is nonbizarre and functioning is intact. In hypochondriasis patients normally are able to briefly accept an alternative explanation and reassurance. However, at the most extreme end in hypochondriasis with poor to absent insight they cannot accept an alternative explanation for their experience and this would also be a reasonable diagnosis to make given the information available. Delusional disorder is made the most likely diagnosis by the delusional perception (smelling dog faeces) which triggered the belief.

8. A. Personality disorder. This man is not delusional as his belief is not fixed. He is suspicious and litigious. The history from the police of multiple previous calls suggests his difficulties are longstanding. This would be consistent with a paranoid personality disorder. However, a fuller background history would be required to make a definite diagnosis.

9. E. Neurosyphilis. This is now a rare diagnosis in the UK but should always be considered in those with work or travel histories that may have placed them at risk of contracting syphilis. Neurosyphilis is a type of tertiary syphilis that emerges several years after initial infection. Clinical features are diverse but can include personality change, grandiose behaviour and dementia, along with upper motor neuron abnormalities such as brisk reflexes and extensor plantars.

Chapter 10 The patient with elated or irritable mood

1. A. Manic episode, with accelerated speech, probable thought disorder, and likely hallucinations. Hypomania and cyclothymia are excluded by the significant functional impairment his symptoms have caused him. An agitated depression could be associated with an increased rate of speech, but the content should be understandable. Schizophrenia can be associated with thought disorder, but very rarely with accelerated rate of speech.

2. B. Bipolar affective disorder. An episode of depression is not necessary to meet criteria for bipolar affective disorder. Recurrent mania and hypomania are not diagnoses. No first-rank symptoms are mentioned, making schizoaffective disorder unlikely. Cyclothymia is excluded by the presence of psychotic symptoms.

3. D. Urine drug screen. This will demonstrate recent use of common recreational drugs (although it will not screen for novel psychoactive substances). The main differentials in a healthy young man are a manic episode or intoxication or mania secondary to psychoactive substance use. Full blood count should be performed to check for evidence of infection, but is likely to be normal. Thyroid function test should be checked to exclude hyperthyroidism but is also likely to be normal. EEG and CT head should only be requested if there are neurological abnormalities.

4. D. Personality disorder. This woman describes a persistent pattern of maladaptive behaviour present since childhood associated with social and occupational dysfunction. This is most likely to be a personality disorder, with prominent impulsivity. It would be important to get a collateral history before making a definite diagnosis. The mood swings are faster than would occur within bipolar affective disorder or cyclothymia and she has never had a period of euthymia, required for a diagnosis of a mood disorder. Dysthymia is prolonged low mood, not mood swings. Although substance use can cause and worsen emotional lability it should not have onset in childhood.

5. C. Hypomanic episode. This man describes elated mood with a decreased need for sleep, poor concentration, increased energy, increased recent expenditure and increased libido. It is interfering with his social and occupational functioning, but these activities are not completely disrupted. We are not given information on past mood abnormalities, so the diagnosis of bipolar affective disorder is not appropriate.

6. A. Manic episode with psychotic features. This patient's presentation is most in keeping with an episode mania with psychotic features. He presents with reduced sleep, reduced appetite, psychomotor agitation and a grandiose delusion which has resulted in marked disruption to his occupational function. It is likely that a diagnosis of bipolar affective disorder will be made, as he has presented with his first episode of mania. Only one episode of mania is required to make a diagnosis of bipolar affective disorder. It is also important to exclude substance use.

Chapter 11 The patient with low mood

1. E. Prednisolone is the only medication listed commonly associated with depression. The others are not.

2. B. The midline neck swelling may represent a goitre. Given the patient's symptoms are mild, there is time to check her thyroid function before commencing treatment. If she is hypothyroid this should be treated first, which may normalize her mood without need for an

antidepressant. Mild depression does not need referral to psychiatry. A neck ultrasound is likely to be needed also, but thyroid function should be checked first. She should not be sent away without investigation as the cause of the midline neck swelling needs to be determined.

3. D. The patient reports symptoms of depression alongside a mood-congruent nihilistic delusion. Therefore, the most likely diagnosis is a severe single depressive disorder with psychotic features. His lack of past psychiatric history makes schizoaffective disorder, schizophrenia and bipolar disorder unlikely, as onset at his age is rare. Early-onset dementia with behavioural and psychological symptoms is an unlikely possibility, but to check for this, his cognition, family history and ability to care for himself should be carefully assessed.

4. D. Suicidal ideation should be checked in everyone with a potential depressive episode. The other areas are all important but can be explored at a later review.

5. D. This patient is in a situational crisis. It is likely that her symptoms will resolve spontaneously. She needs reassurance and to be offered a follow-up appointment to check on her progress. She cannot be diagnosed with depression as her symptoms are present for less than 2 weeks, and she is unlikely to benefit from an antidepressant. However, she may still be at risk of self-harm and should be screened for this. She does not need investigations or a mood diary unless her symptoms persist. Her symptoms are not severe enough to need referral to psychiatry at present.

6. A. Multiple sclerosis. Multiple sclerosis would be an important differential here. This is suggested by her two neurological symptoms separated in time and place. Depression is common in multiple sclerosis.

7. C. Psychomotor agitation. This is a common feature of depression in older adults and describes restlessness and agitation that results in repetitive and unintentional movements.

Chapter 12 The patient with anxiety, fear or avoidance

1. D. Panic attack. This is the most likely diagnosis based on the history. However, it is important to take a full medical history (e.g., asthma, congenital heart disease) and family history (e.g., sudden death in young relatives) and to exclude other causes such as hyperthyroidism and hypoglycaemia, particularly given her repeat attendances. It would also be useful to know whether the attacks appear to have triggers (e.g., substance use/withdrawal, going to the library).

2. C. Blood-injection-injury phobia. This is suggested by his situational paroxysmal anxiety and avoidance. A myocardial infarction is unlikely to occur every time he is due to see the practice nurse. Hypoglycaemia, not hyperglycaemia, could cause these symptoms but is unlikely without a history of diabetes. Panic disorder does not have a specific trigger. Hypochondriasis is fear of having an illness, not fear of being investigated for one.

3. B. Airway, Breathing, Circulation, Disability, Exposure. The first step in management is ABCDE. She is speaking to you, so her airway is maintained independently. The next step is to ascertain her breathing and circulation status. Although the differential includes a panic attack, she could also be experiencing a wide range of acute medical problems requiring urgent management. An ECG, ABG, blood tests and psychiatry referral may all be appropriate in due course.

4. E. Check blood sugar. Someone with type 1 diabetes will be receiving insulin. The description sounds very much like hypoglycaemia. If hypoglycaemia is confirmed it is important to treat the episode by consuming carbohydrate, and then examine his insulin/food/activity regime to reduce further episodes. If his blood sugars are normal, he may be experiencing panic attacks as part of panic disorder. Keeping a diary and deep breathing exercises may help with these (see Chapter 23 for management). Seeing a counsellor may help if he is experiencing a stressful life event, illness or bereavements. Diazepam is only recommended in social anxiety disorder or specific phobia, for infrequent as required use.

5. D. Alcohol withdrawal. This man is drinking at least 60 units/week. He is experiencing physiological withdrawal symptoms after a few hours without alcohol, and the symptoms are relieved by further alcohol. Although anxiety in the morning may be part of diurnal variation in a depressive disorder, this man's mood is generally good, excluding depression. A phobia of something related to work is unlikely as the symptoms have only had onset recently (although enquiring regarding recent changes at work could be helpful). Hypoglycaemia secondary to diabetes is unlikely to present only in the mornings. Panic disorder is excluded by the clear relationship with alcohol.

6. B. Agoraphobia with panic attacks. This lady had a panic attack in a supermarket and has now become increasingly avoidant of crowding and confinement. Her symptoms are restricted to these situations. The weight loss may well be explained by her reduced dietary intake and increased exercise, but other disorders should be

screened for, i.e., hyperthyroidism. All her panic attacks are in the context of going outside in places with lots of people (agoraphobia). If they occurred outwith this context, comorbid panic disorder could be diagnosed too.

7. A. Panic disorder. This man reports repeated nonsituational panic attacks including a sensation of derealization. His symptoms could be due to cardiac problems but his young age, lack of exercise-induced symptoms and normal ECG are reassuring.

8. A. Caffeine. Caffeine has anxiogenic effects. Many soft drinks contain large amounts of caffeine, including tea/coffee, energy drinks and cola.

Chapter 13 The patient with obsessions and compulsions

1. A. No mental illness. Lay people often use 'obsession' loosely. Her thoughts of the show are not obsessional as they are ego-syntonic, pleasurable and not resisted. She describes no compulsions. She is not delusional in that there is no evidence of irrational thinking. She is not socially phobic in that she has not reported anxiety in social situations. There is no evidence of a persistent pattern of perfectionism and rigid thinking, as would be expected in a personality disorder with prominent traits of anankastia. Calling in sick represents unethical behaviour rather than a mental illness.

2. C. Depressive disorder. This man reports obsessions, but they are concurrent with the change in his mood, meeting the criteria for a depressive episode of moderate severity (five depressive symptoms). The obsessions are mood-congruent. Depression rather than obsessive-compulsive disorder is the primary diagnosis. Generalized anxiety disorder is unlikely as he does not report free-floating anxiety about many topics. Hypochondriasis is unlikely as he is not worried about a particular condition, but being dead. A nihilistic delusion is not suggested as he tries to distract himself, suggesting he is resisting the image rather than accepting it as reality.

3. D. OCD with comorbid depressive episode. This man describes obsessions and compulsions associated with functional impairment of greater than 2 weeks duration, giving him a diagnosis of OCD. Superimposed on this he has developed a depressive episode of mild severity. Generalized anxiety disorder is unlikely as he does not report free-floating anxiety about many topics. There is no evidence of a persistent pattern of perfectionism and rigid thinking, as would be expected in a personality disorder with prominent traits of anankastia.

4. B. Mild personality disorder with prominent traits of anankastia. This is suggested by her lifelong history of unusual conscientiousness and perfectionism which has caused some functional impairment (reduction of leisure time and being made redundant). Her thoughts of perfection are ego-syntonic and not resisted, meaning they are not true obsessions. Staying late to check is not a compulsion as it is not an unreasonable way to achieve her goal (assuming she does not check an excessive number of times). There is no evidence of low mood, excluding depressive symptoms. There is no evidence of communication difficulties, making an autism spectrum disorder unlikely.

5. B. Pseudohallucination. She reports a perception in the absence of a stimulus from within internal space. A hallucination would occur in external space. An obsession would be attributed to herself. Thought insertion would be attributed to an external agency. A rumination is not experienced as a voice, but as a thought (see Table 13.1).

6. D. This woman describes classic symptoms of body dysmorphic disorder. She is concerned with her appearance as opposed to an underlying disease (hypochondriasis). If she did hold the over-valued idea with delusional intensity, somatic delusional disorder should be considered. Note that some patients may exaggerate (or even feign) psychological sequelae of imagined or minor flaws in their appearance to receive medical care (factitious disorder) or cosmetic surgery paid for by the state, which would be malingering.

7. E. No mental illness. This woman is not experiencing obsessions or compulsions. She is responding to external influences and her handwashing may realistically reduce the feared outcome of infection transmission.

8. A. Delusion (strictly, a delusional perception). This belief is fixed, was arrived at illogically, and is not amenable to reason. The patient experienced a normal perception but interpreted it with delusional meaning, termed a 'delusional perception'. This is a first rank symptom of schizophrenia.

Chapter 14 The patient with a reaction to a stressful event

1. D. It is vital to robustly exclude physical aetiology prior to attributing symptoms to psychological causes. In this case, excluding intracranial haemorrhage secondary to head injury should take priority. This should include a history of the mechanism of assault (with corroboration from a witness if possible), full neurological examination

and appropriate investigations (which may include a computed tomography brain scan).

2. C. This describes symptoms of fairly marked psychomotor retardation, which would be suggestive that a depressive illness has developed from the bereavement reaction. The other symptoms (wanting to be dead, poor concentration, intense guilt, hallucinations involving the deceased) are typical of normal bereavement.

3. B. This woman is suffering from an adjustment disorder, characterized by difficulty coping with a significant change in circumstances and preoccupation with the stressor. Feelings of inability to cope are fairly typical of difficult adjustment. Note the duration of onset of symptoms (longer than for an acute stress reaction), and the fact that she has been signed off work, suggesting disruption to occupational functioning (which suggests that a diagnosis is appropriate, as opposed to 'no mental illness'). She does not appear to be suffering from other symptoms that would suggest depression or a dissociative neurological symptom disorder.

4. A. This case is fairly typical of dissociative amnesia. She has no memory of a circumscribed period of her life, with intact memory for her past and the more recent present. While head trauma and Wernicke–Korsakoff syndrome (due to inadequate nutrition) is naturally a concern, she appears to have been able to make her way to the UK and apply for asylum, which would suggest that cognitive impairment has not been global (excluding transient global amnesia), and she has been able to function at a reasonable level. She has no symptoms suggestive of posttraumatic stress disorder at this time, and the memory loss is more prolonged than would be expected in this disorder. In terms of stressful events, while she is unable to recall anything, she is seeking asylum from an area in which human rights violations are widely reported. The fact that she was pregnant with no recollection of conception or termination may suggest that she has been the victim of rape (which would be a traumatic stressor).

5. E. This patient has a most likely diagnosis of complex PTSD (or cPTSD). She has posttraumatic symptoms (such as flashbacks with specific triggers, hypervigilance and avoidance), coupled with affective instability, low self-esteem and difficulty maintaining relationships. Her emotions are volatile rather than being low, making depression less likely. While the images are intrusive, they are not linked to rituals or compulsions. There is no evidence of any psychotic features.

6. C. This is a classic presentation of a dissociative amnesia with dissociative fugue, or 'fugue state'. The man is unable to recount any personal details and appears to have travelled from a distant city. Note the possible severe stressor of being involved with a company that has recently been bankrupted.

7. E. This woman is probably suffering from nonepileptic seizures but epilepsy needs to be excluded. Nonepileptic seizures are suggested by the positive features of prolonged duration, a memory for ictal events and resisting eye opening (see Table 14.2). The chronological association with a significant stressor (being told that she will be left alone when her husband starts work) may also be relevant. These are often more common in those with a family or personal history of epilepsy.

8. B. Temporal lobe epilepsy. These symptoms are fairly typical of temporal lobe epilepsy. Note the history of likely head injury (implied by the fact she was referred from the neurosurgical unit). She should be referred for electroencephalogram.

Chapter 15 The patient with medically unexplained physical symptoms.

1. A. Watchful waiting. These situations are commonly encountered by GPs. The patient may well be developing multiple sclerosis; however, his symptoms are minimal and insufficient to make any diagnosis. Overzealous attempts to take his problems seriously by a well-intentioned doctor (such as referral to neurology, advanced investigations or arranging urgent follow-up) may reinforce his belief that something is wrong. However, dismissal by telling him it is 'all in his head' (or – at this stage – even empathic suggestion of psychiatric illness) is likely to cause him to seek a second opinion, and in any case is irresponsible given the inconclusive evidence. In the first instance, empathic acknowledgement and explanation, and inviting the patient to reattend if further symptoms arise (watchful waiting) is the most balanced option of the above.

2. D. Contact previous centres of care. This history is highly suggestive of factitious disorder imposed on self (female, healthcare professional, symptoms without signs, broad knowledge, specific demands, far from home). It is imperative to contact previous hospitals to get more information; however, asking the patient for such contact details may yield vague answers (in some cases, requesting such details will result in the patient discharging themselves). Details of such patients are often shared between local accident and emergency

departments. It is not safe to prescribe pethidine or arrange a laparoscopy. It is not ethical to tell her she is lying without any definite evidence of this. It is too early to refer to psychiatry, although this may help in due course if she is willing to engage.

3. B. Further physical investigations. Onset of such symptoms in older people with no significant medical or psychiatric history is more likely to be indicative of insidious organic disease. Prior to attribution of symptoms to a psychological origin, physical disease needs to be thoroughly excluded. In this case, physical investigations have been inappropriate to exclude likely physical illnesses. At minimum he requires an electrocardiogram.

4. C. Bodily distress disorder. Note the multiple and changing symptoms, refusal to accept the absence of physical cause and duration of more than 2 years. Multiple sclerosis is possible, but more weight than normal should be placed on objective evidence before this is investigated. There is no evidence she is lying about her experiences, making factitious disorder unlikely. She is concerned about her symptoms rather than an underlying disorder, excluding hypochondriasis. Generalized anxiety disorder is possible if she also reports anxiety about things other than physical symptoms.

Chapter 16 The patient with eating, feeding or weight problems

1. A. Significantly low body weight. This occurs in anorexia nervosa, not bulimia nervosa. Patients with bulimia nervosa are of normal or increased weight. Preoccupation with being thin, as well as a dread of fatness and a distorted perception of being too fat are associated with both anorexia and bulimia nervosa. Again, use of medication and exercise as means of controlling weight can occur in both disorders.

2. C. Investigate for physical causes of growth restriction. While patients with eating disorders often deny their symptoms, it is very important to exclude insidious physical illness as a cause of weight loss before attributing it to a psychiatric disorder. Physical causes can include malignancy, inflammatory disorders, infection and endocrine abnormalities. It would also be important to take a collateral history from his main caregiver, including psychosocial stressors.

3. E. Alcohol dependence. Self-neglect due to alcohol or substance use is a common cause of weight loss. Dependence is suggested by her withdrawal symptoms when she does not have access to alcohol (which are

not panic attacks). Low mood is commonly associated with alcohol excess as alcohol is a depressant: the treatment is to stop alcohol. Anorexia and bulimia nervosa are excluded by the fact that she is worried she has lost weight. Her vomiting sounds more likely to relate to gastritis secondary to alcohol excess, not purging.

4. E. Potassium 2.1 mmol/L. She requires an electrocardiogram and cautious intravenous replacement of potassium. Hypoglycaemia, anaemia, hypercholesterolaemia and hypophosphatemia are all common in anorexia nervosa but the values given here are not dangerously low.

5. D. Anorexia nervosa. This woman is dangerously underweight. While all of the listed mental illnesses can cause weight loss, they are differentiated from specific eating disorders by the presence of dread of fatness, distortion of body image and subsequent restriction of her dietary intake. The diagnosis of bulimia is excluded given her low body mass index.

6. E. Unable to rise from squatting without assistance. His blood pressure and heart rate place him at moderate risk but his capillary refill time and temperature are within the normal range. See The Royal College of Psychiatrists 'Medical Emergencies in Eating Disorders' guidance for more details on physical risk assessment in anorexia nervosa.

Chapter 17 The patient with alcohol or substance use problems

1. D. Alcoholic hallucinosis. This is a classic history of alcoholic hallucinosis. Note the absence of memory or attentional problems, excluding delirium tremens or Wernicke – Korsakoff syndrome. Late-onset schizophrenia should be in the differential diagnosis, but is unlikely in this case. Social isolation is often a cause or consequence of alcohol misuse. Hepatic encephalopathy is excluded by her otherwise normal physical examination.

2. D. Neck of femur repair. This man is delirious, and the history of heavy alcohol use suggests this is likely to be an alcohol withdrawal delirium. Note the visual 'Lilliputian hallucinations' of small figures (in his case, a horse), which are typical of alcohol withdrawal. Any surgical intervention should be delayed pending improvement in his delirium, unless it is felt that the fracture itself is a significant contributor to his presentation. The other options are all interventions which should be offered in delirium tremens. Benzodiazepines are used for alcohol withdrawal but

should be avoided in other sorts of delirium. He should be empirically treated with parenteral thiamine as it is very difficult to exclude Wernicke–Korsakoff syndrome in delirious patients, and the consequences of missing it can be severe. A full physical exam may highlight evidence of Wernicke–Korsakoff (ophthalmoplegia, ataxia) or highlight other contributors to the delirium (e.g., chest infection). Consistent nursing care will help to calm and orientate him.

3. C. Obtain a urine sample for drug testing. Oral test strips are an alternative. Before starting opioid replacement establishing that the patient is currently using opioids is essential. Prescribing methadone to someone who is not opioid-tolerant can be fatal. Similarly, prescribing his previous dose of methadone could be fatal as he may be less opioid-tolerant now than he was previously. It is necessary for methadone doses to be initiated at a low level and gradually increased if required (titrated against withdrawal symptoms). Referring him to a drug counselling service may well be appropriate if he wishes to engage. Contacting the police is not appropriate.

4. B. A 'half bottle' (350 mL) of premium gin (40% ABV) per week. To calculate alcohol units, take the % ABV and multiply by volume (in litres): e.g., 40 × 0.350 = 14 units; 350 mL of a 40% ABV spirit contains 14 units. Six pints (3.408 L) of continental lager (5.3% ABV) contains 18 units; two bottles (1.5 L) of red wine (12.5% ABV) contains 18.75 units; 3 L of strong white cider (8.4% ABV) contains 25.2 units; and six bottles (1.980 L) of alcopops (4.9% ABV) contains 9.7 units. She should also be told that there is no 'safe' level at which to drink alcohol, merely lower to higher risk levels. If she plans to drink the full 14 units, it should be recommended that she spreads her alcohol consumption over around 3 days per week.

5. E. Drowsiness. Hyper alertness, tachycardia, hyperthermia, hypertension and psychotic symptoms arise commonly during cocaine use. Chest pain is a very concerning symptom suggesting arrhythmia or cardiac ischaemia due to coronary artery spasm. He should be advised to seek emergency medical care if this occurs after consumption.

6. C. Ketamine. Ketamine is a potent glutamatergic (NMDA receptor) channel blocker, and is a potent short-acting dissociative anaesthetic. It is legitimately used in veterinary surgery as an anaesthetic agent. It can also be used as an anaesthetic analgesic agent in human medicine. The patient's symptoms are in keeping with dissociation, with ketamine being the most likely to cause this of the drugs listed.

Chapter 18 The patient with personality problems

1. B. Mild personality disorder. This lady likely has a mild personality disorder. She describes longstanding issues with personality which manifest in difficulties with relationships and poor self-esteem, however is managing well with her work and with her family. She does have evidence of impairment in managing mutually satisfying relationships. She does describe difficulties in regulating her emotions which would also support a diagnosis of personality disorder.

2. E. Severe personality disorder. This man is likely to have a severe personality disorder. He describes longstanding difficulties with emotional regulation and impulsive behaviour which impact multiple areas of functioning, being unable to sustain relationships, having difficulties with his family, holding down a job and being arrested multiple times. There is insufficient information given to determine whether he also has polysubstance dependence. In any case this would be unlikely to explain his lifelong difficulties and his feelings of self-loathing, although it may be a contributing factor.

3. D. Personality disorder with prominent traits of anankastia. The most prominent personality trait for this patient is anankastia, as she describes difficulties with others when they are unable to meet her standards, perfectionism, and behavioural constraint, having lost a relationship because of lack of spontaneity.

4. C. Personality disorder with prominent traits of dissociality. This patient presents with features of dissociality, describing lack of empathy for the patient he pushed down the stairs, and a self-centred idea that he was more important than this patient. There is evidence this is longstanding and not merely a 'one-off' incident.

5. E. Personality disorder with a borderline pattern and prominent traits of disinhibition. The patient describes a pattern of impulsive actions (including recurrent self-harm) that are often related to her emotional state at the time, and struggles with planning her time. She also describes a fear of abandonment and an unclear sense of self.

Chapter 19 The patient with impairment of consciousness, memory or cognition

1. D. Delirium. This is suggested by her acute onset objective cognitive impairment associated with sleep–wake cycle disturbance. Suspicion and visual hallucinations are common in delirium. Although Lewy body dementia is commonly associated with visual hallucinations it is

excluded by the acute onset. Similarly, Alzheimer dementia is excluded by the acute onset. Late-onset schizophrenia remains a possibility but is far less likely than delirium. Charles Bonnet syndrome would not account for all the features here, e.g., persecutory beliefs, sleep–wake cycle disturbance and cognitive impairment.

2. A. Korsakoff syndrome. This man has an isolated long-term anterograde and retrograde memory impairment, with significant difficulty forming new memories, with intact working memory and other cognitive function. He is confabulating. A history of alcohol excess raises the possibility of Korsakoff syndrome as the cause. He does not have dementia because the impairment is not global or progressive.

3. A. Computed tomography (CT) of the head. This gentleman has a likely diagnosis of dementia. NICE CKS (2022) recommends the blood tests this man has already received plus structural neuroimaging as a minimum assessment for reversible causes of dementia. However, there is some clinical judgement involved. Practice varies locally and some centres would not request a CT head unless there are neurological signs. There is no reason to think this man needs syphilis and HIV serology but for other patients it may be appropriate. EEG, chest X-ray and lumbar puncture are not recommended routinely in assessment of dementia but may be indicated in particular circumstances (e.g., if frontotemporal dementia or Creutzfeldt-Jakob disease is suspected). See Table 19.7.

4. A. Delirium. This woman has recently been extremely unwell. Even though her UTI has been successfully treated, the brain can often lag behind the rest of the body when recovering from a serious illness. The fluctuation in her mental state may reflect a resolving or a new delirium. It would be wise to reassess for other causes that may have been missed initially or occurred since admission, e.g., a hospital-acquired pneumonia. It may be that she will not regain her premorbid cognitive functioning and in due course will be diagnosed with dementia, but it is too early to make this diagnosis.

5. A. Amitriptyline. This man has a delirium. Anticholinergic medication is a common cause of delirium, as are opioids. Amitriptyline is sometimes used to reduce insomnia, although this is extremely inadvisable in an older adult, so this may be the precipitant. Starting or stopping any medication can potentially cause delirium but this does not occur commonly with the other medications listed.

6. E. Subdural haematoma. This woman has atrial fibrillation and so is likely to be on warfarin. There should therefore be a low threshold for suspecting an intracranial bleed after minor or no injury. A chronic subdural haematoma as opposed to neurodegenerative cause of dementia is suggested by her relatively quick cognitive deterioration, possible fluctuating conscious level (uncharacteristic afternoon naps), neurological signs and history of head injury. It is not uncommon for there to be a latent period of days to weeks between injury and symptoms. The next step should be brain imaging.

7. A. Lewy body dementia. The patient has the triad of symptoms of parkinsonism, hallucinations and fluctuating cognition, so Lewy body dementia is the most likely diagnosis.

8. B. Mild neurocognitive impairment. This woman has a below-normal score on standardized cognitive assessment but no impairment in activities of daily living. This low score is quite concerning in view of her young age and high educational attainment and she should be referred to a young onset memory clinic for comprehensive investigation.

Chapter 20 Dementia and delirium

1. A. Assess for changes in physical health. This woman has symptoms of stress and distress in dementia. Reviewing for any potential physical causes of this is recommended first line by NICE (2018), unless there is immediate risk of harm or severe distress. In the event of these risks, antipsychotics would be first line (after consideration of risk of stroke) and cholinesterase inhibitors second line. Antidepressants are only indicated if there is evidence of depression. Referral to speech and language therapy is unlikely to be of benefit given her severe dementia.

2. A. Antipsychotics. Antipsychotics can cause irreversible severe parkinsonian reactions in patients with Lewy body dementia. They are not absolutely contraindicated but should be used with even more caution than in other types of dementia and ideally under specialist advice. The other options may all potentially be of benefit – if his delusion is due to concurrent infection (antibiotics), depression (antidepressants) or worsening dementia – cholinesterase inhibitors can improve behavioural and psychological symptoms of dementia. Nutritional supplements may be of benefit, whatever the cause, if he is losing weight.

3. C. Co-codamol. This contains both codeine and paracetamol. Opioids are very common causes of delirium in older adults, both in their own right and due to their side effect of constipation. Opioids are often started during acute admissions for pain or surgery. Any

medication can potentially precipitate delirium, but opioids, benzodiazepines and anticholinergics are the commonest.

4. D. Acute medical ward. This lady is delirious. This is a medical emergency. She needs to be fully physically investigated. Her acute-onset psychotic symptoms are almost certainly due to her delirium, not a primary psychotic disorder.

5. B. Memantine. This woman has mild to moderate dementia for which cholinesterase inhibitors are recommended. However, she has a number of relative contraindications to cholinesterase inhibitor use. Their cholinergic effects can induce bradycardia, which may be particularly problematic in those with conduction defects. Similarly, cholinergic drugs can cause bronchoconstriction, which may be problematic in COPD and asthma. Cholinergic drugs can also increase gastric acid secretions, which could worsen peptic ulceration. Overall, it would probably be better to try memantine first for this woman.

6. A. No treatment recommended by current guidelines. Unfortunately, no medications have yet been found to slow the progression of frontotemporal dementia.

Chapter 21 Older adult psychiatry

1. A. Antidepressant. The key issue here is the diagnosis. She presents with a common triad in older adults: depressive symptoms, cognitive impairment and functional impairment. It is often difficult to tease out whether someone is experiencing depression manifesting with cognitive impairment or an early dementia leading to comorbid depression. Ideally, depression is treated first, then cognition reassessed once mood is euthymic. An antidepressant would be first line in view of her cognitive impairment, but counselling or psychological therapy could still be considered in someone with this level of cognitive impairment.

2. C. Depressive episode. It is common for depression to manifest with prominent features of anxiety, psychomotor agitation and hypochondriacal ideas in older adults. Mild neurocognitive impairment is the next most likely differential – although her MOCA score of 29/30 is reassuring, a more sensitive test such as the Addenbrooke's Cognitive Examination (ACE-III) may still show an objective impairment. Generalized anxiety disorder or hypochondriasis is unlikely to have onset so late in life, and diagnosis would require a longer duration of symptoms. There are no psychotic features to suggest schizophrenia.

3. A. ECT. All of the suggested management strategies are reasonable, but ECT is preferable because of this man's potentially life-threatening poor fluid intake and poor medication concordance. Depot medication would get around the concordance problem but there are no depot medications licensed as antidepressants. ECT is the quickest and most effective treatment for depression known and seems to work particularly well in older adults.

4. B. All of these patients could potentially have late-onset schizophrenia. However, symptoms of late-onset schizophrenia are predominantly delusional, rather than bizarre or negative symptoms (as in patients A and C). Patient A has some possible features of delirium. Patient D is more likely to have Charles Bonnet syndrome. Late-onset schizophrenia is far more common in women than in men, and social deprivation and hearing impairment are also risk factors. 'Impending sense of doom' as in patient E can be a symptom of MI.

5. D. Continue mirtazapine for at least 8 weeks. Older adults can take longer to show response to antidepressants, so an adequate trial is at least 8 weeks. Augmentation is not necessary at this stage and increases the risk of drug interactions. Tricyclics are not recommended as first line in older adults due to their side-effect profile.

6. E. Delirium. This lady has acute-onset cognitive impairment: delirium until proven otherwise. The history is concerningly suggestive of a focal seizure. She needs to be admitted to a medical ward for investigation. A manic or hypomanic episode would be highly unlikely to have such a rapid onset. Were she on lithium, it would be crucial to check a random lithium level as her presentation could also be due to lithium toxicity.

7. B. This is the simplest and easiest of the options. If concordance remains poor despite this, prompting by a carer could be considered. A depot could be useful if the patient wishes it, or his insight reduces and he requires compulsory treatment. Daily dispensing is normally reserved for methadone or for those at high risk of overdose. In general, simplifying medication regimes to once daily is a good idea, but unfortunately olanzapine is likely to be too sedating to allow use in the mornings. Potentially, his other once-daily medication could be changed to the evening.

8. A. Ask her to attend A&E. It is unclear what dose of trazodone she has taken, or whether she has taken any other tablets. She needs examination, blood samples tested and an electrocardiogram. The next step would be for her to receive an urgent psychiatric review. This lady has recently attempted suicide. Older adults are at high risk of completed suicide. She may perceive taking

extra trazodone as far more harmful than it actually is, as she may have memories of barbiturates – highly toxic sleeping tablets, which are fatal in minor overdose. Her ongoing intent is unclear from the vignette. She may require admission or urgent community support from mental health services.

Chapter 22 Alcohol and substance-related disorders

1. B. Contemplation of change. This man is currently contemplating changing his behaviour. He recognizes the need for change (he wants to give up), but he is ambivalent about it (worrying he will lose all his friends). Motivational interviewing may be helpful to allow him to progress to the next stage of preparation for change.

2. E. Urine drug test to confirm the presence of opioids. Prior to prescribing methadone, it is essential to confirm the use of opioids. A urine or oral drug test can be used to do this. Admission to psychiatric hospital is not necessary, although dose titration should be undertaken in a controlled clinical environment with facilities to measure physiological response to opioids, and with emergency treatment for opioid toxicity (i.e., naloxone) close to hand. Viral serology testing and physical examination is important screening for health complications from intravenous drug use, but it is not necessary for a methadone prescription. Forcing a patient to identify a confidant for the purposes of corroboration can lead to problems, either placing false security in a possibly inaccurate historian or causing disengagement with services.

3. C. Naltrexone. Naltrexone is an opioid receptor antagonist. This may control cravings and reduces the pleasurable effects of drinking alcohol, reducing 'reward' and – by operant conditioning – can 'extinguish' the desire to drink (the 'Sinclair method'). Disulfiram causes an unpleasant reaction when taken with alcohol. Acamprosate may be helpful in controlling cravings. Long-term antidepressants or benzodiazepines are not recommended for the sole purpose of maintaining abstinence. However, antidepressants may be helpful for treating comorbid depression.

4. C. Buprenorphine. Buprenorphine (either oral or subcutaneous) is a partial opioid agonist and can be used for substitution therapy. The other drugs can be used in treating various stages of opioid dependence; however, none are true 'substitutes'.

5. A. Methadone. Methadone is the first-choice agent in substitute prescribing for opioid dependence. Unless there is a strong patient preference for an alternative

agent, patients would usually be titrated onto a methadone prescription by addiction services. Buvidal could be an option, but it is usually used for patients who struggle to attend the chemist regularly to collect their substitute prescriptions, e.g., because of a more chaotic lifestyle.

Chapter 23 The psychotic disorders

1. B. 12.5%. If one parent has schizophrenia, the probability of their offspring having schizophrenia is 13%. The population lifetime risk is 1%.

2. E. 50%. If both parents have schizophrenia, the probability of their offspring having schizophrenia is 50%. The population lifetime risk is 1%.

3. C. 1 to 2 years. This is a difficult question as there is little solid evidence about the optimum period of treatment for a first episode of psychosis. Without prophylactic antipsychotics following a first episode of schizophrenia, over half of patients will relapse within a year. The current recommendation is to continue antipsychotics for 1 to 2 years after a first episode. However, many patients wish to stop sooner. In this case, a gradual reduction over a few weeks reduces the risk of relapse. Alternatively, this man may prefer to switch to an antipsychotic less associated with weight gain.

4. D. Cognitive-behavioural therapy. The other modalities are not recommended in schizophrenia. Interpersonal therapy and cognitive-behavioural therapy are indicated in depression. Dialectical behavioural therapy is indicated in emotionally unstable personality disorder. Cognitive analytic therapy is indicated in eating disorders. Family therapy is also recommended if the patient lives with or is in close contact with their family.

5. C. Commence olanzapine. This patient has schizoaffective disorder which is managed very similarly to schizophrenia, with the possibility of antidepressants or mood stabilizers depending on presentation. An antipsychotic such as olanzapine would be an appropriate first-choice medication. She is under 55, and in particular of childbearing potential, so sodium valproate would be contraindicated. Lithium could be considered as an adjunct. She is clearly unwell so watching and waiting is not appropriate. ECT would only be indicated if she had a treatment-resistant illness or there were life-threatening features.

6. C. Aripiprazole. This is the antipsychotic least likely to be associated with weight gain and the metabolic syndrome. First-generation antipsychotics would be the next best choice.

7. A. Chlorpromazine. The 'rash' is consistent with sunburn, likely due to a photosensitivity reaction from chlorpromazine. Chlorpromazine is often used as an 'as required' medication for agitation.

8. B. Switch to clozapine. This woman has treatment-resistant schizophrenia as she has had two trials of antipsychotic at adequate doses for adequate durations, including at least one second-generation drug.

Chapter 24 The mood (affective) disorders

1. A. Someone who is not eating or drinking. ECT is indicated in options A–D, but not E. Treatment-resistant depression is an indication for ECT but if the patient has capacity and does not wish it, it is not given. No information is given to suggest s/he lacks capacity, which is presumed to be present in adults unless proven otherwise. Life-threatening reduction in oral intake, psychotic depression and previous good response to ECT are all other indications for ECT. If a prioritization has to be made, a life-threatening reduction in oral intake presents the highest risk and so should be treated first.

2. C. Admission under mental health legislation. This man is experiencing a manic episode with psychotic features. His psychotic beliefs place him at high risk of injury or death and are impairing his ability to make decisions regarding management of his mental health. It is not safe to let him go home and police custody is not appropriate given his behaviour is driven by illness. He may be persuadable to be admitted informally but if not, he would meet criteria for detention under mental health legislation (see Chapter 4).

3. D. Citalopram and quetiapine. This man has a severe depressive episode with psychotic features. A combination of an antidepressant and an antipsychotic is indicated. Citalopram is normally tried before amitriptyline as it has fewer side effects. In addition, amitriptyline is more toxic than citalopram in overdose. Given his suicidal ideation it is best to choose the less toxic medication. Quetiapine or any other second-generation antipsychotic would be reasonable to treat his psychosis.

4. B. Olanzapine. Olanzapine, risperidone, quetiapine or haloperidol are the first-line antimanic agents recommended by NICE (2014). Lithium should not be started in the acute situation in someone with a history of nonconcordance. Sodium valproate should not be prescribed in people under the age of 55. Lamotrigine is not recommended during acute mania as it is

ineffective. Citalopram, or any other antidepressant, should be discontinued in a manic patient. This woman is likely also to need rapid tranquillization with a benzodiazepine (see Fig. 7.1).

5. C. Individual CBT. Self-help CBT and structured group physical activity are recommended by NICE for mild depression (2022). Dialectical behaviour therapy is a psychological therapy for borderline pattern personality disorder. Graded exposure therapy is used to treat obsessive-compulsive disorder and phobias.

6. E. Commence fluoxetine. The next step for this man is to consider an antidepressant (typically an SSRI first line), which can be done in primary care.

Chapter 25 The anxiety, stress related, OCD related and bodily distress disorders

1. B. She should be seen on a planned, regular schedule. Seeing patients with anxiety about their physical health on a regular basis can help contain their anxieties and reduce the total number and number of urgent appointments they need. However, this does not mean they should not be allowed access to urgent appointment slots – they will still experience urgent or serious physical health problems at least as commonly as the general population. Similarly, investigations should be carefully considered and avoided if possible, but some are likely to still be required to safely exclude other disorders. Benzodiazepines are not indicated for bodily distress disorder but may be indicated for some other reason. The nature of bodily distress disorder should be explained to patients, but it should not be done in a confrontational manner. Phrases such as 'all in the mind' should be avoided as patients are genuinely experiencing symptoms.

2. B. CBT with desensitization. CBT with desensitization is recommended for phobias with mild to severe functional impairment. Trauma-focused CBT is for posttraumatic stress disorder. PRN diazepam would not be advisable given she is likely to come into contact with bodily fluids on a daily basis. SSRIs are not recommended for specific phobias.

3. C. Selective serotonin reuptake inhibitor (SSRI). An SSRI is the first-line drug therapy for obsessive-compulsive disorder. Clomipramine is usually a second-line drug therapy, or if the patient has had a previously good response to it. Mirtazapine and pregabalin are not recommended by current guidelines. Self-help is recommended for mild symptoms but this woman's symptoms are associated with marked functional impairment. Talking therapies are first line for

moderate to severe OCD and she should be encouraged to reconsider a talking therapy if a SSRI is ineffective.

4. C. CBT with a trauma focus. This would be an appropriate first step in management as suggested by NICE (2018). If the person prefers drug treatment an SSRI could be offered. Long-term prescribing of benzodiazepines should be avoided.

5. E. Applied relaxation. This and CBT are the two psychological therapies recommended for moderate to severe generalized anxiety disorder.

Chapter 26 Feeding and eating disorders

1. B. Family therapy. This is the first-line psychological therapy for adolescents recommended by NICE (2017). The other therapies are all used in adults with anorexia.

2. E. Individual eating disorder-focused CBT. This is one of the three psychotherapeutic modalities recommended first line by NICE (2017) for anorexia in adults. Family therapy is first line for treating anorexia and bulimia in young people. Focal psychodynamic psychotherapy is a second-line treatment in anorexia. Interpersonal therapy is used to treat depression and exposure-response prevention is used to treat obsessive-compulsive disorder.

3. C. Binge–purge symptoms. The presence of binge–purge symptoms is associated with a poorer prognosis in sufferers of anorexia nervosa, as is late age of onset, very low weight (not rapid weight loss), long duration of illness, personality difficulties and difficult family relationships. The presence of a family history of anorexia is not necessarily indicative of poor prognosis, neither is the rate of engagement with psychotherapy.

4. C. Multivitamin. NICE (2017) recommends that people with anorexia nervosa should be encouraged to take a multivitamin and multimineral supplement. Selective serotonin reuptake inhibitors are no longer recommended in the management of eating disorders unless there is comorbid depression or anxiety, and these disorders are most likely to resolve with weight gain alone.

5. C. Phosphate 0.3 mmol/L. All the other blood results are in the normal range. Hypophosphataemia is the hallmark of refeeding syndrome and a low level indicates that replacement is required, along with frequent monitoring of phosphate, magnesium, sodium and potassium levels. Calcium levels are not generally affected in refeeding syndrome.

Chapter 27 The sleep–wake disorders

1. E. Pramipexole. Dopamine agonists such as pramipexole and ropinirole are recommended as first-line treatment for restless legs syndrome. The other medications listed are all potential causes of the syndrome.

2. D. Neuropathy. A peripheral neuropathy is suggested by her history of diabetes. Restless legs syndrome is unlikely as the pain is not brought on by inactivity. Iron deficiency is a cause of restless legs syndrome. Intermittent claudication is unlikely as exercise would worsen symptoms. Akathisia would not be limited to her legs.

3. D. Sleep hygiene advice. Everyone who is struggling with sleep should be given sleep hygiene advice, particularly those with depression. Her insomnia is likely secondary to depression and should improve over time as her mood improves. It is too early to increase the dose of fluoxetine. Hypnotics should be avoided where possible as patients can suffer from daytime drowsiness and develop tolerance. A sleep diary or referral is not indicated.

Chapter 28 Sex and gender Identity

1. A. Caressing without genital contact can improve sex. This is the kind of advice which may be given during sex therapy or in self-help materials related to sexual dysfunction. All the other pieces of advice are the opposite of what should be given: sexual dysfunction is common at all ages, physical problems are a rare cause of anorgasmia, medication may cause sexual dysfunction but should not be stopped immediately (a substitution may be required) and good communication with a partner about sex is associated with fewer sexual difficulties.

2. B. Check blood glucose. Erectile dysfunction is a common presenting symptom in diabetes, as is weight loss. Excluding diabetes is the priority here. All of the other options can also be appropriate management options in erectile dysfunction depending on the context (see Box 28.2).

3. B. Olanzapine. All the other agents are dopaminomimetic agents: levodopa is metabolized to dopamine, pergolide and pramipexole are dopamine receptor agonists and selegiline is a monoamine oxidase B inhibitor, reducing the breakdown of dopamine. High doses of dopaminomimetic agents have rarely been associated with new paraphilias in Parkinson disease, typically younger men with a long duration of illness. Olanzapine is a dopamine receptor antagonist which has been used to treat paraphilias in Parkinson disease.

4. D. Sertraline. Selective serotonin reuptake inhibitors are commonly associated with anorgasmia. Mirtazapine is the antidepressant least likely to be associated with sexual side effects.

Chapter 29 Disorders relating to the menstrual cycle, pregnancy and the puerperium

1. A. Encourage exercise. This woman has mild premenstrual syndrome (PMS). One argument with her boyfriend is not evidence of significant functional impairment. For mild PMS, the National Institute for Health and Care Excellence (NICE; 2014) recommends healthy eating, stress reduction, regular sleep and regular exercise, particularly during the luteal phase. They also recommend smoking cessation and reducing alcohol intake where applicable. The oral contraceptive pill, ibuprofen and CBT are all options in managing moderately severe PMS. SSRIs are reserved for severe PMS.

2. E. Psychological therapy. While the woman in the case description attributes her symptoms to the menopause, the duration of the symptoms accompanied by the presence of suicidal thoughts are more suggestive of a depressive illness. The functional impact and suicidal thoughts suggest an episode of at least moderate severity. The National Institute for Health and Care Excellence (NICE; 2022) recommends a combination of an antidepressant and psychological therapy (cognitive-behavioural therapy or interpersonal therapy) as first line for treating moderate-to-severe depression. Counselling may also be useful if she has issues relating to relationships or bereavements she would like to reflect on, but it is not usually a treatment for depression. Dietary and lifestyle advice (avoiding alcohol, tobacco, eating a balanced diet, exercising) should be offered to everyone with mood symptoms but are unlikely to be sufficient in this case. Around the menopausal years, there can be an increase in psychosocial stressors (children leaving home, 'facing up' to growing older, changes in personal relationships, etc.), which may increase the risk of developing depression independently of the hormonal changes that arise during the menopause. Hormone replacement therapy can be useful in certain circumstances; however, it does not suit everyone, and should not be used as a substitute for recognized treatments in the management of major depression. Omega-3 fish oils may reduce menopausal vasomotor symptoms (hot flushes) but are not recommended as a treatment for depression.

3. E. Refer to perinatal psychiatry. This is a complex risk–benefit scenario that needs to be carefully discussed with the patient and which draws on the latest available evidence. Her history of bipolar disorder places this woman at high risk of postpartum psychosis, even with prophylactic treatment. Discontinuing treatment increases her risk of relapse at any time. A mentally unwell mother is harmful for the child in utero and once born. However, all the mood stabilizers are associated with teratogenic effects to various degrees (valproate > carbamazepine > lithium). The absolute risk of congenital abnormalities remains low with lithium but is unacceptably high with valproate or carbamazepine, so switching to them would not be helpful. Discontinuing lithium and remaining without prophylaxis may be an option depending on the severity of her previous mood episodes. Switching to olanzapine is also a reasonable option as it is thought to be safe in pregnancy but would depend on her past experience with this drug.

4. E. Refer to perinatal mental health team. Reassurance that she will not become unwell cannot be given. This lady has a history of severe postnatal depression and is at greatly increased risk of suffering a further episode. She should be referred to the perinatal mental health team. Given this history, and her good response to medications in the past, commencing antidepressant treatment later in pregnancy or early postpartum may be beneficial. The perinatal mental health team would explore the risks versus benefits of this option. When choosing an agent, consideration should be given to previously effective drugs, and the mother's choice to breastfeed.

5. A. Detention in hospital under mental health act. This woman is experiencing a postpartum psychosis and is at very high risk of infanticide given the severity of her illness, the content of her delusion and the active steps she has taken towards killing her son. This risk is too high to be managed at home, however supportive of her family. She lacks capacity to make decisions about her treatment due to her absent insight, therefore requiring admission under detention rather than informally. This should be to a mother-and-baby unit if available. Transfer to police cells is not appropriate as she requires intensive psychiatric care which cannot be provided there and she has not committed a crime. Outpatient follow-up is not sufficient to manage her acute risk. A referral to social workers is likely to be

helpful in due course as they may be able to identify additional supports for the patient, but the priority at the moment is to maintain her and her child's safety in hospital.

Chapter 30 The personality disorders

1. E. Drug treatment is not the main intervention. NICE (2009) does not recommend drug treatment for the core symptoms of personality disorders with a borderline pattern. However, some medications can be helpful in reducing agitation during crises and in treating comorbid mental illness. The main intervention is psychological therapy.

2. A. Dialectical behaviour therapy. All of the options have evidence supporting their use in personality disorder with a borderline pattern, but dialectical behaviour therapy is the 'gold standard' and recommended by NICE (2009).

3. E. Suggest weekly dispensing of medication. This woman is probably suffering from a comorbid depressive episode. Management of this should be discussed with the patient – she may opt for 'watchful waiting' or it may be appropriate to start an antidepressant. As her risk of suicide has increased, it is sensible to reduce her access to means of suicide by suggesting weekly dispensing. Her risk is not so high that she needs admission. A urine drug screen may be helpful in excluding a substance-induced acute change in mood, but substance use (with the exception of alcohol) is unlikely to account for a month of low mood. Benzodiazepines should be avoided where possible given the risks of dependence, particularly high in someone with persistent symptoms. Dialectical behaviour therapy is recommended for treatment of personality disorder with a borderline pattern in the long term but will not help depression in the short–medium term.

4. C. Alert the police and the intended victim. Given the significant risk to another person, confidentiality needs to be broken in this case. The psychiatrist has a duty to immediately warn the police. In addition, the specific and detailed content of the threat necessitates that the intended victim be warned (see the Tarasoff case for further details). The responsibility for this falls on the doctor; however, in practice the police will usually be happy to facilitate this. Detention under mental health legislation would not be appropriate, as the threat should be addressed by law enforcement agencies in the first instance. Meticulous notes would need to be kept. It is likely that he would be held criminally responsible for his actions. Review in 1 week is too late. Anger management may be appropriate in due course but does not deal with the acute risk. Diazepam should be avoided given risks of dependence and absence of an indication.

Chapter 31 The neurodevelopmental disorders

1. C. None. There is no pharmacological treatment for the core symptoms of autism spectrum disorder. The first-line treatment is social skills training. The medications listed may be indicated to manage common comorbidities of autism spectrum disorder, anxiety or depression (fluoxetine), attention deficit hyperactivity disorder (methylphenidate), psychosis (risperidone) or epilepsy (sodium valproate).

2. D. Methylphenidate. NICE (2018) recommends this as first-line drug treatment for severe ADHD in school-age children. Dexamphetamine and atomoxetine are second line. Parent-training/education programs are recommended as first line for school-age children with mild to moderate impairment, but his parents have already tried this. Severe impairment is suggested by the fact this boy is at risk of losing his school place. Cognitive-behavioural therapy is recommended for older adolescents with mild to moderate ADHD.

3. D. Psychoeducation. This boy has Tourette syndrome. Psychoeducation is first-line treatment for this: speaking to him, his family and his teachers to explain the diagnosis and that the majority of cases improve by adulthood. The other options are all drug treatments that can reduce tics. However, as the tics are causing little interference with day-to-day activities, he may find the side effects outweigh the benefits.

Chapter 32 Intellectual Disability

1. B. A physical examination. It is important not to fall into the trap of 'diagnostic overshadowing'. When there is a significant change in an individual's behaviour, it is important to exclude a physical cause for this, such as constipation; pain; indigestion or another physical illness. It is also important to be aware of the possibility of physical or sexual abuse in vulnerable adults and young people, and this should be.

2. D. Ask the support worker to leave the room so you can speak to the patient alone. People with intellectual disabilities are at greater risk of abuse than the general population, including from carers. It is important to see this woman independently to sensitively enquire about the possibility of abuse. You

could consider seeking the advice of an Intellectual Disability Liaison Nurse if there are any at the hospital, or speak to Speech and Language Therapy about communication aids.

Chapter 33 Child and adolescent psychiatry

1. B. Conduct-dissocial disorder. This is suggested by his major violations of societal norms (arson and severe aggression). Oppositional defiant disorder is often considered to be a 'milder' variant of conduct disorder, where defiant behaviour is characteristic, but this tends not to involve criminality or violating the rights of others. Conduct-dissocial disorder is associated with the development of personality disorder with dissociality, criminality and substance misuse in later life. He is too young to diagnose a personality disorder. Substance misuse is a possibility which should be explored but is unlikely to present with oppositional behaviour in isolation. Reactive attachment disorder presents under the age of 5 years with disordered social interaction.

2. E. The duty social worker and on-call paediatrician should be alerted. Vaginal trauma and genital warts are not normal in an 8-year-old girl, and the findings should immediately raise suspicions of sexual abuse. The safety of the child is paramount, and steps should be taken to maintain this. While protocols vary slightly between areas, child protection procedures usually advise contacting the duty social worker and/or the local paediatrician on-call for child protection. If in any doubt about a possible child protection concern, either of these parties will usually be more than happy to offer guidance. The child should not be directly asked about what happened at this stage: a formal interview needs to be arranged involving the police, social workers and paediatric staff. Police will not question the girl just now. Parents should never be 'confronted' by medical staff; however, it is obviously courteous (if possible) to let them know what is going on and what will happen next. The child should not be allowed home until all relevant agencies are involved and safety at home can be ensured. This may not be possible, and an alternative place of safety may have to be sought. Should the parent remove the child from safety, it would be appropriate to contact the police given the magnitude of the concerns.

3. B. Cognitive-behavioural therapy. This girl has a probable diagnosis of depression, of moderate severity (based on her functional impairment). NICE (2019) recommends individual psychological therapy first line. Fluoxetine is the first-line antidepressant, sertraline and citalopram

are second line. Watchful waiting is recommended only in mild cases.

4. D. Personality disorder with a borderline pattern and prominent traits of negative affectivity. This is suggested by her long-term rapidly fluctuating mood, difficulties in relationships, self-harm, pseudohallucinations (the voice inside her head) and disturbed self-image (feeling empty). Childhood adversity is a risk factor for borderline pattern personality disorders and suggested by a parental overdose. Bipolar affective disorder or a depressive episode would be associated with episodes of altered mood which lasted for days, not hours. However, borderline pattern is a risk factor for comorbid depression. Disordered eating is also common in this personality disorder. Bulimia is unlikely given the rest of the history, but it would be useful to check what her weight-related cognitions are to definitely exclude this. Schizophrenia is unlikely as she is not reporting any psychotic symptoms (she reports pseudohallucinations, not hallucinations).

5. A. Selective mutism. This is suggested by the child's normal language development and ability to speak in some situations. Selective mutism often follows emotional trauma (such as separation from parents, war, severe illness) and situations where there is conflict at home.

6. E. Reactive attachment disorder. This is suggested by the child's history of abuse, marked fearfulness and social withdrawal. The diagnosis is not child abuse alone, as not all children who are abused respond in this way or go on to experience mental disorder.

Chapter 34 Forensic psychiatry

1. C. Previous violence. The best predictor of future violence is past violence. The other options also increase his risk of future violence, particularly substance use.

2. E. He is able to give a coherent account of events leading up to the offence but denies memory of the offence itself. An individual being considered unfit to plead through mental illness is relatively uncommon. The mental state findings given in A–D are all fairly extreme abnormalities suggesting that he would struggle to understand the difference between a plea of guilty and not guilty (D), understand the nature of the charge (D), instruct counsel (A and C), follow the evidence brought before the court (C) or challenge a juror (B and C). Amnesia (real or reported) for the offence itself does not necessarily impact on fitness to plead.

3. E. Murder. This is the only charge for which diminished responsibility may apply. If the accused is found to have

diminished responsibility, the conviction is reduced to manslaughter (or culpable homicide in Scotland). This was particularly important historically when murder carried the death penalty.

4. B. ADHD. This is a typical history for someone with ADHD symptoms of impulsivity and emotional instability leading to offending behaviour. It may be that treatment for ADHD helps this young man. However, it would be crucial to gain collateral history from someone who knew him well during his development before making this diagnosis. The other options are also consistent with the majority of the vignette and are important to consider. The final diagnosis that is imperative to explore is his use of substances.

5. A. Delusional disorder (delusional jealousy). This man is convinced that his partner is being unfaithful, despite extensive reassurances and evidence to the contrary. The name 'Othello syndrome' is derived from the play Othello by William Shakespeare, in which the protagonist murders his wife (Desdemona. which means 'the unfortunate' in Greek). Othello syndrome is associated with alcohol misuse and violence. Treatment includes antipsychotic medication and psychotherapy; however, given the very poor prognosis, it is often said that the most effective treatment is 'geographical' (i.e., relocation of the spouse to a distant area).

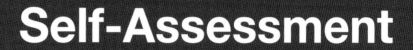

Self-Assessment

UKMLA High Yield Association Table

Presentations

Key Findings	Diagnoses
A female with normal development until 5 months, with gradual loss of skills/functioning after 6 months	Rett syndrome
A child with an intellectual disability, a long face, prominent ears and jaw, and machroorchidism (if male)	Fragile X
A child with an intellectual disability, congenital cardiac defects, a high-pitched voice, a cleft palette	22q11.2 deletion syndrome (DiGeorge/velocardiofacial syndrome)
A child with a narrow face, almond-shaped eyes, excessive weight gain and hunger, hypogonadism	Prader-Willi syndrome
Lifelong difficulties in social interactions and rigid/inflexible patterns of behaviour	Autism spectrum disorder
Lifelong difficulties with inattentiveness and hyperactivity	Attention deficit hyperactivity disorder
A patient with an intellectual disability, microcephaly, growth restriction, executive functioning problems	Foetal alcohol syndrome
Irritability, disinhibition, pressured speech, grandiosity, increased energy	Mania
Low mood, early morning wakening, impaired concentration and anhedonia	Depression
Persistent delusions, auditory hallucinations, thought disorder, experiences of external control, disorganized behaviour WITHOUT mood symptoms	Schizophrenia
Persistent delusions, auditory hallucinations, thought disorder, experiences of external control, disorganized behaviour WITH mood symptoms	Schizoaffective disorder
Anxiety symptoms when in a situation from which escape might be difficult, e.g., crowded shop	Agoraphobia
Anxiety symptoms in social situations or when expected to perform in front of others (e.g., giving a speech)	Social anxiety disorder
Anxiety symptoms when exposed to one specific stimulus (e.g., spiders, heights)	Specific phobia
Panic symptoms unrelated to a particular situation	Panic disorder
Free-floating anxiety	Generalised anxiety disorder
Ego-dystonic intrusive thoughts, compulsive rituals/behaviours	Obsessive-compulsive disorder
Preoccupation with a perceived defect in personal appearance	Body dysmorphic disorder
Reexperiencing a previous traumatic event in the present, avoidant behaviour and persistent perceptions of heightened threat	Post traumatic stress disorder
Reexperiencing a previous traumatic event in the present, avoidant behaviour and persistent perceptions of heightened threat AND with affect regulation difficulties, low self-worth and difficulties in interpersonal relationships	Complex post traumatic stress disorder
Pervasive grief, intense emotional pain, longing for deceased individual, symptoms lasting longer than cultural norms	Prolonged grief disorder
Significant distress related to physical symptoms that have no identified physical cause	Bodily distress disorder
Concern about having a serious illness with associated excessive health-related behaviours	Hypochondriasis

Continued

Key Findings	Diagnoses
Low body weight, amenorrhea, lanugo hair	Anorexia nervosa
Normal or increased body weight, binge-purging	Bulimia
Normal or increased body weight, binging without purging	Binge eating disorder
Tremors, nausea, vomiting, tachycardia, increased anxiety, seizures/hallucinations	Alcohol withdrawal
Altered conscious level, confusion and hallucinations approximately 48 hours after admission	Delirium tremens
Ataxia, ophthalmoplegia and acute cognitive impairment	Wernicke encephalopathy
Acute and fluctuating confusion with impaired cognition and sleep/wake cycle	Delirium
Gradual onset, executive functioning and progressive memory problems, word finding difficulties and functional impairment	Alzheimer dementia
Stepwise deterioration in memory and functioning	Vascular dementia
Parkinsonism, visual hallucinations, fluctuating cognition	Lewy body dementia
Significant personality and behaviour change, language problems, apathy, emotional blunting	Frontotemporal dementia

Management

Key Findings	Management
Attention deficit hyperactivity disorder (ADHD) in <18s	Parent training programme (1st line) Methylphenidate (2nd line)
Attention deficit hyperactivity disorder (ADHD) in >18s	Methylphenidate or lisdexamfetamine
Acute mania in >18s	Haloperidol, olanzapine, risperidone or quetiapine
Bipolar affective disorder – long-term management	Lithium (1st line) Valproate (2nd line if patient >55/not of childbearing potential)
Choosing an antidepressant in <18s	Fluoxetine
Treatment of less severe depression in >18s	Psychological therapy
Treatment of more severe depression in >18s	Psychological therapy + SSRI
Schizophrenia	Atypical antipsychotic
Schizoaffective disorder	Atypical antipsychotic
Obsessive-compulsive disorder with mild functional impairment	CBT with ERP
Obsessive-compulsive disorder with moderate/severe functional impairment	CBT with ERP + SSRI
Post traumatic stress disorder	Trauma-focused CBT
Anorexia nervosa in <18s	Family-based treatment (FBT; 1st line), individual eating-disorder-focused cognitive behavioural therapy (CBT-ED; 2nd line)
Anorexia nervosa in >18s	Individual eating-disorder-focused cognitive behavioural therapy (CBT-ED), Maudsley anorexia nervosa treatment for adults (MANTRA) or specialist supportive clinical management (SSCM)
Bulimia nervosa in <18s	FBT
Bulimia nervosa in >18s	CBT-ED

Key Findings	Management
Alcohol withdrawal	Supportive management, benzodiazepines, Pabrinex
Wernicke encephalopathy	Pabrinex
Opioid dependence	Harm reduction, methadone or buprenorphine
Opioid overdose	Naloxone
Alcohol dependence	Psychological intervention, acamprosate, naltrexone – 1st line, disulfiram – 2nd line
Delirium	Identify and treat underlying cause
Distress in delirium	Identify and treat underlying cause, verbal and nonverbal de-escalation if distressed – 1st line, short-term low dose haloperidol – 2nd line
Alzheimer dementia	Acetylcholinesterase inhibitors, e.g., donepezil/rivastigmine/galantamine – 1st line, memantine – 2nd line
Vascular dementia	No specific pharmacological treatment
Dementia with Lewy bodies	Rivastigmine or donepezil
Frontotemporal dementia	No specific pharmacological treatment
Symptoms of stress and distress in dementia	Exclude physical or environmental cause, verbal, and nonverbal de-escalation – 1st line, risperidone – 2nd line (except in Lewy body dementia or Parkinson dementia)

UKMLA Single Best Answer (SBA) Questions

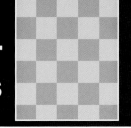

Chapter 2 Pharmacological therapy and electroconvulsive therapy

1. A 37-year-old woman with treatment-resistant schizophrenia is considering commencing clozapine. What should she be advised regarding haematological monitoring that is initially required?
   A. Weekly renal function checks.
   B. Weekly liver function tests.
   C. Weekly full blood counts.
   D. Weekly lipid profiles.
   E. Weekly fasting glucose assays.

2. A 45-year-old woman has recently started phenelzine. She is out for lunch with her friend who is a doctor. She asks her friend which of these options can she safely eat from the menu?
   A. Broccoli and stilton soup.
   B. Pickled herring on a bed of salad.
   C. Marmite and sesame toast.
   D. Smoked mackerel pâté.
   E. Egg mayonnaise toastie.

3. Which of the following is an indication for ECT?
   A. A patient with body dysmorphic disorder not responding to SSRI medication.
   B. A patient presenting with first-episode psychosis and associated acute behavioural disturbance.
   C. A patient with a severe depressive episode with significant weight loss and no oral intake for the past 3 days.
   D. A patient with established bipolar affective disorder on lithium presenting with depressive symptoms and a subtherapeutic lithium level.
   E. A patient with no past psychiatric history who has been admitted after jumping from a local bridge with suicidal intent.

4. Which of these mood stabilizers should NOT be used in people under the age of 55?
   A. Lithium
   B. Carbamazepine
   C. Quetiapine
   D. Sodium valproate
   E. Topiramate

5. A 22-year-old woman recently commenced on an antipsychotic is pacing her bedroom and says she feels very restless. What would be the most appropriate pharmacological agent to trial to manage her symptoms?
   A. Procyclidine
   B. Olanzapine
   C. Propranolol
   D. Quinine
   E. Haloperidol

6. A 26-year-old man commenced antipsychotics a month ago. You review him in your outpatient clinic. His face shows little expression, and he does not swing his arms when he walks. He does not have a tremor, and his gait is not shuffling. What would be the most appropriate medication to manage his side effects?
   A. Intramuscular procyclidine
   B. Oral procyclidine
   C. Oral diazepam
   D. Oral propranolol
   E. Oral quinine

7. A 34-year-old man has been on an intramuscular zuclopenthixol decanoate depot and regular procyclidine for over a decade. His mother contacts you as she has become concerned about unusual facial movements, she has noticed the patient making. When you review him in clinic, you notice that he makes frequent darting movements with his tongue but seems unaware of this. Which of the following would be the most appropriate management option?
   A. Increase the dose of his zuclopenthixol decanoate depot – he is responding to unseen stimuli.
   B. Watch and wait.
   C. Stop procyclidine.
   D. Commence low dose aripiprazole in addition to his zuclopenthixol decanoate depot.
   E. Refer to neurology.

8. Which of the following describes the mechanism of action of venlafaxine?
   A. 5-HT 2C receptor antagonist and melatonin receptor agonist.
   B. Inhibits serotonin and noradrenaline reuptake pumps; does not affect acetylcholine receptors.
   C. Inhibits serotonin and noradrenaline reuptake pumps; also blocks acetylcholine receptors.

D. Reversible inhibition of monoamine oxidase A.
E. Inhibits dopamine and noradrenaline reuptake pumps.

Chapter 3 Psychological therapy

1. A 49-year-old man has been struggling to move on with his life after his son died in a car accident 8 months ago. Which of the following would be the most appropriate psychological therapy in the first instance?
   A. Psychodynamic therapy
   B. Cognitive-behavioural therapy
   C. Person-centred counselling
   D. Exposure and response prevention
   E. Mindfulness-based cognitive therapy

2. A 35-year-old man is undergoing psychodynamic psychotherapy, and a letter from his therapist describes his 'transference'. Which of the following is the most accurate description of transference?
   A. The level of trust in the patient-therapist relationship.
   B. Good eye contact throughout sessions.
   C. Patient response towards the therapist based on previous relationships.
   D. The level of empathy in the patient–therapist relationship.
   E. Therapist attitude towards the patient based on previous relationships.

3. A 25-year-old male student has a history of depression and has been referred for cognitive-behavioural therapy. He reports that 'my life is over because I failed my final exams.' Which of the following most accurately describes this cognitive distortion?
   A. Emotional reasoning
   B. Fortune telling
   C. Personalization
   D. Labelling
   E. Magnification

4. A 57-year-old teacher attends her general practitioner requesting a referral for interpersonal therapy after reading about it in a magazine. In which of the following conditions has interpersonal therapy proven to be of benefit?
   A. Alzheimer disease
   B. Moderate depression
   C. Generalized anxiety disorder
   D. Paranoid schizophrenia
   E. Panic disorder

5. A 57-year-old lady has a depressive disorder of moderate severity. She attributes her symptoms to the fact that her father has been taken into a nursing home, her daughter has left home to attend university and she was recently made redundant from her job in a bank. Which of the following would be the most appropriate modality of psychological therapy to suggest?
   A. Dialectical behavioural therapy (DBT)
   B. Counselling
   C. Psychoanalysis
   D. Interpersonal therapy (IPT)
   E. Eye movement desensitization and reprocessing (EMDR)

6. A 42-year-old gentleman has a diagnosis of obsessive-compulsive disorder and is mainly troubled by having to check switches and locks in his home. He feels that a therapy that is 'more practical than talking' would be helpful. Which of the following would be the most appropriate modality of psychological therapy to suggest?
   A. Cognitive behavioural therapy with exposure and response prevention
   B. Cognitive behavioural therapy
   C. Mindfulness-based cognitive therapy
   D. Interpersonal therapy
   E. Art therapy

Chapter 4 Mental health and the law

1. A 72-year-old woman has recently been diagnosed with dementia. She continues to drive and gets shopping for her and her partner every week. He says there are no problems with her driving. What should she be advised?
   A. She should stop driving immediately.
   B. She should stop driving once she feels her driving is not as good as it used to be.
   C. She should stop driving once her partner feels her driving is not as good as it used to be.
   D. She should continue driving but notify the Driver and Vehicle Licencing Agency (DVLA).
   E. She should continue driving but her general practitioner will notify the DVLA.

2. A 23-year-old man has suffered a head injury in a road traffic accident and has a Glasgow Coma Scale (GCS) score of 8. A decision needs to be made as to whether he

should be ventilated or not. What is the best description of his capacity to make this decision?

A. Capacity should be assumed to be present.
B. Capacity is absent because of impaired communication.
C. Capacity is absent because of impaired understanding.
D. Capacity is absent because of impaired retention of information.
E. Capacity is absent because of impaired ability to balance and weigh up information.

3. A 59-year-old man has suffered from Wernicke encephalopathy and now cannot remember any new information. A decision needs to be made regarding which accommodation option he should choose. What is the best description of his capacity to make this decision?

A. Capacity should be assumed to be present.
B. Capacity is absent because of impaired communication.
C. Capacity is absent because of impaired understanding.
D. Capacity is absent because of impaired retention of information.
E. Capacity is absent because of impaired ability to balance and weigh up information.

4. A 34-year-old woman is experiencing a manic episode with psychotic features. She broke her leg jumping off a bus shelter but denies the need for surgery as she thinks she can heal her leg herself. The decision is whether she needs surgery or not. What is the best description of her capacity to make this decision?

A. Capacity should be assumed to be present.
B. Capacity is absent because of impaired communication.
C. Capacity is absent because of impaired understanding.
D. Capacity is absent because of impaired retention of information.
E. Capacity is absent because of impaired ability to balance and weigh up information.

5. A 55-year-old man has schizophrenia with chronic auditory hallucinations and negative symptoms. The decision is whether he should take a statin or not. What is the best description of his capacity to make this decision?

A. Capacity should be assumed to be present.
B. Capacity is absent because of impaired communication.

C. Capacity is absent because of impaired understanding.
D. Capacity is absent because of impaired retention of information.
E. Capacity is absent because of impaired ability to balance and weigh up information.

Chapter 5 Mental health service provision

1. Which patient is MOST likely to need secondary mental health services?

A. A 34-year-old woman with a first episode of depression, responding well to cognitive behavioural therapy
B. A 34-year-old woman with a first episode of depression, who has not responded to cognitive behavioural therapy or two antidepressants
C. A 34-year-old woman with generalized anxiety symptoms, on the waiting list for cognitive behavioural therapy.
D. A 34-year-old woman who is frequently tearful following the death of her mother 2 months ago
E. A 34-year-old woman who says she has been depressed for years but objectively seems euthymic

2. A 21-year-old man with no past psychiatric history is experiencing odd beliefs that he has some special power and that things around him are of special significance. He struggles to explain these beliefs further and says they cannot be true. He has stopped going out with his friends and his personal hygiene has deteriorated. He has no thoughts of harm to himself or others. Which team should he be referred to?

A. Community mental health team
B. Early intervention in psychosis team
C. Assertive outreach team
D. Home treatment team
E. Inpatient unit

Chapter 6 The patient with thoughts of suicide or self-harm

1. A 45-year-old policeman with a history of self-harm, depression and alcohol dependence discloses that he has been thinking about ways of killing himself since his wife left him a month ago. Which ONE of the following preparatory measures would suggest strong suicidal intent?

A. Internet research
B. Contacting the Samaritans
C. Telling his ex-wife of his plans
D. Making a will and paying bills
E. Telling his general practitioner of his plans

2. A 29-year-old builder with a diagnosis of depression states that he is considering various methods of suicide. Which ONE of the following plans places him at highest risk of suicide?

   A. Jumping from a height
   B. Paracetamol overdose
   C. Suspension hanging
   D. Making cuts to wrists
   E. Carbon monoxide poisoning

3. Which of the following mental disorders is associated with the highest relative risk compared to the general population of completed suicide?

   A. Personality disorders
   B. Generalised anxiety disorder
   C. Anorexia nervosa
   D. Schizophrenia
   E. Obsessive-compulsive disorder

4. A 19-year-old woman states that she is going to kill herself because 'the voices in my head are telling me to'. These started troubling her this morning after an argument with her mother. Yesterday, she felt fine with no voices. She has no symptoms of depression. She insists that 'it will be all your fault when I commit suicide' and demands admission to a psychiatric ward. She has a history of self-harm by cutting and is well known to mental health services from previous emergency presentations. What is the most likely diagnosis?

   A. Schizophrenia
   B. Personality disorder with prominent features of disinhibition and a borderline pattern
   C. Bipolar affective disorder, current episode manic with psychotic symptoms
   D. Single episode depressive disorder
   E. Personality disorder with prominent features of detachment

5. A 50-year-old female bank manager who tried to gas herself in her car is found in a remote forest clearing at 4:30 a.m. by a dog walker. Typed letters to her wife and children (currently on holiday) were found on the passenger seat. She has no psychiatric history. She appeared intoxicated; however, she states she is not a big drinker. She described recent weight loss and wakening early in the morning. She is also convinced that a recent financial crisis is all her fault. What is the most likely diagnosis?

   A. Alcohol dependency
   B. Schizophrenia

C. Single episode depressive disorder, severe with psychotic symptoms
D. Single episode depressive disorder, moderate without psychotic symptoms
E. Severe personality disorder with prominent traits of negative affectivity

Chapter 7 Psychiatric Emergencies

1. A 23-year-old woman presents at the accident and emergency department stating that she is feeling suicidal and has taken an overdose of paracetamol several hours ago. What is the most appropriate initial management step?

   A. History of circumstances leading to overdose
   B. Mental state examination
   C. Physical health assessment including serum paracetamol levels
   D. Determination of suicidal intent
   E. Evaluation of current social supports

2. Nursing staff ask for you to urgently review a 24-year-old man who is a psychiatric inpatient and is hypertensive, tachycardic and pyrexial. He is very drowsy and has rigid limbs. What action will most help distinguish between neuroleptic malignant syndrome and serotonin syndrome?

   A. Checking serum creatinine kinase levels.
   B. Looking at his prescription.
   C. Checking his past medical history.
   D. Formally assessing his cognition.
   E. Monitoring his condition over time.

3. Nursing staff ask for you to urgently review a 24-year-old man who is a psychiatric inpatient and is hypertensive, tachycardic and pyrexial. He is very drowsy and has rigid limbs. He was admitted a week ago with a first episode of psychosis and has received large doses of haloperidol since. What is the most appropriate first management step?

   A. Discontinue all antipsychotics.
   B. Work up for electroconvulsive therapy.
   C. Give dantrolene.
   D. Give bromocriptine.
   E. Assess ABCDE.

4. A 37-year-old woman who takes lithium for bipolar affective disorder has recently completed a course of ibuprofen for a knee injury. She now feels very tired and weak. She is unsteady on her feet and has a coarse tremor. A random lithium level is assessed. What is the

lowest result that would suggest her symptoms are due to lithium toxicity?

A. 0.2 mmol/L
B. 0.4 mmol/L
C. 0.8 mmol/L
D. 1.0 mmol/L
E. 1.8 mmol/L

5. A 23-year-old woman has been admitted to the general adult psychiatry ward due to experiencing persecutory delusional ideas about the NHS and a belief that health professionals are trying to steal her DNA in order to perform experiments on her. She has been detained under the mental health act at the time of admission. She has become acutely distressed, has barricaded herself in the nurse's office and is threatening to hit anyone who tries to enter with a fire extinguisher. Which of these options would be the most appropriate first step to manage the situation

A. I.M. lorazepam
B. Ask security to restrain the patient and return her to her room
C. Contact the police and ask that the patient be taken to custody
D. Verbal de-escalation techniques
E. Oral haloperidol

6. A 35-year-old woman experiencing a manic episode with psychotic features had been attempting to make the voices go away by repeatedly banging her head against her sink. De-escalation techniques had not worked, and she had refused oral medication, so in view of the significant risk to herself she received intramuscular rapid tranquillization. She has no past medical history. It is now 30 minutes post administration and she is sitting dozing peacefully in the quiet room. What monitoring does she now require?

A. No monitoring is required
B. General observations
C. Temperature, pulse, blood pressure, respiratory rate, hydration status and consciousness level every hour
D. Temperature, pulse, blood pressure, respiratory rate, hydration status and consciousness level every 15 minutes
E. Continuous monitoring of pulse, blood pressure and respiratory rate with regular temperatures

7. A 35-year-old woman has received intramuscular rapid tranquillization. Which of the following complications is least important to monitor for?

A. Respiratory depression
B. Inability to protect her own airway
C. Hyperglycaemia
D. Acute arrhythmia
E. Life-threatening hypotension

8. A 22-year-old woman was recently commenced on an antipsychotic. You are called to review her as the nurses are concerned as she has been staring at the ceiling and clenching her jaw tightly. After completing an ABCDE assessment, what would be the most appropriate pharmacological management?

A. Intramuscular procyclidine
B. Oral procyclidine
C. Propranolol
D. Quinine
E. Intramuscular haloperidol

Chapter 8 The patient with neurodevelopmental differences

1. A 7-year-old boy keeps getting up at school and walking to the front of the classroom. His mother is worried he has attention deficit hyperactivity disorder (ADHD). He is not restless at home and sits calmly during the interview. What is the most appropriate initial step in management?

A. Check thyroid function
B. Collateral history from teacher
C. Ensure he has an up-to-date eye test
D. Genetic testing to exclude ADHD
E. Refer for ADHD assessment

2. A 1-year-old girl has stopped crawling. She used to cry a lot but is now calm and placid. She had developed a social smile but has not done this for a few weeks. She also makes less eye contact than she used to. What is the most likely diagnosis?

A. Autism spectrum disorder
B. Heller syndrome
C. Intellectual disability
D. Muscular dystrophy
E. Rett syndrome

3. A 23-year-old man reports he is very anxious in social situations. He recently lost his job because he talked too much in the office. Now he is worried about talking to others at all. He says he 'doesn't get the rules' and he thought his workmates were enjoying what he was telling them about the history of photocopiers. What is the most likely diagnosis?

   A. Personality disorder with prominent traits of anankastia
   B. Autism spectrum disorder
   C. Depressive episode
   D. Generalized anxiety disorder
   E. Social anxiety disorder

4. A 24-year-old woman lives alone with input from a support worker twice a week and works in a bakery. She required extra induction sessions at the bakery before she could independently serve customers as she found it very difficult to use the cash register or give the correct change. She needed extra help at school with reading and writing and did not achieve any qualifications. What would her most likely diagnosis be?

   A. No diagnosis
   B. Mild intellectual disability
   C. Moderate intellectual disability
   D. Severe intellectual disability
   E. Profound intellectual disability

5. A 22-year-old man lives with his family, who are his main carers. He requires some assistance getting dressed and tending to his personal hygiene; however, he can do this by himself on good days. He can feed himself and spends his days watching children's television programmes and playing with Lego. What would his most likely diagnosis be?

   A. No diagnosis
   B. Mild intellectual disability
   C. Moderate intellectual disability
   D. Severe intellectual disability
   E. Profound intellectual disability

6. A 39-year-old man struggles to concentrate on tasks such as paying his bills. He has started gambling. At interview his speech is hard to interrupt and his thought form is tangential. He has had to give up his job as an accountant following involvement in a road traffic accident. What is the most likely driver of his difficulties?

   A. ADHD
   B. Intellectual disability
   C. Traumatic brain injury
   D. Generalized anxiety disorder
   E. Substance misuse

Chapter 9 The patient with psychotic symptoms

1. A 78-year-old widow with macular degeneration is brought to her general practitioner by her daughter who is concerned that her mother has been asking her to move nonexistent dogs and cats off her couch. Her mother is otherwise alert, orientated and in good health. What is the most likely diagnosis?

   A. Brain tumour
   B. Charles Bonnet syndrome
   C. Delirium
   D. Dementia
   E. Schizophrenia

2. A 62-year-old man with schizophrenia attends his general practitioner. He is dishevelled and smells strongly of tobacco. He reports feeling that someone is pressing on his chest, particularly when he approaches the church at the top of the hill. He wonders if it is the devil. What is the most probable cause of the sensation in his chest?

   A. Delusion of control
   B. Ischaemic heart disease
   C. Persecutory delusion
   D. Tactile hallucination
   E. Thought disorder

3. A 43-year-old man tells his general practitioner, 'I think my wife is having an affair'. When asked about why he thinks this, he tells his GP that 2 weeks ago his wife had her hair cut, and since then he has realized that she is being unfaithful to him. He is very upset by this and determined to get conclusive evidence to confront her with. He has quit his job to follow her and taken out a personal loan to purchase cameras to place in her car, workplace and handbag. He becomes annoyed when his GP suggests an alternative explanation for his belief. What is the psychopathology described here?

   A. Delusions of infidelity
   B. Erotomania
   C. Visual hallucination
   D. Obsession
   E. Over-valued idea

4. A 19-year-old man is brought to accident and emergency by his flatmates because for the last fortnight, he has been complaining the neighbours are talking about him and tonight stated 'enough was enough' and picked up his cricket bat to go and confront them. His friends cannot hear the neighbours. The man has smoked cannabis every day for the last 6 months and has recently been experimenting with some 'stimulant medication' he bought online. What is the most likely diagnosis?

A. Delusional disorder
B. Depressive episode, severe, with psychotic features
C. Substance-induced psychotic disorder
D. Schizophrenia
E. Acute and transient psychotic disorder

5. A 43-year-old woman is referred to the community mental health team because she has been seeing shadowy figures in her room at night as she is going to sleep. She denies experiencing auditory hallucinations, and she reports that the figures are only present in this specific setting. What is the most likely explanation for her symptoms?

A. Schizophrenia
B. Hypnogogic hallucination
C. Severe depressive episode with psychotic symptoms
D. Hypnopompic hallucination
E. Pseudohallucination

6. A 45-year-old man has recurrent episodes of low mood associated with third-person auditory hallucinations in the form of an abusive running commentary. These symptoms do not occur separately. What is the most likely diagnosis?

A. Personality disorder
B. Single episode depressive disorder with psychotic symptoms
C. Schizophrenia
D. Schizoaffective disorder
E. Delusional disorder

7. A 47-year-old teacher presents to his GP for the 25th time in 6 months convinced he has bowel cancer, despite having had a normal colonoscopy and abdomen/pelvis computed tomography. His conviction arose after he smelt some dog faeces on the pavement and felt this was a sign. He tells his GP he knows logically he cannot have bowel cancer but at the same time he is certain he does. His mood is normal and he is still working. What is the most likely diagnosis?

A. Hypochondriasis
B. Single episode depressive disorder with psychotic symptoms
C. Schizophrenia
D. Schizoaffective disorder
E. Delusional disorder

8. A 37-year-old man is brought to accident and emergency by the police for assessment after he called them to say his neighbour is persecuting him by refusing to move her wheelie-bin. The police note multiple previous calls over the last decade about previous neighbours. The man

agrees it is possible the neighbour has some other reason for not wanting to move the wheelie-bin, but thinks it is most likely because she wants to spite him. He is angry with the police for bringing him to see a doctor, stating he plans to contact his lawyer about their behaviour. What is the most likely diagnosis?

A. Personality disorder
B. Single episode depressive disorder with psychotic symptoms
C. Schizophrenia
D. Schizoaffective disorder
E. Delusional disorder

9. A woman requests a GP home visit for her 78-year-old father who has no previous psychiatric history. She is concerned that he has told her he can hear his mother and sister, who are both dead, talking. She is also concerned that he seems very forgetful and does not seem to be looking after himself properly. He is quite cheerful and enjoys speaking with his relatives. What is the most likely diagnosis?

A. Huntington disease
B. Vitamin B12 deficiency
C. Cocaine use
D. Hyperthyroidism
E. Neurosyphilis

Chapter 10 The patient with elevated or irritable mood

1. Reception staff ask the general practitioner to see a 29-year-old man with a history of bipolar disorder who has arrived 2 hours late for his appointment. He is speaking very quickly and the words don't make sense. He also appears to be talking to someone who the reception staff cannot see. What is the most likely cause for his presentation?

A. Manic episode with psychotic symptoms
B. Hypomanic episode
C. Single episode depressive disorder
D. Cyclothymia
E. Schizophrenia

2. A 55-year-old man has had several admissions to hospital with elated episodes when he believes he is Jesus Christ but has never been depressed. What is the diagnosis?

A. Recurrent hypomania
B. Bipolar disorder
C. Schizoaffective disorder
D. Cyclothymia
E. Recurrent mania

3. A 25-year-old farmer is brought to accident and emergency by the police after he tried to steal a tractor. He is agitated, but shows no remorse, stating loudly that it rightfully belongs to him as he is the King of Tractors. He has no past psychiatric history, past medical history or previous criminal offences. Which investigation will be most important diagnostically?

A. Computed tomography (CT) scan
B. Electroencephalogram (EEG)
C. Full blood count
D. Urine drug screen
E. Thyroid function

4. A 24-year-old unemployed woman presents to her general practitioner asking to be treated for bipolar disorder. She has looked it up on the internet and thinks it may explain why she is always losing her temper with people. Her mood swings frequently, sometimes several times in a day. She often does things she later regrets and has never managed to maintain a long-term relationship or job. She has had these mood swings from when she was a child. What is the most likely diagnosis?

A. Bipolar disorder
B. Dysthymia
C. Cyclothymia
D. Personality disorder
E. Substance use

5. A 40-year-old lawyer attends his general practitioner (GP) asking for a medication to reduce his sex drive because his wife is complaining. He is smartly dressed in a new suit and says he feels 'on top of the world'. He has been finding it hard to stay focused at work but so far no one has commented. Fortunately, he is able to stay up late catching up on work without feeling tired the next day. He denies any drug or alcohol use. What is the most likely diagnosis?

A. Manic episode with psychotic features
B. Manic episode without psychotic features
C. Hypomanic episode
D. Acute and transient psychotic disorder
E. No mental illness

6. A 28-year-old doctor is brought to A&E by his flatmates. He has recently started a stressful new job and his flatmates are worried because he doesn't seem to be eating or sleeping well, despite seeming quite cheerful. He paces the flat at night talking about new operative techniques he is designing, at times they wondered if he was on the phone as this sounded like a conversation, but they soon realized he was alone in his room. His

consultant sent him home from work because he refused to scrub for theatre, stating 'I'm pristine already'. What is the most likely diagnosis?

A. Manic episode with psychotic features
B. Manic episode without psychotic features
C. Hypomanic episode
D. Acute and transient psychotic disorder
E. No mental illness

Chapter 11 The patient with low mood

1. A 40-year-old woman who was started on a new medication a month ago presents with a 4-week history of depression. Which of the following might account for her presentation?

A. Paracetamol
B. Omeprazole
C. Salbutamol
D. Verapamil
E. Prednisolone

2. A 35-year-old woman presents with mild depression. On examination you notice a midline neck swelling. What is the most appropriate initial step in patient care?

A. Refer to psychiatry
B. Check thyroid function
C. Start an antidepressant
D. Request a neck ultrasound
E. Advise her to return if the symptoms persist

3. A 55-year-old man with no previous psychiatric history presents with low mood, anhedonia and fatigue. He has come for help as he believes his organs are rotting away. What is the most likely diagnosis?

A. Bipolar disorder
B. Schizoaffective disorder
C. Schizophrenia
D. Single episode depressive disorder with psychotic features
E. Dementia

4. A 25-year-old student turns up late for her appointment. She gives a 1-month history of low mood, anhedonia and fatigue. What is the most important area to cover in what remains of the appointment time?

A. Presence of neurovegetative symptoms of depression
B. Drug history
C. Family history of mood disorder
D. Suicidal ideation
E. Past medical history

5. A 19-year-old shop assistant presents in tears because her boyfriend broke up with her the day before. She did not sleep well last night and did not feel like having breakfast. She feels hopeless about the future and thinks she will never meet anyone else. She says she feels really depressed. She denies suicidal ideation. What is the most appropriate initial step in patient care?
    A. Start an antidepressant
    B. Refer to psychiatry
    C. Ask her to complete a mood diary
    D. Watchful waiting
    E. Check full blood count, urea and electrolytes, liver function test and thyroid function test

6. A 26-year-old veterinary student presents with tingling in her left arm. She becomes tearful during the consultation, admitting she is finding the fourth year of her studies much more difficult than the previous years. You see she attended 3 months ago with a sore eye and blurred vision which resolved spontaneously. What is the most likely diagnosis?
    A. Multiple sclerosis
    B. Thrombocytopenia
    C. Cushing syndrome
    D. Systemic lupus erythematosus
    E. Hypothyroidism

7. A 76-year-old widowed retired headmistress is brought to accident and emergency by her family who are concerned she has not been eating. She paces the cubicle, keeps buttoning and unbuttoning her coat and does not sit down when offered a chair. Which term best describes the observed finding in the mental state examination?
    A. Poor self-care
    B. Psychomotor retardation
    C. Psychomotor agitation
    D. Reduced range of reactivity
    E. Incongruous affect

Chapter 12 The patient with anxiety, fear or avoidance

1. A 21-year-old student calls an ambulance because of chest pain, shortness of breath and a feeling she is about to die. This settles by the time she reaches the accident and emergency department. On all occasions, her examination, electrocardiogram and cardiac enzymes are normal. She has her final exams in a fortnight and admits she is very worried. What is the most likely diagnosis?
    A. Acute coronary syndrome
    B. Thyrotoxicosis

C. Hypoglycaemia
D. Panic attack
E. Asthma

2. A 57-year-old obese man keeps cancelling appointments with the practice nurse to have bloods taken for cholesterol and glucose. Although he is normally very cheerful and relaxed, he becomes pale, sweaty and tremulous when you offer to take his bloods during the consultation. What is the most likely diagnosis?
    A. Myocardial infarction
    B. Hyperglycaemia
    C. Blood-injection-injury phobia
    D. Panic disorder
    E. Hypochondriasis

3. A 63-year-old woman with a history of depression presents to the accident and emergency department and tells you she has a dry mouth, a choking sensation, butterflies in her stomach, palpitations and shortness of breath. She tells you she had some bad news recently. What is the most appropriate first step in management?
    A. Electrocardiogram (ECG)
    B. Airway, breathing, circulation, disability, exposure (ABCDE)
    C. Psychiatry referral
    D. Bloods: full blood count, urea and electrolytes, liver function tests and troponin
    E. Arterial blood gas (ABG)

4. A 24-year-old man who was recently diagnosed with type 1 diabetes attends his general practitioner (GP). Over the last month he has experienced recurrent attacks of anxiety associated with sweating and tachycardia. The episodes do not seem to have any triggers, last for about 20 minutes, and resolve when he sits down with his girlfriend and has a cup of tea and a biscuit. What should the GP advise the patient to do next time it happens?
    A. Deep breathing exercises
    B. Note it in a diary
    C. Take diazepam
    D. See a counsellor
    E. Check blood sugar

5. A 44-year-old businessman presents to his general practitioner (GP) because for the last month he has felt anxious, sweaty and shaky in the mornings. He feels better when he has lunch and generally his mood is good. He admits to drinking a bottle of red wine every night, and

usually having champagne during business lunches. What is the most likely diagnosis?

A. Depressive episode
B. Diabetes
C. Panic disorder
D. Alcohol withdrawal
E. Work phobia

6. A 28-year-old secretary presents to her general practitioner with weight loss. Six months ago in a supermarket she suddenly felt like she was going to die. She had pain in her chest, was short of breath and her arms and lips tingled. She rushed outside and the feeling subsided, but now she does not like to go into any large shops and is eating less well. She is still going to work but now walks 5 miles each way as she does not want to be on a bus and have another attack. As long as she is in her house or with her friends she is relaxed. What is the most likely diagnosis?

A. Agoraphobia without panic attacks
B. Agoraphobia with panic attacks
C. Social phobia with panic attacks
D. Generalized anxiety disorder with panic attacks
E. Panic disorder

7. Over the last 3 months, a 35-year-old builder has experienced several episodes of sudden onset shortness of breath, palpitations, sweatiness, nausea, feeling that the world is unreal and feeling he is about to die. These feelings resolve spontaneously over 20 minutes. He cannot identify any triggers. In particular, they are not brought on by exercise and he can continue to do his active job. His electrocardiogram (ECG) is normal. What is the most likely diagnosis?

A. Panic disorder
B. Social phobia
C. Agoraphobia without panic attacks
D. Agoraphobia with panic attacks
E. Generalized anxiety disorder

8. A 23-year-old man has started a new job with a finance company. He has noticed that he gets very irritable and anxious by the end of the day and has had to go home early a couple of times. He drinks a lot of his favourite soft drink, 'Go-Man'. What substance is the most likely driver of his anxiety?

A. Caffeine
B. Cocaine
C. Cannabis
D. Alcohol
E. Amphetamine

Chapter 13 The patient with obsessions and compulsions

1. A 29-year-old woman mentions she is obsessed with a TV talent show. She watches each episode multiple times and has pictures of all the contestants on her bedroom wall. She called in sick the day of the final as her shift clashed with the showing. She enjoys watching and thinking about the show and thinks she might audition next year. What is the most likely diagnosis?

A. No mental illness
B. Social anxiety disorder
C. Personality disorder with prominent traits of anankastia
D. Obsessive-compulsive disorder
E. Delusional disorder

2. A 36-year-old man keeps thinking about his own death. He sees repetitive images of his body in a coffin. He tries to distract himself, but it does not work. The images started about 3 months ago, around the time he started to feel low in mood associated with fatigue, less pleasure in life, insomnia and anorexia. What is the most likely diagnosis?

A. Obsessive-compulsive disorder
B. Generalised anxiety disorder
C. Depressive disorder
D. Hypochondriasis
E. Nihilistic delusion

3. A 44-year-old man has had intrusive thoughts for several years regarding security. He keeps thinking his house is unlocked and has developed a routine of checking every door and window nine times before leaving the premises. This means he has to get up half an hour early and sometimes come home from work early to recheck. This has caused friction with a new manager at work and over the last month he has noticed his mood is lower. He no longer enjoys playing football, is very tired all the time, and is struggling to concentrate at work. What is the most likely diagnosis?

A. Depressive disorder
B. Obsessive-compulsive disorder (OCD)
C. Generalised anxiety disorder
D. OCD with comorbid depressive episode
E. Personality disorder with prominent features of anankastia

4. A 33-year-old graphic designer is driven to produce perfect images. She has always been very conscientious,

even at primary school. The thought of a mistake in one of her designs makes her feel so anxious she often stays late at work checking them through. She is proud of the quality of work, and feels her colleagues are sloppy and should work harder. She had to leave her last two companies because she told the manager this. She has recently separated from her partner as they said she was not 'spontaneous enough'. What is the most likely diagnosis?

A. Obsessive-compulsive disorder
B. Mild personality disorder with prominent features of anankastia
C. No mental illness
D. Autistic spectrum disorder
E. Obsessive-compulsive disorder with comorbid depressive episode

5. A 23-year-old woman reports a voice inside her head telling her to harm herself. She is not sure where it comes from as no one is around when she hears it. What is the psychopathology she displays?

A. Obsession
B. Pseudohallucination
C. Rumination
D. Thought insertion
E. Hallucination

6. A 25-year-old woman insists that she wants plastic surgery on her nose, as she feels it is crooked and deformed. She has stopped leaving the house for fear of other people noticing. She cannot stop thinking about how ugly it is, and this often keeps her awake at night. On examination, her nose is entirely normal, and she does appear slightly reassured when told this. Which of the following is the most likely diagnosis?

A. Somatic delusional disorder
B. Factitious disorder
C. Malingering
D. Body dysmorphic disorder
E. Hypochondriasis

7. For the last few years, a 27-year-old nurse has been influenced by an NHS advertising campaign featuring soiled hands spreading COVID-19. Washing her hands reduces her fear that they are contaminated. Now she washes her hands before and after every patient contact, up to 100 times a day, and is developing contact dermatitis. What is the most likely diagnosis?

A. Phobia
B. Panic disorder
C. Obsessive-compulsive disorder

D. Hypochondriasis
E. No mental illness

8. During an assessment a patient discloses that 'When I saw a picture on TV of germs crawling on someone's skin, I knew that I was fatally ill. The doctor told me I was fine, but I know my days are numbered'. What is the mostly accurate descriptor for this experience?

A. Delusion
B. Obsession
C. Over-valued idea
D. Rumination
E. Hallucination

Chapter 14 The patient with a reaction to a stressful event

1. A 23-year-old man with a history of schizophrenia appears confused and withdrawn the morning after he was severely assaulted by a group of youths in the local park. He has no recollection of the event. Which of the following diagnoses should be initially considered?

A. Acute stress reaction
B. Adjustment disorder
C. Relapse of schizophrenia
D. Intracranial haemorrhage
E. Posttraumatic stress disorder

2. A 57-year-old woman has been referred urgently by her general practitioner for symptoms of low mood, weight loss and insomnia. These have been troublesome for the past 10 weeks, since she watched her husband drown while on a yachting holiday. Which of the following would be suggestive of a diagnosis of depression rather than a normal bereavement reaction?

A. Thinking that she would be better off dead
B. Difficulty concentrating on watching the television
C. Inability to tend to her self-care or get out of bed
D. Extreme guilt for not making her late husband wear a lifejacket
E. Hearing the voice of her late husband while lying alone in bed

3. A 28-year-old woman was signed off her job in a call centre 2 weeks ago with 'work-related stress', a month after she was promoted to a supervisory position in a new department. She has no psychiatric history and denies substance misuse. At interview, she tells you she feels 'unable to cope' with the demands of her new role. She is sleeping well, and continues to enjoy jogging on a daily

basis. Which of the following would be the most appropriate diagnosis?

A. Depressive disorder
B. Adjustment disorder
C. Dissociative neurological symptom disorder
D. Acute stress reaction
E. No mental illness

4. A 19-year-old female asylum seeker is brought to hospital by a social worker regarding concerns with her memory. She recalls her entire life until 3 months ago when she received news that government militia were coming towards her former hometown in Sierra Leone. She has memory of the last 4 weeks of her life in the UK and is able to tell you about her current address, social circle and circumstances. You see from her medical notes that she had a termination of pregnancy 6 weeks ago; however, she has no recollection of either the conception or the procedure. Physical examination and investigations reveal no abnormalities, and she seems indifferent to her difficulties. Which ONE of the following is the most likely diagnosis?

A. Dissociative amnesia
B. Anterograde amnesia following head trauma
C. Transient global amnesia
D. Posttraumatic stress disorder
E. Wernicke–Korsakoff syndrome

5. A 19-year-old woman presents to A&E for the seventh time in the past year after taking an overdose with suicidal intent. She has a history of repeated childhood sexual abuse. She re-experiences the abuse in the form of vivid, intrusive images, triggered by the smell of certain aftershaves. She is easily startled by loud noises in the department and tries to avoid being alone with male members of staff. She describes difficulties since the event with controlling her emotions, maintaining friendships and with feelings of worthlessness. What is the most likely diagnosis?

A. Depressive disorder
B. Post traumatic stress disorder
C. Acute and transient psychotic disorder
D. Obsessive-compulsive disorder
E. Complex post traumatic stress disorder

6. A 46-year-old businessman from a distant city is brought to hospital by the police, after apparently trying to withdraw money from a building society and being unable to remember his name. At interview, he seems unable to recall any personal details about himself and has no idea where he is. He is carrying a bundle of business cards for a company that was recently reported to have gone bankrupt. What is the most likely diagnosis?

A. Dissociative identity disorder
B. Depersonalization disorder
C. Dissociative amnesia with dissociative fugue
D. Posttraumatic stress disorder
E. Trance disorder

7. A 29-year-old mother of two, with a history of depression and a family history of epilepsy, has recently started having episodes, during which she falls to the floor, moving all her limbs, with her eyes squeezed tight shut. The episodes last at least 5 minutes. They do not cause tongue-biting, incontinence or postictal confusion. She can remember 'shaking all over'. She denies alcohol or drug use. Her husband tells you that this started when he told his wife of his new job on an oil rig. He now feels he cannot leave home for fear that she will be seriously harmed by the seizures. What is the most likely diagnosis?

A. Dissociative amnesia
B. Dissociation secondary to psychoactive substance use
C. Epilepsy
D. Functional paralysis
E. Nonepileptic seizures

8. A 27-year-old woman is referred from the neurosurgical unit 4 months after a fall from a first-floor balcony. She reports episodes of derealization, followed by visual hallucinations, loss of memory and extreme tiredness

A. Posttraumatic stress disorder
B. Temporal lobe epilepsy
C. Adjustment disorder
D. Musculoskeletal injury
E. Dissociative neurological disorder

Chapter 15 The patient with medically unexplained physical symptoms

1. A 26-year-old male teacher attends his general practitioner requesting tests to confirm that he is suffering from multiple sclerosis. He thinks that he has this because he had some stabbing pain in his upper arm last week. The pain has now resolved and examination is unremarkable. Which ONE of the following should the GP do?

A. Watchful waiting
B. Refer for urgent neurology appointment
C. Organize magnetic resonance imaging scan and lumbar puncture
D. Tell the patient that he is worrying too much
E. Organize another appointment in 3 days

2. A 32-year-old former nurse complains of pelvic pain. Despite the apparent severity of the pain and the presence of multiple abdominal surgical scars, her physical appearance, examination and basic investigations are entirely normal. She tells you in detail about her previous diagnoses and invasive investigations, and requests pethidine and a diagnostic laparoscopy. She is visiting from a distant town. Which of the following should be the next step in her management?
   A. Urgent diagnostic laparoscopy
   B. Prescribe pethidine
   C. Tell her that she is lying
   D. Contact previous centres of care
   E. Refer to psychiatry

3. A 72-year-old man is referred to psychiatry because of dyspnoea and stabbing pain in his chest. He has not seen a general practitioner for years, and examination and routine blood tests are normal. The medical doctor feels that he has panic attacks. Which ONE of the following should be the next step in his management?
   A. Cognitive-behavioural therapy
   B. Further physical investigations
   C. Explanation of functional illness
   D. Antidepressant medication
   E. Watchful waiting

4. A 41-year-old woman is a frequent visitor to her general practitioner. She has had numerous investigations over several years for a multitude of physical symptoms, including abdominal pain, dysmenorrhoea, dysuria and difficulty swallowing. She refuses to accept her GP's explanation that there is no physical cause for her symptoms. She is now requesting a referral to a neurologist because she has a persistent tingling sensation in her legs. Which of the following is the most likely diagnosis?
   A. Multiple sclerosis
   B. Factitious disorder
   C. Bodily distress disorder
   D. Hypochondriasis
   E. Generalised anxiety disorder

Chapter 16 The patient with eating, feeding or weight problems

1. A 22-year-old female medical student is brought to your clinic by her mother, who discovered she was making herself vomit after meals. Which of the following is suggestive of a diagnosis of anorexia nervosa rather than bulimia nervosa?
   A. Significantly low body weight
   B. A dread of fatness and a distorted image of being too fat
   C. Use of herbal dieting medications
   D. Tendency to exercise excessively
   E. A preoccupation with being thin

2. The weight of a 13-year-old boy is 25% lower than expected, having previously been on the 50th percentile for both height and weight. He has not started puberty. He reports that he eats well and denies any concerns regarding body image. What is the most appropriate next management step?
   A. Refer for psychiatric assessment
   B. Refer for cognitive-behavioural therapy
   C. Investigate for physical causes of growth restriction
   D. Try to establish rapport to facilitate assessment
   E. Ask him to keep a food diary

3. A 32-year-old barmaid is worried that she has lost a great deal of weight recently (body mass index 17). She describes feeling tired all the time and having no appetite. Her mood has been low for the last 3 months, and she is anhedonic. She drinks six vodkas and cokes when she is working, and three on her days off. If she doesn't have a drink she feels anxious and gets palpitations. She is sometimes sick, not always after meals. Physical examination and investigations reveal no abnormalities. What is the most likely diagnosis?
   A. Bulimia nervosa
   B. Depressive episode
   C. Panic disorder
   D. Anorexia nervosa
   E. Alcohol dependence

4. A 25-year-old female lawyer has a diagnosis of anorexia nervosa, with a body mass index of 14.5 kg/m^2. Which of the following investigation results requires urgent treatment?
   A. Glucose 3.7 mmol/L
   B. Haemoglobin 95 g/L
   C. Total cholesterol 7 mmol/L
   D. Phosphate 0.7 mmol/L
   E. Potassium 2.1 mmol/L

5. A 19-year-old female accountant describes a dread of fatness and feels that she is overweight despite having a body mass index of 13.6 kg/m^2. She describes a 1-year

history of severely restricting her dietary intake. She reports amenorrhoea (secondary) and has lanugo hair. Which of the following is the most likely diagnosis?

A. Depressive episode
B. Bulimia nervosa
C. Schizophrenia
D. Anorexia nervosa
E. Obsessive-compulsive disorder

6. A 19-year-old boy has anorexia nervosa and is receiving weekly weights and physical examination. Which of the findings below places him at high physical risk?

A. Blood pressure 95/65 mm Hg supine, 88/60 mm Hg erect
B. Capillary refill time <2 seconds
C. Heart rate 58 bpm, regular
D. Temperature 36.5°C
E. Unable to rise from squatting without assistance

Chapter 17 The patient with alcohol or substance use problems

1. A 57-year-old woman described auditory hallucinations telling her that she was evil. These started a week ago, after several months of heavy alcohol use. She is socially isolated. Her mood, concentration and memory were normal. Other than slightly abnormal liver function tests, physical examination and investigations were normal, and breath alcohol was undetected. What is the most likely diagnosis?

A. Delirium tremens
B. Late-onset schizophrenia
C. Hepatic encephalopathy
D. Alcoholic hallucinosis
E. Wernicke–Korsakoff syndrome

2. A 62-year-old salesman is admitted to an orthopaedic ward following a fractured neck of femur. Two days later (before surgery to repair his hip), he appears shaky, confused and disorientated, and tells you that he can see a small horse on the table. His wife discloses that he had been drinking a bottle of whisky per day in the 3 months prior to admission. Which of the following aspects of his management should be delayed?

A. Benzodiazepines
B. Parenteral thiamine
C. Full physical exam
D. Neck of femur repair
E. Consistent nursing care

3. A 27-year-old man comes to your outpatient clinic and tells you that he has been injecting heroin on a daily basis for several months and wants you to restart his methadone to help him stop. What is the most appropriate initial step in patient care?

A. Prescribe his previous dose of methadone
B. Give him some dihydrocodeine to use first
C. Obtain a urine sample for drug testing
D. Refer him to the drug counselling service
E. Contact the police because he has been using illegal drugs

4. A 35-year-old woman asks you about 'safe' limits for drinking alcohol. You know the answer is 14 units per week; however, she asks you to explain this in terms of how many drinks she can safely take. What would you tell her?

A. Six pints (568 mL) of continental lager (5.3% alcohol by volume (ABV)) per week
B. A 'half bottle' (350 mL) of premium gin (40% ABV) per week
C. Two bottles (2 × 750 mL) of red wine (12.5% ABV) per week
D. A large (3 L) bottle of strong white cider (8.4% ABV) per week
E. Six bottles (6 × 330 mL) of 'alcopops' (4.9% ABV) per week

5. A 24-year-old accountant confides in you that he has tried cocaine on a work night out. He experienced some strange feelings and wants to know whether these were likely to be due to cocaine, or whether he was sold something else. Which of the following symptoms is not suggestive of cocaine intoxication?

A. Chest pain
B. Fast heart rate
C. Fever
D. Hallucinations
E. Drowsiness

6. A 34-year-old musician presents to the ED asking to speak to a psychiatrist. He reports feeling like he is not real and that he is floating outside of his body. He does report some substance use earlier in the day but cannot remember what he has taken. What is the most likely drug he has used

A. Cocaine
B. Buprenorphine
C. Ketamine
D. MDMA
E. LSD

Chapter 18 The patient with personality problems

1. A 20-year-old woman frequently attends her GP reporting low mood and difficulties maintaining romantic relationships due to frequent arguments and fear of abandonment from her partner. She reports that she has poor self-esteem. She has a successful job but has few friends. She has a good relationship with her parents. She also describes difficulties in managing confrontation and feels as though she is quick to anger. These difficulties with friendships and relationships have been present throughout her adolescence. What is the most likely diagnosis?
   A. No mental disorder
   B. Mild personality disorder
   C. Moderate personality disorder
   D. Severe personality disorder
   E. Social anxiety disorder

2. A 35-year-old man is assessed in police custody after he has been arrested following an assault. He reports longstanding difficulties with experiencing intense, and at times unbearable emotions, being extremely quick to anger and being prone to making impulsive and often later regretted decisions. He has been arrested several times before for assault and breach of the peace, with his first arrest at the age of 13. He describes a sense of self-loathing that has been present since his teenage years and he frequently uses alcohol and drugs to help him manage his emotions. He has been in several short-term relationships, but struggles to maintain friendships and is no longer in touch with his family. He is unemployed. He also has a history of self-harm and previous presentations to A&E following impulsive overdoses with suicidal intent. What is the most likely diagnosis?
   A. Social anxiety disorder
   B. Polysubstance dependence
   C. Mild personality disorder
   D. Moderate personality disorder
   E. Severe personality disorder

3. A 55-year-old librarian attends a psychiatric outpatient clinic. She reports that she has, since her teenage years, been a 'perfectionist'. She describes finding it difficult to tolerate her new colleague, who she feels does 'half a job' as they do not follow the extensive guidelines she prepared for them. She lives alone after separating from her partner of 2 years, as they argued too frequently about cleaning tasks in the household and the patient's lack of spontaneity. What is the most likely prominent personality trait?
   A. Personality disorder with prominent features of detachment
   B. Personality disorder with prominent features of negative affectivity
   C. Personality disorder with prominent features of dissociality
   D. Personality disorder with prominent features of anankastia
   E. Personality disorder with prominent features of disinhibition

4. A 25-year-old prisoner is reviewed in clinic after pushing a fellow prisoner down a flight of stairs. When challenged about this, he stated that the person had been walking too slowly and was preventing them from getting dinner. He states that he does not feel guilty, as the fellow prisoner is not as important as him, and his needs are more important than theirs. You look back through their medical records and can see that this is not the first time they have done something like this, with the earliest entry being from when they were 17 and had punched their social worker for suggesting they would not be entitled to increased benefits. What is the most likely diagnosis?
   A. Personality disorder with prominent features of detachment
   B. Personality disorder with prominent features of negative affectivity
   C. Personality disorder with prominent features of dissociality
   D. Personality disorder with prominent features of anankastia
   E. Personality disorder with prominent features of disinhibition

5. A 21-year-old woman is seen in the emergency department. This is her fourth presentation with a paracetamol overdose in the past 2 months. At assessment, she describes difficulties with maintaining relationships, constantly worrying that people are going to abandon her. She describes feeling 'empty' and feels as though she does not know who she is as a person. She has a history of self-harm dating back to the age of 11, and states she uses self-harm as a way to deal with her emotions going 'all over the place' and manage her distress after arguments. She also describes making impulsive decisions and acting based on immediate emotional responses to situations, rather than thinking through her actions. She 'never' plans anything and

becomes distracted by what is going on around her during the assessment. What is the most likely diagnosis?

A. Personality disorder with prominent features of detatchment and a borderline pattern
B. Personality disorder with prominent features of negative affectivity and a borderline pattern
C. Personality disorder with a prominent features of dissociality and a borderline pattern
D. Personality disorder with prominent features of anankastia and a borderline pattern
E. Personality disorder with prominent traits of disinhibition and a borderline pattern

Chapter 19 The patient with impairment of consciousness, memory or cognition

1. An 82-year-old woman is brought to A&E by her family. They are concerned that over the last couple of days she has been very suspicious of them, has mentioned seeing wolves in her kitchen and has been pacing her sitting room all night. She scores 4/10 on the Abbreviated Mental Test. She normally functions well, living alone with no carers. What is the most likely diagnosis?

A. Late onset schizophrenia
B. Lewy body dementia
C. Alzheimer dementia
D. Delirium
E. Charles Bonnet syndrome

2. A woman brings her 62-year-old father to register at a new GP practice as he has recently moved to the area to be closer to her. He tells the GP about upcoming events and occasions he has planned, but his daughter says none of this is true, and that for some years now he has had a very poor memory for new information. He can spell 'WORLD' backwards and draw a clock face without difficulty. By the end of the consultation, he is not able to recall what you said to him or why he is in the practice. He used to be a heavy drinker. What is the most likely diagnosis?

A. Korsakoff syndrome
B. Dementia
C. Alcohol excess
D. Malingering
E. Fugue state

3. A 75-year-old retired fisherman presents to his general practitioner with a 12-month history of gradual onset, gradually worsening memory impairment confirmed by his wife. He is no longer able to cook or help mend nets like he used to. ACE-III is 76/100. He has a past medical history of hypertension and is an ex-smoker. Physical

examination is normal. He has had normal full blood count, U&Es, calcium, HbA1c, vitamin B12, folate CRP, ESR and thyroid function tests in the last month. Which of these investigations would be the most appropriate next step?

A. Computed tomography (CT) of the head
B. Chest X-ray
C. Syphilis and HIV serology
D. Electroencephalogram (EEG)
E. Cerebrospinal fluid examination

4. A 77-year-old woman is an inpatient on a general medical ward. She was admitted 2 weeks ago with a severe urinary tract infection (UTI) requiring intravenous antibiotics. In A&E her Abbreviated Mental Test (AMT) was 2/10. Since admission she has been disorientated and hallucinating. Her antibiotics finished a week ago and her inflammatory markers returned to normal. Four days ago she was almost discharged, but became very confused and agitated the night before going. Repeat AMT was 4/10. Prior to admission she functioned well and was cognitively normal. What is the most likely diagnosis?

A. Delirium
B. Late-onset schizophrenia
C. Lewy body dementia
D. Alzheimer dementia
E. Charles Bonnet syndrome

5. A 74-year-old man is admitted to hospital because he has acute cognitive impairment and is hypervigilant and agitated. Past medical history is of insomnia and ischaemic heart disease. His medications are amitriptyline 50 mg nocte, aspirin 75 mg mane, lisinopril 5 mg, omeprazole 20 mg mane, simvastatin 20 mg nocte. His daughter thinks he has recently started a new medication. Physical examination, blood tests, electrocardiogram, chest X-ray and head computed tomography are normal. What is the most likely cause of his presentation?

A. Amitriptyline
B. Aspirin
C. Lisinopril
D. Omeprazole
E. Simvastatin

6. A 74-year-old woman presents to her general practitioner (GP) with her husband who is concerned that over the last 8 weeks she has become increasingly forgetful and disorientated. She has burnt a couple of pans after leaving them unattended. Some days she takes afternoon naps, which is new for her. When pressed he recalls she was hit on the head by a football around 3 months ago while watching her grandson's team but seemed fine

afterwards. Past medical history includes atrial fibrillation and asthma. ACE-III is 70/100 and neurological exam shows normal conscious level and a subtle right hemiparesis. What is the most likely diagnosis?

A. Hypothyroidism
B. Vitamin B12 deficiency
C. Space occupying lesion
D. Addison disease
E. Chronic subdural haematoma

7. An 81-year-old man has an 18-month history of fluctuating cognitive impairment on a background of a gradual cognitive deterioration. He has been investigated for delirium but no cause found. Sometimes he is very drowsy during the day. He is increasingly stiff and finds it hard to roll over in bed. He also finds it hard to keep his balance and has had a lot of falls recently. Sometimes he experiences visual hallucinations of cats and mice. Head CT shows generalized cerebral atrophy. Which is the most likely diagnosis?

A. Lewy body dementia
B. Alzheimer dementia
C. Alcohol-related brain damage
D. Vascular dementia
E. Frontotemporal dementia

8. A 62-year-old teacher presents to her GP because she feels she is not remembering the names of the children in her class as well as she used to. She is worried she has dementia like her mother. She has no difficulties in activities of daily living and her mood is normal. She scores 82/100 on ACE-III.

A. Alzheimer dementia
B. Mild neurocognitive impairment
C. Vascular dementia
D. Factitious Disorder
E. Delirium

Chapter 20 Dementia and delirium

1. A 91-year-old nursing home resident with severe Alzheimer dementia frequently shouts unintelligible words. Physical examination and investigations are normal, and she does not seem low in mood. Staff can detect no pattern or triggers to her shouting. She appears mildly distressed by it. What option should be tried first to reduce her shouting?

A. Assess for changes to physical health
B. Antipsychotic
C. Antidepressant
D. Cholinesterase inhibitor
E. Referral to speech and language therapy

2. A 75-year-old man has Lewy body dementia. His carers are worried that he is not eating well. He tells his general practitioner that he is certain his carers are trying to poison him. What management strategy should be avoided if possible?

A. Antipsychotics
B. Nutritional supplements
C. Cholinesterase inhibitors
D. Antibiotics
E. Antidepressants

3. A 77-year-old man was admitted 3 days ago with abdominal pain of uncertain aetiology. Initially he was alert and orientated but nurses are concerned that he is now acutely disorientated and agitated. Which medication is most likely to explain his behaviour?

A. Paracetamol
B. Metoclopramide
C. Co-codamol
D. Omeprazole
E. Cyclizine

4. A general practitioner (GP) is asked to visit a 71-year-old woman in her home. She is disorientated in time, does not recognize the GP (whom she has known for years) and is very drowsy. She is plucking at her bedclothes and refuses to let the GP examine her because she thinks he wants to hurt her. Her husband states she was fine until 2 days ago, but now he cannot cope with her. Where should the GP manage this lady with acute onset psychotic symptoms?

A. Her own home
B. Day hospital
C. Emergency respite via social work
D. Acute medical ward
E. Acute psychiatric ward

5. A 78-year-old woman has a recent diagnosis of Alzheimer dementia. She continues to live at home with support workers visiting daily. Her past medical history includes sick sinus syndrome, chronic obstructive pulmonary disease (COPD) and an active peptic ulcer. Which of the following is the most appropriate treatment to try and maintain her current level of cognitive functioning?

A. Donepezil
B. Memantine
C. Fluoxetine
D. Quetiapine
E. Rivastigmine

6. A 67-year-old man presents with a change in his personality, trouble communicating and his wife has concerns that he has been making sexually inappropriate comments to their cleaner. He is diagnosed with frontotemporal dementia. Which of the following options would be the most appropriate treatment to try and maintain his current level of cognition?
   A. No medication recommended by current guidelines
   B. Memantine
   C. Donepezil
   D. Trazodone
   E. Olanzapine

Chapter 21 Older adult psychiatry

1. A 74-year-old woman gives a 6-month history of low mood, anhedonia and fatigue associated with difficulty concentrating and remembering. Neighbours have noticed she is forgetting to put her bins out and no longer cooks meals for herself. Her score on the Addenbrooke's Cognitive Examination (ACE-III) is 72/100. What is the best management option?
   A. Antidepressant
   B. Cholinesterase inhibitor
   C. Memantine
   D. Refer for cognitive reminiscence therapy and occupational therapy
   E. Refer for counselling

2. A 72-year-old widow has presented to her general practitioner 20 times in the last month with minor physical concerns. Previously she attended infrequently. During consultations she is restless, wrings her hands and seems to struggle to remember advice given to her. Her friends are struggling to cope as she telephones them throughout the night to check they are alright. Her score on the Montreal Cognitive Assessment (MoCA) is 29/30. What is the most likely diagnosis?
   A. Mild neurocognitive impairment
   B. Generalised anxiety disorder
   C. Single episode depressive disorder
   D. Late-onset schizophrenia
   E. Hypochondriasis

3. A 71-year-old widower has a 3-month history of low mood, fatigue and anhedonia associated with anorexia. He was transferred from a general hospital to a psychiatric hospital 4 weeks ago after an episode of acute kidney injury precipitated by poor oral intake. He has been commenced on an antidepressant but is poorly concordant and his presentation has changed little. His kidney function has not returned to baseline as he continues to drink little fluid. What is the best management option?
   A. Electroconvulsive therapy (ECT)
   B. Continue current oral antidepressant
   C. Commence depot medication with antidepressant properties
   D. Change to an alternative oral antidepressant
   E. Change to lithium

4. An out-of-hours general practitioner calls for advice about a patient who has been 'behaving oddly'. The computer system is down, so their past psychiatric history is unknown. Which of the patients below is most likely to have late-onset schizophrenia?
   A. A diabetic man who reports that the police are stealing his thoughts. He cannot say what day it is or where he is
   B. A deaf woman who lives alone and reports that the police are trying to rob her
   C. A woman who lives alone and is seeing 'shadow figures'
   D. A blind woman who lives alone and reports seeing policemen in her living room every night
   E. A man with ischaemic heart disease who feels like he is going to die

5. A 76-year-old woman who started mirtazapine for a depressive episode 4 weeks ago attends her general practitioner. Her son also has depression and noticed improvement after 2 weeks of an antidepressant. She has not noticed any benefit or side effects from mirtazapine and is wondering if she should change treatment. What would be the best management option?
   A. Change to the antidepressant that worked for her son
   B. Augment mirtazapine with the antidepressant that worked for her son
   C. Change to a tricyclic antidepressant
   D. Continue mirtazapine for at least 8 weeks
   E. Discontinue mirtazapine and observe without antidepressant

6. A 77-year-old lady with a history of bipolar affective disorder no longer requiring medication is brought to the accident and emergency department by her family. In the past 24 hours she has started behaving very oddly – getting dressed in the middle of the night, dropping to the ground and shaking her leg about and shouting irritably at

people when she is asked questions about her orientation. Her Abbreviated Mental Test score is 2/10. What is the most likely diagnosis?

A. Lithium toxicity
B. Manic episode
C. Hypomanic episode
D. Bodily distress disorder
E. Delirium

7. A general practitioner (GP) pays a home visit to a 74-year-old man with a long history of schizophrenia. The man mentions that he is more bothered by auditory hallucinations than normal. The GP notices little piles of olanzapine tablets on saucers in the kitchen and living room. The man admits that he is struggling to keep track of whether he has taken his medication or not. What would be the best way to improve concordance?

A. Start a depot antipsychotic
B. Dispense medication weekly in a labelled compliance aid
C. Refer for a support worker to prompt medication
D. Arrange daily dispensing at the local pharmacy
E. Change the time of olanzapine so he can take it in the morning with his other medication

8. An 82-year-old widow with no past psychiatric history presents to her general practitioner (GP) requesting a repeat prescription of trazodone. Her supply should not have run out yet, and she admits she took six extra tablets last night in the hope of 'going to sleep and not waking up'. In the event she just overslept, and no harm was done. She feels foolish now and would just like to go home and stop wasting the GP's time. What is the best management option?

A. Ask her to attend accident and emergency (A&E)
B. Review by GP in a week
C. Refer to the local lunch club
D. Refer to psychiatric outpatients
E. Refer for urgent, same day, psychiatric review

Chapter 22 Alcohol and substance-related disorders

1. A 29-year-old man with alcohol dependence syndrome tells you that he wants to give up drinking, but he is worried that he will lose all his friends from the pub. At which stage of the Prochaska and DiClemente

Transtheoretical Model of Change would you consider him to be?

A. Precontemplation of change
B. Contemplation of change
C. Preparation for change
D. Action for change
E. Maintenance of change

2. A 21-year-old homeless woman tells you that she uses £20 of heroin per day via intravenous injection. She is keen to be prescribed methadone. Which of the following measures would be essential prior to starting methadone?

A. History from a friend to corroborate her usage
B. Viral serology for HIV and hepatitis B and C
C. Thorough physical examination with focus on injection sites
D. Admission to psychiatric hospital
E. Urine drug test to confirm presence of opioids

3. A 45-year-old man is being treated by the alcohol problems team. He has successfully been 'detoxified' using chlordiazepoxide. Which of the following is true regarding his future pharmacological treatment?

A. Trazodone can be prescribed to treat his alcohol dependence
B. Long-term, low-dose chlordiazepoxide is the treatment of choice
C. Naltrexone can be helpful even if he relapses to drinking
D. Acamprosate causes an unpleasant reaction when taken with alcohol
E. Disulfiram should control his cravings for alcohol

4 A 26-year-old woman asks you for help with her heroin dependence. She does not want to receive methadone, as she feels this is more addictive than heroin. Which of the following drugs might she prefer to try as substitution therapy?

A. Lofexidine
B. Diazepam
C. Buprenorphine
D. Clonidine
E. Naltrexone

5. A 21-year-old former gymnast presents to addiction services for support with her excessive use of dihydrocodeine. She was prescribed this following an injury three years ago, and her use has escalated to the

degree she is buying dihydrocodeine from street dealers. She has tried to stop 'cold turkey' but experienced significant withdrawal symptoms. She is willing to attend the chemist regularly if required. What would be the first-line treatment?

A. Methadone prescription
B. Ongoing dihydrocodeine prescription
C. Disulfiram
D. Naltrexone
E. Subcutaneous buprenorphine (Buvidal)

Chapter 23 The psychotic disorders

1. A pregnant woman with schizophrenia asks how likely her child is to develop schizophrenia. Her partner does not have a mental illness.

A. 1%
B. 12.5%
C. 2.5%
D. 37.5%
E. 50%

2. A pregnant woman with schizophrenia asks how likely her child is to develop schizophrenia. Her partner also has schizophrenia.

A. 1%
B. 12.5%
C. 25%
D. 37.5%
E. 50%

3. A 22-year-old man was started on olanzapine 4 months ago for a first episode of schizophrenia. He is now symptom free, but troubled by weight gain. He asks how long in total he needs to stay on an antipsychotic.

A. 6 months
B. 9 months
C. 1–2 years
D. 3–5 years
E. Lifelong

4. A 27-year-old woman has developed schizophrenia. She is interested in talking therapies. What type of psychological therapy does NICE (2014) recommend to her?

A. Psychodynamic psychotherapy
B. Interpersonal therapy
C. Dialectical behaviour therapy
D. Cognitive-behavioural therapy
E. Cognitive analytic therapy

5. A 32-year-old woman with an established diagnosis of schizoaffective disorder is admitted to hospital. She describes grandiose delusional beliefs that she is the wife of a prominent religious figure and has healing powers. She has pressured speech and is not sleeping. She is noted to be very irritable in her interactions with staff and fellow patients on the ward. She is not currently prescribed any medication as she has had a long period of stability in the community. What would be the most appropriate first management step?

A. Commence lithium
B. Commence sodium valproate
C. Commence olanzapine
D. Electroconvulsive therapy (ECT)
E. Watch and wait approach

6. A 28-year-old model has been admitted to an inpatient ward with a first episode of psychosis. She is very keen to avoid weight gain and states she would not be concordant with any treatment that causes her to gain weight. Which would be the most appropriate antipsychotic to trial first?

A. Olanzapine
B. Risperidone
C. Aripiprazole
D. Quetiapine
E. Zuclopenthixol

7. A 43-year-old woman with a diagnosis of schizophrenia presents to her GP complaining of a new 'rash' on her face, hands and upper chest. She was recently prescribed an 'as required' medication by her psychiatrist to help with periods of agitation in the context of a resolving psychotic episode. On examination she has widespread redness to the skin which is painful to touch. Which of the following medications is the most likely to have been prescribed and has cause of her symptoms?

A. Chlorpromazine
B. Olanzapine
C. Quetiapine
D. Risperidone
E. Diazepam

8. A 26-year-old woman with a diagnosis of schizophrenia remains troubled by distressing psychotic experiences associated with functional impairment. Her pharmacological management so far has included a 3-month trial of olanzapine and a 3-month trial of

risperidone at optimum doses. What would be the most appropriate next management step?

A. Switch to aripiprazole
B. Switch to clozapine
C. Work up for consideration of ECT treatment
D. Argument risperidone with lithium
E. Augment risperidone with amisulpride

Chapter 24 The mood (affective) disorders

1. Which of the following patients with depression would be the highest priority for electroconvulsive therapy (ECT)?
   A. Someone who is not eating or drinking
   B. Someone who believes they are already dead, so there is no point taking medication, but they are drinking fluids
   C. Someone who has experienced no benefit from two antidepressants
   D. Someone who has benefited from ECT in the past
   E. Someone who has experienced no benefit from several antidepressants but does not want ECT

2. A 24-year-old man is brought to accident and emergency by the police. He has a 1-week history of irritable mood, insomnia and grandiose delusions that he has superpowers. The police found him about to jump off some scaffolding to prove he is invincible. He does not believe he is unwell and says there is no way he is coming into hospital. What is the best initial step in management?
   A. Appointment with general practitioner later that day
   B. Informal admission
   C. Admission under mental health legislation
   D. Urgent outpatient psychiatric review
   E. Police custody after arrest for breach of the peace

3. A 45-year-old man is admitted to hospital with a 6-week history of low mood. He plans to kill himself at the first opportunity because he believes the world is going to end soon and wants to die quickly. He is not currently on any medication. What would be the best management option?
   A. Citalopram
   B. Amitriptyline
   C. Quetiapine
   D. Citalopram and quetiapine
   E. Amitriptyline and quetiapine

4. A 29-year-old postgraduate student with a diagnosis of bipolar affective disorder is admitted with a manic episode after stopping medication. She is very agitated on the ward, pacing, being verbally aggressive to staff and fellow patients, and punching her wardrobe. What is the best medication to commence?
   A. Lithium
   B. Olanzapine
   C. Citalopram
   D. Sodium valproate
   E. Lamotrigine

5. A 36-year-old lecturer with moderate to severe depression wants to try a psychological therapy for depression. Which of the following should be offered?
   A. Self-help cognitive-behavioural therapy (CBT)
   B. Structured group physical activity
   C. Individual CBT
   D. Dialectical behaviour therapy
   E. Graded exposure therapy

6. A 55-year-old man with a mild depressive episode has not benefited from self-help CBT. He is not keen to try further psychological therapies. What would be the next most appropriate management step?
   A. Refer to secondary care mental health services
   B. Commence venlafaxine
   C. Refer for psychodynamic psychotherapy
   D. Commence clomipramine
   E. Commence fluoxetine

Chapter 25 The anxiety, stress related, OCD related and bodily distress disorders

1. A 35-year-old woman has been recently diagnosed with bodily distress disorder. How should this diagnosis change her management by her general practitioner?
   A. She should not be allowed access to urgent appointment slots
   B. She should be seen on a planned, regular schedule
   C. She should not be investigated for physical complaints
   D. She should never be prescribed benzodiazepines
   E. She should be reassured that her symptoms do not really exist

2. A 17-year-old school pupil has a phobia of bodily fluids but aspires to be a nurse. What treatment can she be offered?
   A. None – she should change her career plans
   B. Cognitive-behavioural therapy (CBT) with desensitization
   C. CBT focused on trauma
   D. Diazepam when necessary (PRN) – to be taken before any possible contact with bodily fluids
   E. Selective serotonin reuptake inhibitor (SSRI)

3. A 29-year-old chemist has obsessive-compulsive disorder (OCD) regarding orderliness. She has been tidying up her colleagues' laboratory benches and spoilt some experiments. She has been threatened with dismissal. She does not want to try any talking therapies. What treatment can she be offered?
   A. Clomipramine
   B. Mirtazapine
   C. Selective serotonin reuptake inhibitor (SSRI)
   D. Pregabalin
   E. Self-help

4. A 35-year-old former soldier has been diagnosed with post traumatic stress disorder. He does not have a preference for either pharmacological or psychological therapy. What would be the most appropriate first step in his management?
   A. Inpatient admission
   B. Selective serotonin reuptake inhibitor (SSRI)
   C. CBT with a trauma focus
   D. Quetiapine
   E. Diazepam

5. A 44-year-old zookeeper has generalised anxiety disorder and is unable to work. He has tried CBT in the past and would now like to try a different talking therapy. Which would be the next most appropriate management option?
   A. Interpersonal therapy (IPT)
   B. Dialectical behavioural therapy (DBT)
   C. Mindfulness-based cognitive therapy (MBT)
   D. Psychodynamic psychotherapy
   E. Applied Relaxation

Chapter 26 Feeding and eating disorders

1. A 17-year-old boy has a median percentage body mass index (m% BMI) of 80%, wears baggy clothes, and states that he is worried about being overweight. He is diagnosed with anorexia nervosa, although he does not feel that he has a problem. However, he is agreeable to meeting a therapist, mainly to please his mother. Which of the following modalities of psychotherapy would be recommended in the first instance?
   A. Maudsley model of anorexia treatment for adults
   B. Family therapy
   C. Focal psychodynamic psychotherapy
   D. Cognitive-behavioural therapy
   E. Specialist supportive clinical management

2. A 20-year-old man has a body mass index of 16 kg/m^2, wears baggy clothes, and states that he is worried about

being overweight. He was diagnosed with anorexia nervosa as a 17-year-old. After a period of treatment and remission his symptoms have returned. Which of the following modalities of psychotherapy would be recommended in the first instance?
   A. Exposure-response prevention therapy
   B. Family therapy
   C. Focal psychodynamic psychotherapy
   D. Interpersonal therapy
   E. Individual eating-disorder-focused cognitive behavioural therapy (CBT-ED)

3. A 29-year-old female actuary is diagnosed with anorexia nervosa. Which of the following factors is associated with a poor prognosis?
   A. Early age of onset
   B. Rapid weight loss
   C. Binge–purge symptoms
   D. Family history of anorexia
   E. Slow to engage with psychotherapy

4. A 17-year-old woman has been diagnosed with anorexia nervosa. Which medication should she be advised to take until she regains a healthy nutritional intake?
   A. Citalopram
   B. Fluoxetine
   C. Multivitamin
   D. Paroxetine
   E. Sertraline

5. A 21-year-old woman with severe anorexia nervosa was found collapsed in the street secondary to heart failure due to malnutrition. She has subsequently been admitted to a specialist eating disorder unit to receive nasogastric feeding under mental health legislation. Which of the following blood test results raises concern that she is experiencing refeeding syndrome?
   A. Calcium 2.4 mmol/L
   B. Magnesium 1.7 mEq/L
   C. Phosphate 0.3 mmol/L
   D. Potassium 3.7 mmol/L
   E. Sodium 141 mmol/L

Chapter 27 The sleep–wake disorders

1. A 33-year-old woman describes creeping, burning sensations in her legs which keep her awake at night. She finds getting up and walking around eases them. Her mother had the same problem. She has tried nonpharmacological management and would like to try

medication. Which medication is recommended first line?

A. Fluoxetine
B. Haloperidol
C. Lithium
D. Metoclopramide
E. Pramipexole

2. A 33-year-old woman describes creeping, burning sensations in her legs which keep her awake at night. The pain also affects her throughout the day. She finds getting up and walking around makes little difference. She has poorly controlled type one diabetes. What is the most likely diagnosis?

A. Akathisia
B. Intermittent claudication
C. Iron deficiency
D. Neuropathy
E. Restless legs syndrome

3. A 33-year-old woman describes trouble sleeping at night, with early morning wakening. She has recently been diagnosed with depression and started on fluoxetine (20 mg) 2 weeks ago. Her mood is slightly better, but she is worried that her sleep is not. What is the next best management step?

A. Increase fluoxetine dose
B. Keep a sleep diary
C. Refer for polysomnography
D. Sleep hygiene advice
E. Short course of temazepam

Chapter 26 Sexual problems and disorders

1. A 24-year-old woman presents to her general practitioner concerned that she achieves orgasm infrequently during penetrative sex with her partner. What should she be advised?

A. Caressing without genital contact can improve sex
B. Sexual dysfunction is rare in young people
C. She is likely to have a physical problem preventing orgasm
D. She should stop any medication which could be contributing
E. Talking about sexual problems with her partner is likely to increase anxiety in the bedroom

2. A 57-year-old man tells his general practitioner he is unable to have an erection, even when masturbating. He occasionally found it hard to achieve an erection as a younger man but it has got much worse recently. He was

previously obese but has lost weight recently. What is the most important next management step?

A. Advise to lose more weight and return if problem persists
B. Check blood glucose
C. Direct to self-help resources regarding sexual dysfunction
D. Prescribe sildenafil
E. Refer to urology

3. A 63-year-old man with Parkinson disease has recently started making obscene phone calls. He becomes sexually aroused during this. He has been working his way through his wife's address book and several of her friends have been very distressed. Which of the medications below is least likely to have caused this behaviour?

A. Levodopa
B. Olanzapine
C. Pergolide
D. Pramipexole
E. Selegiline

4. A 23-year-old woman with obsessive-compulsive disorder attends her GP reporting that she is having difficulty achieving orgasm during sex with her long-term partner. Which of the following medications is the most likely to have contributed to this problem?

A. Mirtazapine
B. Pregabalin
C. Propranolol
D. Sertraline
E. Bupropion

Chapter 29 Disorders relating to the menstrual cycle, pregnancy and the puerperium

1. A 27-year-old schoolteacher reports increased irritability in the week prior to menstruation. This quickly resolves within a day of starting her period. Most of the time the irritability does not cause her any problems apart from when she recently had an argument with her boyfriend. What is the best management option?

A. Encourage exercise
B. Prescribe combined oral contraceptive pill
C. Prescribe ibuprofen
D. Prescribe selective serotonin reuptake inhibitor (SSRI)
E. Refer for cognitive-behavioural therapy (CBT)

2. A 53-year-old company director reports low mood, increased fatigability and early morning wakening for the past 2 months, accompanied by increased suicidal thoughts. She has had to take some time off work. She

attributes her symptoms to her menopause. What is the best management option?

A. Hormone replacement therapy
B. Dietary and lifestyle advice
C. Omega-3 fish oils
D. Counselling
E. Psychological therapy

3. A 25-year-old artist has a history of bipolar disorder. She has been taking lithium and has been well for the past 3 years. She presents to her GP and explains that she wants to start a family with her partner and has heard that lithium can cause problems with foetal malformations. What is the most appropriate management?

A. Switch to semisodium valproate
B. Switch to carbamazepine
C. Discontinue lithium and continue without treatment
D. Switch to olanzapine
E. Refer to perinatal mental health team

A. A 33-year-old woman previously experienced a protracted episode of postnatal depression following the birth of her first child, which necessitated admission to a mother-and-baby unit. The episode responded well to antidepressant medication. She has recently become pregnant and is incredibly anxious that she will become unwell again postnatally. What is the most appropriate management?

A. Reassure that becoming unwell again would be unlikely
B. Restart antidepressant treatment immediately
C. Referral to psychologist to identify relapse signature
D. Watchful waiting
E. Referral to perinatal mental health team

5. A 22-year-old lady is found by the police. She was found walking near a river with her 2-week-old baby boy. She reported that the infant was possessed by the devil, and that she had thoughts that she needed to drown him to save humanity. At interview, she appears perplexed and is openly responding to auditory hallucinations. She does not want to be admitted to hospital as she does not think she is unwell. She has a very supportive family who are keen to look after her at home. What is the most appropriate initial management option?

A. Detention in hospital under mental health act
B. Treatment at home under care of crisis team
C. Transfer to police cells
D. Urgent referral for outpatient follow-up by perinatal mental health team
E. Urgent referral to social work

Chapter 30 The personality disorders

1. A 19-year-old hairdresser has a diagnosis of a moderate personality disorder with prominent features of negative affectivity and disinhibition and a borderline pattern. She requests information on drug treatment that may be beneficial. What should she be advised?

A. Sodium valproate is effective for reducing interpersonal problems
B. Omega-3 fatty acids are effective in reducing impulsivity
C. Risperidone is effective for reducing anger
D. Amitriptyline reduces chronic feelings of emptiness
E. Drug treatment is not the main intervention

2. A 34-year-old man has a diagnosis of a personality disorder with prominent features of disinhibition and dissociality, and requests information on different types of psychotherapy that may be beneficial. Which of the following psychological treatments does NICE (2009) recommend?

A. Dialectical behaviour therapy
B. Mentalization-based therapy
C. Psychodynamic
D. Cognitive-analytical therapy
E. Therapeutic communities

3. A 27-year-old female postgraduate student has a diagnosis of a personality disorder with prominent features of negative affectivity and a borderline pattern. She reported low mood and insomnia for the past month and has subsequently been absent from university (which is unusual for her). Normally, she is easily angered, but relatively cheerful. At assessment she reports increased thoughts of suicide, but no immediate plans. What is the most appropriate next step in management?

A. Refer for dialectical behaviour therapy
B. Request a urine drug screen
C. Prescribe diazepam
D. Admit to an acute psychiatric ward
E. Suggest 'weekly dispensing' of medication

4. A 29-year-old man has a diagnosis of a severe personality disorder with prominent features of dissociality. He coldly tells his psychiatrist of his intention to kill his landlord following an argument about rent arrears, before describing a detailed plan on how he would stab him in the throat. What is the most appropriate next management step?

A. Ask him to return for review in 1 week
B. Prescribe diazepam
C. Alert the police and the intended victim
D. Admit to psychiatric hospital under detention
E. Refer for anger management

Chapter 31 The neurodevelopmental disorders

1. A 23-year-old man is diagnosed with an autism spectrum disorder. Which medication can be prescribed to reduce the core symptoms of his disorder?
   A. Fluoxetine
   B. Methylphenidate
   C. None
   D. Risperidone
   E. Sodium valproate

2. A 7-year-old boy has recently been diagnosed with attention deficit hyperactivity disorder (ADHD). It is having a substantial impact on his behaviour at school, and he is at risk of expulsion. His parents have already attended a parent-training programme. What should be the next management option trialled?
   A. Atomoxetine
   B. Cognitive-behavioural therapy
   C. Dexamphetamine
   D. Methylphenidate
   E. Referral to social work for consideration of a place at a special educational needs school

3. A 12-year-old boy has multiple motor tics and repeatedly shouts 'Batman!' when he is stressed or excited. He had to leave the cinema once because of this but is otherwise not troubled by his symptoms. What is the first-line treatment for this disorder?
   A. Clonidine
   B. No treatment
   C. Pimozide
   D. Psychoeducation
   E. Risperidone

Chapter 32 Intellectual Disability

1. A 24-year-old man with a moderate intellectual disability is referred to his local Community Learning Disability team by the manager of his care home. He has become increasingly distressed at mealtimes, and is at times hitting out at staff. What would be the appropriate first step in management?
   A. Commence risperidone 0.5 mg twice daily
   B. A physical examination
   C. Arrange care in a secure facility
   D. Suggest he is placed under 1:1 supervision
   E. Contact the police to report the assaults on staff

2. A 32-year-old woman with a mild learning disability who lives in supported accommodation is admitted to hospital following an overdose of paracetamol. She is reviewed with her support worker, and presents as very withdrawn and appears to startle easily when her support worker moves closer to her. The support worker has requested that they are present to 'help with communication'. You notice some unusual bruising on her arms. What would be the most appropriate first step?
   A. Discharge her home
   B. Refer to the community learning disability team
   C. Continue trying to assess her with her support worker present
   D. Ask the support worker to leave the room so you can speak to the patient alone
   E. Admit to an inpatient psychiatric ward for further assessment

Chapter 33 Child and adolescent psychiatry

1. For the past 6 months, a 12-year-old boy has repeatedly been in trouble with the police. Recently, he has been violent towards his sister and has killed her pet hamster. His mother sought help after he deliberately set the garden shed on fire. What is the most likely diagnosis?
   A. Personality disorder with prominent traits of dissociality
   B. Conduct-dissocial disorder
   C. Oppositional defiant disorder
   D. Reactive attachment disorder
   E. Substance misuse

2. An 8-year-old girl presents with encopresis. During examination by the junior doctor, genital warts and vaginal trauma are noted. What is the next most appropriate step in management?
   A. The child should be sent home and seen in outpatients
   B. The parents should be confronted by the nurses
   C. The child should be directly asked what happened
   D. Police should be contacted to question the girl
   E. The duty social worker and on-call paediatrician should be alerted

3. A 16-year-old girl presents with a 2-month history of low mood and fatigue. She no longer enjoys playing netball and feels her friends do not like her anymore. She is still attending school but is no longer doing well academically. What treatment should she be offered first line?
   A. Citalopram
   B. Cognitive-behavioural therapy
   C. Fluoxetine
   D. Sertraline
   E. Watchful waiting

4. A 16-year-old girl presents with low mood. She has had episodes of low mood for most of her life, often varying from good to bad and back again within a day. She has never had any close friends because she feels her peers have always rejected her. She has self-harmed by cutting since the age of 13 years, and often makes herself sick after meals. She says she feels angry and empty at the same time. After her father took an overdose she started hearing his voice inside her head telling her to do it too. Her body mass index is 22 kg/m². What is the most likely diagnosis?

   A. Bipolar disorder
   B. Bulimia nervosa
   C. Depressive episode
   D. Personality disorder prominent features of negative affectivity and a borderline pattern
   E. Schizophrenia

5. A 4-year-old boy has recently been adopted by his aunt and uncle after his parents died in a road traffic accident. He had normal language development and initially he seemed to settle in well to his new home. However, he gradually stopped speaking at home. Nursery staff report he speaks normally there. During the consultation he initially does not speak but does so when his adoptive parents leave the room. His adoptive parents appear caring but anxious and unsure what to do. They have been arguing recently. What is the most likely diagnosis?

   A. Selective mutism
   B. Posttraumatic stress disorder
   C. Social anxiety disorder
   D. Autism spectrum disorder
   E. Reactive attachment disorder

6. A 4-year-old girl watches other children playing at nursery but does not attempt to join in. When she falls over in the playground she cowers away when an adult offers first-aid. She has a sad demeanour but otherwise shows little emotion. She has been taken into care after experiencing physical abuse from both parents. What is the most likely diagnosis?

   A. Selective mutism
   B. Posttraumatic stress disorder
   C. Social anxiety disorder
   D. Autism spectrum disorder
   E. Reactive attachment disorder

Chapter 34 Forensic psychiatry

1. A 32-year-old man with substance misuse problems reports he is thinking of taking up mugging to fund his habit. Which of the following factors in his history places him at highest risk of future violence?

   A. Having a mental disorder
   B. Using substances
   C. Previous violence
   D. Experiencing command hallucinations
   E. Childhood abuse

2. A 19-year-old gentleman has been charged with a serious assault. He appears incredibly distracted and distressed and is openly responding to auditory hallucinations. The forensic psychiatrist has been asked to assess his fitness to plead. What finding on mental state exam would suggest he was fit to plead?

   A. He is unable to say why he is in custody
   B. He asks for most questions to be repeated as he is distracted by hallucinations
   C. He is thought disordered, with loosening of associations such that his answers are very hard to follow
   D. He believes he has been abducted by aliens and his answers will determine the fate of the universe
   E. He is able to give a coherent account of events leading up to the offence but denies memory of the offence itself

3. A 36-year-old man with schizophrenia has committed a crime. He asks his lawyer if he can be considered to have had diminished responsibility. What is the only charge diminished responsibility applies to?

   A. Arson
   B. Rape
   C. Theft
   D. Grievous bodily harm
   E. Murder

4. A 21-year-old man has been charged with assaulting a police officer. He has a lengthy history of police contacts from adolescence onwards, mainly for impulsive acts of aggression. He dropped out of school at 14 years of age because he struggled to concentrate. He is angry with himself for getting into trouble with the police again and is

asking for help in controlling his bursts of anger. What diagnosis should he be further assessed for?

A. Personality disorder with prominent features of dissociality

B. Attention deficit hyperactivity disorder (ADHD)

C. Autism spectrum disorder

D. Bipolar disorder

E. Personality disorder prominent features of disinhibition and a borderline pattern

5. A 35-year-old man was arrested after he assaulted a bus driver. He believed that the driver was trying to procure the services of his wife, who he is convinced is working as a prostitute. He has dismissed extensive reassurances from his wife and his own siblings. He reports that he has a sword in the back of his car and intended to 'get the truth out of her'. He has a history of alcohol abuse. What is the most likely diagnosis?

A. Delusional disorder (delusional jealousy)

B. Schizophrenia

C. Schizoaffective disorder

D. Personality disorder with a borderline pattern and prominent traits of dissociality

E. Single episode depressive disorder

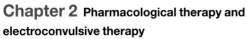

Chapter 2 Pharmacological therapy and electroconvulsive therapy

1. C. Weekly full blood counts (FBCs). Without monitoring, just under 3% of patients treated with clozapine develop neutropenia (low neutrophil count), and just under 1% develop agranulocytosis (negligible neutrophil count). This is most likely to occur early in treatment. Therefore, weekly FBCs are advised initially. As for all antipsychotics, she will also require regular checks of blood pressure, liver function, lipid profile and glucose. These parameters should be checked every 1 to 3 months initially, then annually.

2. E. Egg mayonnaise toastie is the only safe option, given the dietary restrictions required for irreversible monoamine oxidase inhibitors such as phenelzine. See Box 2.2. She should also avoid drinking Chianti wine with lunch.

3. C. This patient is at significant risk of harm related to their severe depression due to their lack of oral intake. Due to the life-threatening nature of this presentation ECT would be indicated.

4. D. Sodium valproate must not be used in women or men of childbearing potential due to the risks of congenital abnormalities in an unborn foetus (neurodevelopmental disorders including malformation of the spinal cord) and risks of infertility in men.

5. C. Propranolol. This woman is probably experiencing akathisia. This is hard to treat, but propranolol or benzodiazepines can help. Procyclidine does not help akathisia and may make it worse as it is an alerting medication. Ideally, the dose of antipsychotic is reduced. Quinine can be used for restless leg syndrome when in bed. The differential includes agitation secondary to psychosis.

6. B. Oral procyclidine. This man has drug-induced parkinsonism. In the early stages, the features are different to idiopathic parkinsonism. Anticholinergics such as procyclidine can help, but ideally the dose of antipsychotic would be reduced or an alternative antipsychotic trialled.

7. C. Stop anticholinergics, such as procyclidine. This man has tardive dyskinesia. This is hard to treat but stopping anticholinergics and reducing or withdrawing antipsychotics, if possible, can help.

8. B. Venlafaxine is an SNRI. SNRIs work by inhibiting reuptake of serotonin and noradrenaline back into cells and do not affect acetylcholine. Duloxetine is another of the SNRIs.

Chapter 3 Psychological therapy

1. C. This man is likely suffering from prolonged grief disorder. In the first instance, it would be helpful to direct him to bereavement counselling, which most commonly takes the form of person-centred counselling. In the United Kingdom, Cruse is a large voluntary sector service offering bereavement counselling. Psychodynamic therapy, cognitive-behavioural therapy and mindfulness-based cognitive therapy have little evidence to support their use in this instance. Exposure and response prevention is a behavioural therapy used in the treatment of obsessive-compulsive disorder.

2. C. Transference is the theoretical process by which the patient transfers feelings or attitudes experienced in an earlier significant relationship onto the therapist. Counter-transference refers to the feelings that are evoked in the therapist during the course of therapy. The therapist pays attention to these feelings, as they may be representative of what the patient is feeling, and so helps the therapist to empathize with the patient. Often, the therapist has undergone therapy themselves as part of their training; this helps the therapist to separate out what feelings belong to them, and what feelings belong to the patient.

3. E. This cognitive distortion is an example of magnification (also known as 'catastrophization or catastrophizing'), where things get 'blown out of proportion.' An example of emotional reasoning in this context would be 'I feel so miserable, so I must have failed my exam.' An example of fortune telling would be 'I failed my exam, so in the future no one will employ me.' An example of personalization would be 'It is all my fault: I failed my exams.' An example of labelling would be 'I am stupid.' Note that more than one type of cognitive distortion can exist in the same patient in the same circumstances. See Table 3.3.

4. B. There is a strong evidence base to support the use of interpersonal therapy in the treatment of mild to

moderate depression. See Table 3.5 for modalities of benefit in the other conditions listed.

5. D. Interpersonal therapy is based on the assumptions that problems with interpersonal relationships and social functioning contribute significantly to mental illness. Main areas of focus include role disputes, role transitions, interpersonal deficits and grief. She may also find cognitive-behavioural therapy of benefit, for example, if interpersonal therapy is not available.

6. A. Exposure and response prevention is a type of cognitive-behavioural therapy in which the patient is encouraged not to respond to the obsessional thought with a compulsive act. Relaxation techniques are used instead to overcome the anxiety associated with not carrying out the compulsion.

Chapter 4 Mental health and the law

1. D. She needs to notify the DVLA of her diagnosis. They will then ask for a doctor's report and potentially a driving assessment and are likely to arrange more frequent reviews of the licence than otherwise (e.g., annually). It is the DVLA's decision as to whether she is fit to drive or not. Many patients with mild dementia are found fit to continue to drive. Patient and partner reports of driving can be unreliable as patients can have poor insight and partners may not want to act in a way they perceive as harming the patient, or themselves. It is the patient's responsibility to notify the DVLA although doctors may need to do so if patients ignore this advice and present a significant risk to others through driving.

2. B. The patient lacks capacity as his low GCS means he will not be able to communicate his decision. He is also unlikely to be able to understand, to retain and to weigh up information, but this cannot be assessed in the absence of communication.

3. D. He is likely to lack capacity for any decisions requiring more consideration than is available in working memory as he will not be able to retain information for long enough to weigh it up. As a guide, someone should be able to retain information for as long as necessary to make a decision. A quick decision, e.g., meal choice, does not require a long time to make. A big decision, e.g., where to live, would normally be something that a person would consider and mull over for a few days at least.

4. C. She lacks capacity for the decision about surgery, as she does not believe the information because of a delusion. However, she is likely to have the capacity to make decisions about which she does not have delusions.

5. A. He should be assumed to have the capacity to make a decision about a statin, unless his psychotic symptoms relate to cholesterol (which is unusual) or he is very thought disordered.

Chapter 5 Mental health service provision

1. B. Patient B has evidence of treatment resistance, and would be most appropriate for CMHT input.

2. B. Early intervention in psychosis team. This man may be experiencing prodromal psychosis. He does not currently appear to be at high enough risk to require home treatment or admission. As he does not have an established diagnosis of mental illness, an assertive outreach team is not appropriate. A community mental health team could manage him, but early intervention teams are expert at identifying early psychosis and are therefore best placed to monitor him.

Chapter 6 The patient with thoughts of suicide or self-harm

1. D. While researching methods is also worrying, acts of closure (such as making a will, organizing finances, writing suicide notes) are the most worrying signs and suggest strong suicidal intent. Contacting voluntary support agencies (such as the Samaritans) suggests emotional distress but also a degree of ambivalence. Telling his wife of his plans may be a way of communicating his feelings to her but is not necessarily a final act. Disclosing plans to a healthcare professional does not reduce his risk.

2. C. Suspension hanging is the most common method of completed suicide in England, Wales and many other countries. Means are widely available and lethality is high. Paracetamol is the most common drug of overdose in the UK; however, advances in medical treatment and public health measures have reduced mortality associated with this. Jumping from height is a fairly 'public' method of suicide and thus is often reported in the news (although media coverage of all suicides has reduced in recent years due to campaigns to reduce 'advertising' of suitable locations). Carbon monoxide poisoning used to be fairly common; however, catalytic converters on modern motor vehicles has reduced fatality of this method.

3. A. Personality disorders with a borderline pattern carries a 45-fold risk of completed suicide compared to the general population. Personality disorders without a borderline pattern are also associated with elevated, but lower, risk. Anxiety disorders carry a 3-fold risk, anorexia

carries an 8-fold risk, schizophrenia has a 13-fold risk and OCD is not associated with increased risk of completed suicide. There is some variation in these figures depending on the source.

4. B. Personality disorder with a borderline pattern and prominent traits of disinhibition. She is a young woman with a long history of self-harm, difficulties with interpersonal relationships and auditory pseudohallucinations at times of stress. She has no symptoms suggestive of a depressive illness.

5. C. This woman has made a serious suicide attempt. Note that she went to some effort to prevent discovery (remote location, unsocial hour) and made acts of closure (typed letters imply that some thought had gone into these). She has neurovegetative and psychotic symptoms of depression. She may have intoxicated herself to reduce her inhibitions prior to the act and is not necessarily alcohol dependent.

Chapter 7 Psychiatric emergencies

1. C. Physical health assessment including measurement of serum paracetamol levels (plus INR, liver function, other baseline bloods) to determine the requirement for potentially life-saving treatment is the priority in this case. This can be measured from 4 hours postingestion although levels become harder to interpret after 15 hours. The other options are all important aspects of psychiatric evaluation and risk assessment but are not urgent.

2. B. Looking at his prescription. Although the two syndromes have features in common, they can nearly always be easily distinguished by medication history (see Table 2.8). Clonus is another useful distinguishing factor, as it is present in serotonin syndrome but absent in neuroleptic malignant syndrome (where lead-pipe rigidity is common).

3. E. Assess ABCDE. This man is likely to be experiencing neuroleptic malignant syndrome. After ABCDE has been addressed, all antipsychotics should also be discontinued. The other answers are all possible treatment options, but none are first line. Before they are considered, he needs initial resuscitation, and then is likely to need transfer to a general hospital for investigation and monitoring. See Table 2.8.

4. E. 1.8 mmol/L. Her symptoms are consistent with lithium toxicity in the 1.5–2.0 mmol/L range. However, symptoms of toxicity can manifest at lower levels, particularly in older adults. Toxicity is likely to have been precipitated by the recent course of nonsteroidal antiinflammatory drugs. See Table 2.3.

5. D. If safe to do so verbal de-escalation techniques should always be attempted in the first instance. If these fail more restrictive measures such as oral/IM medication or restraint can be considered. As this patient believes staff are trying to perform experiments on her, touching her against her will (such as during a restraint or IM) may escalate the situation rather than diffuse it.

6. D. Temperature, pulse, blood pressure, respiratory rate, hydration status and consciousness level should be checked every 15 minutes following parenteral administration of rapid tranquillization (until there are no further concerns about the patient's physical health status) where any of the following apply (NICE 2015):

Patient appears to be asleep or sedated

Patient has recently taken recreational drugs or alcohol

BNF maximum doses for medication have been exceeded

Patient has a preexisting physical health problem

Patient experienced any harm as a result of the intervention

If none of the above have occurred, observations should be hourly until the patient is able to walk and interact normally. If the patient refuses or remains too behaviourally disturbed to allow observations, they should be regularly observed for respiratory effort, airway and consciousness level. See Fig. 21.2.

7. C. Transient hyperglycaemia secondary to stress may arise but is unlikely to be clinically important. All the other options are potentially life-threatening: benzodiazepines can cause respiratory depression, oversedation by any means can cause loss of airway, antipsychotics and hyperarousal increase the risk of arrhythmia, and benzodiazepines and antipsychotics can both cause hypotension. Additional life-threatening complications of antipsychotic use include seizures and dystonias. All these complications can occur with oral formulations also, but are more likely when large doses are given via a fast-acting method.

8. A. Intramuscular procyclidine. This woman is experiencing a dystonia with an oculogyric crisis and trismus (sustained contraction of muscles of mastication). Her clenched jaw means administering oral procyclidine is not possible. Baclofen and dantrolene should be used for chronic spasticity.

Chapter 8 Patient with neurodevelopmental differences

1. C. Ensure he has an eye test. This boy may not be able to see the blackboard. Children can be embarrassed to admit this. ADHD and thyroid dysfunction are unlikely given that the symptoms are only present in one setting. Genetic testing is not yet indicated in ADHD and certainly cannot be used to exclude it. A collateral history from the teacher would be helpful if his eye test comes back normal.

2. E. Rett syndrome. The fact that she initially developed normally, then regressed, excludes autism and intellectual disability. Heller syndrome (childhood disintegrative disorder) is possible but unlikely as it is more common in males and usually has onset after the age of 2 years. Muscular dystrophy is also possible, but the child would be more likely to present with generalized muscle weakness, rather than only a reduced use of those muscles important for social interaction. It also mainly affects boys.

3. B. Autism spectrum disorder. This is suggested by his poor understanding of social cues and the hint that he has an unusually intense interest. To make this diagnosis definitive, a much fuller history would be required. Social anxiety is unlikely as the problem is his poor social understanding, not him feeling that others are critical of him. Social anxiety is nonetheless common as a consequence of autism. A personality disorder with prominent traits of anankastia is unlikely as this does not impair the ability to interact socially. A depressive episode might follow his redundancy but it is not the primary problem. Generalized anxiety is unlikely as he has not mentioned worrying about anything except social situations.

4. B. This woman has a mild intellectual disability. It will take her longer to learn tasks than her peers without an intellectual disability, but she is able to work and live independently with appropriate support in place. Individuals in this group represent the majority (85%) of all people with intellectual disabilities.

5. D. This man has a severe intellectual disability. He lives with his family, who are his main carers and is able to perform simple tasks under supervision. His self-care skills are limited, but sometimes he seems able to contribute to these.

6. C. Traumatic brain injury. This would need to be confirmed by checking the details of his injuries in the road traffic accident. ADHD is excluded by the lack of significant difficulties prior to the accident (suggested by his ability to work as an accountant). He may be suffering neuropsychological sequelae post damage to his frontal lobes.

Chapter 9 The patient with psychotic symptoms

1. B. Charles Bonnet syndrome. Based on the information given here, Charles Bonnet syndrome is the most likely diagnosis. However, it is crucial to exclude delirium with a physical examination and cognitive assessment.

2. B. Ischaemic heart disease. This man has risk factors for ischaemic heart disease (age, male, smoker) and gives a description of exercise-induced chest pain with a classic 'weight on chest' description typical of cardiac ischaemia. People with schizophrenia are at increased risk of cardiovascular disease. Although this symptom could also be a tactile hallucination, it is important to exclude a physical origin before making this attribution.

3. A. Delusions of infidelity. This man has developed a delusion that his wife is having an affair based on a seemingly illogical factor (in this case how she is doing her hair), and this is fixed, as shown by his upset when questioned by his GP. The impact of this delusion on this man's life is substantial as he has become preoccupied with it to an unreasonable extent.

4. B. Substance-induced psychotic disorder. Substance intoxication is also a differential, particularly if he has been using the new stimulants every day or nearly every day – more information is needed as to timing and pattern of his substance use. A definite diagnosis of substance-induced psychotic disorder is the most likely diagnosis but requires a longitudinal assessment. The diagnosis would be confirmed if he stops using substances and his symptoms resolve. However, chronic cannabis use is a risk factor for developing schizophrenia and if his symptoms persist despite abstaining from substances this may emerge as the diagnosis. At present he has not had the symptoms long enough to meet criteria for schizophrenia in any case.

5. B. Hypnogogic hallucinations are hallucinations that occur as a person is falling asleep. A hypnopompic hallucination occurs as a person is waking up. These hallucinations do not occur at any times other than when she is falling asleep, so schizophrenia or a severe depression with psychotic symptoms are unlikely. A pseudohallucination is an abnormal perception that the patient is able to recognize as being from their own mind.

6. D. Schizoaffective disorder is the most likely diagnosis. This man has concurrent mood symptoms and first-rank symptoms of schizophrenia. His mood and psychotic symptoms are equally prominent, making a recurrent psychotic depression unlikely.

7. E. Delusional disorder is the most likely diagnosis. This man has a longstanding unshakeable belief arrived at through faulty reasoning: a delusion. He has insight into this. Schizophrenia is unlikely because the delusion is nonbizarre and functioning is intact. In hypochondriasis patients normally are able to briefly accept an alternative explanation and reassurance. However, at the most extreme end in hypochondriasis with poor to absent insight they cannot accept an alternative explanation for their experience and this would also be a reasonable diagnosis to make given the information available. Delusional disorder is made the most likely diagnosis by the delusional perception (smelling dog faeces) which triggered the belief.

8. A. Personality disorder. This man is not delusional as his belief is not fixed. He is suspicious and litigious. The history from the police of multiple previous calls suggests his difficulties are longstanding. This would be consistent with a paranoid personality disorder. However, a fuller background history would be required to make a definite diagnosis.

9. E. Neurosyphilis. This is now a rare diagnosis in the UK but should always be considered in those with work or travel histories that may have placed them at risk of contracting syphilis. Neurosyphilis is a type of tertiary syphilis that emerges several years after initial infection. Clinical features are diverse but can include personality change, grandiose behaviour and dementia, along with upper motor neuron abnormalities such as brisk reflexes and extensor plantars.

Chapter 10 The patient with elated or irritable mood

1. A. Manic episode, with accelerated speech, probable thought disorder, and likely hallucinations. Hypomania and cyclothymia are excluded by the significant functional impairment his symptoms have caused him. An agitated depression could be associated with an increased rate of speech, but the content should be understandable. Schizophrenia can be associated with thought disorder, but very rarely with accelerated rate of speech.

2. B. Bipolar affective disorder. An episode of depression is not necessary to meet criteria for bipolar affective disorder. Recurrent mania and hypomania are not diagnoses. No first-rank symptoms are mentioned, making schizoaffective disorder unlikely. Cyclothymia is excluded by the presence of psychotic symptoms.

3. D. Urine drug screen. This will demonstrate recent use of common recreational drugs (although it will not screen for novel psychoactive substances). The main differentials in a healthy young man are a manic episode or intoxication or mania secondary to psychoactive substance use. Full blood count should be performed to check for evidence of infection, but is likely to be normal. Thyroid function test should be checked to exclude hyperthyroidism but is also likely to be normal. EEG and CT head should only be requested if there are neurological abnormalities.

4. D. Personality disorder. This woman describes a persistent pattern of maladaptive behaviour present since childhood associated with social and occupational dysfunction. This is most likely to be a personality disorder, with prominent impulsivity. It would be important to get a collateral history before making a definite diagnosis. The mood swings are faster than would occur within bipolar affective disorder or cyclothymia and she has never had a period of euthymia, required for a diagnosis of a mood disorder. Dysthymia is prolonged low mood, not mood swings. Although substance use can cause and worsen emotional lability it should not have onset in childhood.

5. C. Hypomanic episode. This man describes elated mood with a decreased need for sleep, poor concentration, increased energy, increased recent expenditure and increased libido. It is interfering with his social and occupational functioning, but these activities are not completely disrupted. We are not given information on past mood abnormalities, so the diagnosis of bipolar affective disorder is not appropriate.

6. A. Manic episode with psychotic features. This patient's presentation is most in keeping with an episode mania with psychotic features. He presents with reduced sleep, reduced appetite, psychomotor agitation and a grandiose delusion which has resulted in marked disruption to his occupational function. It is likely that a diagnosis of bipolar affective disorder will be made, as he has presented with his first episode of mania. Only one episode of mania is required to make a diagnosis of bipolar affective disorder. It is also important to exclude substance use.

Chapter 11 The patient with low mood

1. E. Prednisolone is the only medication listed commonly associated with depression. The others are not.

2. B. The midline neck swelling may represent a goitre. Given the patient's symptoms are mild, there is time to check her thyroid function before commencing treatment. If she is hypothyroid this should be treated first, which may normalize her mood without need for an

antidepressant. Mild depression does not need referral to psychiatry. A neck ultrasound is likely to be needed also, but thyroid function should be checked first. She should not be sent away without investigation as the cause of the midline neck swelling needs to be determined.

3. D. The patient reports symptoms of depression alongside a mood-congruent nihilistic delusion. Therefore, the most likely diagnosis is a severe single depressive disorder with psychotic features. His lack of past psychiatric history makes schizoaffective disorder, schizophrenia and bipolar disorder unlikely, as onset at his age is rare. Early-onset dementia with behavioural and psychological symptoms is an unlikely possibility, but to check for this, his cognition, family history and ability to care for himself should be carefully assessed.

4. D. Suicidal ideation should be checked in everyone with a potential depressive episode. The other areas are all important but can be explored at a later review.

5. D. This patient is in a situational crisis. It is likely that her symptoms will resolve spontaneously. She needs reassurance and to be offered a follow-up appointment to check on her progress. She cannot be diagnosed with depression as her symptoms are present for less than 2 weeks, and she is unlikely to benefit from an antidepressant. However, she may still be at risk of self-harm and should be screened for this. She does not need investigations or a mood diary unless her symptoms persist. Her symptoms are not severe enough to need referral to psychiatry at present.

6. A. Multiple sclerosis. Multiple sclerosis would be an important differential here. This is suggested by her two neurological symptoms separated in time and place. Depression is common in multiple sclerosis.

7. C. Psychomotor agitation. This is a common feature of depression in older adults and describes restlessness and agitation that results in repetitive and unintentional movements.

Chapter 12 The patient with anxiety, fear or avoidance

1. D. Panic attack. This is the most likely diagnosis based on the history. However, it is important to take a full medical history (e.g., asthma, congenital heart disease) and family history (e.g., sudden death in young relatives) and to exclude other causes such as hyperthyroidism and hypoglycaemia, particularly given her repeat attendances. It would also be useful to know whether the attacks appear to have triggers (e.g., substance use/withdrawal, going to the library).

2. C. Blood-injection-injury phobia. This is suggested by his situational paroxysmal anxiety and avoidance. A myocardial infarction is unlikely to occur every time he is due to see the practice nurse. Hypoglycaemia, not hyperglycaemia, could cause these symptoms but is unlikely without a history of diabetes. Panic disorder does not have a specific trigger. Hypochondriasis is fear of having an illness, not fear of being investigated for one.

3. B. Airway, Breathing, Circulation, Disability, Exposure. The first step in management is ABCDE. She is speaking to you, so her airway is maintained independently. The next step is to ascertain her breathing and circulation status. Although the differential includes a panic attack, she could also be experiencing a wide range of acute medical problems requiring urgent management. An ECG, ABG, blood tests and psychiatry referral may all be appropriate in due course.

4. E. Check blood sugar. Someone with type 1 diabetes will be receiving insulin. The description sounds very much like hypoglycaemia. If hypoglycaemia is confirmed it is important to treat the episode by consuming carbohydrate, and then examine his insulin/food/activity regime to reduce further episodes. If his blood sugars are normal, he may be experiencing panic attacks as part of panic disorder. Keeping a diary and deep breathing exercises may help with these (see Chapter 23 for management). Seeing a counsellor may help if he is experiencing a stressful life event, illness or bereavements. Diazepam is only recommended in social anxiety disorder or specific phobia, for infrequent as required use.

5. D. Alcohol withdrawal. This man is drinking at least 60 units/week. He is experiencing physiological withdrawal symptoms after a few hours without alcohol, and the symptoms are relieved by further alcohol. Although anxiety in the morning may be part of diurnal variation in a depressive disorder, this man's mood is generally good, excluding depression. A phobia of something related to work is unlikely as the symptoms have only had onset recently (although enquiring regarding recent changes at work could be helpful). Hypoglycaemia secondary to diabetes is unlikely to present only in the mornings. Panic disorder is excluded by the clear relationship with alcohol.

6. B. Agoraphobia with panic attacks. This lady had a panic attack in a supermarket and has now become increasingly avoidant of crowding and confinement. Her symptoms are restricted to these situations. The weight loss may well be explained by her reduced dietary intake and increased exercise, but other disorders should be

screened for, i.e., hyperthyroidism. All her panic attacks are in the context of going outside in places with lots of people (agoraphobia). If they occurred outwith this context, comorbid panic disorder could be diagnosed too.

7. A. Panic disorder. This man reports repeated nonsituational panic attacks including a sensation of derealization. His symptoms could be due to cardiac problems but his young age, lack of exercise-induced symptoms and normal ECG are reassuring.

8. A. Caffeine. Caffeine has anxiogenic effects. Many soft drinks contain large amounts of caffeine, including tea/coffee, energy drinks and cola.

Chapter 13 The patient with obsessions and compulsions

1. A. No mental illness. Lay people often use 'obsession' loosely. Her thoughts of the show are not obsessional as they are ego-syntonic, pleasurable and not resisted. She describes no compulsions. She is not delusional in that there is no evidence of irrational thinking. She is not socially phobic in that she has not reported anxiety in social situations. There is no evidence of a persistent pattern of perfectionism and rigid thinking, as would be expected in a personality disorder with prominent traits of anankastia. Calling in sick represents unethical behaviour rather than a mental illness.

2. C. Depressive disorder. This man reports obsessions, but they are concurrent with the change in his mood, meeting the criteria for a depressive episode of moderate severity (five depressive symptoms). The obsessions are mood-congruent. Depression rather than obsessive-compulsive disorder is the primary diagnosis. Generalized anxiety disorder is unlikely as he does not report free-floating anxiety about many topics. Hypochondriasis is unlikely as he is not worried about a particular condition, but being dead. A nihilistic delusion is not suggested as he tries to distract himself, suggesting he is resisting the image rather than accepting it as reality.

3. D. OCD with comorbid depressive episode. This man describes obsessions and compulsions associated with functional impairment of greater than 2 weeks duration, giving him a diagnosis of OCD. Superimposed on this he has developed a depressive episode of mild severity. Generalized anxiety disorder is unlikely as he does not report free-floating anxiety about many topics. There is no evidence of a persistent pattern of perfectionism and rigid thinking, as would be expected in a personality disorder with prominent traits of anankastia.

4. B. Mild personality disorder with prominent traits of anankastia. This is suggested by her lifelong history of unusual conscientiousness and perfectionism which has caused some functional impairment (reduction of leisure time and being made redundant). Her thoughts of perfection are ego-syntonic and not resisted, meaning they are not true obsessions. Staying late to check is not a compulsion as it is not an unreasonable way to achieve her goal (assuming she does not check an excessive number of times). There is no evidence of low mood, excluding depressive symptoms. There is no evidence of communication difficulties, making an autism spectrum disorder unlikely.

5. B. Pseudohallucination. She reports a perception in the absence of a stimulus from within internal space. A hallucination would occur in external space. An obsession would be attributed to herself. Thought insertion would be attributed to an external agency. A rumination is not experienced as a voice, but as a thought (see Table 13.1).

6. D. This woman describes classic symptoms of body dysmorphic disorder. She is concerned with her appearance as opposed to an underlying disease (hypochondriasis). If she did hold the over-valued idea with delusional intensity, somatic delusional disorder should be considered. Note that some patients may exaggerate (or even feign) psychological sequelae of imagined or minor flaws in their appearance to receive medical care (factitious disorder) or cosmetic surgery paid for by the state, which would be malingering.

7. E. No mental illness. This woman is not experiencing obsessions or compulsions. She is responding to external influences and her handwashing may realistically reduce the feared outcome of infection transmission.

8. A. Delusion (strictly, a delusional perception). This belief is fixed, was arrived at illogically, and is not amenable to reason. The patient experienced a normal perception but interpreted it with delusional meaning, termed a 'delusional perception'. This is a first rank symptom of schizophrenia.

Chapter 14 The patient with a reaction to a stressful event

1. D. It is vital to robustly exclude physical aetiology prior to attributing symptoms to psychological causes. In this case, excluding intracranial haemorrhage secondary to head injury should take priority. This should include a history of the mechanism of assault (with corroboration from a witness if possible), full neurological examination

and appropriate investigations (which may include a computed tomography brain scan).

2. C. This describes symptoms of fairly marked psychomotor retardation, which would be suggestive that a depressive illness has developed from the bereavement reaction. The other symptoms (wanting to be dead, poor concentration, intense guilt, hallucinations involving the deceased) are typical of normal bereavement.

3. B. This woman is suffering from an adjustment disorder, characterized by difficulty coping with a significant change in circumstances and preoccupation with the stressor. Feelings of inability to cope are fairly typical of difficult adjustment. Note the duration of onset of symptoms (longer than for an acute stress reaction), and the fact that she has been signed off work, suggesting disruption to occupational functioning (which suggests that a diagnosis is appropriate, as opposed to 'no mental illness'). She does not appear to be suffering from other symptoms that would suggest depression or a dissociative neurological symptom disorder.

4. A. This case is fairly typical of dissociative amnesia. She has no memory of a circumscribed period of her life, with intact memory for her past and the more recent present. While head trauma and Wernicke–Korsakoff syndrome (due to inadequate nutrition) is naturally a concern, she appears to have been able to make her way to the UK and apply for asylum, which would suggest that cognitive impairment has not been global (excluding transient global amnesia), and she has been able to function at a reasonable level. She has no symptoms suggestive of posttraumatic stress disorder at this time, and the memory loss is more prolonged than would be expected in this disorder. In terms of stressful events, while she is unable to recall anything, she is seeking asylum from an area in which human rights violations are widely reported. The fact that she was pregnant with no recollection of conception or termination may suggest that she has been the victim of rape (which would be a traumatic stressor).

5. E. This patient has a most likely diagnosis of complex PTSD (or cPTSD). She has posttraumatic symptoms (such as flashbacks with specific triggers, hypervigilance and avoidance), coupled with affective instability, low self-esteem and difficulty maintaining relationships. Her emotions are volatile rather than being low, making depression less likely. While the images are intrusive, they are not linked to rituals or compulsions. There is no evidence of any psychotic features.

6. C. This is a classic presentation of a dissociative amnesia with dissociative fugue, or 'fugue state'. The man is unable to recount any personal details and appears to have travelled from a distant city. Note the possible severe stressor of being involved with a company that has recently been bankrupted.

7. E. This woman is probably suffering from nonepileptic seizures but epilepsy needs to be excluded. Nonepileptic seizures are suggested by the positive features of prolonged duration, a memory for ictal events and resisting eye opening (see Table 14.2). The chronological association with a significant stressor (being told that she will be left alone when her husband starts work) may also be relevant. These are often more common in those with a family or personal history of epilepsy.

8. B. Temporal lobe epilepsy. These symptoms are fairly typical of temporal lobe epilepsy. Note the history of likely head injury (implied by the fact she was referred from the neurosurgical unit). She should be referred for electroencephalogram.

Chapter 15 The patient with medically unexplained physical symptoms.

1. A. Watchful waiting. These situations are commonly encountered by GPs. The patient may well be developing multiple sclerosis; however, his symptoms are minimal and insufficient to make any diagnosis. Overzealous attempts to take his problems seriously by a well-intentioned doctor (such as referral to neurology, advanced investigations or arranging urgent follow-up) may reinforce his belief that something is wrong. However, dismissal by telling him it is 'all in his head' (or – at this stage – even empathic suggestion of psychiatric illness) is likely to cause him to seek a second opinion, and in any case is irresponsible given the inconclusive evidence. In the first instance, empathic acknowledgement and explanation, and inviting the patient to reattend if further symptoms arise (watchful waiting) is the most balanced option of the above.

2. D. Contact previous centres of care. This history is highly suggestive of factitious disorder imposed on self (female, healthcare professional, symptoms without signs, broad knowledge, specific demands, far from home). It is imperative to contact previous hospitals to get more information; however, asking the patient for such contact details may yield vague answers (in some cases, requesting such details will result in the patient discharging themselves). Details of such patients are often shared between local accident and emergency

departments. It is not safe to prescribe pethidine or arrange a laparoscopy. It is not ethical to tell her she is lying without any definite evidence of this. It is too early to refer to psychiatry, although this may help in due course if she is willing to engage.

3. B. Further physical investigations. Onset of such symptoms in older people with no significant medical or psychiatric history is more likely to be indicative of insidious organic disease. Prior to attribution of symptoms to a psychological origin, physical disease needs to be thoroughly excluded. In this case, physical investigations have been inappropriate to exclude likely physical illnesses. At minimum he requires an electrocardiogram.

4. C. Bodily distress disorder. Note the multiple and changing symptoms, refusal to accept the absence of physical cause and duration of more than 2 years. Multiple sclerosis is possible, but more weight than normal should be placed on objective evidence before this is investigated. There is no evidence she is lying about her experiences, making factitious disorder unlikely. She is concerned about her symptoms rather than an underlying disorder, excluding hypochondriasis. Generalized anxiety disorder is possible if she also reports anxiety about things other than physical symptoms.

Chapter 16 The patient with eating, feeding or weight problems

1. A. Significantly low body weight. This occurs in anorexia nervosa, not bulimia nervosa. Patients with bulimia nervosa are of normal or increased weight. Preoccupation with being thin, as well as a dread of fatness and a distorted perception of being too fat are associated with both anorexia and bulimia nervosa. Again, use of medication and exercise as means of controlling weight can occur in both disorders.

2. C. Investigate for physical causes of growth restriction. While patients with eating disorders often deny their symptoms, it is very important to exclude insidious physical illness as a cause of weight loss before attributing it to a psychiatric disorder. Physical causes can include malignancy, inflammatory disorders, infection and endocrine abnormalities. It would also be important to take a collateral history from his main caregiver, including psychosocial stressors.

3. E. Alcohol dependence. Self-neglect due to alcohol or substance use is a common cause of weight loss. Dependence is suggested by her withdrawal symptoms when she does not have access to alcohol (which are

not panic attacks). Low mood is commonly associated with alcohol excess as alcohol is a depressant: the treatment is to stop alcohol. Anorexia and bulimia nervosa are excluded by the fact that she is worried she has lost weight. Her vomiting sounds more likely to relate to gastritis secondary to alcohol excess, not purging.

4. E. Potassium 2.1 mmol/L. She requires an electrocardiogram and cautious intravenous replacement of potassium. Hypoglycaemia, anaemia, hypercholesterolaemia and hypophosphatemia are all common in anorexia nervosa but the values given here are not dangerously low.

5. D. Anorexia nervosa. This woman is dangerously underweight. While all of the listed mental illnesses can cause weight loss, they are differentiated from specific eating disorders by the presence of dread of fatness, distortion of body image and subsequent restriction of her dietary intake. The diagnosis of bulimia is excluded given her low body mass index.

6. E. Unable to rise from squatting without assistance. His blood pressure and heart rate place him at moderate risk but his capillary refill time and temperature are within the normal range. See The Royal College of Psychiatrists 'Medical Emergencies in Eating Disorders' guidance for more details on physical risk assessment in anorexia nervosa.

Chapter 17 The patient with alcohol or substance use problems

1. D. Alcoholic hallucinosis. This is a classic history of alcoholic hallucinosis. Note the absence of memory or attentional problems, excluding delirium tremens or Wernicke – Korsakoff syndrome. Late-onset schizophrenia should be in the differential diagnosis, but is unlikely in this case. Social isolation is often a cause or consequence of alcohol misuse. Hepatic encephalopathy is excluded by her otherwise normal physical examination.

2. D. Neck of femur repair. This man is delirious, and the history of heavy alcohol use suggests this is likely to be an alcohol withdrawal delirium. Note the visual 'Lilliputian hallucinations' of small figures (in his case, a horse), which are typical of alcohol withdrawal. Any surgical intervention should be delayed pending improvement in his delirium, unless it is felt that the fracture itself is a significant contributor to his presentation. The other options are all interventions which should be offered in delirium tremens. Benzodiazepines are used for alcohol withdrawal but

should be avoided in other sorts of delirium. He should be empirically treated with parenteral thiamine as it is very difficult to exclude Wernicke–Korsakoff syndrome in delirious patients, and the consequences of missing it can be severe. A full physical exam may highlight evidence of Wernicke–Korsakoff (ophthalmoplegia, ataxia) or highlight other contributors to the delirium (e.g., chest infection). Consistent nursing care will help to calm and orientate him.

3. C. Obtain a urine sample for drug testing. Oral test strips are an alternative. Before starting opioid replacement establishing that the patient is currently using opioids is essential. Prescribing methadone to someone who is not opioid-tolerant can be fatal. Similarly, prescribing his previous dose of methadone could be fatal as he may be less opioid-tolerant now than he was previously. It is necessary for methadone doses to be initiated at a low level and gradually increased if required (titrated against withdrawal symptoms). Referring him to a drug counselling service may well be appropriate if he wishes to engage. Contacting the police is not appropriate.

4. B. A 'half bottle' (350 mL) of premium gin (40% ABV) per week. To calculate alcohol units, take the % ABV and multiply by volume (in litres): e.g., 40 × 0.350 = 14 units; 350 mL of a 40% ABV spirit contains 14 units. Six pints (3.408 L) of continental lager (5.3% ABV) contains 18 units; two bottles (1.5 L) of red wine (12.5% ABV) contains 18.75 units; 3 L of strong white cider (8.4% ABV) contains 25.2 units; and six bottles (1.980 L) of alcopops (4.9% ABV) contains 9.7 units. She should also be told that there is no 'safe' level at which to drink alcohol, merely lower to higher risk levels. If she plans to drink the full 14 units, it should be recommended that she spreads her alcohol consumption over around 3 days per week.

5. E. Drowsiness. Hyper alertness, tachycardia, hyperthermia, hypertension and psychotic symptoms arise commonly during cocaine use. Chest pain is a very concerning symptom suggesting arrhythmia or cardiac ischaemia due to coronary artery spasm. He should be advised to seek emergency medical care if this occurs after consumption.

6. C. Ketamine. Ketamine is a potent glutamatergic (NMDA receptor) channel blocker, and is a potent short-acting dissociative anaesthetic. It is legitimately used in veterinary surgery as an anaesthetic agent. It can also be used as an anaesthetic analgesic agent in human medicine. The patient's symptoms are in keeping with dissociation, with ketamine being the most likely to cause this of the drugs listed.

Chapter 18 The patient with personality problems

1. B. Mild personality disorder. This lady likely has a mild personality disorder. She describes longstanding issues with personality which manifest in difficulties with relationships and poor self-esteem, however is managing well with her work and with her family. She does have evidence of impairment in managing mutually satisfying relationships. She does describe difficulties in regulating her emotions which would also support a diagnosis of personality disorder.

2. E. Severe personality disorder. This man is likely to have a severe personality disorder. He describes longstanding difficulties with emotional regulation and impulsive behaviour which impact multiple areas of functioning, being unable to sustain relationships, having difficulties with his family, holding down a job and being arrested multiple times. There is insufficient information given to determine whether he also has polysubstance dependence. In any case this would be unlikely to explain his lifelong difficulties and his feelings of self-loathing, although it may be a contributing factor.

3. D. Personality disorder with prominent traits of anankastia. The most prominent personality trait for this patient is anankastia, as she describes difficulties with others when they are unable to meet her standards, perfectionism, and behavioural constraint, having lost a relationship because of lack of spontaneity.

4. C. Personality disorder with prominent traits of dissociality. This patient presents with features of dissociality, describing lack of empathy for the patient he pushed down the stairs, and a self-centred idea that he was more important than this patient. There is evidence this is longstanding and not merely a 'one-off' incident.

5. E. Personality disorder with a borderline pattern and prominent traits of disinhibition. The patient describes a pattern of impulsive actions (including recurrent self-harm) that are often related to her emotional state at the time, and struggles with planning her time. She also describes a fear of abandonment and an unclear sense of self.

Chapter 19 The patient with impairment of consciousness, memory or cognition

1. D. Delirium. This is suggested by her acute onset objective cognitive impairment associated with sleep–wake cycle disturbance. Suspicion and visual hallucinations are common in delirium. Although Lewy body dementia is commonly associated with visual hallucinations it is

excluded by the acute onset. Similarly, Alzheimer dementia is excluded by the acute onset. Late-onset schizophrenia remains a possibility but is far less likely than delirium. Charles Bonnet syndrome would not account for all the features here, e.g., persecutory beliefs, sleep–wake cycle disturbance and cognitive impairment.

2. A. Korsakoff syndrome. This man has an isolated long-term anterograde and retrograde memory impairment, with significant difficulty forming new memories, with intact working memory and other cognitive function. He is confabulating. A history of alcohol excess raises the possibility of Korsakoff syndrome as the cause. He does not have dementia because the impairment is not global or progressive.

3. A. Computed tomography (CT) of the head. This gentleman has a likely diagnosis of dementia. NICE CKS (2022) recommends the blood tests this man has already received plus structural neuroimaging as a minimum assessment for reversible causes of dementia. However, there is some clinical judgement involved. Practice varies locally and some centres would not request a CT head unless there are neurological signs. There is no reason to think this man needs syphilis and HIV serology but for other patients it may be appropriate. EEG, chest X-ray and lumbar puncture are not recommended routinely in assessment of dementia but may be indicated in particular circumstances (e.g., if frontotemporal dementia or Creutzfeldt-Jakob disease is suspected). See Table 19.7.

4. A. Delirium. This woman has recently been extremely unwell. Even though her UTI has been successfully treated, the brain can often lag behind the rest of the body when recovering from a serious illness. The fluctuation in her mental state may reflect a resolving or a new delirium. It would be wise to reassess for other causes that may have been missed initially or occurred since admission, e.g., a hospital-acquired pneumonia. It may be that she will not regain her premorbid cognitive functioning and in due course will be diagnosed with dementia, but it is too early to make this diagnosis.

5. A. Amitriptyline. This man has a delirium. Anticholinergic medication is a common cause of delirium, as are opioids. Amitriptyline is sometimes used to reduce insomnia, although this is extremely inadvisable in an older adult, so this may be the precipitant. Starting or stopping any medication can potentially cause delirium but this does not occur commonly with the other medications listed.

6. E. Subdural haematoma. This woman has atrial fibrillation and so is likely to be on warfarin. There should therefore be a low threshold for suspecting an intracranial bleed after minor or no injury. A chronic subdural haematoma as opposed to neurodegenerative cause of dementia is suggested by her relatively quick cognitive deterioration, possible fluctuating conscious level (uncharacteristic afternoon naps), neurological signs and history of head injury. It is not uncommon for there to be a latent period of days to weeks between injury and symptoms. The next step should be brain imaging.

7. A. Lewy body dementia. The patient has the triad of symptoms of parkinsonism, hallucinations and fluctuating cognition, so Lewy body dementia is the most likely diagnosis.

8. B. Mild neurocognitive impairment. This woman has a below-normal score on standardized cognitive assessment but no impairment in activities of daily living. This low score is quite concerning in view of her young age and high educational attainment and she should be referred to a young onset memory clinic for comprehensive investigation.

Chapter 20 Dementia and delirium

1. A. Assess for changes in physical health. This woman has symptoms of stress and distress in dementia. Reviewing for any potential physical causes of this is recommended first line by NICE (2018), unless there is immediate risk of harm or severe distress. In the event of these risks, antipsychotics would be first line (after consideration of risk of stroke) and cholinesterase inhibitors second line. Antidepressants are only indicated if there is evidence of depression. Referral to speech and language therapy is unlikely to be of benefit given her severe dementia.

2. A. Antipsychotics. Antipsychotics can cause irreversible severe parkinsonian reactions in patients with Lewy body dementia. They are not absolutely contraindicated but should be used with even more caution than in other types of dementia and ideally under specialist advice. The other options may all potentially be of benefit – if his delusion is due to concurrent infection (antibiotics), depression (antidepressants) or worsening dementia – cholinesterase inhibitors can improve behavioural and psychological symptoms of dementia. Nutritional supplements may be of benefit, whatever the cause, if he is losing weight.

3. C. Co-codamol. This contains both codeine and paracetamol. Opioids are very common causes of delirium in older adults, both in their own right and due to their side effect of constipation. Opioids are often started during acute admissions for pain or surgery. Any

medication can potentially precipitate delirium, but opioids, benzodiazepines and anticholinergics are the commonest.

4. D. Acute medical ward. This lady is delirious. This is a medical emergency. She needs to be fully physically investigated. Her acute-onset psychotic symptoms are almost certainly due to her delirium, not a primary psychotic disorder.

5. B. Memantine. This woman has mild to moderate dementia for which cholinesterase inhibitors are recommended. However, she has a number of relative contraindications to cholinesterase inhibitor use. Their cholinergic effects can induce bradycardia, which may be particularly problematic in those with conduction defects. Similarly, cholinergic drugs can cause bronchoconstriction, which may be problematic in COPD and asthma. Cholinergic drugs can also increase gastric acid secretions, which could worsen peptic ulceration. Overall, it would probably be better to try memantine first for this woman.

6. A. No treatment recommended by current guidelines. Unfortunately, no medications have yet been found to slow the progression of frontotemporal dementia.

Chapter 21 Older adult psychiatry

1. A. Antidepressant. The key issue here is the diagnosis. She presents with a common triad in older adults: depressive symptoms, cognitive impairment and functional impairment. It is often difficult to tease out whether someone is experiencing depression manifesting with cognitive impairment or an early dementia leading to comorbid depression. Ideally, depression is treated first, then cognition reassessed once mood is euthymic. An antidepressant would be first line in view of her cognitive impairment, but counselling or psychological therapy could still be considered in someone with this level of cognitive impairment.

2. C. Depressive episode. It is common for depression to manifest with prominent features of anxiety, psychomotor agitation and hypochondriacal ideas in older adults. Mild neurocognitive impairment is the next most likely differential – although her MOCA score of 29/30 is reassuring, a more sensitive test such as the Addenbrooke's Cognitive Examination (ACE-III) may still show an objective impairment. Generalized anxiety disorder or hypochondriasis is unlikely to have onset so late in life, and diagnosis would require a longer duration of symptoms. There are no psychotic features to suggest schizophrenia.

3. A. ECT. All of the suggested management strategies are reasonable, but ECT is preferable because of this man's potentially life-threatening poor fluid intake and poor medication concordance. Depot medication would get around the concordance problem but there are no depot medications licensed as antidepressants. ECT is the quickest and most effective treatment for depression known and seems to work particularly well in older adults.

4. B. All of these patients could potentially have late-onset schizophrenia. However, symptoms of late-onset schizophrenia are predominantly delusional, rather than bizarre or negative symptoms (as in patients A and C). Patient A has some possible features of delirium. Patient D is more likely to have Charles Bonnet syndrome. Late-onset schizophrenia is far more common in women than in men, and social deprivation and hearing impairment are also risk factors. 'Impending sense of doom' as in patient E can be a symptom of MI.

5. D. Continue mirtazapine for at least 8 weeks. Older adults can take longer to show response to antidepressants, so an adequate trial is at least 8 weeks. Augmentation is not necessary at this stage and increases the risk of drug interactions. Tricyclics are not recommended as first line in older adults due to their side-effect profile.

6. E. Delirium. This lady has acute-onset cognitive impairment: delirium until proven otherwise. The history is concerningly suggestive of a focal seizure. She needs to be admitted to a medical ward for investigation. A manic or hypomanic episode would be highly unlikely to have such a rapid onset. Were she on lithium, it would be crucial to check a random lithium level as her presentation could also be due to lithium toxicity.

7. B. This is the simplest and easiest of the options. If concordance remains poor despite this, prompting by a carer could be considered. A depot could be useful if the patient wishes it, or his insight reduces and he requires compulsory treatment. Daily dispensing is normally reserved for methadone or for those at high risk of overdose. In general, simplifying medication regimes to once daily is a good idea, but unfortunately olanzapine is likely to be too sedating to allow use in the mornings. Potentially, his other once-daily medication could be changed to the evening.

8. A. Ask her to attend A&E. It is unclear what dose of trazodone she has taken, or whether she has taken any other tablets. She needs examination, blood samples tested and an electrocardiogram. The next step would be for her to receive an urgent psychiatric review. This lady has recently attempted suicide. Older adults are at high risk of completed suicide. She may perceive taking

extra trazodone as far more harmful than it actually is, as she may have memories of barbiturates – highly toxic sleeping tablets, which are fatal in minor overdose. Her ongoing intent is unclear from the vignette. She may require admission or urgent community support from mental health services.

agent, patients would usually be titrated onto a methadone prescription by addiction services. Buvidal could be an option, but it is usually used for patients who struggle to attend the chemist regularly to collect their substitute prescriptions, e.g., because of a more chaotic lifestyle.

Chapter 22 Alcohol and substance-related disorders

1. B. Contemplation of change. This man is currently contemplating changing his behaviour. He recognizes the need for change (he wants to give up), but he is ambivalent about it (worrying he will lose all his friends). Motivational interviewing may be helpful to allow him to progress to the next stage of preparation for change.

2. E. Urine drug test to confirm the presence of opioids. Prior to prescribing methadone, it is essential to confirm the use of opioids. A urine or oral drug test can be used to do this. Admission to psychiatric hospital is not necessary, although dose titration should be undertaken in a controlled clinical environment with facilities to measure physiological response to opioids, and with emergency treatment for opioid toxicity (i.e., naloxone) close to hand. Viral serology testing and physical examination is important screening for health complications from intravenous drug use, but it is not necessary for a methadone prescription. Forcing a patient to identify a confidant for the purposes of corroboration can lead to problems, either placing false security in a possibly inaccurate historian or causing disengagement with services.

3. C. Naltrexone. Naltrexone is an opioid receptor antagonist. This may control cravings and reduces the pleasurable effects of drinking alcohol, reducing 'reward' and – by operant conditioning – can 'extinguish' the desire to drink (the 'Sinclair method'). Disulfiram causes an unpleasant reaction when taken with alcohol. Acamprosate may be helpful in controlling cravings. Long-term antidepressants or benzodiazepines are not recommended for the sole purpose of maintaining abstinence. However, antidepressants may be helpful for treating comorbid depression.

4. C. Buprenorphine. Buprenorphine (either oral or subcutaneous) is a partial opioid agonist and can be used for substitution therapy. The other drugs can be used in treating various stages of opioid dependence; however, none are true 'substitutes'.

5. A. Methadone. Methadone is the first-choice agent in substitute prescribing for opioid dependence. Unless there is a strong patient preference for an alternative

Chapter 23 The psychotic disorders

1. B. 12.5%. If one parent has schizophrenia, the probability of their offspring having schizophrenia is 13%. The population lifetime risk is 1%.

2. E. 50%. If both parents have schizophrenia, the probability of their offspring having schizophrenia is 50%. The population lifetime risk is 1%.

3. C. 1 to 2 years. This is a difficult question as there is little solid evidence about the optimum period of treatment for a first episode of psychosis. Without prophylactic antipsychotics following a first episode of schizophrenia, over half of patients will relapse within a year. The current recommendation is to continue antipsychotics for 1 to 2 years after a first episode. However, many patients wish to stop sooner. In this case, a gradual reduction over a few weeks reduces the risk of relapse. Alternatively, this man may prefer to switch to an antipsychotic less associated with weight gain.

4. D. Cognitive-behavioural therapy. The other modalities are not recommended in schizophrenia. Interpersonal therapy and cognitive-behavioural therapy are indicated in depression. Dialectical behavioural therapy is indicated in emotionally unstable personality disorder. Cognitive analytic therapy is indicated in eating disorders. Family therapy is also recommended if the patient lives with or is in close contact with their family.

5. C. Commence olanzapine. This patient has schizoaffective disorder which is managed very similarly to schizophrenia, with the possibility of antidepressants or mood stabilizers depending on presentation. An antipsychotic such as olanzapine would be an appropriate first-choice medication. She is under 55, and in particular of childbearing potential, so sodium valproate would be contraindicated. Lithium could be considered as an adjunct. She is clearly unwell so watching and waiting is not appropriate. ECT would only be indicated if she had a treatment-resistant illness or there were life-threatening features.

6. C. Aripiprazole. This is the antipsychotic least likely to be associated with weight gain and the metabolic syndrome. First-generation antipsychotics would be the next best choice.

7. A. Chlorpromazine. The 'rash' is consistent with sunburn, likely due to a photosensitivity reaction from chlorpromazine. Chlorpromazine is often used as an 'as required' medication for agitation.

8. B. Switch to clozapine. This woman has treatment-resistant schizophrenia as she has had two trials of antipsychotic at adequate doses for adequate durations, including at least one second-generation drug.

Chapter 24 The mood (affective) disorders

1. A. Someone who is not eating or drinking. ECT is indicated in options A–D, but not E. Treatment-resistant depression is an indication for ECT but if the patient has capacity and does not wish it, it is not given. No information is given to suggest s/he lacks capacity, which is presumed to be present in adults unless proven otherwise. Life-threatening reduction in oral intake, psychotic depression and previous good response to ECT are all other indications for ECT. If a prioritization has to be made, a life-threatening reduction in oral intake presents the highest risk and so should be treated first.

2. C. Admission under mental health legislation. This man is experiencing a manic episode with psychotic features. His psychotic beliefs place him at high risk of injury or death and are impairing his ability to make decisions regarding management of his mental health. It is not safe to let him go home and police custody is not appropriate given his behaviour is driven by illness. He may be persuadable to be admitted informally but if not, he would meet criteria for detention under mental health legislation (see Chapter 4).

3. D. Citalopram and quetiapine. This man has a severe depressive episode with psychotic features. A combination of an antidepressant and an antipsychotic is indicated. Citalopram is normally tried before amitriptyline as it has fewer side effects. In addition, amitriptyline is more toxic than citalopram in overdose. Given his suicidal ideation it is best to choose the less toxic medication. Quetiapine or any other second-generation antipsychotic would be reasonable to treat his psychosis.

4. B. Olanzapine. Olanzapine, risperidone, quetiapine or haloperidol are the first-line antimanic agents recommended by NICE (2014). Lithium should not be started in the acute situation in someone with a history of nonconcordance. Sodium valproate should not be prescribed in people under the age of 55. Lamotrigine is not recommended during acute mania as it is

ineffective. Citalopram, or any other antidepressant, should be discontinued in a manic patient. This woman is likely also to need rapid tranquillization with a benzodiazepine (see Fig. 7.1).

5. C. Individual CBT. Self-help CBT and structured group physical activity are recommended by NICE for mild depression (2022). Dialectical behaviour therapy is a psychological therapy for borderline pattern personality disorder. Graded exposure therapy is used to treat obsessive-compulsive disorder and phobias.

6. E. Commence fluoxetine. The next step for this man is to consider an antidepressant (typically an SSRI first line), which can be done in primary care.

Chapter 25 The anxiety, stress related, OCD related and bodily distress disorders

1. B. She should be seen on a planned, regular schedule. Seeing patients with anxiety about their physical health on a regular basis can help contain their anxieties and reduce the total number and number of urgent appointments they need. However, this does not mean they should not be allowed access to urgent appointment slots – they will still experience urgent or serious physical health problems at least as commonly as the general population. Similarly, investigations should be carefully considered and avoided if possible, but some are likely to still be required to safely exclude other disorders. Benzodiazepines are not indicated for bodily distress disorder but may be indicated for some other reason. The nature of bodily distress disorder should be explained to patients, but it should not be done in a confrontational manner. Phrases such as 'all in the mind' should be avoided as patients are genuinely experiencing symptoms.

2. B. CBT with desensitization. CBT with desensitization is recommended for phobias with mild to severe functional impairment. Trauma-focused CBT is for posttraumatic stress disorder. PRN diazepam would not be advisable given she is likely to come into contact with bodily fluids on a daily basis. SSRIs are not recommended for specific phobias.

3. C. Selective serotonin reuptake inhibitor (SSRI). An SSRI is the first-line drug therapy for obsessive-compulsive disorder. Clomipramine is usually a second-line drug therapy, or if the patient has had a previously good response to it. Mirtazapine and pregabalin are not recommended by current guidelines. Self-help is recommended for mild symptoms but this woman's symptoms are associated with marked functional impairment. Talking therapies are first line for

moderate to severe OCD and she should be encouraged to reconsider a talking therapy if a SSRI is ineffective.

4. C. CBT with a trauma focus. This would be an appropriate first step in management as suggested by NICE (2018). If the person prefers drug treatment an SSRI could be offered. Long-term prescribing of benzodiazepines should be avoided.

5. E. Applied relaxation. This and CBT are the two psychological therapies recommended for moderate to severe generalized anxiety disorder.

Chapter 26 Feeding and eating disorders

1. B. Family therapy. This is the first-line psychological therapy for adolescents recommended by NICE (2017). The other therapies are all used in adults with anorexia.

2. E. Individual eating disorder-focused CBT. This is one of the three psychotherapeutic modalities recommended first line by NICE (2017) for anorexia in adults. Family therapy is first line for treating anorexia and bulimia in young people. Focal psychodynamic psychotherapy is a second-line treatment in anorexia. Interpersonal therapy is used to treat depression and exposure-response prevention is used to treat obsessive-compulsive disorder.

3. C. Binge–purge symptoms. The presence of binge–purge symptoms is associated with a poorer prognosis in sufferers of anorexia nervosa, as is late age of onset, very low weight (not rapid weight loss), long duration of illness, personality difficulties and difficult family relationships. The presence of a family history of anorexia is not necessarily indicative of poor prognosis, neither is the rate of engagement with psychotherapy.

4. C. Multivitamin. NICE (2017) recommends that people with anorexia nervosa should be encouraged to take a multivitamin and multimineral supplement. Selective serotonin reuptake inhibitors are no longer recommended in the management of eating disorders unless there is comorbid depression or anxiety, and these disorders are most likely to resolve with weight gain alone.

5. C. Phosphate 0.3 mmol/L. All the other blood results are in the normal range. Hypophosphataemia is the hallmark of refeeding syndrome and a low level indicates that replacement is required, along with frequent monitoring of phosphate, magnesium, sodium and potassium levels. Calcium levels are not generally affected in refeeding syndrome.

Chapter 27 The sleep–wake disorders

1. E. Pramipexole. Dopamine agonists such as pramipexole and ropinirole are recommended as first-line treatment for restless legs syndrome. The other medications listed are all potential causes of the syndrome.

2. D. Neuropathy. A peripheral neuropathy is suggested by her history of diabetes. Restless legs syndrome is unlikely as the pain is not brought on by inactivity. Iron deficiency is a cause of restless legs syndrome. Intermittent claudication is unlikely as exercise would worsen symptoms. Akathisia would not be limited to her legs.

3. D. Sleep hygiene advice. Everyone who is struggling with sleep should be given sleep hygiene advice, particularly those with depression. Her insomnia is likely secondary to depression and should improve over time as her mood improves. It is too early to increase the dose of fluoxetine. Hypnotics should be avoided where possible as patients can suffer from daytime drowsiness and develop tolerance. A sleep diary or referral is not indicated.

Chapter 28 Sex and gender Identity

1. A. Caressing without genital contact can improve sex. This is the kind of advice which may be given during sex therapy or in self-help materials related to sexual dysfunction. All the other pieces of advice are the opposite of what should be given: sexual dysfunction is common at all ages, physical problems are a rare cause of anorgasmia, medication may cause sexual dysfunction but should not be stopped immediately (a substitution may be required) and good communication with a partner about sex is associated with fewer sexual difficulties.

2. B. Check blood glucose. Erectile dysfunction is a common presenting symptom in diabetes, as is weight loss. Excluding diabetes is the priority here. All of the other options can also be appropriate management options in erectile dysfunction depending on the context (see Box 28.2).

3. B. Olanzapine. All the other agents are dopaminomimetic agents: levodopa is metabolized to dopamine, pergolide and pramipexole are dopamine receptor agonists and selegiline is a monoamine oxidase B inhibitor, reducing the breakdown of dopamine. High doses of dopaminomimetic agents have rarely been associated with new paraphilias in Parkinson disease, typically younger men with a long duration of illness. Olanzapine is a dopamine receptor antagonist which has been used to treat paraphilias in Parkinson disease.

4. D. Sertraline. Selective serotonin reuptake inhibitors are commonly associated with anorgasmia. Mirtazapine is the antidepressant least likely to be associated with sexual side effects.

Chapter 29 Disorders relating to the menstrual cycle, pregnancy and the puerperium

1. A. Encourage exercise. This woman has mild premenstrual syndrome (PMS). One argument with her boyfriend is not evidence of significant functional impairment. For mild PMS, the National Institute for Health and Care Excellence (NICE; 2014) recommends healthy eating, stress reduction, regular sleep and regular exercise, particularly during the luteal phase. They also recommend smoking cessation and reducing alcohol intake where applicable. The oral contraceptive pill, ibuprofen and CBT are all options in managing moderately severe PMS. SSRIs are reserved for severe PMS.

2. E. Psychological therapy. While the woman in the case description attributes her symptoms to the menopause, the duration of the symptoms accompanied by the presence of suicidal thoughts are more suggestive of a depressive illness. The functional impact and suicidal thoughts suggest an episode of at least moderate severity. The National Institute for Health and Care Excellence (NICE; 2022) recommends a combination of an antidepressant and psychological therapy (cognitive-behavioural therapy or interpersonal therapy) as first line for treating moderate-to-severe depression. Counselling may also be useful if she has issues relating to relationships or bereavements she would like to reflect on, but it is not usually a treatment for depression. Dietary and lifestyle advice (avoiding alcohol, tobacco, eating a balanced diet, exercising) should be offered to everyone with mood symptoms but are unlikely to be sufficient in this case. Around the menopausal years, there can be an increase in psychosocial stressors (children leaving home, 'facing up' to growing older, changes in personal relationships, etc.), which may increase the risk of developing depression independently of the hormonal changes that arise during the menopause. Hormone replacement therapy can be useful in certain circumstances; however, it does not suit everyone, and should not be used as a substitute for recognized treatments in the management of major depression. Omega-3 fish oils may reduce menopausal vasomotor symptoms (hot flushes) but are not recommended as a treatment for depression.

3. E. Refer to perinatal psychiatry. This is a complex risk–benefit scenario that needs to be carefully discussed with the patient and which draws on the latest available evidence. Her history of bipolar disorder places this woman at high risk of postpartum psychosis, even with prophylactic treatment. Discontinuing treatment increases her risk of relapse at any time. A mentally unwell mother is harmful for the child in utero and once born. However, all the mood stabilizers are associated with teratogenic effects to various degrees (valproate > carbamazepine > lithium). The absolute risk of congenital abnormalities remains low with lithium but is unacceptably high with valproate or carbamazepine, so switching to them would not be helpful. Discontinuing lithium and remaining without prophylaxis may be an option depending on the severity of her previous mood episodes. Switching to olanzapine is also a reasonable option as it is thought to be safe in pregnancy but would depend on her past experience with this drug.

4. E. Refer to perinatal mental health team. Reassurance that she will not become unwell cannot be given. This lady has a history of severe postnatal depression and is at greatly increased risk of suffering a further episode. She should be referred to the perinatal mental health team. Given this history, and her good response to medications in the past, commencing antidepressant treatment later in pregnancy or early postpartum may be beneficial. The perinatal mental health team would explore the risks versus benefits of this option. When choosing an agent, consideration should be given to previously effective drugs, and the mother's choice to breastfeed.

5. A. Detention in hospital under mental health act. This woman is experiencing a postpartum psychosis and is at very high risk of infanticide given the severity of her illness, the content of her delusion and the active steps she has taken towards killing her son. This risk is too high to be managed at home, however supportive of her family. She lacks capacity to make decisions about her treatment due to her absent insight, therefore requiring admission under detention rather than informally. This should be to a mother-and-baby unit if available. Transfer to police cells is not appropriate as she requires intensive psychiatric care which cannot be provided there and she has not committed a crime. Outpatient follow-up is not sufficient to manage her acute risk. A referral to social workers is likely to be

helpful in due course as they may be able to identify additional supports for the patient, but the priority at the moment is to maintain her and her child's safety in hospital.

Chapter 30 The personality disorders

1. E. Drug treatment is not the main intervention. NICE (2009) does not recommend drug treatment for the core symptoms of personality disorders with a borderline pattern. However, some medications can be helpful in reducing agitation during crises and in treating comorbid mental illness. The main intervention is psychological therapy.

2. A. Dialectical behaviour therapy. All of the options have evidence supporting their use in personality disorder with a borderline pattern, but dialectical behaviour therapy is the 'gold standard' and recommended by NICE (2009).

3. E. Suggest weekly dispensing of medication. This woman is probably suffering from a comorbid depressive episode. Management of this should be discussed with the patient – she may opt for 'watchful waiting' or it may be appropriate to start an antidepressant. As her risk of suicide has increased, it is sensible to reduce her access to means of suicide by suggesting weekly dispensing. Her risk is not so high that she needs admission. A urine drug screen may be helpful in excluding a substance-induced acute change in mood, but substance use (with the exception of alcohol) is unlikely to account for a month of low mood. Benzodiazepines should be avoided where possible given the risks of dependence, particularly high in someone with persistent symptoms. Dialectical behaviour therapy is recommended for treatment of personality disorder with a borderline pattern in the long term but will not help depression in the short–medium term.

4. C. Alert the police and the intended victim. Given the significant risk to another person, confidentiality needs to be broken in this case. The psychiatrist has a duty to immediately warn the police. In addition, the specific and detailed content of the threat necessitates that the intended victim be warned (see the Tarasoff case for further details). The responsibility for this falls on the doctor; however, in practice the police will usually be happy to facilitate this. Detention under mental health legislation would not be appropriate, as the threat should be addressed by law enforcement agencies in the first instance. Meticulous notes would need to be kept. It is likely that he would be held criminally

responsible for his actions. Review in 1 week is too late. Anger management may be appropriate in due course but does not deal with the acute risk. Diazepam should be avoided given risks of dependence and absence of an indication.

Chapter 31 The neurodevelopmental disorders

1. C. None. There is no pharmacological treatment for the core symptoms of autism spectrum disorder. The first-line treatment is social skills training. The medications listed may be indicated to manage common comorbidities of autism spectrum disorder, anxiety or depression (fluoxetine), attention deficit hyperactivity disorder (methylphenidate), psychosis (risperidone) or epilepsy (sodium valproate).

2. D. Methylphenidate. NICE (2018) recommends this as first-line drug treatment for severe ADHD in school-age children. Dexamphetamine and atomoxetine are second line. Parent-training/education programs are recommended as first line for school-age children with mild to moderate impairment, but his parents have already tried this. Severe impairment is suggested by the fact this boy is at risk of losing his school place. Cognitive-behavioural therapy is recommended for older adolescents with mild to moderate ADHD.

3. D. Psychoeducation. This boy has Tourette syndrome. Psychoeducation is first-line treatment for this: speaking to him, his family and his teachers to explain the diagnosis and that the majority of cases improve by adulthood. The other options are all drug treatments that can reduce tics. However, as the tics are causing little interference with day-to-day activities, he may find the side effects outweigh the benefits.

Chapter 32 Intellectual Disability

1. B. A physical examination. It is important not to fall into the trap of 'diagnostic overshadowing'. When there is a significant change in an individual's behaviour, it is important to exclude a physical cause for this, such as constipation; pain; indigestion or another physical illness. It is also important to be aware of the possibility of physical or sexual abuse in vulnerable adults and young people, and this should be.

2. D. Ask the support worker to leave the room so you can speak to the patient alone. People with intellectual disabilities are at greater risk of abuse than the general population, including from carers. It is important to see this woman independently to sensitively enquire about the possibility of abuse. You

could consider seeking the advice of an Intellectual Disability Liaison Nurse if there are any at the hospital, or speak to Speech and Language Therapy about communication aids.

Chapter 33 Child and adolescent psychiatry

1. B. Conduct-dissocial disorder. This is suggested by his major violations of societal norms (arson and severe aggression). Oppositional defiant disorder is often considered to be a 'milder' variant of conduct disorder, where defiant behaviour is characteristic, but this tends not to involve criminality or violating the rights of others. Conduct-dissocial disorder is associated with the development of personality disorder with dissociality, criminality and substance misuse in later life. He is too young to diagnose a personality disorder. Substance misuse is a possibility which should be explored but is unlikely to present with oppositional behaviour in isolation. Reactive attachment disorder presents under the age of 5 years with disordered social interaction.

2. E. The duty social worker and on-call paediatrician should be alerted. Vaginal trauma and genital warts are not normal in an 8-year-old girl, and the findings should immediately raise suspicions of sexual abuse. The safety of the child is paramount, and steps should be taken to maintain this. While protocols vary slightly between areas, child protection procedures usually advise contacting the duty social worker and/or the local paediatrician on-call for child protection. If in any doubt about a possible child protection concern, either of these parties will usually be more than happy to offer guidance. The child should not be directly asked about what happened at this stage: a formal interview needs to be arranged involving the police, social workers and paediatric staff. Police will not question the girl just now. Parents should never be 'confronted' by medical staff; however, it is obviously courteous (if possible) to let them know what is going on and what will happen next. The child should not be allowed home until all relevant agencies are involved and safety at home can be ensured. This may not be possible, and an alternative place of safety may have to be sought. Should the parent remove the child from safety, it would be appropriate to contact the police given the magnitude of the concerns.

3. B. Cognitive-behavioural therapy. This girl has a probable diagnosis of depression, of moderate severity (based on her functional impairment). NICE (2019) recommends individual psychological therapy first line. Fluoxetine is the first-line antidepressant, sertraline and citalopram

are second line. Watchful waiting is recommended only in mild cases.

4. D. Personality disorder with a borderline pattern and prominent traits of negative affectivity. This is suggested by her long-term rapidly fluctuating mood, difficulties in relationships, self-harm, pseudohallucinations (the voice inside her head) and disturbed self-image (feeling empty). Childhood adversity is a risk factor for borderline pattern personality disorders and suggested by a parental overdose. Bipolar affective disorder or a depressive episode would be associated with episodes of altered mood which lasted for days, not hours. However, borderline pattern is a risk factor for comorbid depression. Disordered eating is also common in this personality disorder. Bulimia is unlikely given the rest of the history, but it would be useful to check what her weight-related cognitions are to definitely exclude this. Schizophrenia is unlikely as she is not reporting any psychotic symptoms (she reports pseudohallucinations, not hallucinations).

5. A. Selective mutism. This is suggested by the child's normal language development and ability to speak in some situations. Selective mutism often follows emotional trauma (such as separation from parents, war, severe illness) and situations where there is conflict at home.

6. E. Reactive attachment disorder. This is suggested by the child's history of abuse, marked fearfulness and social withdrawal. The diagnosis is not child abuse alone, as not all children who are abused respond in this way or go on to experience mental disorder.

Chapter 34 Forensic psychiatry

1. C. Previous violence. The best predictor of future violence is past violence. The other options also increase his risk of future violence, particularly substance use.

2. E. He is able to give a coherent account of events leading up to the offence but denies memory of the offence itself. An individual being considered unfit to plead through mental illness is relatively uncommon. The mental state findings given in A–D are all fairly extreme abnormalities suggesting that he would struggle to understand the difference between a plea of guilty and not guilty (D), understand the nature of the charge (D), instruct counsel (A and C), follow the evidence brought before the court (C) or challenge a juror (B and C). Amnesia (real or reported) for the offence itself does not necessarily impact on fitness to plead.

3. E. Murder. This is the only charge for which diminished responsibility may apply. If the accused is found to have

diminished responsibility, the conviction is reduced to manslaughter (or culpable homicide in Scotland). This was particularly important historically when murder carried the death penalty.

4. B. ADHD. This is a typical history for someone with ADHD symptoms of impulsivity and emotional instability leading to offending behaviour. It may be that treatment for ADHD helps this young man. However, it would be crucial to gain collateral history from someone who knew him well during his development before making this diagnosis. The other options are also consistent with the majority of the vignette and are important to consider. The final diagnosis that is imperative to explore is his use of substances.

5. A. Delusional disorder (delusional jealousy). This man is convinced that his partner is being unfaithful, despite extensive reassurances and evidence to the contrary. The name 'Othello syndrome' is derived from the play Othello by William Shakespeare, in which the protagonist murders his wife (Desdemona. which means 'the unfortunate' in Greek). Othello syndrome is associated with alcohol misuse and violence. Treatment includes antipsychotic medication and psychotherapy; however, given the very poor prognosis, it is often said that the most effective treatment is 'geographical' (i.e., relocation of the spouse to a distant area).

OSCEs and Short Clinical Cases

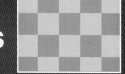

OVERVIEW OF SAMPLE QUESTIONS

1. History of cognitive decline from a relative
2. History of low mood
3. Risk assessment following self-harm
4. Alcohol history and brief alcohol intervention
5. Explanation and advice on schizophrenia
6. History of anxiety

HISTORY OF COGNITIVE DECLINE FROM A RELATIVE

Candidate instructions

You are a medical student attached to a GP practice. Mrs Jones attends alone to discuss concerns she has about her mother (Margaret) who has been found wandering and more confused lately. You are asked to take a history from them, then report your findings and discuss management with a more senior doctor.

There are two parts to this station:

1. Take a collateral history focussing on Margaret's cognitive decline and possible contributing factors.
   Do not take a full psychiatric history.
2. With 2 minutes remaining, the examiner will ask you to:
   • Suggest your differential diagnosis
   • Explain your reasoning based on your findings from the history
   • Suggest an initial management plan, including investigations

You have 8 minutes for this station.

CHECKLIST

Communication

- Introduce yourself
- Confirm to whom you are speaking and their relationship with patient
- Use open questions to elicit their concerns

History

- Clarify key features of cognitive decline
  - Nature of problems (memory and/or other domains)?
  - Acute, chronic, acute on chronic?
  - Associated with functional impairment?
  - Associated with risk? (e.g., wandering, cooking)
- Screen for precipitants of decline
  - Medication changes
  - Physical health changes
  - Depression

Differential diagnosis is of delirium, dementia or depression.

Initial management should include:

- Same-day review (GP home visit or A&E attendance).
- Initial investigations to include a full physical exam, urine dipstick and blood tests.

A good student would specify most of the required blood tests (FBC, U&E, LFT, TFT, glucose, Ca, PO_4, Mg, B_{12}/folate), an excellent student would specify them all. An excellent student would also suggest other investigations that may be indicated by the patient's physical symptoms/signs (e.g., MSU, ECG, CXR, CT head).

A good student would also suggest a structured cognitive assessment. A very good student would specify an appropriate test (4AT, AMT, ACE-III, MOCA).

Discriminating viva questions

1. What are the causes of delirium?
   (see Table 19.1)
2. Where should delirium be managed?
   (see Chapter 20, Delirium: management)
3. What medication can be of benefit in delirium?
   (see Chapter 20, Delirium: management and Fig. 20.2)
4. What environmental modifications can be of benefit in delirium?
   (see Chapter 20, Delirium: management and Fig. 20.2)
5. What is the prognosis of delirium?
   (see Chapter 20, Delirium: course and prognosis)

HISTORY OF LOW MOOD

Candidate instructions

You are a medical student attached to a General Practice. Your next patient is Mr Smith, a 57-year-old man with COPD. His sister has booked him an appointment because she is concerned about his mood.

There are two parts to this station:

1. Take a history of the presenting complaint and relevant background from Mr Smith in order to establish the most likely diagnosis.
   Do not take a full psychiatric history.
2. Conduct a mental state examination alongside taking a history.
3. With 2 minutes remaining, the examiner will ask you to:
   - Suggest your differential diagnosis
   - Explain your reasoning based on your findings from the history
   - Suggest an initial management plan

You have 8 minutes for this station.

CHECKLIST

Communication

- Introduce yourself
- Clarify to whom you are speaking
- Communicate sensitively with someone who is depressed

History

- The three clusters of depression symptoms:
  - Affective: Depressed mood, anhedonia
  - Cognitive-behavioural: Impaired concentration, low self-esteem/guilt, hopelessness, thoughts of death or suicide
  - Neurovegetative: Sleep disturbance, appetite changes, psychomotor agitation/ retardation, fatigue
- Screen for psychotic symptoms
- Possible triggers (e.g., stress, chronic pain, social circumstances)
- Substance use
- Past psychiatric history
- Family psychiatric history
- Past medical history

Initial management.

This will depend on severity of depressive episode and patient preference.

- Lifestyle advice (sleep hygiene, physical activity, avoid substances)
- Psychological therapies
- Pharmacological treatments

Discriminating viva questions

1. How common is depression?
   (see Table 24.1)

2. What is the heritability of depression?
   (see Chapter 24, Depressive disorders: aetiology, genetics)
3. What would a first-line antidepressant be?
   (see Chapter 24, Depressive disorders: management, pharmacological treatment)
4. What would a first-line high-intensity psychological intervention be?
   (see Fig. 24.2)
5. How would you distinguish mild from moderate-severe depression?
   (see Chapter 11, Depressive episode specifiers)

ASSESSING RISK TO SELF

Candidate instructions

You are a medical student in A&E. A 37-year-old patient is in the department after taking an overdose. The A&E team have assessed them and they do not require any medical treatment. You are asked to assess whether they are safe to go home, then report your findings to a senior doctor.

There are three parts to this station:

1. Take a history focusing on their recent overdose, and relevant background information.
   Do not take a full psychiatric history.
2. Conduct a mental state examination alongside taking a history.
3. With 2 minutes remaining, the examiner will ask you to:
   - Estimate the patient's risk to themselves
   - Explain your reasoning based on findings from your history and mental state examination
   - Present a brief initial management plan

You have 8 minutes in total for this station.

CHECKLIST

Communication

- Introduce yourself
- Clarify to whom you are speaking
- Communicate sensitively with someone who is distressed

History

- Assess the presence of ongoing suicidal intent or not (pass/fail)
  - Circumstances of the overdose
    - Planning
    - Final acts
    - Intent
    - Method used
    - Perceived lethality
    - Circumstances of discovery
    - Whether regretful
    - Role of substances
- Assess for contributory factors (stress, relationships, employment, physical illness)
- Assess for protective factors
- Assess for current social support
- Past psychiatric history (including previous self-harm)
- Evidence for current mental disorder

Initial management

Initial management will depend greatly on the severity of risk the patient presents, and on the contributing and positive factors. Consider a short- and long-term plan which may include:

- Crisis contact details (e.g., helplines, mental health services)
- Reducing access to means of self-harm (e.g., removal of unnecessary medication)
- Involvement of existing social supports
- Low-intensity support (e.g., GP review, referral to psychiatric outpatients)
- High-intensity support (e.g., crisis team, hospital admission)

Discriminating viva questions

1. What are the risk factors for suicide?
   (see Box 6.1)
2. Which methods of suicide place the patient at highest risk of death?
   (see Chapter 6, Assessment of patients who have inflicted harm upon themselves: suicidal intent)
3. What mental disorders are associated with an increased risk of suicide?
   (see Table 6.1)
4. How many times more likely is someone with a borderline pattern personality disorder to end their life via suicide?
   (see Table 6.1)
5. Are people who self-harm at increased risk of suicide?
   (see Chapter 6, Assessment of patients who have inflicted harm upon themselves: introductory paragraph)

BRIEF ALCOHOL INTERVENTION

Candidate instructions

You are a medical student attached to a general practice. Your next patient is Mr Brown, a 47-year-old man who had abnormal liver function tests (mildly elevated gamma GT and transaminases) noted as part of a routine medical exam for insurance purposes. You have been asked to meet with him to take an alcohol history and offer a brief alcohol intervention if indicated.

There are two parts to this station:

1. Take an alcohol history, establishing how many units Mr Brown drinks per week and any harm caused by alcohol.
   Do not take a full psychiatric history.
   Do not take a full history regarding causes of abnormal liver function tests.
2. Provide a brief alcohol intervention, covering Mr Brown's motivation to change and options for how to do so.
   You have 8 minutes for this station. You are advised to spend around 4 minutes on each part.

CHECKLIST

Communication

- Check patient's understanding, e.g., are they aware of the abnormal LFTs? What do they think caused them?
- Use non-judgemental tone and language
- Demonstrate empathy
- Encourage self-efficacy of patient: express confidence in their ability to change. An excellent student would elicit confident statements from patient
- Use a mixture of open and closed questions

History

- Use of alcohol
  - Typical weekly alcohol consumption in sufficient detail to allow calculation of units (e.g., size of bottles, typical strength of beer or wine)
  - Pattern of drinking: every day? Binges?
  - Duration of drinking
  - Used alongside any other substances?
- Harm caused by drinking
  - Livelihood – problems with employment?
  - Liver – health: physical or mental harm?
  - Love – problems with relationships?
  - Law – criminal charges?
- Features of dependence.
- *Impaired control* over substance use, including how often, how much, and when to stop.

Continued

- *Increasing priority* given to substances, over, e.g., relationships, work, school, or activities of daily living.
- *Physiological features* of dependence such as increasing tolerance or withdrawal symptoms.

Initial management (provision of a brief alcohol intervention using aspects of FRAMES)

(Appropriate feedback, advice and menu will depend on history. The below is appropriate if Mr Jones is a harmful drinker but not dependent)

- Feedback – the harm caused by alcohol (abnormal LFT, potentially other harms from history).
- Responsibility – emphasize to the patient the decision is theirs. Ask the patient what they would like to do.
- Advice – advise to cut back on use to within low-risk drinking guidelines (see Fig. 17.2).
- Menu – offer a range of patient-centred practical steps. An excellent candidate would come up with options collaboratively with the patient, including options to circumvent things the patient sees as barriers to change. Potential next steps are:
  - Alcohol diary
  - Alcohol-free days
  - Putting money that would have been spent on alcohol aside for a treat
  - Alternative activity to alcohol, e.g., going to sports class on Friday night instead of pub
  - Attending third-sector alcohol counselling or mutual aid

Empathy and self-efficacy are covered under communication.

Discriminating viva questions

1. What are maximum weekly units for men and for women advised by the low-risk drinking guidelines? (see Fig. 17.2)
2. What type of cancers is Mr Brown at increased risk of? (see Box 17.2)
3. What stage is Mr Brown at in the Prochaska and DiClemente model of change? (see Fig. 22.3)
4. If Mr Brown decides he wishes to become abstinent, will he need a detoxification with benzodiazepines? (see Chapter 22, Management: treatment of alcohol withdrawal)
5. If Mr Brown decides he wishes to become abstinent, what medication could help him? (see Chapter 22, Management: maintenance after detoxification, pharmacological therapy)

SCHIZOPHRENIA EXPLANATION AND ADVICE

Candidate instructions

Background

You are a 5th-year medical student on your Psychiatry attachment where you meet Alex White, a 23-year-old man who has recently been diagnosed with schizophrenia. For a year he has experienced auditory hallucinations of three CIA agents talking about him amongst themselves. He holds the delusional belief that the CIA have placed a brain chip in him that broadcasts his thoughts to them. He has made a cut in his scalp to try to remove the chip. He does not believe he is unwell and last week was admitted to hospital using the mental health act. He has not yet received any treatment. He has never used recreational substances.

You have been asked to speak to Alex's mother about his diagnosis and what treatment may be available.

Your task is to explore her understanding of schizophrenia and answer her questions. Alex has given permission for you to share information with his mother.

You have 8 minutes in total for this station.

CHECKLIST

Communication

- Check mother's initial understanding – of Alex's symptoms, diagnosis and treatment options
- Demonstrate empathy
- An excellent student will summarize information
- An excellent student will check mother's understanding at end

Explanation and advice

Likely questions to cover would be:

- What is schizophrenia?
- What are the symptoms of schizophrenia?
- What is a hallucination?
- What causes schizophrenia?
- Why has the mental health act been used to keep Alex in hospital?

(Note risk and poor insight highlighted in history)

- How can schizophrenia be treated?
- What are the common side effects of medication?
- What happens if Alex refuses medication?
- What is the long-term outcome likely to be for Alex?
- If Alex has a child, what is their chance of having schizophrenia?

Discriminating viva questions

1. What is the mechanism of action of antipsychotics?
   (see Chapter 2, Antipsychotics: mechanism of action)
2. What is the management of treatment-resistant schizophrenia?
   (see Chapter 21, Management, pharmacological treatments, treatment-resistant schizophrenia)
3. Does Alex have any first-rank symptoms of schizophrenia?
   (see Box 9.3)
4. What psychological therapies are used in schizophrenia?
   (see Chapter 23, Management, psychological treatments)
5. What physical health monitoring should Alex receive if he remains on antipsychotics?
   (see Chapter 23, Management, physical health monitoring)

HISTORY OF ANXIETY

Candidate instructions

You are a medical student attached to a General Practice. Your next patient is Lisa Johnson, a 27-year-old woman with anxiety. There are two parts to this station:

1. Take a history of the presenting complaint and relevant background from Lisa in order to establish the most likely diagnosis.
   Do not take a full psychiatric history.
2. Conduct a mental state examination alongside taking a history.
3. With 2 minutes remaining, the examiner will ask you to:
   - Suggest your differential diagnosis
   - Explain your reasoning based on your findings from the history
   - Suggest an initial management plan

   You have 8 minutes for this station.

CHECKLIST

Communication

- Introduce yourself
- Clarify to whom you are speaking
- Communicate sensitively with someone who is anxious

History

Check for core symptoms of range of anxiety disorders.

- Onset after life event?
(Adjustment disorder, acute stress reaction, PTSD – if considering PTSD, screen for hypervigilance, re-experiencing and avoidance)

- Onset unrelated to life event?
  - Anxious only following clear trigger?
  - Particular situations? (specific phobia, social anxiety, agoraphobia)
  - Intrusive thought or image? (OCD or related disorder – check for compulsions)
  - Anxious unpredictably, in range of situations?
  - Panic attacks (panic disorder)
  - Free-floating, multiple topics (GAD – check for motor tension and autonomic overactivity)
- Assess for low mood
- Check for thoughts of self-harm or suicide
- Screen for psychotic symptoms
- Possible triggers (e.g., stress, chronic pain, social circumstances)
- Substance use
- Past psychiatric history
- Family psychiatric history
- Past medical history

Initial management:

This will depend on severity of anxiety and patient preference.

- Lifestyle advice (sleep hygiene, avoid substances).
- Psychological therapies – these are first line for all anxiety disorders. Primarily self-help for milder cases and CBT for moderate-severe cases.
- Pharmacological treatments – second line. SSRIs are recommended first.

Discriminating viva questions

1. What investigations would you perform in someone presenting with anxiety for the first time? (see Chapter 12, Investigations)
2. Which anxiety disorders have the highest heritability? (see Chapter 25, Anxiety disorders, aetiology)
3. What would a first-line medication be for GAD? (see Chapter 25, Anxiety disorders, management)
4. What would a first-line high-intensity psychological intervention be for OCD? (see Chapter 25, Obsessive-compulsive disorders, management)
5. What is the role of benzodiazepines in managing anxiety disorders? (see Chapter 25, Anxiety disorders, management)

CLINICAL CASES

CASE 1 – First episode psychosis in a young person

A 22-year-old man presents with auditory hallucinations.

Q1. What differential diagnoses would you consider for this patient?

- Psychosis secondary to a general medical condition
- Substance intoxication
- Substance withdrawal
- Substance-induced psychotic disorder
- Schizophrenia
- Acute and transient psychotic disorder
- Other primary psychotic disorder
- Schizoaffective disorder
- Mania with psychotic symptoms
- Depressive episode with psychotic symptoms

Psychosis secondary to a general medical condition – suggested by presence of a physical health problem associated with psychosis (e.g., temporal lobe epilepsy, Huntington's, HIV) or presence of severe systemic disease leading to delirium. Treatment of the physical health problem (where possible) should improve the psychosis.

Substance intoxication/withdrawal/substance-induced psychotic disorder – use of a psychoactive substance prior to onset of symptoms, particularly one known to be associated with psychotic symptoms (cocaine, amphetamines, cannabis, extensive alcohol use) or withdrawal from a psychoactive substance (e.g., alcohol withdrawal).

Schizophrenia – suggested by *gradual onset associated with social and occupational decline*. Symptoms lasting longer than 1 month. Must have at least two of the key diagnostic features, which include persistent delusions, persistent hallucinations, disorganized thinking, experiences of influence, passivity or control or negative symptoms. First-rank symptoms are highly suggestive of schizophrenia but not essential to diagnosis.

Acute and transient psychotic disorder – *acute onset without a prodrome, with symptoms typically lasting less than 1 month*. Symptoms change rapidly and negative symptoms are not present. Often follow acute stress. If symptoms are not polymorphic or negative symptoms are present consider other primary psychotic disorder.

Schizoaffective disorder – prominent mood symptoms (sufficient to diagnose mania or depression) and symptoms typical of schizophrenia (bizarre delusions or hallucinations) arise around the same time and within the same episode of illness.

Mania with psychotic symptoms – presence of manic symptoms (e.g., elated or irritable mood, reduced sleep, reduced appetite, increased energy, poor concentration). Mood congruent psychotic symptoms (e.g., grandiose delusions, encouraging auditory hallucinations).

Depression with psychotic symptoms – presence of core depressive symptoms (low mood, fatigue, anhedonia). Mood congruent psychotic symptoms (e.g., nihilistic delusions, derogatory second-person auditory hallucinations)

Q2. What information would you seek in the clinical examination?

a. Mental state examination

Appearance and behaviour:

- Poor self-care suggests an insidious onset with social decline, suggesting schizophrenia.
- Abnormal movements may suggest catatonia.
- Agitation can suggest intoxication, withdrawal, mania or psychosis.

Speech: pressured speech or wordplay suggests mania, delayed speech or poverty of speech in single-episode depressive disorder with psychotic symptoms.

Mood: lowered or elated mood suggests depression or mania.

Thought form: flight of ideas suggests mania, loosening of associations suggests psychosis.

Thought content: bizarre delusions (e.g., thought insertion/withdrawal/broadcast or passivity phenomena) suggest schizophrenia. Grandiose delusions suggest mania with psychotic symptoms. Nihilistic delusions suggest single-episode depressive disorder with psychotic symptoms.

Perception: visual hallucinations are more common in psychosis secondary to a medical condition/delirium.

Cognition: distractibility suggests mania or delirium.

b. General examination

Inspection:

- Injection sites suggestive of substance use
- Intoxication with a substance, e.g., constricted pupils, slurred speech, ataxia

Endocrine: goitre may suggest hypo or hyperthyroidism
Neurological:

- Symptoms of catatonia suggestive of schizophrenia
- Abnormal movements suggestive of Huntington's
- Peripheral neuropathy suggestive of vitamin B_{12}/folate deficiency or prolonged alcohol excess

Q3. What investigations would you request?

a. For everyone

- Full blood count (FBC), urea and electrolytes (U&E), liver function test (LFT), Ca, thyroid function test (TFT), prolactin, glucose, C-reactive protein/erythrocyte sedimentation rate (CRP/ESR) – to screen for potential general medical causes of psychosis and to establish pretreatment baselines.
- Toxicology – typically an oral or urine drug screen, to screen for common psychoactive substances.
- ECG to provide pretreatment baseline, particularly if any cardiac history.

b. Consider

- Consider Computed tomography (CT) or magnetic resonance imaging (MRI) head if case is atypical, not responding to treatment or any neurological abnormalities.
- Syphilis or HIV serology if indicated by history.

CASE 2 – Weight loss in an adolescent

A 16-year-old female presents with weight loss.

Q1. What differential diagnoses would you consider for this patient?

- Weight loss secondary to a general medical condition
- Substance use (including alcohol)
- Psychotic disorder
- Depression
- Obsessive-compulsive disorder
- Anorexia nervosa
- Bulimia nervosa
- Avoidant restrictive food intake disorder

Weight loss secondary to a general medical condition – check for past history and assess for current symptoms of systemic illness, gastrointestinal illness, endocrine disorders (e.g., hyperthyroidism, diabetes) or malignancy.

Substance use – alcohol can lead to weight loss if patients spend money on alcohol rather than food, and through malabsorption. Amphetamines and other stimulants suppress appetite.

Psychotic disorder – this is unlikely in a 16-year old but important not to miss. Psychotic symptoms can lead to weight loss directly (e.g., delusional belief that food is poisoned or that person already dead) or indirectly (distress due to psychotic experiences reducing appetite).

Depression – a severe depression can reduce appetite. In anorexia, appetite is usually maintained until late in illness. Check for core symptoms of depression (*low mood, fatigue, anhedonia*). These symptoms are also caused by severe weight loss, so a longitudinal history is important (low mood then weight loss is more suggestive of depression).

Obsessive-compulsive disorder – obsessions can lead to weight loss directly (e.g., fears of contamination) or indirectly (e.g., time spent on time-consuming rituals around meal times leaving little time to eat).

Anorexia nervosa – *significantly low body weight with persistent pattern of behaviours aimed to prevent restoration of normal body weight.* Commonly used threshold is body mass index (BMI) < 18.5 kg/m^2 for adults and BMI for age under 5th centile for young people under 18. Often accompanied with physical complications of starvation, including amenorrhoea, bradycardia, postural hypotension, hypothermia and biochemical abnormalities.

Bulimia nervosa – *over-valued idea of being fat* coupled with episodes of binge eating and compensatory behaviours, e.g., self-induced vomiting. Behaviours usually result in a normal or increased weight. This diagnosis is unlikely given the presentation with weight loss.

Avoidant restrictive food intake disorder – *avoidance or restriction of food* resulting in significant weight loss *without preoccupation with low body weight*.

Q2. What information would you seek in the clinical examination?

a. Mental state examination

- Mood: lowered mood suggests depression or response to starvation.
- Thought content: overvalued idea about body shape being too fat suggests anorexia nervosa or bulimia nervosa. Obsessions suggest OCD and delusions suggest a psychotic illness.
- Cognition: concentration and memory are likely to be impaired in someone who is significantly underweight.

b. General examination

Inspection:

- Observations, including weight and height (BMI < 18.5 or loss of >20% of body weight in 6 month period suggests anorexia in adults, hypothermia suggests anorexia)
- Lanugo hair (anorexia)
- Callused knuckles (self-induced vomiting (Russel sign))
- Poor dentition (frequent vomiting)
- Signs of puberty (delayed if anorexia of early onset)
- Signs of dehydration (anorexia)

Cardiovascular: pulse, erect and supine blood pressure (dehydration in anorexia).

Gastrointestinal: faecal loading common in anorexia (dehydration).

Musculoskeletal: sit-up, stand-squat (SUSS) test – proximal muscle wasting suggests anorexia.

RED FLAG

See Red Flag box in Chapter 16 for high-risk physical findings in anorexia. When assessing physical risk of eating disorders in people under 18 years old, refer to age-specific guidelines.

Q3. What investigations would you request?

a. For everyone

- FBC, U&E, LFT, amylase, TFT, glucose, lipids, CRP/ESR – to screen for potential general medical causes of weight loss and to assess for complications of weight loss.
- ECG (to assess for conduction changes secondary to starvation).

b. Consider

- DXA scan to assess bone density.
- Toxicology – typically an oral or urine drug screen to screen for common psychoactive substances.

CASE 3 – Inattention in a child

A 7-year-old boy presents with trouble paying attention at school.

Q1. What differential diagnoses would you consider for this patient?

- Normal for age
- Secondary to sensory impairment
- Secondary to mental or physical health problem
- Secondary to psychosocial adversity
- Intellectual disability
- Attention deficit hyperactivity disorder
- Disruptive behaviour disorders
- Specific learning difficulty, e.g., dyslexia

Normal for age – children are less able to sustain attention than adults. Check with the caregivers and teacher as to whether the child's behaviour is different to his peers.

Secondary to sensory impairment – difficulty hearing or seeing can make a child appear inattentive. They may also be bored and stop paying attention if they cannot fully participate in an activity, e.g., cannot hear a story.

Secondary to mental or physical health problem – if a child is preoccupied or distracted by pain, anxiety or any other sort of discomfort, they will be less able to pay attention.

Secondary to psychosocial adversity – if a child is hungry, or worried about a caregiver's behaviour towards them (e.g., abuse) or experiencing illness or bereavement in the family, this may result in them not focussing on schoolwork.

Intellectual disability – if schoolwork is too hard, or too easy, a child will not be able to engage with it.

Attention deficit hyperactivity disorder – the core symptoms are *impaired attention, impulsivity and hyperactivity*. These should be present and persistent in multiple settings.

Disruptive behaviour disorders (oppositional defiant disorder or conduct-dissocial disorder) – a child has the ability to pay attention but something in their life or upbringing is making it hard for them to do so. A history of trauma or attachment problems are very common among children and young people with disruptive behaviour disorders. Associated features are limited expression of emotions, limited remorse or guilt about their behaviour and limited capacity for empathy towards others.

Specific learning difficulty – a child with a specific learning difficulty is able to sustain attention in most areas and at home but may struggle with lessons related to a topic they find particularly difficult, e.g., dyscalculia may lead to inattention during maths, dyslexia to inattention during reading.

Q2. What information would you seek in the clinical examination?

a. Mental state examination

Appearance and behaviour:

- Dysmorphic features suggest an intellectual disability.
- Excess activity (e.g., noisy play, running around) during the consultation suggests ADHD.
- Abnormal caregiver–child interaction (e.g., child appears scared of parent) raises possibility of child abuse.
- Challenging behaviour during consultation suggests disruptive behaviour disorder (e.g., refusing to enter room, running away, assaultative behaviour).

Speech: over-talkativeness and interrupting suggest ADHD.
Cognition:

- Not paying attention to information and asking repetitive questions suggest ADHD.
- Distractibility by external stimuli suggests ADHD.
- Difficulty comprehending questions suggests intellectual disability.

b. General examination

Inspection:

- Dysmorphic signs suggest intellectual disability.
- Signs of general medical disorder may suggest pain or discomfort.
- Signs of malnutrition (e.g., low weight, rickets) suggest child neglect.

Test hearing and vision.

Q3. What investigations would you request?

a. For everyone

- No investigations are mandatory in assessment for neurodevelopmental disorder.

b. Consider

- Genetic testing for known causes of intellectual disability
- Blood tests as indicated if general medical cause suspected
- Structured rating scales for symptoms of ADHD completed by parents and teachers can be useful

CASE 4 – Memory problems in an older adult

A 77-year-old woman presents with trouble remembering names.

Q1. What differential diagnoses would you consider for this patient?

- Delirium
- Dementia
- Mild neurocognitive disorder
- Subjective cognitive impairment
- Stable cognitive impairment post insult
- Depression
- Psychotic disorders
- Amnestic disorder

Delirium – this is important not to miss. Check for its core features: acute or fluctuating cognitive impairment, altered conscious level and inattention.

Dementia – trouble remembering names by itself is not a big problem. If it is associated with objective cognitive impairment which is *generalized*, *progressive* (over several months) and associated with *functional impairment*, consider the diagnosis of dementia. Fluctuations in impairment or consciousness level make delirium more likely.

Mild cognitive impairment – *objective cognitive impairment which is not associated with functional impairment*. This is a risk state for later onset of dementia.

Subjective cognitive impairment – if a patient scores normally on standardized cognitive testing but still feels they have a problem with their cognition.

Stable cognitive impairment post insult – objective impairment on standardized test following a one-off insult to the brain, e.g., stroke, viral encephalitis. Impairment should not be progressive. If affecting memory, it may be termed an amnestic disorder.

Depression – depression impairs concentration and memory. Assess for the core features (low mood, fatigue, anhedonia). These features can occur with advanced dementia but are unlikely to be prominent in early dementia.

Psychotic disorders – negative symptoms in schizophrenia can include marked cognitive deficits but these will have gradually worsened from the time of the onset of the psychotic illness.

Amnestic disorder – suggested if objective cognitive impairment only involves anterograde memory and there is strong evidence of a brain disease known to cause the amnesic disorder (e.g., Korsakoff's, head injury, stroke).

Q2. What information would you seek in the clinical examination?

a. Mental state examination

Appearance and behaviour:

- Poor self-care or poor punctuality suggests functional impairment.
- Disinhibition or abnormal social manner suggests frontotemporal dementia.

Speech: increased latency or word-finding difficulties suggest dementia (particularly frontotemporal dementia).
Mood: low mood suggests depression. Anxiety may precipitate subjective cognitive impairment.
Thought content: negative cognitions suggest depression.
Perceptions: hallucinations suggest Lewy body dementia or delirium.
Cognition:

- Altered conscious level suggests delirium.
- Inattention or distractibility suggests delirium.
- Impairment on standardized cognitive test excludes subjective cognitive impairment.
- Confabulation (plausible recounting of untrue autobiographical information) suggests amnestic syndrome.

b. General examination

Check hearing and vision
Inspection:

- Signs of malnutrition (e.g., low weight) or injury suggest functional impairment.
- Abnormal gait suggests vascular dementia, Parkinsonism (Lewy body dementia), Huntington's.

Cardiovascular:

- Hypertension and atrial fibrillation are risk factors for dementia.

Neurological:

- Focal neurological signs suggest vascular dementia.
- Parkinsonism (bradykinesia, rigidity, tremor) suggests Lewy body dementia.
- Abnormal movements (e.g., dystonia, chorea) suggest Huntington's.

Q3. What investigations would you request?

a. For everyone

If diagnosis is subjective cognitive impairment, psychosis or depression, these investigations are not needed, but if there is any doubt it is safer to perform them.

- U&E, Ca, TFT, glucose, vitamin B_{12}/folate to exclude reversible causes of dementia.

b. Consider

- Structural brain imaging (CT or MRI) to exclude reversible causes of dementia.
- In delirium, further tests as indicated e.g., ECG, CXR, urinalysis.
- Syphilis or HIV screening if indicated by history (can cause dementia).
- Genetic testing in young onset dementia, e.g., Huntington's, Alzheimer's.
- Functional brain imaging to support diagnosis of subtypes of dementia, e.g., hypoactivation of frontal lobes in frontotemporal dementia.

Q4. What potential reversible cause of dementia should be further investigated given these blood results (see table 35.1 below for example blood results)?

Blood test	Result	Normal value
Sodium	129 mmol/L	133–146 mmol/L
Potassium	5.9 mmol/L	3.5–5.3 mmol/L
Calcium (adjusted)	2.4 mmol/L	2.2–2.6 mmol/L
Magnesium	0.89 mmol/L	0.7–1.0 mmol/L
Chloride	99 mmol/ L	98–106 mmol/L
Phosphate	1.2 mmol/ L	0.74–1.4 mmol/L
Urea	6.9 mmol/L	2.5–7.8 mmol/L

Table 35.1 Example blood results

Answer: A ddison's disease.

CASE 5 – Medically unexplained symptoms in an adult

A 37-year-old woman repeatedly presents with extreme concern about tingling in her arm, which has been appropriately investigated with no problems identified.

Q1. What differential diagnoses would you consider for this patient?

- Undiagnosed unknown medical condition
- Undiagnosed known medical condition
- Dissociative neurological symptoms disorder (functional disorder)
- Hypochondriasis
- Bodily distress disorder
- Body dysmorphic disorder
- Factitious disorder/malingering
- Anxiety disorder
- Mood disorder
- Psychotic disorder

Undiagnosed unknown medical condition – this is *impossible to exclude*. Positive features of other conditions (see later) can make this unlikely.

Undiagnosed known medical condition (e.g., systemic lupus erythematosus, multiple sclerosis) – *known conditions should always be excluded* with minimally invasive tests proportionate to the symptom and its associated features.

Dissociative neurological symptom disorder (functional disorder) – this is the most likely diagnosis given the brief details given. It would be supported by a nondermatomal pattern of paraesthesia and positive signs of other functional symptoms (such as Hoover sign and tremor entrainment (see Table 14.1)). The diagnosis would also be supported by past trauma or a recent stressful event, although this is not essential to the diagnosis. 'Functional disorder' is an umbrella term for *presumed dysfunction in high-level cortical processing* of motor and sensory information leading to symptoms which are genuinely experienced and involuntary, even though no structural or physiological abnormality is identified.

Bodily distress disorder – this is suggested by bodily symptoms that are *distressing to the individual, with excessive attention being directed toward the symptoms*. The patient could have had multiple other symptoms from multiple other systems which have also been investigated without finding physiological abnormality (e.g., diarrhoea, urinary frequency, muscle pain).

Hypochondriasis – persistent *preoccupation about the possibility of having a serious illness* suggests hypochondriasis. Associated with repetitive and excessive health-related behaviours, e.g., repeatedly checking body or researching the illness.

Body dysmorphic disorder – concern about one or more *subjectively perceived defects with appearance* with associated *repetitive and excessive behaviours* associated with the body part, e.g., checking in mirror would suggest body dysmorphic disorder. What does the patient think about the appearance of their arm?

Factitious disorder/malingering – these are suggested by evidence that the *symptom is fabricated*. Given the intrinsically subjective nature of paraesthesia, this could only be proven if the patient reported they had been lying about their experiences. If the gain is to receive health care, this is factitious disorder. If the gain is secondary (e.g., access to disability benefits as a result of symptoms) the diagnosis is malingering.

Anxiety disorder – *paraethesia is a common symptom of anxiety*. Screen for other physical symptoms of anxiety (e.g., muscle tension, palpitations) and ask about anxious cognitions. Check if the paraesthesia is continuous or episodic, if episodic, what is the trigger?

Mood disorder – sometimes patients attend GPs regarding minor symptoms when the true problem is a mood problem, or a psychosocial stressor. Check for common symptoms of depression (*low mood, fatigue, anhedonia*) and ask what else is going on in the patient's life.

Psychotic disorder – this is unlikely but important not to miss. Carefully assess the patient's beliefs about the origin of the sensation. It could potentially be a passivity symptom (a delusion that others are controlling what the patient thinks or feels).

Q2. What information would you seek in the clinical examination?

a. Mental state examination

Appearance and behaviour:

- Evidence of functional symptoms, e.g., atypical ataxia?
- Evidence of abnormal illness behaviour, e.g., holding the arm in a sling? (which would not be expected to alleviate paraesthesia).

Mood: low mood suggests depression. Check also for anxiety. Thought content: assess the patient's concerns carefully. Are they worried about the tingling itself (bodily distress disorder), the possibility of a serious underlying illness (hypochondriacal disorder) or about an effect on their appearance (body dysmorphic disorder)? Are they delusional?

b. General examination

A thorough physical examination on the relevant system is required when a patient first presents with a symptom. However, if the symptom is unchanged there is no benefit in repeating the examination.

Consider assessing for positive signs of other functional neurological conditions (see Table 14.2).

Q3. What investigations would you request?

a. For everyone

- No investigations can be used to diagnose a functional or bodily distress disorder.

b. Consider

- Relevant investigation of the symptom in a proportionate and minimally invasive way.

Glossary

Affect Affect refers to the transient ebb and flow of emotion in response to particular stimuli, for example, smiling at a joke or crying at a sad memory. It is assessed by observing the patient's posture, facial expression, emotional reactivity and speech. The two components that should be assessed are the appropriateness of the affect and its range. See Chapter 1.

Anhedonia Anhedonia is a loss of pleasure or joy in usual activities, and is one of two core affective symptoms of depression. See Chapter 11.

Anxiety Anxiety is a mood state. It is a response to an unknown, internal or vague threat. This is distinct from fear, which is defined later. The experience of anxiety consists of both apprehensive or nervous thoughts and the awareness of a physical reaction to anxiety. See Chapter 12.

Apophenia Apophenia is when patients make delusional connections between unrelated things. See Chapter 9.

Attempted suicide An episode of deliberate self-harm, which did not end in death but was driven by suicidal intent. This is in contrast to episodes of nonfatal deliberate self-harm driven by other motivations. See Chapter 6.

Capacity Capacity is the ability of an individual to make their own decisions. See Chapter 4.

Circumstantiality Circumstantiality describes over-inclusive speech that is delayed in reaching its final goal. This is because of excessive detail and diversion. However, the final goal will be reached, which distinguishes it from flight of ideas. Circumstantiality can be found in the normal population but is increased in anxiety disorders and hypomania. See Chapter 9.

Compulsions Compulsions can be defined as repetitive mental operations (such as counting) or physical acts (such as checking) that a patient feels compelled to perform in response to their own obsessions. The motivation for compulsions is the reduction of anxiety generated by an obsession. The compulsion may be either unrelated to the preceding obsession (e.g., counting) or an unnecessarily excessive response to the obsession (e.g., handwashing). See Chapter 13

Delusion A delusion is the most severe form of an abnormal idea. It is a fixed belief arrived at illogically and is not amenable to reason. It is not accepted in the patient's cultural background. The presence of a delusion signifies a psychotic disorder. See Chapter 9.

Delusional perception Experiencing a normal perception but interpreting it with delusional meaning. For example, 'I heard the clock chime and I knew that meant the aliens were planning to kill me'. This is a first-rank symptom of schizophrenia. See Chapter 9.

Depersonalization Depersonalization is feeling yourself to be strange or unreal.

Derealization Derealization is feeling that external reality is strange or unreal.

Depression A depressed mood is when a patient describes feeling depressed, sad, dejected, despondent or low. A depressive disorder is a specific psychiatric condition diagnosed if the mood change is sufficiently severe and chronic and occurs with other symptoms.

Dissociation Dissociation is an altered state of consciousness in which normally integrated experiences or processes are disrupted. For example, walking to work on 'autopilot' and not noticing a new shop front – the sensory information has not been integrated with the conscious experience. Depersonalization and derealization are dissociative symptoms (see definitions above). Extreme dissociative states can be associated with disorders including nonepileptic seizures and fugue. See Chapter 14.

Distress Distress is the experience of emotions that impact a person's ability to function in everyday life. Distress may be caused by a difficult experience, troubling thoughts or a mental illness.

DSM-5 The Diagnostic and Statistical Manual of Mental Disorders, Fifth Edition. This is a 2013 publication by the American Psychiatric Association used to classify mental disorders in the United States of America.

Dysgnosia Dysgnosia is an impairment in the ability to interpret sensory information despite intact sensory organ function. See Chapter 19.

Dysphasia Dysphasia is an impairment of language abilities despite intact sensory and motor function. See Chapter 19.

Dyspraxia Dyspraxia is an impairment of the ability to carry out skilled motor movements despite intact motor function. See Chapter 19.

Dystonia Dystonia is sudden muscle spasming that leads to an unintentional movement. See Chapter 7.

Echolalia Echolalia is when a patient senselessly repeats words or phrases that have been spoken near them. It can be viewed either as a form of disorganized thinking or as an abnormality of speech. It occurs in a range of psychiatric conditions such as schizophrenic catatonia, autism and dementia.

Fear Fear, similar to anxiety, is an alerting signal in response to a potential threat. It differs from anxiety in that it is a response to a known, external or definite object. Anxiety and fear are discussed in Chapter 12.

First-rank symptoms First-rank symptoms were described by Schneider who suggested that the presence of one or more first-rank symptoms, in the absence of organic disease, was sufficient to diagnose schizophrenia. These symptoms still feature strongly in modern diagnostic criteria for schizophrenia. See Chapter 9.

Flight of ideas Flight of ideas can be described as either a disorder of thought form or an abnormality of speech. It describes thinking that is markedly accelerated and results in a stream of loosely connected concepts. The link between concepts can be normal, tenuous or through puns and clanging. It differs from circumstantiality in that the links between concepts are more tenuous and the final goal is less likely to be reached. In its extreme form, speech can become unintelligible or approach the incoherent thought disorder of schizophrenia. See Chapter 9.

Functional symptoms Functional symptoms are physical symptoms without identifiable physiological or structural cause. They may arise due to dysfunction of high-level cortical processing of motor and sensory information. They are genuinely experienced, involuntary and not necessarily related to past or current trauma. See Chapter 14.

Hallucination Hallucinations are perceptions that occur in the absence of external stimuli and are indistinguishable from normal sensation. See Chapter 9.

ICD-10 ICD-10 is the International Statistical Classification of Diseases and Related Health Problems, 10th Revision. This is a publication by the WHO which contains codes and descriptions to classify diseases and is widely used across the world, including the UK. ICD-10 was published in 1994.

ICD-11 ICD-11 is the International Classification of Diseases for Mortality and Morbidity Statistics, 11th Revision and it was published in 2022.

Illusion Illusions are misperceptions of real external stimuli. For example, spots on the carpet are perceived as insects. Illusions can occur in healthy people particularly when tired, not concentrating, experiencing strong emotions or intoxicated with substances.

Insight Insight describes a patient's understanding of the nature and degree of his or her mental illness and the recognition of the need for treatment. An assessment of insight is an integral part of the mental state examination. See Chapter 1.

NICE The National Institute for Health and Care Excellence is an organization that produces guidelines for clinical practice in the UK.

Mood Mood is sustained emotion over a period. This differs from a 'feeling', which is a short-lived experience, and 'affect', which is the external expression of transient emotion.

Neologism Neologism is an example of disorganized thinking. It is a new word created by the patient, often combining syllables. It is classically associated with schizophrenia and can also occur in organic brain disorder. They also arise in popular culture, for example, 'webinar' (a seminar on the Web) or 'staycation' (staying at home for a vacation).

Obsession An obsession is an involuntary thought, image or impulse, which is recurrent, intrusive, unpleasant and enters the mind against conscious resistance. Patients recognize that the thoughts are a product of their own mind even though they are involuntary and repugnant. See Chapter 13.

Over-valued idea An over-valued idea is an incorrect belief that is not impossible (in contrast to some schizophrenic delusions) and is held with marked emotional investment but not with unshakable conviction. See Chapter 9.

Panic attack Panic attacks are discrete episodes of short-lived (usually less than 1 hour), intense anxiety. They have an abrupt onset and rapidly build up to a peak level of anxiety. They are accompanied by strong autonomic symptoms, which may lead patients to believe that they are dying, having a heart attack or going mad. See Chapter 12.

Paranoia Paranoia has a range of meanings. Strictly it means that someone is falsely relating things to themselves (e.g., fears that someone wishes to harm them (persecutory delusions, feelings that the TV/radio/Internet is specifically designed to communicate with them (delusions of reference)). It is used by lay people to mean that someone feels persecuted or at risk 'I've felt awfully paranoid recently, I don't feel safe outside'. Paranoid schizophrenia is a subtype of schizophrenia.

Perseveration Perseveration is when a patient inappropriately repeats an initially correct action. For example, unnecessarily repeating a word or phrase, or applying the rules of one task to a second task.

Pseudohallucinations Pseudohallucinations are perceptions that occur in the absence of external stimuli but are experienced in the internal world rather than the external world. For example, hearing a voice 'inside my head'. See Chapter 9.

Psychosis Psychosis is the presence of hallucinations, delusions or thought disorder.

Psychotherapy Psychotherapy is an umbrella term for psychological or talking therapy. There are a large number of psychological therapies; the most common ones include supportive therapy, cognitive-behavioural therapy, psychodynamic psychotherapy, family therapy and group therapy. It is sometimes used to refer to a subtype of psychological therapies only: psychodynamic psychotherapy and psychoanalysis.

Psychotropic medication Psychotropic medication influences cognition, mood or behaviour. All medications used to treat psychiatric disorders are psychotropic.

Rumination Repeatedly thinking about the causes and experience of previous distress and difficulties. Voluntary thinking is not resisted.

Self-harm Self-harm is a blanket term used to mean any intentional act done in the knowledge that it was potentially harmful. It can take the form of self-poisoning (overdosing) or self-injury (cutting, slashing, burning, etc.). See Chapter 6.

Specifier Additional information can be added to a diagnosis in the ICD-11 to further describe the patient's presentation,

e.g., the addition of a borderline pattern specifier to a diagnosis of personality disorder.

Suicide Suicide is the act of intentionally ending one's own life.

Thought disorder Thought disorder is speech so disorganized that it becomes difficult to understand what is meant. The coherency of patients with disorganized thinking varies from being mostly understandable in patients exhibiting circumstantial thinking to being completely incomprehensible in patients with a word salad phenomenon. See Chapter 9.

Toxidrome A toxidrome is a constellation of signs and symptoms that occur secondary to use of a particular agent, e.g., an anticholinergic toxidrome (blurred vision, tachycardia, hyperthermia, delirium) arising after an atropine overdose. See Chapter 7.